LoBiondo-Wood and Haber's

NURSING RESEARCH
IN CANADA

Methods, Critical Appraisal, and Utilization

MINA D. SINGH, RN, RP, BSc, BScN, MEd, PhD, I-FCNEI
Professor
School of Nursing
Faculty of Health, York University
Toronto, Ontario
Canada

LORRAINE M. THIRSK, RN, PhD
Assistant Professor
Faculty of Health Disciplines
Athabasca University
Athabasca, Alberta

Associate Editors

SARAH STAHLKE, BScN, MHSA, PhD
Adjunct Professor/Associate Lecturer
Department of Sociology
University of Alberta; Edmonton, Alberta
Sessional Instructor
Faculty of Health Disciplines
Athabasca University
Athabasca, Alberta

RAMESH VENKATESA PERUMAL, RN, MSc(N), CCNE, CNCC®, PhD(c)
Professor
School of Community and Health Studies
Centennial College;
Assistant Professor
School of Nursing
Faculty of Health
York University
Toronto, Ontario

US Authors

GERI LOBIONDO-WOOD, PhD, RN, FAAN
Professor, Director of PhD Nursing Program
University of Texas Health Sciences Center
School of Nursing, Nursing Systems and Technology
Houston, Texas

JUDITH HABER, PhD, RN, FAAN
The Ursula Springer Leadership Professor in Nursing
Rory Meyers College of Nursing
New York University
New York, New York

ELSEVIER

Elsevier

LOBIONDO-WOOD AND HABER'S NURSING RESEARCH IN CANADA:
METHODS, CRITICAL APPRAISAL, AND UTILIZATION, FIFTH EDITION   ISBN: 978-0-323-77898-5

Notice

Library of Congress Control Number: 2021946978

Managing Director, Global ERC: Kevonne Holloway
Senior Content Strategist (Acquisitions, Canada): Roberta A. Spinosa-Millman
Content Development Specialist: Theresa Fitzgerald
Publishing Services Managers: Shereen Jameel/Deepthi Unni
Project Managers: Rukmani Krishnan/Manchu Mohan
Design Direction: Renee Duenow

Working together
to grow libraries in
developing countries

www.elsevier.com • www.bookaid.org

Last digit is the print number: 9 8 7 6 5 4 3 2 1

Contents

Appendices

Author Biographies

Mina D. Singh, RN, RP, BSc, BScN, MEd, PhD, I-FCNEI, is a Professor at the School of Nursing, York University. She has a long career in nursing, having worked in acute care, mental health, psychotherapy, and public health. Her expertise is as a research methodologist, statistician, and program evaluator. In addition, she is a psychotherapist. She won the 2012 National Nursing Research Scholar award and the 2014 Accreditation Reviewer Excellence award, both granted by the Canadian Association of Schools of Nursing (CASN). She was an Accreditation Reviewer for CASN for over 18 years and has travelled internationally and nationally reviewing nursing education programs.

Lorraine M. Thirsk, RN, PhD, is an Assistant Professor in the Faculty of Health Disciplines, Athabasca University. Over the last 20 years, she has worked in rural and tertiary hospitals, home care, and palliative care. In advanced practice, she worked as a community therapist, nurse consultant, and a clinical nurse specialist. Her research program focuses on family nursing interventions in adult populations facing serious illness. As an educator, she is interested in supporting undergraduate nursing students to develop competencies in working with families and supporting graduate students from across the health disciplines in the research process. In addition, she is passionate about supporting and advancing evidence-informed nursing practice. Methodologically, she is interested in mixed methods and using qualitative research to understand complex interventions.

Sarah Stahlke, BScN, MHSA, PhD, is a sociologist and a nurse. As a clinician, her experience is in acute care, mainly in the operating room and intensive care. After moving into leadership and administrative roles, she worked in program development, hospital management, and professional regulation. She is currently an adjunct professor and lecturer in sociology at the University of Alberta and an instructor in the nursing/health studies master's degree program at Athabasca University. Her research and teaching interests relate to nursing roles, nursing practice environments, employee engagement, organizational studies, professional regulation, and interprofessional relationships. Sarah is an internationally recognized qualitative methodologist and has taught numerous courses and workshops on qualitative research methods.

Ramesh Venkatesa Perumal, RN, MSc(N), CCNE, CNCC®, PhD(c), is a Professor at Centennial College and an Assistant Professor at York University. In addition to being a Critical Care Nurse, Ramesh has more than 20 years of experience in teaching, research, and community service. He has served on the editorial boards of nursing journals and has been a peer reviewer of nursing journals. He won a prestigious award for the best teacher (Award for Excellence in Teaching) in 2009 at a public university in Muscat, Sultanate of Oman. His research and teaching interests relate to mentorship in nursing, Internationally Educated Nurses (IEN), and Relational Care in intensive care units.

Geri LoBiondo-Wood, PhD, RN, FAAN, is Professor and Director of the PhD in Nursing Program at the University of Texas Health Science Center at Houston, School of Nursing (UTHSC-Houston) and former Director of Research and Evidence-Based Practice Planning and

Development at the MD Anderson Cancer Center, Houston, Texas. She received her Diploma in Nursing at St. Mary's Hospital School of Nursing in Rochester, New York; Bachelor's and Master's degrees from the University of Rochester; and a PhD in Nursing Theory and Research from New York University. Dr. LoBiondo-Wood teaches research and evidence-based practice principles to undergraduate, graduate, and doctoral students. At MD Anderson Cancer Center, she developed and implemented the Evidence-Based Resource Unit Nurse (EB-RUN) Program, a hospital-wide program that involves all levels of nurses in the application of research evidence to practice. She has extensive national and international experience guiding nurses and other health care professionals in the development and utilization of research. Dr. LoBiondo-Wood is an editorial board member of *Progress in Transplantation* and a reviewer for *Nursing Research, Oncology Nursing Forum, Oncology Nursing,* and *Nephrology Nursing Journal.* Her research and publications focus on chronic illness and oncology nursing.

Dr. LoBiondo-Wood has been active locally and nationally in many professional organizations, including the Oncology Nursing Society, Southern Nursing Research Society, the Midwest Nursing Research Society, and the North American Transplant Coordinators Organization. She has received local and national awards for teaching and contributions to nursing. In 1997, she received the Distinguished Alumnus Award from New York University, Division of Nursing Alumni Association. In 2001, she was inducted as a Fellow of the American Academy of Nursing and in 2007 as a Fellow of the University of Texas Academy of Health Science Education. In 2012, she was appointed as a Distinguished Teaching Professor of the University of Texas System.

Judith Haber, PhD, RN, FAAN, is the Ursula Springer Leadership Professor in Nursing at the Rory Meyers College of Nursing, at New York University. She received her undergraduate nursing education at Adelphi University in New York, and she holds a Master's degree in Adult Psychiatric–Mental Health Nursing and a PhD in Nursing Theory and Research from New York University. Dr. Haber is internationally recognized as a clinician and educator in psychiatric–mental health nursing. She has extensive clinical experience in psychiatric nursing, having been an advanced practice psychiatric nurse in private practice for over 30 years, specializing in treatment of families coping with the psychosocial sequelae of acute and chronic catastrophic illness. Her NIH-funded program of research addressed physical and psychosocial adjustment to illness, focusing specifically on women with breast cancer and their partners and, more recently, breast cancer survivorship. Dr. Haber is also committed to an interprofessional program of clinical scholarship related to improving oral-systemic health outcomes and leads the *Oral Health Nursing Education and Practice (OHNEP)* program funded by the DentaQuest Foundation, as well as the HRSA-funded *Teaching Oral Systemic Health (TOSH)* program.

Dr. Haber has been active locally and nationally in many professional organizations, including the American Nurses Association, the American Psychiatric Nurses Association, and the American Academy of Nursing. She has received numerous local, state, and national awards for public policy, clinical practice, and research, including the APNA Psychiatric Nurse of the Year Award in 1998 and 2005 and the APNA Outstanding Research Award in 2005. She received the 2007 NYU College of Nursing Distinguished Alumnus Award, the 2011 NYU Distinguished Teaching Award, and the 2013 NYU Alumni Meritorious Service Award. In 1993, she was inducted as a Fellow of the American Academy of Nursing and in 2012 as a Fellow in the New York Academy of Medicine.

Contributors

Megan Aston, RN, PhD
Professor
School of Nursing
Dalhousie University
Halifax, Nova Scotia

Luisa Barton, NP-PHC, BScN, MN, DNP
Assistant Professor
Faculty of Health Disciplines
Athabasca University
Athabasca, Alberta

Caroline Foster-Boucher, RN, MN
Assistant Professor
Department of Nursing Science
MacEwan University
Edmonton, Alberta

Mélanie Lavoie-Tremblay, BScN, MScN, PhD
Associate Professor
Ingram School of Nursing
McGill University
Montréal, Quebec

Shannon MacDonald, RN, PhD
Assistant Professor
Faculty of Nursing
University of Alberta
Edmonton, Alberta

Martha MacLeod, RN, PhD
Professor
School of Nursing & School of Health Sciences
University of Northern British Columbia
Prince George, British Columbia

Christine Maheu, PN, PhD
Associate Professor
Ingram School of Nursing
McGill University
Montreal, Quebec

Ruth Rodney, RN, PhD
Assistant Professor
School of Nursing
York University
Toronto, Ontario

Evelyn Voyageur, RN, PhD (psychology)
Elder in Residence, Aboriginal Education
North Island College, Comox Valley Campus
Courtney, British Columbia

Reviewers

Miranda Bevilacqua, RN, BScN, MN, PhD(c)
Professor
School of Health, Negahneewin, & Community Services
Confederation College
Thunder Bay, Ontario

Ellen Buck-McFadyen, RN, MScN, PhD
Assistant Professor
Trent/Fleming School of Nursing
Trent University
Peterborough, Ontario

Tracy M. Christianson, RN, BSN, MN, DHEd, CCNE
Assistant Professor
School of Nursing
Thompson Rivers University
Kamloops, British Columbia

Angela J. Gillis, RN, PhD
Professor Emeritus
School of Nursing
Saint Francis Xavier University
Antigonish, Nova Scotia

Tracy Hoot RN, BScN, MSN, DHEd
Associate Dean
School of Nursing
Thompson Rivers University
Kamloops, British Columbia

Laura Anne Killam, BScN, RN, MScN
Professor
Health Sciences, Nursing & Emergency Services
Cambrian College
Sudbury, Ontario

Tsorng-Yeh Lee, RN, PhD
Associate Professor
School of Nursing
York University
Toronto, Ontario

Catherine (Cathy) Doreen MacDonald, BScN, RN, MN, PhD
Associate Dean Academic Affairs, Arts & Science
Arts & Science & Nursing
Rankin School of Nursing
Saint Francis Xavier University
Antigonish, Nova Scotia

Elise J. Matthews, BScN, BA, RN, PhD
Assistant Professor
Faculty of Nursing
University of Regina
Regina, Saskatchewan

Christie Pettipas, BSW, MPA, EdD
Instructor
School of Community Studies
Bow Valley College
Calgary, Alberta

Cheryl Pollard, RPN, RN, PhD
Dean
Faculty of Nursing
University of Regina
Regina, Saskatchewan

Nancy A. Sears, RN, BNSc, MPA, CHE, PhD
Professor
School of Baccalaureate Nursing
St. Lawrence College (Laurentian University collaborative BScN program)
Kingston, Ontario

Candice Waddell, RPN, BScPN, MPN, PhD(c)
Assistant Professor
Department of Psychiatric Nursing
Faculty of Health Studies
Brandon University
Brandon, Manitoba

Karla L. Wolsky, RN, PhD
Nursing Instructor
Nursing Centre for Health and Wellness
Lethbridge College
Lethbridge, Alberta

Acknowledgements

THIS MAJOR UNDERTAKING WAS ACCOMPLISHED WITH the help of many people, some of whom made direct contributions to this new edition and some of whom contributed indirectly. We acknowledge with deep appreciation and our warmest thanks the following people who made this fifth Canadian edition possible:

- The Inuit, First Nations, and Métis people who first lived on these lands and whose ancestors shared their knowledge with the settlers
- Nursing educators across Canada who provided valuable and insightful comments that helped to direct the revisions featured in this edition and contributed to improving the content
- Our students, particularly past and present nursing students at York University, University of Alberta, and Athabasca University, who inspired us with their feedback and ideas
- Roberta A. Spinosa-Millman, Senior Content Strategist, who got us started with encouragement, a sense of humour, and great insight
- Theresa Fitzgerald, Content Development Specialist, who encouraged us with positive feedback, made sense of the process, and understood writing during the pandemic would mean extending deadlines
- Our vignette contributors, whose willingness to share their wisdom and evidence of their innovative research made a unique contribution to this edition
- All of the reviewers, who provided thoughtful feedback not only on the previous four editions but also on the fifth Canadian edition manuscript
- Our families, who supported us and picked up the "loose ends" while we wrote and revised.

To my husband Neranjan, my daughter Sandhya, and my parents Ram and Betty Laljie, for their support and encouragement.

Mina D. Singh

To my husband Reidar Hagtvedt, my sons Benjamin and Alexander, and my parents Theo and Margot Thirsk. Completing this fifth edition, during the pandemic, would not have been possible without your support.

Lorraine M. Thirsk

Preface

THE FOUNDATION OF THE FIFTH CANADIAN edition of *LoBiondo-Wood and Haber's Nursing Research in Canada: Methods, Critical Appraisal, and Utilization* continues to be the belief that nursing research is integral to all levels of nursing education and practice. Since the first edition of this textbook, we have seen the depth and breadth of nursing research grow. More nurses are conducting research and using research evidence to shape clinical practice, education, administration, and health policy.

The Canadian Nurses Association promotes the notion that nurses must provide care that is based on the best available scientific evidence. This is an exciting challenge to meet. Nurses are using the best available evidence, combined with their clinical judgement and patient preferences, to influence the nature and direction of health care delivery and to document outcomes related to the quality and cost-effectiveness of patient care. As nurses continue to develop a unique body of nursing knowledge through research, decisions about clinical nursing practice will be increasingly evidence informed.

As editors, we believe that all nurses not only need to understand the research process but also need to know how to critically read, evaluate, and apply research findings in practice. We realize that understanding research, as a component of evidence-informed practice, is a challenge for every student, but we believe that the challenge can be accomplished in a stimulating, lively, and learner-friendly manner.

Consistent with this perspective is a commitment to advancing implementation of the evidence-informed practice paradigm. Understanding and applying nursing research must be an integral dimension of nursing education, evident not only in the undergraduate nursing research course but also throughout the curriculum. The research role of nurses calls for evidence-informed practice competencies; central to this are critical appraisal skills—that is, nurses should be competent in using research.

Preparing students for this role involves developing their critical thinking and reading skills, thereby enhancing their understanding of the research process and their ability to appraise research critically. An undergraduate course in nursing research should develop this basic level of competence, which is an essential requirement if students are to engage in evidence-informed clinical decision-making and practice. This contrasts with a graduate-level research course, in which the emphasis is on conducting research, as well as understanding and appraising it.

The primary audience for this textbook remains undergraduate students who are learning the steps of the research process, as well as how to develop clinical questions, critically appraise published research literature, and use research findings to inform evidence-informed clinical practice. This book is also a valuable resource for students at the Master's and doctoral levels who want a concise review of the basic steps of the research process, the critical appraisal process, and the principles and tools for evidence-informed practice.

This text is also a key resource for health care leaders who are preparing to be experts at evidence-informed initiatives in clinical settings. Furthermore, it is an important resource for practising nurses who strive to use research evidence as the basis for clinical decision-making and development of evidence-informed policies, protocols, and standards, rather than rely on tradition, authority, or trial and error. It is an important resource for nurses who collaborate with nurse-scientists in the conduct of clinical research and evidence-informed practice.

Building on the success of the fourth edition, we maintain our commitment to introduce evidence-informed practice and research principles to baccalaureate students, thereby providing a cutting-edge research consumer foundation for their clinical practice.

Knowledge and language concerning sex, gender, and identity are fluid and continually evolving. The language and terminology presented in this text endeavours to be inclusive of all people and reflects what is to the best of our knowledge current at the time of publication.

LoBiondo-Wood and Haber's Nursing Research in Canada: Methods, Critical Appraisal, and Utilization prepares nursing students and practising nurses to become knowledgeable nursing research consumers in the following ways:

- Addressing the evidence-informed practice role of the nurse, thereby embedding evidence-informed competence in the clinical practice of every baccalaureate graduate.
- Demystifying research, which is sometimes viewed as a complex process.
- Using an evidence-informed approach to teaching the fundamentals of the research process.
- Teaching the critical appraisal process in a user-friendly but logical and systematic progression.
- Promoting a lively spirit of inquiry that develops critical thinking and critical reading skills, facilitating mastery of the critical appraisal process.
- Developing information literacy, searching, and evidence-informed practice competencies that prepare students and nurses to effectively locate and evaluate the best available research evidence.
- Elevating the critical appraisal process and research appreciation to a position of importance comparable to that of producing research. Before students become research producers, they must become knowledgeable research consumers.
- Emphasizing the role of evidence-informed practice as the basis for informing clinical decision-making and nursing interventions that support nursing practice, demonstrating quality and cost-effective outcomes of nursing care delivery.
- Presenting numerous examples of recently published research studies that illustrate and highlight each research concept in a manner that brings abstract ideas to life for students new to the research and critical appraisal process.
- These examples are a critical link for reinforcement of evidence-informed concepts and the related research and critiquing process.
- Showcasing, in **Research Vignettes,** the work of renowned nurse researchers whose careers exemplify the links among research, education, and practice.
- Providing numerous pedagogical chapter features, including **Learning Outcomes, Key Terms, Key Points,** new **Critical Thinking Challenges, Research Hints, Evidence-Informed Practice Tips,** new **Practical Applications,** revised **Critical Thinking Decision Paths,** and **Critical Judgement Questions,** as well as numerous tables, boxes, and figures. At the end of each chapter that presents a step of the research process, we feature a section titled **Appraising the Evidence,** which reviews how each step of the research process should be evaluated from a consumer's perspective. This section is accompanied by an updated **Critiquing Criteria** box.
- Providing a **Study Guide** that promotes active learning and assimilation of nursing research content.
- Offering an Evolve site presenting free **Evolve Resources for Instructors** that includes a Test Bank, TEACH, PowerPoint slides, critiquing exercises, an Image Collection, and critical appraisal activities. There are also Evolve

resources for both the student and faculty that include an audio glossary.

The fifth Canadian edition of *LoBiondo-Wood and Haber's Nursing Research in Canada: Methods, Critical Appraisal, and Utilization* is organized into seven parts. Each part is preceded by an introductory section and opens with an exciting "Research Vignette" by a renowned nurse researcher.

Part One, Research Overview, contains six chapters. Chapter 1, "The Role of Research in Nursing," provides an excellent overview of research and evidence-informed practice processes that shape clinical practice. This chapter introduces the role that research plays in practice and education, the roles of nurses in research activities, a historical perspective, and future directions in nursing research. The style and content of this chapter are designed to make subsequent chapters more user-friendly. Chapter 2, "Theoretical Framework," focuses specifically on how theoretical frameworks guide and inform knowledge generation through the research process. Chapter 3, "Critical Appraisal Strategies: Reading Research," addresses students directly and highlights critical thinking and critical reading concepts and strategies, thereby facilitating students' understanding of the research process and its relationship to the critical appraisal process. This chapter introduces a model evidence hierarchy that is used throughout the text.

The next two chapters address foundational components of the research process. Chapter 4, "Developing Research Questions, Hypotheses, and Clinical Questions," focuses on how research questions, hypotheses, and evidence-informed practice questions are derived, operationalized, and critically appraised. Numerous clinical examples illustrating different types of research questions and hypotheses maximize student understanding. Students are also taught how to develop clinical questions that are used to guide evidence-informed inquiry. Chapter 5, "Finding and Appraising the Literature," showcases cutting-edge information literacy content, providing students and nurses with the tools necessary to effectively search, retrieve, manage, and evaluate research studies and their findings. This chapter also develops research consumer competencies that prepare students and nurses to critically read, understand, and appraise a study's literature review and framework. The final chapter in this section, Chapter 6, "Legal and Ethical Issues," provides an overview of the increased emphasis on the legal and ethical issues facing researchers in Canada.

Part Two, Indigenous Peoples: Research, Knowledges, and Ways of Knowing, is an exciting, brand-new section in this fifth edition. We were honoured to be able to include an interview with Elder Evelyn Voyageur, and to work with Caroline Foster-Boucher, to develop Chapter 7, "Indigenous Peoples: Research, Knowledges, and Ways of Knowing." This section will introduce students to the history and significance of colonization as it relates to how Indigenous peoples have been affected by, and are affecting, nursing and health research. The chapter highlights the relevant recommendations from the Truth and Reconciliation Commission and offers a beginning exploration of Indigenous Methodologies.

Part Three, Qualitative Research, contains two interrelated qualitative research chapters. Chapter 8, "Introduction to Qualitative Research," provides a framework for understanding qualitative research designs and literature, as well as the significant contribution of qualitative research to evidence-informed practice. Chapter 9, "Qualitative Approaches to Research," presents, illustrates, and, in examples from the literature, showcases major qualitative methods. This chapter highlights the questions most appropriately answered using qualitative methods.

Part Four, Quantitative Research, contains Chapter 10 ("Introduction to Quantitative Research"), 11 ("Experimental and Quasiexperimental Designs"), and 12 ("Nonexperimental Designs"). These chapters delineate the essential steps of the quantitative research process, with published, current clinical research studies used to illustrate each step. Links between the steps and their relationship to the total research process are examined.

Part Five, Processes Related to Research, describes the specific steps of the research process for qualitative and quantitative studies. The chapters make the case for linking an evidence-informed approach with essential steps of the research process by teaching students how to critically appraise the strengths and weaknesses of each step of the research process. Students learn how to select participants (Chapter 13, "Sampling"), gather data (Chapter 14, "Data-Collection Methods"), analyze the results (Chapter 16, "Qualitative Data Analysis," and Chapter 17, "Quantitative Data Analysis"), and present their results (Chapter 18, "Presenting the Findings"). Chapter 15, "Rigour in Research," gives students the tools for assessing the quality and trustworthiness of a study.

Part Six, Critiquing Research, makes the case for linking an evidence-informed approach with essential steps of the research process by teaching students how to critically appraise the strengths and weaknesses of each step of the research process. Each chapter critiques two examples of actual published research. Chapter 19, "Critiquing Qualitative Research Articles," focuses on qualitative research, whereas Chapter 20, "Critiquing Quantitative Research," is based on the quantitative research process.

Part Seven, Application of Research: Evidence-Informed Practice, contains the final chapter in the book. Chapter 21, "Developing an Evidence-Informed Practice," provides a dynamic review of evidence-informed models. These models can be applied—step by step, at the organizational or individual patient level—as frameworks for implementing and evaluating the outcomes of evidence-informed health care.

The Evolve website that accompanies the fifth Canadian edition provides interactive learning activities that promote the development of critical thinking, critical reading, and information literacy skills designed to develop the competencies necessary to produce informed consumers of nursing research. Instructor resources are available at a passcode-protected website that gives faculty access to all instructor materials online, including the TEACH for Nurses Lesson Plans, Image Collection, PowerPoint Slides, a Test Bank that allows faculty to create examinations through the use of the ExamView test generator program, and more.

The development and refinement of an evidence-informed foundation for nursing practice is an essential priority for the future of professional nursing practice. The fifth Canadian edition of *LoBiondo-Wood and Haber's Nursing Research in Canada: Methods, Critical Appraisal, and Utilization* will help students develop a basic level of competence in understanding the steps of the research process that will enable them to critically analyze research studies, evaluate their merit, and judiciously apply evidence in practice. To the extent that this goal is accomplished, the next generation of nursing professionals will include a cadre of clinicians who inform their practice by using theory and research evidence, combined with their clinical judgement, and specific to the health care needs of patients and their families in health and illness.

Mina D. Singh
minsingh@yorku.ca
Lorraine M. Thirsk
lthirsk@athabascau.ca

To the Student

EVIDENCE-INFORMED PRACTICE is integral to meeting the challenge of providing quality health care in partnership with patients and their families and significant others, as well as with the communities in which they live. As you read this fifth Canadian edition of *LoBiondo-Wood and Haber's Nursing Research in Canada: Methods, Critical Appraisal, and Utilization*, we hope you develop an appreciation of the importance of nursing research to practice. Whether you are a student or a practising nurse whose goal is to use research evidence as the foundation of your practice, you will discover that nursing research and a commitment to evidence-informed practice positions our profession at the forefront of change. As you learn about nursing research and evidence-informed practice, you will develop a foundation of knowledge and skills that will equip you for clinical practice today and into the future.

The fifth Canadian edition of *LoBiondo-Wood and Haber's Nursing Research in Canada: Methods, Critical Appraisal, and Utilization* reflects cutting-edge trends for developing evidence-informed nursing practice. The seven-part organization and special features in this text are designed to help you develop your critical thinking, critical reading, information literacy, and evidence-informed clinical decision-making while providing a user-friendly approach to learning that expands your competence to deal with these new and challenging experiences. The companion *Study Guide,* with its chapter-by-chapter activities, will serve as a self-paced learning tool to reinforce the content of the text. The accompanying Evolve website offers "summative" review material to help you reinforce the concepts discussed throughout the book.

Remember that evidence-informed practice skills are used in every clinical setting and can be applied to every patient population or nursing practice issue. Whether your practice involves primary care or specialty care and provides inpatient or outpatient treatment in a hospital, clinic, or home, you will be challenged to use research as the foundation for your evidence-informed practice. The fifth Canadian edition of *LoBiondo-Wood and Haber's Nursing Research in Canada: Methods Critical Appraisal, and Utilization* will guide you as you discover your ability to play a vital role in contributing to the building of an evidence-informed professional nursing practice.

Mina D. Singh
minsingh@yorku.ca

Lorraine M. Thirsk
lthirsk@athabascau.ca

A NOTE ABOUT THE NEXT-GENERATION NCLEX

The National Council for the State Boards of Nursing (NCSBN) is a not-for-profit organization whose members include nursing regulatory bodies. In empowering and supporting nursing regulators in their mandate to protect the public, the NCSBN is involved in the development of nursing licensure examinations, such as the NCLEX-RN®. In Canada, the NCLEX-RN® was introduced in 2015 and is, as of the writing of this text, the recognized licensure exam required for practising RNs in Canada.

The NCLEX-RN® will, as of 2023, be changing in order to ensure that its item types adequately measure clinical judgement, critical thinking, and problem-solving skills on a consistent basis. The

NCSBN will also be incorporating into the examination what they call the Clinical Judgement Measurement Model (CJMM), which is a framework that the NCSBN has created to measure a novice nurse's ability to apply clinical judgement in practice.

These changes to the examination come as a result of research findings that indicated that novice nurses have a much higher than desirable error rate with patients (i.e., errors that cause patient harm) and, upon NCSBN's investigation, the discovery that the overwhelming majority of these errors were caused by failures of clinical judgement.

Clinical judgement has been a foundation underlying nursing education for decades, based on the work of a number of nursing theorists. The theory of clinical judgement that most closely aligns to what NCSBN is basing their CJMM is the work by Christine A. Tanner.

The new version of the NCLEX-RN® is loosely being identified as the "Next-Generation NCLEX" or "NGN" and will feature the following:

- Six key skills in the CJMM: recognizing cues, analyzing cues, prioritizing hypotheses, generating solutions, taking actions, and evaluating outcomes.
- Approved item types as of June 2020: multiple response, extended drag and drop, cloze (dropdown), enhanced hotspot (highlighting), and matrix/grid. More question types may be added.

- All new item types are accompanied by mini case studies with comprehensive patient information—some of it relevant to the question, and some of it not.
- Case information may present a single, unchanging moment in time (a "single-episode" case study) or multiple moments in time as a patient's condition changes (an "unfolding" case study).
- Single-episode case studies may be accompanied by one to six questions; unfolding case studies are accompanied by six questions.

For more information (and detail) regarding the NCLEX-RN® and changes coming to the exam, visit the NCSBNs website: https://www.ncsbn.org/11447.htm and https://ncsbn.org/Building_a_Method_for_Writing_Clinical_Judgment_It.pdf.

For further NCLEX-RN® examination preparation resources, see *Silvestri's Canadian Comprehensive Review for the NCLEX-RN® Examination*, Second Edition, ISBN 9780323709385.

Prior to preparing for any nursing licensure examination, please refer to your provincial or territorial nursing regulatory body to determine which licensure examination is required in order for you to practise in your chosen jurisdiction.

Next-Generation NCLEX™ (NGN)-Style Case Studies can be found on this text's accompanying Evolve site.

Research Overview

RESEARCH **VIGNETTE**

Nursing Research to Improve Immunization in Canada

Shannon MacDonald, PhD, RN
Assistant Professor
Faculty of Nursing
University of Alberta
Edmonton, Alberta

We have all seen social media posts that try to scare people about vaccines. There are claims that vaccines are unnecessary, ineffective, or unsafe. Unfortunately, the average Canadian doesn't see the other side of the story, namely the people who have come to harm because they weren't protected from vaccine-preventable diseases. As nurses, we see both sides because we are the ones caring for people infected with these diseases. We also have the scientific literacy to critically read and evaluate the evidence on this topic. Thus, nurses are in the ideal position to promote vaccine uptake; to advocate for equitable vaccine access; and to ask important research questions that ensure that safe and effective vaccine programs continue to be provided to Canadians.

My own interest in the immunization field started when I worked as a nurse in the Pediatric Intensive Care Unit. I cared for children who were on ventilators as a result of a whooping cough infection contracted because they were too young to be vaccinated; teenagers who lost hands or legs to meningococcemia because the vaccine wasn't yet available to them; and children who had measles encephalopathy because their parents had decided not to give them the vaccine. Later in my nursing career, I travelled to less developed regions of the world, where it wasn't uncommon for mothers to report losing multiple children to vaccine-preventable diseases. In those cases, it wasn't due to a choice not to vaccinate, but instead due to limited access to health services. The cumulative effect of those clinical experiences led to my lifelong passion and program of research focused on improving immunization practices, policies, and parent decision-making.

The World Health Organization (WHO, 2014) has a conceptual framework to explain the influences on vaccine hesitancy and uptake. They identify 'the 3 Cs': **Complacency** (vaccines are not perceived as necessary), **Confidence** (lack of trust in the vaccines/providers/policy-makers), and **Convenience** (physical availability, affordability, geographical accessibility, ability to understand, and appeal/ease of immunization services). Any one, or a combination, of these factors can act as an impediment to someone accepting vaccines for themselves or their children.

When considering the WHO '3 Cs' framework, I have always found it striking that 'convenience' can prevent someone from vaccinating, even if complacency or confidence are not a concern. Thus, I have chosen to focus my research on identifying and improving system-level factors that influence convenience, such as immunization access, accurate immunization records, and reminder systems. Through our research, my team has found that these system-level barriers disproportionately impact vulnerable populations, including children receiving child intervention services (Hermann et al., 2019), First Nations children (MacDonald et al., 2016), and children in single-parent, low-income families that have unstable housing (Bell et al., 2015). Identifying these at-risk populations allows us as nurses to develop strategies to reach them, and to advocate for public health policies to provide system-level supports for these populations. I will share with you two examples of my research that seeks to achieve these goals.

Under-immunization of children receiving child intervention services: Children who receive intervention from the child welfare system (sometimes referred to as "children in care") typically do so to ensure their safety and security (Canadian Child Welfare Research Portal, 2020). However, the circumstances in their home, the processes of removal from their home, and their subsequent placement in one or more other care settings (e.g., foster care homes) may result in interruptions in provision of their immunizations (Hermann et al., 2019). In our study (Hermann et al., 2019), we wanted to assess vaccine coverage (i.e., the proportion of the eligible population who have received a vaccine) of children who had spent time in care of the child welfare system. What we discovered was that children in care have consistently lower vaccine coverage than children who had never been in care. For instance, at age 2, vaccination coverage for children in care ranged from 54.3% to 81.4%, depending on vaccine, while coverage for those not in care ranged from 74.2% to 87.4%. So, our study revealed that vaccine coverage for this already vulnerable population was significantly below the rest of the population and vastly below the target level for vaccine coverage (target levels for most vaccines are >95%). As a result of our study, we have advocated for improvements in tracking immunizations for children in care, as well as increased collaboration between health and children's services ministries to ensure these vulnerable children are better served. We also identified the need to conduct more research on this topic, specifically, qualitative studies to identify the specific barriers that are preventing equitable access to immunizations for this population.

Rotavirus immunization for pre-term infants: Rotavirus vaccine is provided to infants, starting when they are 2 months old, with additional booster doses provided before the child turns 8 months old. Unlike some other vaccines, there is an upper age limit to when children can receive the vaccine, due to safety concerns for older children (Parashar et al., 2018). Our team conducted a study (Rafferty et al., 2019) to determine whether there were some sub-populations of children in Alberta that had lower vaccine

coverage for rotavirus vaccine, in order to identify areas for improved service delivery. What we found was that pre-term infants were less likely to be vaccinated, despite being at higher risk of becoming seriously ill from a rotavirus infection. Other studies from the USA (Fathima et al., 2019; Dahl et al., 2018), found similarly that infants that were pre-term and/or low birth weight had low rotavirus vaccine coverage, and that these infants were more likely to have spent their first days/weeks/months in a Neonatal Intensive Care Unit (NICU). Our study raised a red flag in Alberta regarding whether infants in the NICU were receiving their recommended vaccines while hospitalized. It led us to collaborate with public health and hospital-based clinicians to assess and remedy the situation.

These are just two examples of the type of research that I and my research team have engaged in to improve immunization service delivery, and to improve the convenience for parents seeking immunizations for their children. The fact that I am a nurse leads me to approach this research through a nursing lens. I also approach research from a very applied, rather than theoretical, perspective. I am always eager to move beyond acquisition of knowledge, to identify ways that this new knowledge can improve clinical care and health policies in the real world.

Nurses, and nurse researchers, have the potential to play important roles in supporting immunization best practices, policies, and parent decision-making. As one of

the largest groups of health care providers, and the most trusted by the public (Milton, 2018), we are in a prime position to provide clear, evidence-informed guidance to families who are struggling with the immunization decision. In many provinces and territories of Canada, nurses are also the main provider of immunizations. Thus, the role we can play is significant. Nurses are also ideally positioned to lead research in the field of immunization. We have the clinical perspective, the experience of interacting with families, and the education to engage in critical inquiry. Currently, there are only a handful of nurses in Canada who are working in this field. My dream is for nurses and emerging nurse researchers to accept the challenge to improve the care provided to families in Canada and beyond through improved evidence-informed immunization services. ∎

REFERENCES

Bell, C. A., Simmonds, K. A., & MacDonald, S. E. (2015). Exploring the heterogeneity among partially vaccinated children in a population-based cohort. *Vaccine, 33*(36), 4572–4578.

Canadian Child Welfare Research Portal (2020). *Frequently Asked Questions (FAQs)*. http://cwrp.ca/faqs.

Dahl, R. M., Curns, A. T., Tate, J. E., & Parashar, U. D. (2018). Effect of rotavirus vaccination on acute diarrheal hospitalizations among low and very low birth weight us infants, 2001-2015. *The Pediatric Infectious Disease Journal, 37*(8), 817–822. https://doi.org/10.1097/INF.0000000000001930.

Fathima, P., Gidding, H. F., Snelling, T. L., McIntyre, P. B., Blyth, C. C., Sheridan, S., & Moore, H. C. (2019). Timeliness and factors associated with rotavirus vaccine uptake among Australian Aboriginal and non-Aboriginal children: A record linkage cohort study.

Vaccine, 37(39), 5835–5843. https://doi.org/10.1016/j.vaccine.2019.08.013.

Hermann, J. S., Featherstone, R. M., Russell, M. L., & MacDonald, S. E. (2019). Immunization coverage of children in care of the child welfare system in high-income countries: A systematic review. *American Journal of Preventive Medicine, 56*(2), e55–e63. https://doi.org/10.1016/j.amepre.2018.07.026.

Hermann, J. S., Simmonds, K. A., Bell, C. A., Rafferty, E., & MacDonald, S. E. (2019). Vaccine coverage of children in care of the child welfare system. *Canadian Journal of Public Health, 110*(1), 44–51. https://doi.org/10.17269/s41997-018-0135-5.

MacDonald, S. E., Bell, C. A., & Simmonds, K. A. (2016). Coverage and determinants of uptake for privately funded rotavirus vaccine in a Canadian birth cohort, 2008–2013. *The Pediatric Infectious Disease Journal, 35*(6), e177–e179. https://doi.org/10.1097/INF.0000000000001125.

Milton, C. L. (2018). Will nursing continue as the most trusted profession? An ethical overview. *Nursing Science Quarterly, 31*(1), 15–16. https://doi.org/10.1177/2F0894318417741099.

Parashar, U. D., Cortese, M. M., & Offit, P. A. (2018). *Rotavirus vaccines* (7th ed.). Philadelphia: Elsevier.

Rafferty, E., Guo, X., McDonald, B., Svenson, L. W., & MacDonald, S. E. (2019). Measurement of coverage, compliance and determinants of uptake in a publicly funded rotavirus vaccination programme: A retrospective cohort study. *BMJ Open, 9*(11). http://dx.doi.org/10.1136/bmjopen-2019-031718.

World Health organization (WHO) (2014). *Report of the SAGE working group on vaccine hesitancy*. http://www.who.int/immunization/sage/meetings/2014/october/SAGE_working_group_revised_report_vaccine_hesitancy.pdf?ua=1. Accessed May 14, 2020.

CHAPTER 1

The Role of Research in Nursing

Lorraine Thirsk

LEARNING OUTCOMES

After reading this chapter, you will be able to do the following:

- State the significance of research to the practice of nursing.
- Recognize that theory, research, and practice are related.
- Describe the history of nursing research.
- Identify the roles of the research user and producer.
- Identify trends and priorities in health care research.

KEY TERMS

critical appraisal	evidence-based practice	quality improvement
data	evidence-informed practice	research
dissemination	phenomena	

STUDY RESOURCES

 Go to Evolve at http://evolve.elsevier.com/Canada/LoBiondo/Research for the Audio Glossary.

HOW DO YOU KNOW WHAT YOU know? Is it less painful for a patient if you remove a burn dressing slowly or quickly? What are the challenges that pregnant women face in obtaining prenatal care, and how is this complicated if they lack transportation or housing? How do you assess pain in someone with cognitive impairment like dementia? What is the best way to talk with a family who is hesitant to vaccinate their child? Does cannabis have a therapeutic effect for the treatment of anxiety? These are all questions that can be answered with research and are important to nurses.

Research is a systematic way to acquire knowledge. We also acquire knowledge through our own experiences, from our family, culture, traditions, and authorities. Historically, many nursing practices were based on received wisdom or tradition. Some of the first documentation discussing the importance of research evidence in nursing practice is from Florence Nightingale, who, in the 1850s, noted there was a connection between poor sanitary conditions and death rates among wounded soldiers (Nightingale, 1863).

In Europe, in the early 20th century, a movement began to define criteria that would separate science from non-sciences such as pseudoscience, metaphysics, ideology, and religion (Hansson, 2017). The scientific method was developed as a systematic way to determine knowledge and understand the world. While human beings have an incredible capacity for thinking and understanding the world around them, the mind does sometimes make mistakes and is influenced by beliefs and ideology that do not always reflect reality. Over the last century, psychological studies have revealed that people have biases in their thought processes that can be problematic and give us an incorrect or a skewed view of the world around us (Buetow, 2019; Kahneman, 2011; Paley et al., 2007). Our hunches about patterns and probabilities are insufficient to ensure good decision-making. Health care resources are scarce, and thus it is prudent for nurses and other health care professionals to ensure that scarce resources are used wisely. In other words, we need to know that our decisions are based on the best evidence available (Melnyk & Fineout-Overholt, 2011).

Research is integral to achieving the goal of providing quality outcomes in partnership with patients, their families and significant others, and the communities in which they live. As you progress through your educational program you will be taught how to ensure quality and safety in practice by acquiring knowledge of various sciences and health care principles. Research is a critical foundation of an **evidence-informed** approach to nursing practice, positioning nurses at the cutting edge of change and improvement in patients' outcomes.

The aim of this book is to prepare you to critically appraise research and incorporate research into your practice. Throughout this text you will find special features that will help refine and develop your competence in using research. Each chapter contains a *Critical Thinking Decision Path* related to each step of the research process; these will sharpen your decision-making skills as you critique research articles. *Internet* resources in the chapters will also enhance your research user skills. *Critical Thinking Challenges*, which appear at the end of each chapter, are designed to reinforce your critical thinking and judgment skills in relation to the steps of the research process. *Research Hints*, designed to reinforce your understanding and critical thinking, appear at various points throughout the chapters. *Evidence-Informed Practice Tips* will help you apply evidence-informed practice strategies in your clinical practice. Finally, *Practical Application* boxes offer examples of translating principles and methods of nursing research into real-life nursing situations and interventions.

Your critical thinking, critical reading, and clinical decision-making skills will expand as you develop clinical questions, search the research literature, evaluate the research evidence found in the literature, and make clinical decisions about applying the best available evidence. In this book you will discover the "who, what, where, when, why, and how" of research and develop a foundation of knowledge, evidence-informed practice, and competencies that will equip you for 21st-century nursing practice. To begin, this chapter provides an overview of the importance of research to evidence-informed practice, the role that research plays in practice, the roles of nurses in research activities, and future directions of health care research.

SIGNIFICANCE OF RESEARCH AND EVIDENCE-INFORMED PRACTICE

The health care environment is changing at an increasingly rapid pace. The challenges associated with these changes and with nursing's rapid pace of growth can best be met by integrating evidence-informed knowledge into nursing practice. Nursing research provides scientific knowledge that enables nurses to keep up with these changes.

In learning about research, it is important to differentiate between the terms *research, evidence-based practice,* and *evidence-informed practice.* **Research** is systematic, rigorous, logical investigation with the aim of answering questions about nursing phenomena. **Phenomena** can be defined as occurrences, situations, or facts that are perceptible by the senses. Although the origin of the term *phenomena* refers to events that are observable and/or measurable, nurses are also interested in experiences that are not easily observed, such as the experiences of pain, loss, or anxiety.

In the past 25 years, many health care disciplines have adopted the tenets of evidence-informed practice to provide better health care for their patients. The roots of modern evidence-informed practice stem from Dr. Archie Cochrane's investigation of the efficacy of health care interventions, particularly in medicine. His work resulted in the establishment of the Cochrane Collaboration, which provides systematic reviews of health care interventions.

In 1996, Sackett and colleagues defined "evidence-based medicine" as the "conscientious, explicit, and judicious use of current best evidence in making decisions about the care of individual patients" (p. 312). This was considered the beginning of **evidence-based** practice, which most health professions have now adopted. Research is completed, published in academic journals, and then assessed to determine application to clinical practice—this results in practice that is evidence-based. The evidence-based practice movement has not been without challenges and problems. The strict application of algorithms and guidelines, along with selective trials that overlook multiple morbidities, means that individual patients are not always receiving the most appropriate care (Greenhalgh et al., 2014). Evidence-based practice can become rigid and not consider patient preferences, individuality, and contexts.

Evidence-informed practice extends beyond the early definitions of evidence-based practice. With evidence-informed practice, the methods for gathering evidence are the same as the processes used for evidence-based practice; however, the evidence also incorporates expert opinion, clinical expertise, patient preference, and other resources (CNA, 2018). It is important to remember that evidence-informed practice focuses on a more inclusive and interactive process of decision-making that pertains to all nurses—whether they are clinicians, educators, researchers, administrators, or policy-makers (CNA, 2018). Building on the foundation of evidence-based practice, evidence-informed practice also involves acknowledging and considering the myriad factors that constitute decision-making, taking into account patient preference, culture, history, and local context.

When you first read about the research and the evidence-informed practice process, you will notice that both processes may seem similar. Each begins with a question. The difference is that in a research study, the question is tested with a design appropriate for the question and with specific methods (sample, instruments, procedures, and **data** analysis). In the evidence-informed practice process, a question is used to search the literature for studies already completed and then you critically appraise this literature in order to answer your clinical question.

Broadly, there are two types of research: quantitative and qualitative. Increasingly, many researchers use mixed methods—in other words, they utilize both types of research in one project, or in examination of one phenomenon in a program of research. You will be introduced to these types of research in more depth in Chapter 2. In addition, the *Research Vignettes* included throughout the text will introduce you to nurses who use a variety of research methods to study phenomenon important to health care and nursing practice. The methods used by nurse researchers are the same methods used in other disciplines; the difference is that nurses study questions relevant to nursing practice. Nurse researchers also conduct research collaboratively with researchers from other disciplines. Through the conducting of research, they produce knowledge that is reliable and useful for nursing practice. The methods and findings of studies provide evidence that is evaluated, and their applicability to practice is used to inform decisions.

Throughout this text, the steps of the research and evidence-informed practice processes are described. Understanding the step-by-step process that researchers use will help you develop the assessment skills necessary to judge the soundness of research studies and participate in or lead research projects someday. Chapter 21 will further describe how you can implement evidence into practice to improve patient outcomes.

RESEARCH: THE ELEMENT THAT LINKS THEORY, EDUCATION, AND PRACTICE

Research links theory, education, and practice. Theoretical formulations supported by, or developed from, research findings may become the foundations of theory-informed practice in nursing and inform further research studies. Your educational setting, whether a nursing program or the health care organization where you are employed, provides an environment in which you, as a student or an employee, can learn about the research process. In the setting of a nursing program or a health care organization, you can also explore different theories and practices and begin to evaluate them based on research findings. The knowledge you gain through your educational program, whether theory or research based, will inform the decisions that you make in your practice. See the Practical Application box for an example of how theory and research influence health care practices.

The example in the Practical Application box is an attempt to answer a question that you may have asked before taking this course: "How will the theory and research content of this course relate to my nursing practice?" This example demonstrates how theory informs practice, how knowledge based only on experience can be biased and limited, and how approaching clinical problems with systematic, scientific research methods can improve patient outcomes. Dan Ariely was not a nurse, but this anecdote demonstrates how nursing practice could be drastically changed by research. In this example you can see how theory, research, and practice are connected. Theory is used to explain causal relationships (e.g., if I remove the dressing quickly, it will be less painful). Theory needs to be tested

> ### ⟶ Practical Application
>
> Dan Ariely was badly burned when he was 18 years old (Ariely, 2009)—70% of his body experienced 3rd degree burns. During daily dressing changes, he noticed that most of the nurses would grab the bandages and rip them off as quickly as possible. He recalls thinking the nurses had *theorized* that quick, sharp bursts of pain were better for the patient than slowly pulling off the bandages. In addition, he noticed that there was no rationale as to whether the dressing changes were started at the most painful part of his body or the least painful part. As a patient, he had opinions about which methods were better, but there did not seem to be any *evidence* to help guide the nurses on the best methods. When he later attended university, Ariely began working as a research assistant and eventually started to test some of his theories about pain and the removal of burn dressings. The *research* he conducted showed that slowly removing burn dressings would result in the least amount of pain for the patient. He wondered how these kind and experienced nurses could be so wrong. "I knew that their behaviour was not due to maliciousness, stupidity, or neglect. Rather, they were most likely the victims of inherent biases in their perceptions of their patients' pain—biases that apparently were not altered even by their vast experience" (Ariely, 2009, p. xvi). Interestingly, when he reported his results back to the nurses at the burn unit, one nurse explained that perhaps removing the dressings quickly lessened the nurse's *psychological pain*, which they experienced when they inflicted pain on patients.

Source: Based on Ariely, D. (2009). *Predictably Irrational: The Hidden Forces That Shape Our Decisions.* New York:. Harper Perennial.

through research, and then this new evidence needs to be incorporated into practice. Often in the absence of evidence, theoretical knowledge will guide practice. Research can also be used to generate new theory. The relationships between theory, practice, and research will be further explored in Chapter 2.

🔍 Evidence-Informed Practice Tip

What is the current evidence on how to remove burn dressings? Given that the example provided was over a decade old, has this research been incorporated into practice? Has more recent research been done? Health care leaders have an important role to play in implementing research in practice areas. Implementing research in practice requires support from leaders who are champions of evidence (see Chapter 21 for more about implementing evidence-informed practice).

Learning about research will provide you with an appreciation and understanding of the research process so that you can more easily become a participant in research activities and an intelligent consumer of research. A research user actively uses and applies research. To be a knowledgeable research user, you must have knowledge about the relevant subject matter, the ability to discriminate and to evaluate information logically, and the ability to apply the knowledge gained. You need not actually conduct research to be able to appreciate and use research findings in practice. Rather, you must understand the research process and develop the critical evaluation skills needed to judge the merit and relevance of evidence before applying it to practice. The success of evidence-informed practice depends on your ability to understand the research process and to evaluate the evidence. Nurses in practice, who understand research and its contribution to knowledge, are ideally suited to identify phenomena and issues to be studied by asking relevant research questions.

ROLES OF THE NURSE IN THE RESEARCH PROCESS

Every nurse practising in the 21 century has a role to play in the research process.

The Canadian Nurses Association (2017) declares that "nurses support, use and engage in research and other activities that promote safe, competent, compassionate and ethical care, and they use guidelines for ethical research that are in keeping with nursing values" (p. 9). What does this mean for you? There is a consensus that effective use of research calls for the skills of **critical appraisal**; that is, you can appraise research evidence and use existing standards to determine the merit and readiness of research for use in clinical practice:

> Sources of evidence need to be critically appraised before their findings are incorporated into decision-making and practice. Sources that meet this standard include systematic reviews, research studies and peer-

> reviewed journals that summarize valid and clinically useful published studies. (CNA, 2018, p. 1)

Therefore, to use research for evidence-informed practice, you may not necessarily be conducting research, but you can understand and appraise the steps of the research process in order to read the research literature critically and use it to inform your clinical decisions. Even as students you can participate by completing surveys, attending research conferences, and asking questions.

At a provincial level, each province in Canada has its own standards for entry into nursing practice, and many of these standards have specific related research competencies. For example, the College and Association of Registered Nurses of Alberta (2019) outlined the following competencies for nurses in their role as scholars:

> Registered nurses are scholars who demonstrate a lifelong commitment to excellence in practice through critical inquiry, continuous learning, application of evidence to practice, and support of research activities. (p. 15)

Nurses must be intelligent users of research; that is, they must understand all steps of the research process and their interrelationships. Frisch et al. (2013) have developed a useful description of a *Health Services Researchers Pathway* that explains the five levels of nurses' roles in research (Table 1.1). The nurse interprets, evaluates, and determines the credibility of research findings. The nurse discriminates between interesting findings for which further investigation is required and those that are sufficiently supported by evidence before applying findings to practice. The nurse should then use these competencies to advance nursing or interdisciplinary evidence-informed practice projects (e.g., developing clinical standards, tracking **quality improvement** data, or coordinating implementation of a pilot project to test the efficacy of a new wound care protocol) of the workplace committees to which he or she belongs. Nurses are also responsible for generating clinical questions to identify nursing issues that necessitate

TABLE **1.1**

HEALTH SERVICES RESEARCHER PATHWAY

	RESEARCH PROCESS	DATA ANALYSIS LITERACY	KNOWLEDGE TRANSLATION
Level 1 Research User: Learning about research use in care delivery settings	• Defines and distinguishes between research and quality improvement • Follows agency policy and clinical practice guidelines; collaborates on QI activities • Curious and willing to learn about research	• Understands and values statistics and quantitative and qualitative research methods • Reads research reports	• Identifies credible and reliable resources • Performs literature searches, integrating evidence into EIP • Interested in and advocates for practice improvement
Level 2 Research User: Using research in care delivery settings	• Describes research and QI processes; explains QI processes and models • Interprets protocols for relevancy, conducts literature reviews, participates in policy development and QI • Appreciates relationship between research and practice, values active engagement of front-line staff in QI and research	• Understands application of statistics and steps of research process • Collects and uses accurate data, uses basic statistics and qualitative methods • Appreciates the process of conducting research	• Identifies opportunities for knowledge sharing, understands concept of strength of evidence, distinguishing between single studies and systematic reviews • Collaborates with team to change practice and support KT • Aware of and appreciates research activities in the workplace and willing to lead KT activities
Level 3 Research User: Facilitating and leading research use in care delivery settings	• Describes emerging knowledge, best practices and priorities; facilitates research	• Interprets qualitative and quantitative data and can conduct simple analysis	• Describes KT practices and facilitates KT projects, translates projects
Level 4 Research Producer: Beginning researcher	• Understands research designs and theoretical frameworks, manages research projects, contributes to research teams	• Understands advanced analysis techniques, critically and accurately analyzes research data	• Uses research findings to support policy and practice, carries out KT plans
Level 5 Research Producer: Research scientist leading a program of research	• Expertise in at least one method, understands various research approaches • Leads a program of research	• Expert in analysis methods in own research program, manages and supervises use of data, values rigorous analysis	• Builds and implements KT as part of own research program

Source: Adapted from Frisch & Hamilton (2013). *Health Services Researcher Pathway.* Michael Smith Foundation for Health Research and the BC Nursing Research Initiative.

investigation and for participating in the implementation of scientific studies. Nurses often generate research ideas or questions from hunches, gut-level feelings, intuition, or observations of patients or nursing care. These ideas often become the seeds of research investigations.

Nurses may participate in research projects as members of research teams in one or more phases of a project. For example, a staff nurse may work on a clinical research unit in which a research project is underway to test a new type of nursing care (e.g., for pain management, prevention of falls, or treatment of urinary incontinence). In situations such as these, the nurse administers care according to the format described in the research protocol. The nurse may also be involved in collecting and recording data relevant to the administration of, and the patient's response to, nursing care.

After new knowledge is generated, it is important to share findings widely. This is called **dissemination**. Examples of dissemination include publishing an article or presentation at a conference. It may involve joining a health care agency's research committee or its quality assurance or quality improvement committee, in which research articles, integrative reviews of the literature, and clinical practice guidelines are evaluated for evidence-informed clinical decision-making.

Nurses who have graduate degrees are further prepared to conduct research as co-investigators or primary investigators. With a master's degree, nurses can focus on being more active members of research teams. Although master's degrees may focus on advanced clinical practice, advanced practice nurses are still champions for research. They can assume the role of clinical expert, collaborating with an experienced researcher in proposal development, data collection, data analysis, and interpretation. Nurses with master's degrees enhance the quality and relevance of nursing research by providing clinical expertise and evidence-informed knowledge about the way clinical services are delivered. Nurses with

master's-level training also facilitate the investigation of clinical problems by enabling a climate that is open to nursing research and by engaging in evidence-informed practice projects. A clinical nurse specialist prepared with a master's or doctoral degree in nursing who has clinical expertise in a specific practice area can be the primary researcher or act as a collaborator to "ensure their practice applies evidence-based care most effectively while being a leader in every aspect of research" (CNA, 2020, Roles section).

To achieve the greatest expertise in appraising, designing, and conducting research, nurses must complete PhDs. Nurses with doctoral degrees develop theories for phenomena relevant to nursing, develop methods of scientific inquiry, and use a variety of methods to modify or extend existing knowledge so that it is relevant to nursing (or to other areas of health care). In addition to their role as researchers, nurses with doctoral-level training act as role models and mentors to guide, stimulate, and encourage other nurses who are developing their research skills. Nurses with doctoral degrees also collaborate and consult with social, educational, and health care institutions or governmental agencies in their respective research endeavours. These nurses then disseminate their research findings to the scientific community, clinicians, and—as appropriate—the general public through scientific journal articles and presentations at research conferences.

An essential responsibility of all nurses is to pay special regard to the ethical principles of research, especially the protection of human participants (see Chapter 6). For example, nurses caring for patients who are participating in research on antinausea chemotherapy must ensure that patients have signed the informed consent form and that all their questions are answered by the research team before they begin participation. Furthermore, if patients have an adverse reaction to the medication, nurses must not administer more doses until they have notified an appropriate member of the research team. Regardless of their role, nurses need to view the research process as integral to the growing professionalism in nursing.

As a professional, you must take time to read research studies and evaluate them, using the current standards for scientific research. Also, you will need to use the critiquing process to identify the strengths and weaknesses of each study. Bearing in mind that each study has its limitations, you should consider whether sound and relevant evidence from one study can be used in other settings as well. Chapter 21 will expand on how to bring research into your nursing practice.

HISTORICAL PERSPECTIVE[1]

During the Crimean War, Florence Nightingale's detailed and systematic observation of nursing actions and outcomes resulted in major changes in nursing practice. Her work demonstrated the importance of systematic observational research to nursing practice.

In Canada, the establishment of university nursing courses starting in 1918, followed by master's degree programs in the 1950s and 1970s and by doctoral programs in the 1990s and 2000s, was crucial to the development of nursing research. Since the 1970s and 1980s, the two major factors in the development of nursing research have been the establishment of research training through doctoral programs and the establishment of funding to support nursing research. Throughout the 1970s and 1980s, university faculties and schools of nursing built their research resources so that they could establish doctoral programs. The first provincially approved doctoral nursing program was established at the University of Alberta Faculty of Nursing in

[1]This section (i.e. Historical Perspectives p. 12) is adapted with permission from Duggleby, W., & Astle, B.J. (2019). The development of nursing in Canada. In Potter, P., Duggleby, W., Stockert, P. Astle, B., Perry A., & Hall, A. (Eds.), *Canadian fundamental of nursing* (6th ed., pp. 75–80). Elsevier.

1991. Another was established at the University of British Columbia School of Nursing later that year, and programs at McGill University and the University of Toronto followed in 1993. Now there are many doctoral nursing programs in universities across Canada. In addition, there has been growth of university-based Registered Psychiatric Nursing programs, with the first master's degree established at Brandon University in 2011.

Growing awareness of the importance of nursing research gradually led to the availability of research funds. The year 1964 marked the first time that a federal granting agency funded nursing research in Canada (Good, 1969). In 1999, the Canadian government established the Nursing Research Fund, budgeting $25 million for nursing research ($2.5 million over each of the following 10 years). The research areas targeted for support included nursing policies, management, human resources, and nursing care. Although this funding is no longer available, nurse researchers have been successful at obtaining Tri-Council funding nationally and international funding to support their programs of research. Tri-Council is a term referring to three federal research agencies: Canadian Institutes of Health Research, National Science and Engineering Research Council of Canada, and the Social Sciences and Humanities Research Council.

CURRENT STATE AND FUTURE DIRECTIONS

While the last 30 years has seen an increase in the number of nurse researchers in Canada, there are still challenges. A global shortage of nursing faculty, particularly of nurses who hold PhDs, impacts the education of the next generation of nurses as well as the capacity for nursing research (Vandyk et al., 2017). In Canada, there are numerous faculty vacancies and an insufficient number of PhD graduates every year to fill these spaces; recruitment and retention of faculty is a concern with an aging nursing faculty workforce (Canadian Association of

Schools of Nursing, 2016). Nursing faculty are needed to teach in undergraduate and graduate programs and mentor the new generation of nurse researchers. To further the body of nursing knowledge, nurses will need to develop programs of research, increase research on nursing interventions and outcomes, and be aware of national and international trends and issues in health and health care.

Developing Programs of Research

To build robust research knowledge, nurses need to be recruited early in their careers to pursue graduate education and develop programs of research. Developing a program of research can take years. Researchers need time in their careers to establish their expertise and develop the necessary collaborations and funding streams to support their investigations.

Research programs that include a series of studies in a similar area, each of which builds on a prior investigation, promote depth and credibility in nursing science. An example of a research program can be seen in the Practical Application box. To maximize use of resources and to prevent duplication, researchers must develop intradisciplinary, interdisciplinary, and international networks in similar areas of study. Researchers from a variety of health professions (e.g., medicine, nursing, and respiratory therapy) and other disciplines such as psychology, law, and business can come together to delineate common and unique aspects of patient care. Interdisciplinary health research may be "a team of researchers who come together to research an important and challenging health issue" (Hall et al., 2006, p. 764). Interdisciplinary research is increasingly becoming a mandate of research funders, as it is recognized that expertise is required from many disciplines to solve complex health and social problems (Clarke et al., 2012).

Dr. Stajduhar's work illustrates the value of building a program of research and highlights

 Practical Application

Dr. Kelli Stajduhar is a professor at the Institute for Aging and Lifelong Health and the School of Nursing at the University of Victoria. With a research career spanning more than 20 years, Dr. Stajduhar leads a team of researchers studying palliative and end-of-life care issues. The work of this team of researchers spans from palliative care in vulnerable populations (Stajduhar et al., 2019), supporting family caregivers (Sutherland et al., 2016), and understanding family's experiences (Stajduhar et al., 2017). Dr. Stajduhar collaborates with researchers from around the world, as well as policy makers and health care providers. This work has influenced and will continue to shape a palliative approach to care in Canada.

the importance of research teams. A large cadre of nurse researchers, who begin their research careers at a young age, is important for the development of research programs like Dr. Stajduhar's. The goal is to increase the longevity of research careers, enhance the discipline's scientific development, promote mentoring opportunities, prepare the next generation of researchers, and provide leadership in health care. The *Research Vignettes* included in this book have further examples of Canadian nurse researchers who have developed programs of research addressing a variety of current health care trends and issues.

Interventions and Outcomes

Globally, there is a need for more research on nursing interventions (Richards, Hanssen, & Borglin, 2018) and fundamental nursing care (Kitson et al., 2019). Quality research is still needed to address essential nursing care tasks including managing elimination, hygiene, nutrition, and mobility with patients (Richards, Hilli, et al., 2018).

Strategies that enhance nurses' focus on outcomes management through evidence-informed quality improvement activities and the use of research findings for effective clinical decision making also are being refined and identified as research priorities (see Chapter 21).

Evidence-informed practice guidelines, standards, protocols, decision tools, and critical pathways are becoming benchmarks for cost-effective, high-quality clinical practice. For example, the Registered Nurses' Association of Ontario (RNAO) (2016) has developed 50 best practice guidelines to support nurses in their efforts to provide the best possible patient care.

Evidence-Informed Practice Tip ____

The COVID-19 pandemic in 2020 created many challenges and opportunities for nursing research. While delaying the conduct of some research projects and funding decisions, the pandemic also resulted in a plethora of research on new topics. For example, research is examining the impact of personal protective equipment on nursing workflow in emergency departments (Government of Canada, 2020), standardized nursing care models for COVID-19 patients (Richards, 2020), and nursing leadership in acute and long term care settings during the pandemic (Baxter, 2020).

An International Perspective

The continuing development of a national and international research environment is essential to the nursing profession's mission to "improve the health and well-being of all world citizens" (National Institute of Nursing Research, 2015, n.p.). The CNA has been partnering with many international networks in more than 45 countries to strengthen the nursing profession's contribution to global health through study, research, and practice (CNA, 2012). Because of nursing's emphasis on the cultural aspects of care and the influence of such factors on practice, international research is likely to increase. Access to multiple populations as a function of globalization allows the testing of nursing science from various perspectives.

International research projects are often focused on comparative research in which a phenomenon is studied in more than one country. Ideally, relationships are formed with researchers from the international sites, resulting in collaborative research projects. Despite the financial and logistical limitations of this method, the number of international collaborative research projects has increased. Nurse researchers participating in collaborative international research projects are well positioned to play a large role in improving health care globally (CNA, 2012; Grady, 2015). An example of international collaboration can be seen in Chapter 19 (Harvey et al., 2019).

International organizations committed to the goal of health care for all help create natural research partnerships. For example, the World Health Organization (WHO, n.d.) has established a series of collaboration centres to advance health care for the global community. One such centre works toward maximizing the contribution of nursing and midwifery and provides relevant research and clinical training to nurses worldwide.

Research Priorities Reflecting Trends and Issues

Funding agencies often determine research priorities based on their needs and interests. These priorities are often reflective of trends and issues in health and health care. In 2018, the Canadian Association of Schools of Nursing identified seven priorities for nursing research:

- Indigenous and other vulnerable and/or equity seeking communities
- Chronic disease management and care delivery across space and time
- Home care and primary health care nursing
- Care of older adults across diverse care contexts
- Roles, scopes of practice, and value of RNS, and/or NPs to health care
- Nursing care, quality improvement, and patient safety
- Nursing education outcomes

The Canadian Foundation for Healthcare Improvement (CFHI, 2020a) supports spreading health care innovations throughout Canada by bringing together patients, families, health and social services providers, governments, and other organizations from across the country to solve persistent health care problems. Two priority health challenges that have been identified are improving access to addiction and mental health services, and home and community care (CFHI, 2020b). These two areas were identified by the Government of Canada as shared health priorities between federal, provincial, and territorial governments (Health Canada, 2018).

The Canadian Institute for Health Research (CIHR) is one of the largest funders of health research, although the application process is highly competitive, with as few as 13% of applicants being successful in procuring funding (Semeniuk, 2016).

In 2016, CIHR developed a strategy for patient-oriented research to help engage patients in research as more than just participants and to promote research that addressed patients' concerns (CIHR, 2018). This resulted in research units being developed across the country to help researchers increase and improve patient-oriented research. It has impacted how researchers get funding for research and offers support to help facilitate research that is focused on patient outcomes.

Reducing health disparities in underserviced communities and vulnerable populations is another major topic that will shape the focus of future nursing- and interdisciplinary-related research agendas, particularly among Indigenous peoples. The CIHR (2020) has an Institute of Indigenous Peoples' Health and the health of First Nations, Inuit and Metis Peoples is a priority for the other institutes of CIHR that offer research funding. In 2019, CIHR created six research awards for Indigenous Research Chairs in Nursing. These awards, totalling close to $6 million, support Indigenous and nonindigenous nurses to conduct research focused on Indigenous health.

Health research will continue to occur across the lifespan. For example, the health concerns of mothers and infants will continue to spur research that deals effectively with the maternal–neonatal mortality rate. Individuals of all ages who have

sustained life-threatening illnesses will live with the help of new life-sustaining technology that will in turn create new demands for self-care and family support. Cancer, heart disease, arthritis, asthma, chronic pulmonary disease, diabetes, and Alzheimer's disease, prevalent during middle age and later life, will be responsible for expenditures of large proportions of the available health care resources. The impacts of the COVID-19 pandemic on the health of individuals and communities will likely not be fully understood for years. HIV/AIDS, a chronic illness that affects men, women, and children, will continue to have a significant effect on health care delivery. Access to quality palliative care services and groundbreaking research on medical assistance in dying will be prevalent.

Another vulnerable population, persons with mental health illness and addictions, will be served by a better understanding of mental disorders, which will emerge because of advancements in psychobiological knowledge and research initiatives. Mental health illnesses will continue to be a major public health issue; "depression is a leading cause of disability and a major contributor to the overall global burden of disease" (WHO, 2020, Key Facts). Alcohol and drug abuse will continue to be responsible for significant individual suffering and health care expenses as well as significant social and economic losses (WHO, 2018).

Nurse researchers will have an increasingly strong voice in shaping public policy relating to health care. Disciplines such as nursing—because of its focus on treatment of chronic illness, health promotion, independence in health, and care of the acutely ill, all of which are heavily emphasized values for the future—will be central to the shaping of health care policy in the future. Research evidence that supports or refutes the merit of health care needs and programs focusing on these issues will be timely and relevant. Thus, nursing and its scientific base is well placed to shape health policy decisions (Turale & Kunaviktikul, 2019).

Data analytics has incredible potential to improve health care. Nurse leaders will need competencies in analyzing, managing, and using data analysis tools. Using this unprecedented amount of information, nurses can improve patient care and mitigate risk by informing decisions about patient flow, interventions, workforce modelling, cost drivers, and workplace safety (Solman, 2017). Knowing how to ethically access and successfully analyze this data will be key if nurses—regardless of their role—are to make the best use out of this increase in technology and computing power.

Communication of nursing research has also become increasingly important. Research findings continue to be disseminated in professional arenas (e.g., international, national, regional, and local electronic and print publications and conferences) as well as in consultations and staff development programs implemented on site through webinars and websites. Dissemination of research findings in the public sector has also gained importance.

Increasingly, nurse researchers are being asked to testify at governmental hearings and to serve on commissions and task forces related to health care. Nurses are quoted in the media when health care topics are addressed, and their visibility has expanded significantly.

As opportunities are recognized and gaps in science are observed, nurses will conduct, critique, and use nursing research in ways that publicly demonstrate how nursing care makes a difference in patients' lives. Nurses have a research heritage to be proud of. They also have a challenging and exciting future ahead of them. Both researchers and users of research need to engage in a united effort to gather and assess research findings that make a difference in the care that is provided and in the lives that are touched by their commitment to evidence-informed nursing practice.

CRITICAL THINKING CHALLENGES

- What research roles are you interested in?
- What effects will evidence-informed patient outcome studies have on the practice of nursing?
- Have you had any experiences, like Dan Ariely's, that make you question nursing practice?
- Why is it important to have interdisciplinary and international research perspectives?
- What topics in nursing do you think require further research?

CRITICAL JUDGEMENT QUESTIONS

1. What is the most appropriate source of information for evidence-informed practice?
   A. Charge nurse
   B. Attending physician
   C. Clinical practice guideline
   D. Nightingale's notes on nursing

2. Why are interdisciplinary networks important in research?
   A. Collaboration can help solve complex problems
   B. Nurses do not do independent research
   C. Research funding needs to be spread across disciplines
   D. There is overlap in the scopes of practice

3. What drives the priorities for health care research?
   A. Political agenda
   B. Changes in values in society
   C. Trends and issues in health care
   D. The United Nations

KEY POINTS

- Nursing research expands the body of scientific knowledge that forms the foundation of evidence-informed nursing practice.
- Nurses gain research literacy through education and practical experience. As users of

research, nurses must have a basic understanding of the research process and must demonstrate critical appraisal skills to evaluate the strengths and weaknesses of research before applying the research to clinical practice.

- All nurses, whether they possess baccalaureate, master's, or doctoral degrees, have a responsibility to participate in the research process.
- Programs of research studies and replication of studies will become increasingly valuable.
- Research studies will emphasize clinical issues, problems, and outcomes. Priority will be given to research studies that focus on health promotion, care for the health needs of vulnerable groups, and the development of cost-effective health care systems.
- Both users of research and nurse researchers will engage in a collaborative effort to further the growth of nursing research and accomplish the profession's research objectives.

📶 FOR FURTHER STUDY

Go to Evolve at http://evolve.elsevier.com/Canada/LoBiondo/Research for the Audio Glossary.

REFERENCES

Ariely, D. (2009). *Predictably irrational*. New York: Harper.

Baxter, P. (2020). *Nursing leadership during the pandemic*. McMaster University School of Nursing. Retrieved from https://nursing.mcmaster.ca /news-events/news/news-item/2020/09/08 /nursing-leadership-during-the-pandemic.

Buetow, S. (2019). Apophenia, unconscious bias and reflexivity in nursing qualitative research. *International Journal of Nursing Studies, 89*, 8–13. https://doi .org/10.1016/j.ijnurstu.2018.09.013.

Canadian Association of Schools of Nursing [CASN]. (2016). *Registered nurses education in Canada statistics*. Retrieved from http://www.casn.ca/wp-content /uploads/2016/11/2014-2015-SFS-FINAL-REPORT -suppressed-updated.pdf.

Canadian Association of Schools of Nursing [CASN]. (2018). *National research priorities for nursing*. Retrieved from https://www.casn.ca/wp-content /uploads/2018/12/Research-Priorities-2018-EN.pdf.

Canadian Foundation for Healthcare Improvement [CFHI]. (2020a). About us. Retrieved from https:// www.cfhi-fcass.ca/AboutUs.aspx.

Canadian Foundation for Healthcare Improvement [CFHI]. (2020b). *Priority health innovation challenge*. Retrieved from https://www.cfhi-fcass.ca /WhatWeDo/challenges/priority-challenge.

Canadian Institutes of Health Research [CIHR]. (2018). *About SPOR*. Retrieved from https://cihr-irsc .gc.ca/e/51036.html.

Canadian Institutes of Health Research [CIHR]. (2020). *Indigenous health research at CIHR*. Retrieved from https://cihr-irsc.gc.ca/e/50339.html.

Canadian Nurses Association [CNA]. (2012). CNA global health partnerships retrospective. Retrieved from https:// nurseone.ca/, http://media/cna/page-content/pdf-fr /global_health_partnership_program_2012_e.pdf?la=en.

Canadian Nurses Association [CNA]. (2017). Code of ethics for registered nurses. Retrieved from https:// www.cna-aiic.ca/html/en/Code-of-Ethics-2017 -Edition/files/assets/basic-html/page-1.html.

Canadian Nurses Association [CNA]. (2018). Evidence-informed decision-making and nursing practice. Retrieved from https://www.cna-aiic.ca/-/media/cna /page-content/pdf-en/evidence-informed-decision -making-and-nursing-practice-position-statement _dec-2018.pdf.

Canadian Nurses Association [CNA]. (2020). *Clinical nurse specialists,*.Retrieved from https://www.cna -aiic.ca/en/nursing-practice/the-practice-of-nursing /advanced-nursing-practice/clinical-nurse-specialists.

Clarke, D., Hawkins, R., Sadler, E., Harding, G., Forster, A., McKevitt, C., Godfrey, M., Monaghan, J., & Farrin, A. (2012). Interdisciplinary health research: perspectives from a process evaluation research team. *Quality in primary care, 20*(3), 179–189. https:// pubmed.ncbi.nlm.nih.gov/22828672/.

College and Association of Registered Nurses of Alberta. (2019). *Entry-level competencies for the practice of registered nurses*. Retrieved from https://nurses.ab.ca /docs/default-source/document-library/standards /entry-to-practice-competencies-for-the-registered -nurses-profession.pdf?sfvrsn=15c1005a_16.

Frisch, N., Hamilton, S., Borycki, E., Lawrie, B., MacPhee, M. Mallidou, A., Mickelson, G., Redekopp, M., & Young, L. (2013). *Health services researcher pathway*. Retrieved from https://www.msfhr.org /health-services-researcher-pathway-0.

Good, S. R. (1969). *Submission to the study of support of research in universities for the Science Secretariat of the Privy Council*. Ottawa: Canadian Nurses Association and Canadian Nurses Foundation.

Government of Canada. (2020). *Government of Canada funds 49 additional COVID-19 research projects – details of the funded projects.* Retrieved from https://www.canada.ca/en/institutes-health-research /news/2020/03/government-of-canada-funds-49 -additional-covid-19-research-projects-details-of-the -funded-projects.html.

Grady, P. (2015). Questions and answers. *Global Health Matters, 14*(1), 5.

Hall, J. G., Bainbridge, L., Buchan, A., et al. (2006). A meeting of the minds: Interdisciplinary research in the health sciences in Canada. *Canadian Medical Association Journal, 175*(7), 753–761.

Greenhalgh, T., Howick, J., & Maskrey, N. (2014). Evidence based medicine: A movement in crisis? *BMJ, 348,* g3725.

Hansson, S. O. (2017). Science and pseudo-science. In E. N. Zalta (Ed.), *The Stanford Encyclopedia of Philosophy* (Summer 2017 Edition). Stanford, CA: Stanford University. https://plato.stanford.edu /archives/sum2017/entries/pseudo-science.

Harvey, G., Gifford, W., Cummings, G., Kelly, J., Kislov, R., Kitson, A., Pettersson, L., Wallin, L., Wilson, P., & Ehrenberg, A. (2019). Mobilising evidence to improve nursing practice: A qualitative study of leadership roles and processes in four countries. *International Journal of Nursing Studies, 90,* 21–30. https://doi .org/10.1016/j.ijnurstu.2018.09.017.

Health Canada. (2018). *A common statement of principles on shared health priorities.* Retrieved from https://www.canada.ca/en/health-canada/corporate /transparency/health-agreements/principles-shared -health-priorities.html.

Kahneman, D. (2011). *Thinking, fast and slow.* New York: Macmillan.

Kitson, A., Carr, D., Conroy, T., et al. (2019). Speaking up for fundamental care: The ILC Aalborg Statement. *BMJ Open, 9*(12). http://dx.doi.org/10.1136 /bmjopen-2019-033077.

Melnyk, B. M., & Fineout-Overholt, E. (Eds.). (2011). *Evidence-based practice in nursing & healthcare: A guide to best practice.* Philadelphia, PA: Lippincott Williams & Wilkins.

National Institute of Nursing Research. (2015). *Overview of global health research.* Retrieved from https://www .ninr.nih.gov/researchandfunding/globalhealth.

Nightingale, F. (1863). *Notes on hospitals.* London: Longman Group.

Paley, J., Cheyne, H., Dalgleish, L., Duncan, E. A., & Niven, C. A. (2007). Nursing's ways of knowing and dual process theories of cognition. *Journal of Advanced Nursing, 60*(6), 692–701. https://doi .org/10.1111/j.1365-2648.2007.04478.x.

Potter, P., Duggleby, W., Stockert, P., Astle, B., Perry, A., & Hall, A. (Eds.). (2019). *Canadian fundamentals of nursing* (6th ed.). Toronto: Elsevier Canada.

Registered Nurses' Association of Ontario [RNAO]. (2016). *Best practice guidelines.* Retrieved from http:// rnao.ca/bpg.

Richards, D. A. (2020). *COVID-NURSE.* Retrieved from http://blogs.exeter.ac.uk/covid-nurse/.

Richards, D. A., Hanssen, T. A., & Borglin, G. (2018). The second triennial systematic literature review of European nursing research: Impact on patient outcomes and implications for evidence-based practice. *Worldviews on Evidence-Based Nursing, 15*(5), 333–343. https://doi10.1111/wvn.12320.

Richards, D. A., Hilli, A., Pentecost, C., Goodwin, V. A., & Frost, J. (2018). Fundamental nursing care: A systematic review of the evidence on the effect of nursing care interventions for nutrition, elimination, mobility and hygiene. *Journal of Clinical Nursing, 27*(11-12), 2179–2188. https://doi.org/10.1111/jocn.14150.

Sackett, D. L., Rosenberg, W., Gray, J. A., et al. (1996). Editorial: Evidence based medicine: What it is and what it isn't. *British Medical Journal, 312*(7023), 71.

Semeniuk, I. (2016). Pushback from scientists forces rethink of grant competition process. *The Globe and Mail.* Retrieved from http://www.theglobeandmail .com/news/national/pushback-from-scientists-forces -overhaul-of-funding-system/article30931215/.

Solman, A. (2017). Nursing leadership challenges and opportunities. *Journal of Nursing Management, 25*(6), 405–406. https://doi.org/10.1111/jonm.12507.

Stajduhar, K., Mollison, A., Giesbrecht, M., et al. (2019). "Just too busy living in the moment and surviving": Barriers to accessing health care for structurally vulnerable populations at end-of-life. *BMC Palliative Care, 18*(11). https://doi.org/10.1186 /s12904-019-0396-7.

Stajduhar, K., Sawatzky, R., Cohen, S. R., et al. (2017). Bereaved family members' perceptions of the quality of end-of-life care across four types of inpatient care settings. *BMC Palliative Care, 16*(1), 59. https://doaj .org/article/d2caf13917824bc58502028154915d72.

Sutherland, N., Ward-Griffin, C., McWilliam, C., & Stajduhar, K. (2016). Structural impact on gendered expectations and exemptions for family caregivers in hospice palliative home care. *Nursing Inquiry, 24*(1), e12157. https://doi.org/10.1111/nin.12157.

Turale, S., & Kunaviktikul, W. (2019). The contribution of nurses to health policy and advocacy requires leaders to provide training and mentorship. *International Nursing Review, 66*(3), 302–304. https:// onlinelibrary .wiley.com/doi/full/10.1111/inr.12550.

Vandyk, A., Chartrand, J., Beké, É., Burlock, L., & Baker, C. (2017). Perspectives from academic leaders of the nursing faculty shortage in Canada. *International Journal of Nursing Education Scholarship, 14*(1). https://doi.org/10.1515 /ijnes-2017-0049.

World Health Organization. (n.d.). *Networks of WHO collaborating centres.* Retrieved from http://www.who .int/collaboratingcentres/networks/networksdetails/en /index1.html.

World Health Organization. (2018). *Alcohol.* Retrieved from https://www.who.int/news-room/fact-sheets /detail/alcohol.

World Health Organization. (2020). *Depression.* Retrieved from https://www.who.int/en/news-room /fact-sheets/detail/depression.

CHAPTER 2

Theoretical Frameworks

Sarah Stahlke

LEARNING OUTCOMES

After reading this chapter, you will be able to do the following:

- Define key concepts in the philosophy of science.
- Identify and differentiate between theoretical/empirical, aesthetic, personal, sociopolitical, and ethical ways of knowing.
- Identify assumptions underlying the post-positivist, critical social, and interpretive/constructivist views of research.
- Compare inductive and deductive reasoning.
- Describe how a framework guides research.
- Differentiate between conceptual and operational definitions.
- Describe the relationships among theory, research, practice, and leadership.
- Discuss levels of abstraction related to frameworks guiding research.
- Describe the points of critical appraisal used to evaluate the appropriateness, cohesiveness, and consistency of a framework guiding research.

KEY TERMS

aim of inquiry	epistemology	post-positivism
concept	hypothesis	qualitative research
conceptual definition	inductive reasoning	quantitative research
conceptual framework	methodology	text
constructivism	model	theoretical framework
constructivist paradigm	ontology	theory
context	operational definition	values
critical social theory	paradigm	worldview
critical social thought	philosophical beliefs	
deductive reasoning	positivism	

STUDY RESOURCES

Go to Evolve at http://evolve.elsevier.com/Canada/LoBiondo/Research for the Audio Glossary.

THE NATURE OF KNOWLEDGE

AS YOU LEARNED IN CHAPTER 1, NURSES DEVISE clinical questions, based on their daily practice experiences, that, if answered, can improve the care they provide to individuals, families, and communities. Each question requires that clinicians and nurse researchers engage in a knowledge development process (Fig. 2.1). The process begins with the identification of *knowledge gaps:* the absence of theoretical or scientific knowledge relevant to the phenomenon of interest. *Knowledge generation* occurs next, with the conduct of research that provides answers to well-thought-out research questions. This *knowledge* is then *distributed* through journal articles, textbooks, and public presentations to nurses. Next, the *knowledge* is *adopted,* as nurses alter their practice based on published information or as health care organizations develop policies and protocols that are informed by newly generated knowledge. Finally, *knowledge is reviewed and revised* as new health issues arise, advances in clinical practice occur, or knowledge becomes outdated. In this chapter, we focus specifically on theoretical frameworks and how they guide and inform *knowledge generation.*

Nursing knowledge is created and interpreted at various **levels of abstraction**, ranging from the most abstract to the most concrete thinking (Butts, 2015). Fawcett has identified five components of nursing knowledge, which span a range of abstraction levels. These include metaparadigm, philosophy, conceptual model, theory, and empirical indicator (Butts, 2015). The metaparadigm is the most abstract level of knowledge in nursing. It is the worldview of the discipline, which distinguishes its focus (Butts, 2015). Philosophy addresses questions about existence, reality, knowing, and ethics as they pertain to nursing (Butts, 2015). Conceptual models are a set of concepts that address broad, general ideas of interest to the discipline, while theories translate concepts into testable questions that can be explored using empirical indicators such as instruments, experiments, or procedures (Butts, 2015).

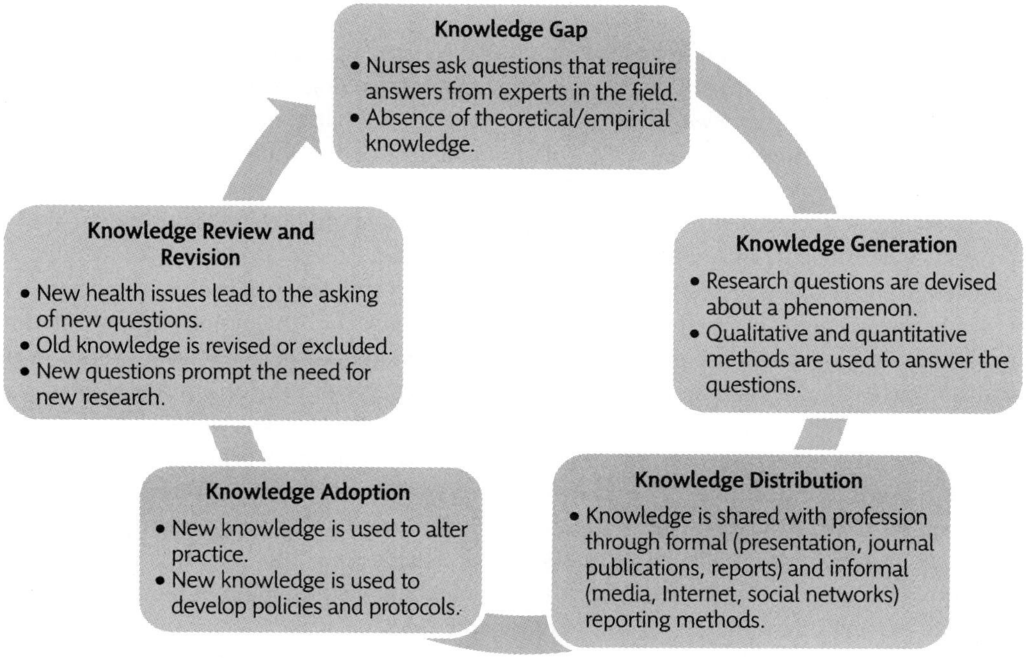

Knowledge Gap
- Nurses ask questions that require answers from experts in the field.
- Absence of theoretical/empirical knowledge.

Knowledge Generation
- Research questions are devised about a phenomenon.
- Qualitative and quantitative methods are used to answer the questions.

Knowledge Distribution
- Knowledge is shared with profession through formal (presentation, journal publications, reports) and informal (media, Internet, social networks) reporting methods.

Knowledge Adoption
- New knowledge is used to alter practice.
- New knowledge is used to develop policies and protocols.

Knowledge Review and Revision
- New health issues lead to the asking of new questions.
- Old knowledge is revised or excluded.
- New questions prompt the need for new research.

FIG. 2.1 Knowledge development process.

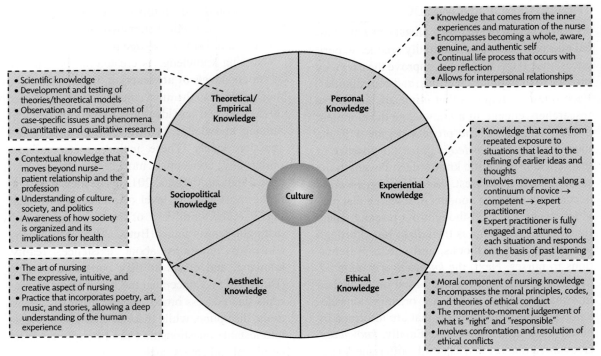

• Scientific knowledge
• Development and testing of theories/theoretical models
• Observation and measurement of case-specific issues and phenomena
• Quantitative and qualitative research

• Knowledge that comes from the inner experiences and maturation of the nurse
• Encompasses becoming a whole, aware, genuine, and authentic self
• Continual life process that occurs with deep reflection
• Allows for interpersonal relationships

• Contextual knowledge that moves beyond nurse–patient relationship and the profession
• Understanding of culture, society, and politics
• Awareness of how society is organized and its implications for health

• Knowledge that comes from repeated exposure to situations that lead to the refining of earlier ideas and thoughts
• Involves movement along a continuum of novice → competent → expert practitioner
• Expert practitioner is fully engaged and attuned to each situation and responds on the basis of past learning

• The art of nursing
• The expressive, intuitive, and creative aspect of nursing
• Practice that incorporates poetry, art, music, and stories, allowing a deep understanding of the human experience

• Moral component of nursing knowledge
• Encompasses the moral principles, codes, and theories of ethical conduct
• The moment-to-moment judgement of what is "right" and "responsible"
• Involves confrontation and resolution of ethical conflicts

Theoretical/Empirical Knowledge — Personal Knowledge — Sociopolitical Knowledge — Culture — Experiential Knowledge — Aesthetic Knowledge — Ethical Knowledge

FIG. 2.2   Nursing knowledge.
(Adapted from Chapter 2 of the previous edition of this book, written by Cherylyn Cameron.)

Figure 2.2 outlines the various ways by which nurses inform their practice. These include *theoretical/empirical, personal, experiential, ethical, aesthetic,* and *sociopolitical/cultural* ways of knowing (Chinn & Kramer, 2015; Zander, 2007). Empirical knowing is acquired through the scientific process, which results in tested and justifiable knowledge for practice (Zander, 2007). In contrast, aesthetics is the art of nursing in which the nurse interprets the patient's behaviour and needs and addresses the bigger picture of patient care (Zander, 2007). Ethical knowing is the moral component of nursing and is concerned with justifying and judging actions. This knowing depends on an understanding of philosophical concepts about what is good as well as rights and obligations (Zander, 2007). Personal knowing involves an existential awareness of self and others in relationship (Zander, 2007). Experience and intuition constitute other forms of knowing

in nursing (Zander, 2007). Understanding the sociopolitical context of practice is an overarching way of knowing; nurses can situate their practice and knowledge within a societal context (Zander, 2007).

It is important to remember that the way we understand these aspects of knowledge is based on our cultural perspectives, such as Western ideologies or Indigenous ways of knowing. Indigenous perspectives are covered in depth in Chapter 7, but a brief introduction is warranted here. Indigenous knowledge is "a learned way of looking at the world that may have very different forms of acquisitions, transmission, and manifestation for Indigenous peoples" (Battiste & Henderson, 2000, p. 48). Indigenous knowledge is transmitted through oral traditions, which provides a way of understanding Indigenous people's experiences and promotes a continued existence of their culture. Battiste (2000) rightly notes that Indigenous knowledge is essential for transformation toward a just society that will "engage with and react to multiple circumstances and shapes of oppression, exploitation, assimilation, colonization, racism, genderism, ageism, and the many other strategies of marginalization" (p. xxi). Battiste (2002) claimed that Indigenous epistemology is located in theories, philosophies, histories, ceremonies, and stories as ways of knowing. The guiding tenets of Indigenous epistemology encompass a legitimate way of knowing, storytelling as a method for sharing knowledge, and the relationship between the researcher and participants as a natural component of the research process (Kovach, 2005). Indigenous epistemology is derived from multiple sources including traditional knowledge from previous generations, empirical knowledge from careful observation, personal knowledge and experiences, oral transmission, holistic knowledge, and experimental knowledge (Castellano, 2000).

From the Western perspective that is common in Canada, theoretical/empirical knowledge is most commonly referred to as *scientific knowledge*. Recently, theoretical/empirical knowledge has gained prominence in nursing with the increasing focus on evidence-informed practice. Theoretical and empirical knowledge really cannot be separated; however, theoretical knowing is concerned with developing or testing theories (possible explanations or ideas) that nurse researchers have about how the world operates. Theoretical knowing is informed by empirical knowing, which involves observations of reality. Observations may include the following:

1. Speaking with people about their life experiences (e.g., living with Alzheimer's disease) and using their responses to specific and general questions to understand the phenomenon
2. Observing social or cultural interactions (e.g., homeless individuals interacting with service providers) as they naturally occur, interpreting what the interactions might mean for both parties, and using those inter-

pretations to develop theories about health service delivery for that population
3. Delivering an intervention (e.g., a school health program for obese children) and assessing changes in health care–related behaviours (e.g., type of foods consumed, amount of daily exercise, weight and other biomedical parameters) after the delivery of the intervention
4. Using surveys or a questionnaire to ask a large group of people questions about health experiences or their current symptom levels with regard to, for example, pain, digestive problems, or depression.

Taking an example of published work, Nahm and colleagues (2010) hypothesized that using social cognitive theory (involving self-efficacy, mastery, and modelling) as the foundation for a hip fracture prevention website would be more effective in changing individuals' health behaviours than conventional educational strategies; this **hypothesis** is an example of *theoretical knowing*. However, it was only through developing a clinical trial that tested the intervention that Nahm and colleagues could observe the effectiveness of the theory-based educational website (e.g., differences in knowledge and health behaviours) compared to the effectiveness of a conventional prevention website. Their results provided support for the hypothesis; this support is an example of *empirical knowing*.

PHILOSOPHIES OF RESEARCH

Thus far, we have used a number of terms that may be new to you. Every discipline has characteristic terminology for communicating important features of the work in that field. Learning new terminology is part of what nursing students do when they learn research methods and skills. Each research method and all philosophies of science have specialized language that nursing students will encounter in the literature. Thus, to help you comprehend the research you will read, it is important to clarify a few terms.

All research is based on **philosophical beliefs** about the world; these beliefs are the motivating values, concepts, principles, and the nature of human knowledge of an individual, group, or culture, and they are the basis of a **worldview**, or **paradigm**. *Paradigm* is from the Greek word *paradeigma,* meaning "pattern." Paradigms are "different ways of viewing the world and often form the foundation from which research is undertaken. They consist of a set of assumptions about what is reality, how knowledge is created and what is valuable to learn" (Davies & Fisher, 2018, p. 21). Therefore, knowing and comprehending these views and practices is important in understanding and using research findings. They are not right or wrong; rather, they represent different ways of viewing the world and the way things operate within it. Nursing researchers may tend to gravitate toward a particular worldview but it is important to remember that different kinds of research questions call for different approaches to understanding and studying reality, so it is possible for researchers to value different worldviews at different times. For example, a researcher can know that a certain drug has side effects or that turning bedridden patients regularly will reduce the risk of skin breakdown but also understand that people's narratives about their experiences will yield multiple and sometimes conflicting explanations. This shows how different paradigms can be held simultaneously.

It is important to note that there can be overlap between paradigms and they are not always exclusive of one another (Davies & Fisher, 2018), although categorizations can simplify learning about the basic worldviews. In nursing, there are three key paradigmatic perspectives that are commonly held and that generally underpin various approaches to research. These are positivism/post-positivism, constructivism, and critical theory. These three paradigms are compared in Table 2.1; however, first you need to understand the philosophical language used in the table. **Ontology** (from the Greek word *onto,* meaning "to be") is the science or study of being or existence and its relationship to nonexistence. Ontology addresses two primary questions: (1) What exists or what is real? and (2) Into what categories can existing things be sorted? **Epistemology** addresses four key questions: (1) What is knowledge? (2) What are the sources of knowledge? (3) What are the ways we come to know something, in contrast to believing, wondering, guessing, or imagining? and (4) What is truth and what role does it play in knowledge? **Methodology** refers to the principles, rules, and procedures that guide the process through which knowledge is acquired. The **aim of inquiry** refers to the goals or specific objectives of the research. **Context** refers to the personal, social, organizational, cultural and/or political environment in which a phenomenon of interest (that "thing of interest") occurs. The context of research studies can include physical settings, such as the hospital or home, or less concrete "environments," such as the context that cultural understandings bring to an experience. **Values** are the things that the nurse researcher holds to be important.

Positivism is a philosophical orientation that arose in the 18th century, as part of a movement away from religious knowing to reasoning and science. Positivistic research aims for objectivity and impartiality, with a goal of producing unbiased, generalizable research. **Post-positivism** emerged in response to the realization that such objectivity is usually not possible and our observations cannot always be relied upon because they are subject to error and human bias—we all have different values, cultures, and life experiences and, thus, generate different interpretations.

Constructivism, which is also referred to as interpretivism or relativism, points to the centrality of human experiences, social and cultural constructs, values, perspectives, and language (Clark, 2008). It is a philosophical orientation that suggests that reality and the way in which we understand our world are largely dependent on our perceptions and context. Truth about life experience is regarded as relative and multiple rather than absolute. The value of knowledge development lies in the ability to understand how people perceive their world. Knowledge development occurs through observation, dialogue with people, or both, and as a result of paying attention to the language people use to describe life experiences. Constructivists tap into personal experience rather than seeking measurement and elusive objectivity. This form of research is aimed at creating an understanding of people and their life experiences from their point of view.

Critical realism is a philosophical orientation that has become of great interest in nursing research.

It harnesses the strengths and addresses the weaknesses of positivism and constructivism (Clark, 2008) by acknowledging that, although there is a single reality, we cannot know it for sure (Davies & Fisher, 2018). This perspective offers a middle ground that "does not reduce the world to unknowable chaos [as might be the case with relativism] or a positivistic universal order" (Clark, 2008, p. E68). In critical realism, social entities exist independently of human understanding. For example, discrimination and power imbalances exist regardless of whether humans recognize their influence.

TABLE **2.1**

BASIC RESEARCH PARADIGMS

ITEM/QUESTIONS	POST-POSITIVISM	CRITICAL THEORY	CONSTRUCTIVISM
ONTOLOGY			
What can be said to exist? Into what categories can we sort existing things?	A material world exists. Not all things can be understood, sensed, or placed into a cause-and-effect relationship. The senses provide us with an imperfect understanding of the external/material world.	Reality is constructed by those with the most power at particular points in history. Over time, reality is shaped by numerous social, political, economic, and cultural forces. Stories/discourses shaped by the powerful become accepted reality.	Reality is constructed by individual perception within a social context. Truth is relative and based on perception or some particular frame of reference.
EPISTEMOLOGY			
What is knowledge? How is knowledge acquired? How do we know what we know?	Researchers are naturally biased. Objectivity (controlled bias) is the ultimate goal, although pure objectivity is not attainable. Uses triangulation and replication of findings across multiple perspectives.	Research is a transaction that occurs between the researcher and research participant. The perceptions (standpoint) of the researcher and the research participants naturally influence knowledge generation/creation. Perceptions (standpoints) are determined by context, and so contextual awareness and its relationship to the participant's understanding of reality is the focus of the research.	Research is a transaction that occurs between the researcher and research participant. Research emphasizes the meaning ascribed to human experiences. Objectivity is not possible; knowledge is co-created.
RESEARCHER'S VALUES			
How do the researcher's values influence the knowledge development process?	All attempts are made to exclude researcher bias. Influence is denied.	Researcher perspectives are acknowledged and recognized as influential. Researcher values drive research questions and purpose; researcher manages own perspectives.	Researcher perspectives, values, experiences are recognized as potentially influential. Influence is managed with reflection and bracketing.

Continued

TABLE **2.1**

BASIC RESEARCH PARADIGMS—cont'd

ITEM/QUESTIONS	POST-POSITIVISM	CRITICAL THEORY	CONSTRUCTIVISM
METHODOLOGY Within a particular discipline, what principles, rules, and procedures guide the process through which knowledge is acquired?	Inquiry generally involves quantitative methods and is viewed as a series of logically related steps. Research questions/hypotheses are proposed and subjected to empirical testing. Research is characterized by careful accounting for and control of factors that may influence research findings. Qualitative research may be used to develop hypotheses.	Inquiry requires dialogue between the investigator and research participant. Research purposes are transformative, emancipatory, or consciousness raising. Dialogue brings to the forefront the historical context behind experiences of suffering, conflict, and collective struggles. Dialogue increases participants' awareness of actions required to incite change.	Inquiry requires dialogue between the investigator and research participant. Focus is on interpretation of interview data, documents, and artifacts, including written texts, art, pictures. Interpretation brings to the forefront the varying ways in which people construct their understanding of their social world and how their interpretation shifts as they interact with others.
AIM OF INQUIRY What is the goal of research?	Explanation, prediction, and control.	Critique, change, reconstructed reality, and emancipation.	Understanding of social realities and interpretations of meaning.
CONTEXT What biographical, life, social, and political factors may influence the research findings?	Attempt is made to set aside researcher histories, politics, ideologies, and experiences.	Focus is on historical, social, and political context. *Context* refers to the social and political climate in which an event or process occurred. Social context highlights how structural, economic, representational, and institutional factors of the past influence how people understand an issue today. Political context highlights how political dialogue and opinions, legal directives, and government policies of the past influence how people understand an issue.	Focus is on life context, including significant conditions and demands that provide greater understanding of the phenomena being studied; focus also emphasizes time and place.
SUB-PARADIGMS/ THEORIES/ METHODS	Critical realism Mixed methods	Feminism Critical Race Theory Intersectionality Disability Studies Critical Policy Analysis	Symbolic Interactionism Philosophy Qualitative approaches

Adapted from Denzin, N. K., & Lincoln, Y. S. (2000). *Handbook of Qualitative Research.* SAGE Publications Inc.

However, human perceptions and experiences can still be incorporated into an understanding of reality (Clark, 2008). From a research perspective, truth and reality are ascertained through varied approaches to data collection and analysis to increase the accuracy with which social phenomena are understood (Davies & Fisher, 2018).

Critical social theory emphasizes that reality and our understanding of reality are constructed by people with the most power in a particular time and place. This perspective supports the understanding that health and other aspects of reality are shaped by numerous social, political, economic, and cultural factors. Such factors include gender, sexual orientation, class and economic status, race and ethnicity, ability, and geographic location. In nursing research, a strong emphasis is placed on understanding how power imbalances associated with these factors influence health and well-being, access to health care, and patient experiences and outcomes. The goal of critical research is emancipation and social change (Davies & Fisher, 2018).

Some specific types of critical theory include feminist theory, critical race theory, queer theory, disability theory, and intersectionality. Feminist theories are numerous and varied (e.g., Marxist, poststructuralist, cultural, eco) but generally focus on the experiences of women, although this can be broadened to study the experiences and perspectives of all genders, especially in terms of stereotyping, marginalization (exclusion), and emancipation. The primary intent of feminist theories is to dismantle systems of oppression and to raise awareness of gender disparities in a more meaningful way. Rolls and Young (2012) assert that feminist nursing research ought to benefit women; value women's experiences, ideas, and needs; recognize the structural, interpersonal, and ideological conditions that oppress women; and include a portrayal of women's strengths (p. 18). To apply this, they conducted a review of the research literature about older women's experiences of heart failure. They found that there were very few studies on this topic because men have been the subjects of most research about cardiovascular disease; they call for more women-focused studies to inform nursing practice more broadly.

Critical race theory provides a foundation for "studying and transforming the relationship among race, racism, and power" (Delgado & Stefancic, 2001, p. 2). Critical race theorists point out that racism is an everyday experience that is difficult to address because it is not acknowledged. They also note that race is an idea that benefits the dominant group so they have no incentive to eliminate racism (Wesp et al., 2018). Wesp and colleagues (2018) evaluated models and guidelines for cultural competency in nursing from a critical race perspective. They noted that most nurses would agree that there is a need to reduce culturally based disparities in health care, which cultural competency guidelines seek to address. However, they show that these guidelines are flawed because they fail to consider the prejudicial attitudes and imbalances of power that affect patient care and nursing practice. Instead of promoting cultural competence, these guidelines can ironically perpetuate stereotypes and fail to produce change.

Queer theory offers a critique of normative understandings of sex, gender, and sexuality, combining these with other aspects of social difference such as race and class (Hall & Jagose, 2013). Disability theory critiques the medical view of disability as an individual defect that requires cure or elimination. Critical disability theories allow scholars to explore and challenge social injustice and oppression, which equate ability with human worth (Siebers, 2008). Intersectionality is a critical theoretical perspective that combines various critical theories. This shifts the focus from single aspects of identity (such as gender or race) toward a recognition that these aspects work together in people's lived experience. The way that these social forces, identities, and ideologies combine in people's lives has an impact on how much power they have or lack (Crenshaw, 2017). This has implications for people's expectations and experiences of care and for the ways that nurses relate to patients/clients (Van Herk et al., 2011).

Van Herk and colleagues (2011) point out that nurses do not use intersectionality and critical theories as much as they should. They point out that nurses need to have a critical awareness of how power works to create privilege for some and oppression for others in order to provide safe, meaningful, and high-quality care.

Research Hint

Values are involved in all research. For the positivist/post-positivist, it is assumed that values will be held at a distance to minimize their influence. For critical social and constructivist researchers, values and their potential influences on the research results are incorporated more overtly in the research process. However, it is important to remember that all researchers have values and these influence research, regardless of whether they are acknowledged or made explicit.

RESEARCH METHOD\S: QUALITATIVE AND QUANTITATIVE

Research methods are the techniques, procedures, and processes used by researchers to organize a study so that it provides answers to the research question. Research methods can be classified into two major categories: qualitative and quantitative. A researcher chooses between these categories primarily on the basis of the question the researcher is asking. If a researcher wishes to test a cause-and-effect relationship, such as how different levels of social support (cause) leads to high blood pressure (effect), quantitative methods are most appropriate. If, however, a researcher wishes to discover and understand the meaning of an experience or process, such as death and dying, a qualitative approach would be appropriate. A researcher can also design a study that combines both categories, which is known as mixed-methods.

Qualitative research is a systematic, inter-active research method used to describe and interpret life experiences. The emphasis is on capturing the personal perceptions of the study participants. Figure 2.3 outlines the qualitative research process. A researcher would choose to conduct a qualitative research study if the question to be answered concerns the illumination and understanding of human experience, such as illness, loss, or life change.

A study by Smith and colleagues (2018) demonstrates the qualitative research process. They investigated mothers' experiences of supporting their adolescent children though treatment for substance use disorder. The research process as described in Figure 2.3 was used in this study as follows:

Step 1: The researchers began with a broad research question so that they could freely explore the experience rather than narrow it from the start. They state that "the purpose of this study was to gain insights into the women's experiences, to explore how they composed themselves as mothers in the midst of dominant and competing stories of motherhood, family, and substance abuse" (p. 512). The researchers supported their research question with a literature review that covered statistics about the prevalence of substance abuse, the impact of substance abuse on families, and the perceptions and self-perceptions that exist about mothers of children with substance use disorders.

Step 2: A purposive sample of four mothers was selected from one family-oriented, long-term treatment centre for adolescents with alcohol and/or drug addictions. Mothers from different stages of the treatment program were included to explore their experiences at different stages.

Step 3: Each of the mothers participated in six one-on-one interviews as well as six group conversations. Meeting locations included the treatment centre, restaurants, and participants' homes. Data collection strategies were varied, "including conversations, genograms, talking about items of significance, telling personal and family stories, reviewing photos, and writing Haikus, journals, and letters" (p. 514).

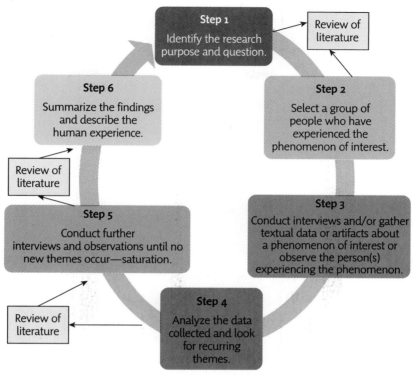

FIG. 2.3 Qualitative research process.

Step 4: After the interviews, "narrative accounts were co-composed with each participant" (p. 515). Four narrative threads (like themes) were theorized from the narratives.

Step 5: Several interviews were held with each participant over a year-long period to generate rich stories of the experience over time.

Step 6: The findings are presented and then linked to the existing literature.

As illustrated by this study, qualitative research is generally conducted in natural settings. Data are usually words and/or images rather than numbers. Sample sizes are often relatively small when compared to quantitative research because the goal is to study a phenomenon in depth with people who can speak knowledgeably about an experience. Thus, data from qualitative studies help nurses understand experiences or phenomena that affect patients, and this information in turn leads to improved care and stimulates further research. Chapters 8 and 9 provide an in-depth overview of the underpinnings, designs, and methods of qualitative research.

Where the purpose of qualitative research is to explore, describe, and/or explain a phenomenon or generate theory, a researcher would choose to conduct a **quantitative** research study if the question to be answered concerned testing for the presence of specific relationships, assessing for group differences, clarifying cause-and-effect interactions, or explaining how effective a nursing intervention was. Quantitative methods entail the use of precise and controlled measurement techniques to gather data that can be analyzed and summarized statistically. Figure 2.4 outlines the quantitative research process. Like the qualitative research process, the quantitative research process begins with the development of a research question and a purpose statement that highlight a relationship between two things.

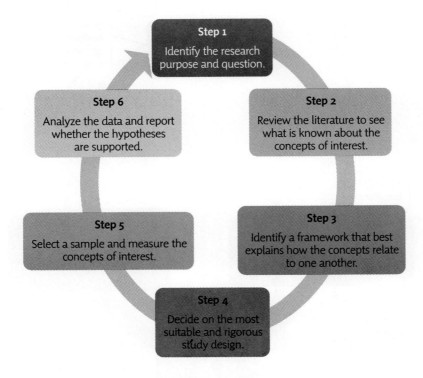

FIG. 2.4   Quantitative research process.

A study completed by El-Masri and colleagues (2014) demonstrates the quantitative research process. They explored the impact of cancer radiation treatment on men with prostate cancer. The research process as described in Figure 2.4 was used in this study as follows:

Step 1: They defined the purpose of the study as being "to compare the effects of 3 types of radiation treatment on functions, bother, and well-being in men with prostate cancer at 1, 6, and 12 months after completion of treatment" (p. 42).

Step 2: The research process began with a review of the literature, which can include journal articles, books, government documents, and even Internet sources, to determine what is known about the phenomenon of interest and theories that explain the phenomenon. In their introduction and review of the literature, the authors noted that although there were several studies on urinary, sexual, and bowel func-

tion after treatment for prostate cancer, there was a dearth of studies that followed patients through the first year of recovery after the radiation treatments. They noted that studies focusing on the well-being and psychosocial impacts were inconsistent.

Step 3: The study was to compare the effect of three different types of radiation on the functions, bother, and well-being of men with prostate cancer.

Step 4: The researchers established a baseline survey prior to treatment, followed by a series of subsequent surveys to measure patients' self-perceived functions, bother, and well-being. The surveys, with the exception of the demographic data collected during the baseline survey (i.e., age), were identical. The authors described the survey tool in detail and provided rationale for the choice of the surveys, including reliability and validity.

Step 5: The researchers recruited participants during an orientation class that all patients attended before commencement of their radiation treatment. To be considered for inclusion, patients had to (1) have a confirmed case of localized prostate cancer; (2) be about to undergo radiation treatment (one of the three types identified); (3) be able to read and understand English; and (4) be able to provide consent.

Step 6: After conducting the statistical analysis, the authors concluded that there were "no differences among the three radiation treatments with regard to any of the outcome variables" (p. 50). They found that there was improvement over time in all of the variables measured; however, the researchers noted that although sexual function improved over time, sexual function continued to be a concern at one year post-treatment.

An important part of the quantitative research process is to decide which design is most appropriate for answering the research question. The numerous choices include descriptive, correlational, longitudinal, quasi-experimental, and experimental designs. El-Masri and colleagues chose a longitudinal design, specifically a repeated survey method, to compare the function, bother, and well-being in men with prostate cancer who had undergone three different radiation regimens.

As demonstrated in the article by El-Masri and colleagues (2014), quantitative research techniques are systematic, and the methodology emphasizes control of the research process, the environment in which the study is conducted, and how each variable is measured. In contrast to qualitative approaches—in which a question is asked and the participant is responsible for providing an in-depth response—quantitative responses are restricted to a preselected set of responses.

When you read research articles, remember that researchers may vary the steps slightly, depending on the nature of the research problem, but all of the steps should be addressed systematically.

INTRODUCTION TO FRAMEWORKS FOR RESEARCH

Frameworks provide a general orientation to understanding a phenomenon of interest and identify what factors are most significant as we examine various aspects of health. A **concept** is an image or symbolic representation of an abstract idea. Chinn and Kramer (2015, p. 160) define concept as a "complex mental formulation of experience." Concepts offer ways to convey abstract ideas. A **conceptual framework** is a structure or assembly of concepts that is used as a map or a scaffolding of ideas for the study. Generally, a conceptual framework is a synthesis or integration of existing views and knowledge on a topic, developed from a review of the literature (Imenda, 2014). It defines the main ideas and the network of relationships between them, grounding the study in the knowledge bases that are relevant to the study. A specific theory may not be guiding the study but concepts always are (Rocco & Plakhotnik, 2009).

A **theoretical framework** is similar but distinct; a **theory** is a unified set of interrelated concepts that serves the purpose of explaining or predicting phenomena. A theory is like a blueprint, which depicts the elements of a structure and the relationship of each element to the other, just as a theory unifies and depicts both the concepts that compose it and how they are related (Imenda, 2014). Chinn and Kramer (2015) define theory as an "expression of knowledge... the creative and rigorous structuring of ideas that project a tentative, purposeful, and systematic view of phenomena" (p. 255). Theory guides practice and research; practice enables testing of theory and generates questions for research; and research contributes to theory building. Thus, what is learned through practice, theory, and research constitutes the knowledge of the discipline of nursing. When a researcher uses a theoretical framework, they are presenting a specific, unified, highly developed theory, such as systems theory or self-efficacy, and any previous empirical work about or development of that theory (Imenda, 2014; Rocco & Plakhotnik, 2009).

The social determinants of health framework is one example that is often used in nursing, based on the understanding that the primary factors that shape the health of Canadians are not medical treatments or lifestyle choices but rather the inequitable living conditions they experience (Mikkonen & Raphael, 2010). This framework depicts how people's health and well-being are determined by 14 factors:

1. Aboriginal status
2. Gender
3. Disability
4. Housing
5. Early childhood development
6. Income and income distribution
7. Education
8. Race
9. Employment and working conditions
10. Social exclusion
11. Food insecurity
12. Social safety net
13. Health services
14. Unemployment and job security

A framework does not necessarily reveal how every possible factor relates to one another. The social determinants of health framework guides the researcher in addressing the relationship between health and any of the 14 factors just listed. The researcher can determine how many factors to focus on and in what way the factors are related to each other and, in turn, to health. In some cases, the researcher may develop a diagram or a pictorial representation of these relationships.

A **model** is a symbolic representation of a set of concepts that is created to depict relationships. Figure 2.5 shows Stewart et al.'s (2009) model of social support. It highlights the process through which support from peers and professionals influences the stressful life situations, coping behaviours, and health care–related behaviours of homeless youths. In this model, arrows are used to depict a process that explains how social support is related to the social network, stress, and health functioning. For example, the arrow from "social support" to "processes" suggests that social support has an effect on social network comparison, exchange, and learning. Whether this is positive or negative is unknown; however, the social network then influences coping behaviours (problem focused, support seeking, and emotion focused), which in turn influence health care–related functioning (loneliness, depression, drug use, and health behaviours).

Qualitative and quantitative research rely on different forms of reasoning to arrive at their conclusions. Inductive reasoning is the pattern of "figuring out what is there" from the details of the nursing practice experience and is the foundation for most qualitative inquiry. Research questions related to the issue of the meaning of experience for the patient can be addressed with the inductive reasoning of qualitative inquiry. Inductive reasoning is a process of starting with the details of experience and building toward a general picture. Deductive reasoning, followed by quantitative researchers, involves a process of starting with the general picture—in this case, the theory—and moving toward the specific. In deductive reasoning, the researcher measures concepts that, when combined, enable the researcher to suggest relationships between the concepts. Deductive reasoning begins with a structure that guides searching for "what is there." Inductive and deductive reasoning can both be used within a field of study or even within a single study to explore concepts and test variables, thereby building a comprehensive body of knowledge within a topic area.

Variables are factors that can take on a range of values (e.g., temperature, heart rate, pain, job satisfaction). The key empirical aspects of a study—its concepts and variables—are generally articulated through conceptual and operational definitions. A **conceptual definition** is much like a dictionary

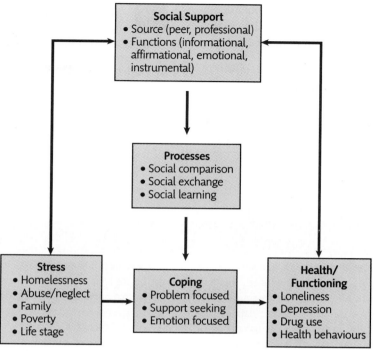

FIG. 2.5 Conceptual model.
(From Stewart, M. et al. (2009). A support intervention to promote health and coping among homeless youths. *Canadian Journal of Nursing Research, 41*(2), 54–77.) SAGE Publications Inc.

definition, conveying the general meaning of the concept. However, for research, the conceptual definition goes beyond the general meaning found in the dictionary; the concept is defined as it is rooted in the theoretical literature. The **operational definition** specifies how the concept will be measured—that is, what instruments will be used to capture the features of the variable.

The Critical Thinking Decision Path on p. 34 takes you through the thinking of a researcher who is about to begin conducting research. You can expect to find some, but not all, of the phases of decision making addressed in a research publication. Beginning with the research question, the researcher is inclined to approach a research problem from the perspective of inductive or deductive reasoning. Qualitative researchers, who pursue an inductive reasoning approach, generally do not present a framework before beginning the

discussion of methods. This is not to say that the literature will not be reviewed before the methods are introduced. Qualitative researchers may use a conceptual or theoretical framework to inform or sensitize them to existing thinking and theorizing about their topic (Bowen, 2006) but avoid using a framework to structure their analysis so that they are able to see freely what their data contain.

Conversely, researchers who use deductive reasoning must choose between a conceptual and a theoretical framework. In the theory literature, these terms are used interchangeably (Chinn & Kramer, 2015), although, in the case presented in the Critical Thinking Decision Path, each term is distinguished from the other on the basis of whether the researcher is creating the structure or whether the structure has already been created by someone else. In general, each of these terms refers to a structure that provides guidance for research by assisting the researcher in determining study variables and operational definitions. *In other words, conceptual and then operational definitions will emerge from the framework.*

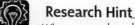

Research Hint

Some research reports embed conceptual definitions in the literature review. The reader should find the conceptual definitions so that the logical fit between the conceptual and the operational definitions can be determined.

Research Hint

When researchers have used conceptual frameworks to guide their studies, you can expect to find a system of ideas, synthesized for the purpose of organizing thinking and providing study direction.

APPRAISING THE EVIDENCE

The Framework

The framework for research provides guidance for the researcher as study questions are fine-tuned, methods for measuring variables are selected (for quantitative research), and analyses are planned. Once data are collected and analyzed, the framework is used as a basis for comparison. The reader of research needs to know how to critically appraise a framework for research (see the Critiquing Criteria box below).

Evaluating frameworks for research requires skill that can be acquired only through repeated critique and discussion with other nurses who have critiqued the same publication. The novice reader of research must be patient while developing these skills. With continuing education and a broader knowledge of potential frameworks, you will build a repertoire of knowledge to enable you to judge the foundation of a research study, the framework for research.

CRITIQUING CRITERIA

1. Is the framework for research clearly identified?
2. Is the framework consistent with a nursing perspective?
3. Is the framework appropriate to guide research on the subject of interest?
4. Are the concepts and variables (if doing a quantitative study) clearly and appropriately defined?
5. Did the study present sufficient literature to support the selected concepts?
6. Is there a logical, consistent link between the framework, the concepts being studied, and the data collection strategies?
7. Are the study findings examined in relation to the framework?

CRITICAL THINKING CHALLENGES

- Explain the difference between research that is based on a constructivist paradigm and research that is based on a positivist paradigm.
- Discuss how a researcher's values can influence the results of a study. Include an example in your answer.
- You are taking an elective course in advanced pathophysiology. The professor compares the knowledge of various disciplines and states that nursing is an example of a nonscientific discipline, declaring in support of this position that nursing's knowledge has been generated with unstructured methods, such as intuition, trial and error, tradition, and authority. What assumptions has this professor made? How would you counter or support this position?
- How would you argue against the following statement: "As a beginning consumer of research, it is ridiculous to expect me to determine whether a researcher's study has an appropriate theoretical framework."

CRITICAL JUDGEMENT QUESTIONS

1. Nurses inform their practice through various ways of knowing. Which of the following is NOT true about how nurses use forms of knowledge in practice?
   a. Theoretical knowing is relevant for practice.
   b. Empirical knowing is acquired through the scientific process.
   c. Personal knowing is based on opinion rather than fact.
   d. Ethical knowing depends on an understanding of what is good.

2. Which of the following statements about research methods is true?
   a. Qualitative research is not systematic.
   b. Quantitative research eliminates bias.
   c. Quantitative research always produces better evidence.
   d. Qualitative research is more appropriate than quantitative research for questions about the meaning of an experience.

3. Critical social theory influences nursing because it:
   a. Shows nurses how power imbalances influence health.
   b. Focuses on women at the expense of men.
   c. Makes nurses view things negatively.
   d. Brings theories into nursing research that are interesting but not directly relevant to nursing practice.

KEY POINTS

- The scientific approaches used to generate nursing knowledge reflect both inductive and deductive reasoning.
- The interaction among theory, practice, and research is central to knowledge development in the discipline of nursing.
- Conceptual and theoretical frameworks can be created by the researcher as a result of the study findings or found in the existing literature and used to support the study.
- The use of a framework for research is important as a guide to systematically identify concepts and, for quantitative research, study variables.
- Conceptual and operational definitions are critical in the evolution of a study, regardless of whether they are explicitly stated in a research report.
- In developing or selecting a framework for research, knowledge may be acquired from other disciplines or directly from nursing. In either case, that knowledge is used to answer specific nursing questions.
- When you critique a framework for research, examine the logical, consistent link between the framework, the concepts for study, and the methods of data collection.

🔊 FOR FURTHER STUDY

Go to Evolve at http://evolve.elsevier.com/Canada/LoBiondo/Research for the Audio Glossary.

REFERENCES

Battiste, M. (2000). *Reclaiming indigenous voice and vision*. Vancouver, BC, Canada: UBC Press.

Battiste, M. (2002). *Indigenous knowledge and pedagogy in First Nations education: A literature review with recommendations*. Ottawa, ON, Canada: National Working Group on Education and the Minister of Indian Affairs, Indian and Northern Affairs Canada.

Battiste, M., & Henderson, J. Y. (2000). *Protecting indigenous knowledge and heritage*. Saskatoon, SK, Canada: Purich Publishing Ltd.

Bowen, G. A. (2006). Grounded theory and sensitizing concepts. *International Journal of Qualitative Methods, 5*(3), 12–23.

Butts, J. B. (2015). Components and levels of abstraction in nursing knowledge. In J. B. Butts, & K. L. Rich (Eds.), *Philosophies and theories for advanced nursing practice* (pp. 87–108). Burlington, MA: Jones & Bartlett Learning.

Castellano, M. (2000). Updating Aboriginal traditions of knowledge. In G. Dei, B. Hall, & D. Rosenberg (Eds.), *Indigenous knowledges in global contexts* (pp. 21–36). Toronto, ON, Canada: University of Toronto Press.

Chinn, P. L., & Kramer, M. K. (2015). *Knowledge development in nursing. Theory and process* (9th ed.). St. Louis, MO: Elsevier.

Clark, A. (2008). Complex critical realism: Tenets and application in nursing research. *Advances in Nursing Science, 31*(4), E67–E79.

Crenshaw, K. (2017). *On intersectionality: Essential writings*. New York: The New Press.

Davies, C., & Fisher, M. (2018). Understanding research paradigms. *Journal of the Australasian Rehabilitation Nurses' Association, 21*(3), 21–25.

Delgado, R., & Stefancic, J. (2001). *Critical race theory: An introduction*. New York: New York University Press.

El-Masri, M. M., Fox-Wasylyshyn, S. M., Springer, C. D., et al. (2014). Exploring the impact of prostate cancer radiation treatment on functions, bother, and well-being. *Canadian Journal of Nursing Research, 46*(2), 42–56.

Hall, D. E., & Jagose, A. (Eds.). (2013). *The Routledge queer studies reader*. Abingdon: Routledge.

Imenda, S. (2014). Is there a conceptual difference between theoretical and conceptual frameworks? *Journal of Social Sciences, 38*(2), 185–195.

Kovach, M. (2005). *Emerging from the margins: Indigenous methodologies*. Toronto, ON: Canadian Scholars' Press/Women's Press.

Mikkonen, J., & Raphael, D. (2010). *Social determinants of health: The Canadian facts*. Toronto: York University School of Health Policy and Management.

Nahm, E., Barker, B., Resnick, B., Covington, B., Magaziner, J., & Brennan, P. F. (2010). Effects of a social cognitive theory-based hip fracture prevention website for older adults. *Computers, Informatics, Nursing, 28*(6), 371–379.

Rocco, T. S., & Plakhotnik, M. S. (2009). Literature reviews, conceptual frameworks, and theoretical frameworks: Terms, functions, and distinctions. *Human Resource Development Review, 8*(1), 120–130.

Rolls, T. P., & Young, L. E. (2012). Disrupting the biomedical discourse: Older women's lived experiences with heart failure: A feminist review of the literature. *Canadian Journal of Cardiovascular Nursing, 22*(1), 18–25.

Siebers, T. (2008). *Disability theory*. Ann Arbor, MI: University of Michigan Press.

Smith, J. M., Estefan, A., & Caine, V. (2008). Mothers' experiences of supporting adolescent children through long-term treatment for substance use disorder. *Qualitative Health Research, 28*(4), 511–522.

Stewart, M., Reutter, L., Letourneau, N., & Makwarimba, E. (2009). A support intervention to promote health and coping among homeless youths. *Canadian Journal of Nursing Research, 41*(2), 54–77.

Van Herk, K. A., Smith, D., & Andrew, C. (2011). Examining our privileges and oppressions: Incorporating an intersectionality paradigm into nursing. *Nursing Inquiry, 18*(1), 29–39.

Wesp, L. M., Scheer, V., Ruiz, A., Walker, K., Weitzel, J., Shaw, L., Kako, P. M., & Mkandawire-Valhmu, L. (2018). An emancipatory approach to cultural competency: The application of critical race, postcolonial, and intersectionality theories. *Advances in Nursing Science, 41*(4), 316–326.

Zander, P. E. (2007). Ways of knowing in nursing: The historical evolution of a concept. *Journal of Theory Construction and Testing, 11*(1), 7–11.

CHAPTER 3

Critical Appraisal Strategies: Reading Research

Lorraine Thirsk

LEARNING OUTCOMES

After reading this chapter, you will be able to do the following:

- Explain the importance of critical appraisal of research articles.
- Summarize the steps associated with appraising research articles.
- Use identified strategies to critically read research articles.
- Identify the format and style of research articles.
- Develop a strategy to read research articles effectively.

KEY TERMS

abstract	critical reading	critiquing criteria
assumptions	critical thinking	reliability
critical appraisal	critique	validity

STUDY RESOURCES

 Go to Evolve at http://evolve.elsevier.com/Canada/LoBiondo/Research for the Audio Glossary.

AS YOU READ THIS TEXT, YOU will learn details of how the steps of the research process unfold. The steps are systematic and orderly, and they relate to the development of nursing knowledge. Understanding the step-by-step process that researchers use will help you develop the critiquing skills necessary to judge the soundness of research studies you will encounter in the literature. Throughout the chapters in this book, research terms pertinent to each step are identified, defined, and illustrated with many examples from the research literature. Five published research studies are featured in the appendices (A–E), and they are used as examples to illustrate significant points in each chapter. Judging not only a study's soundness but also its applicability to practice is a key skill. This chapter provides an overview of the format of research articles. It also introduces you to the critical appraisal skills you will need to be a knowledgeable research user. The chapter is designed to help you begin to read research articles more effectively and with greater understanding.

Before you can assess a study, you need to understand the differences between and among studies. As you read the chapters and the appendices, you will encounter many different study designs, as well as standards for critiquing the soundness of each step of a study and for judging both the strength of evidence provided by a study and its applicability to practice. While the presentation of the research may vary between articles and types of research, all the steps should be addressed systematically. In general, the steps of the research process are reflected in the layout of the research article. The sections of the research article where these steps of the research process are described are presented in Table 3.1 for qualitative research and Table 3.2 for quantitative research.

As you continue to use and perfect your critical appraisal skills, remember that these very skills are an expected competency for delivering evidence-informed nursing practice.

CRITICAL APPRAISAL SKILLS

Your critical appraisal, also called a critique of the literature, is an organized, systematic approach to evaluating a research study or group of research studies. It involves the use of a set of established critical appraisal criteria to objectively determine the strength, quality, and consistency of evidence; these characteristics help you determine the applicability of the evidence to research, education, or practice. As a research user, you will become skilled at critically appraising research studies, combining the evidence with your clinical experience and the patient population you are caring for, to make an evidence-informed decision about the applicability of a particular nursing intervention for your patient or for the patient population in your practice setting.

TABLE **3.1**

STEPS OF THE RESEARCH PROCESS AND JOURNAL FORMAT: QUALITATIVE RESEARCH

RESEARCH PROCESS STEPS OR FORMAT ISSUES	USUAL LOCATION IN JOURNAL HEADING OR SUBHEADING
Identification of the phenomenon	In abstract, introduction, or both
Purpose of research study	In abstract, at beginning or end of introduction, or in more than one of these locations
Literature review	In introduction, discussion, or both
Design	In abstract, "Introduction" section, "Methods" subsection titled "Design," "Methods" section in general, or more than one of these locations
Sample	In "Methods" subsection titled "Sample," "Subjects," or "Participants"
Legal–ethical issues	In section on data collection, in "Procedures" section, or in description of sample
Data-collection procedure	In "Data Collection" or "Procedures" section
Data analysis	In "Methods" subsection titled "Data Analysis" or "Data Analysis and Interpretation"
Results	In abstract (briefly), in separate section titled "Results" or "Findings"
Discussion and recommendations	In separate "Discussion" or "Discussion and Implications" section
References	At end of article

TABLE **3.2**

STEPS OF THE RESEARCH PROCESS AND JOURNAL FORMAT: QUANTITATIVE RESEARCH

RESEARCH PROCESS STEPS OR FORMAT ISSUES	USUAL LOCATION IN JOURNAL HEADING OR SUBHEADING
Research problem	In abstract, introduction (not labelled as a research problem), or separate subsection titled "Problem"
Purpose	In abstract or introduction or both; at end of literature review or discussion of theoretical framework; or in separate section titled "Purpose"
Literature review	At end of introduction but not labelled as a literature review; in separate section titled "Literature Review," "Review of the Literature," or "Related Literature"
	Variables reviewed may appear as titles of sections or subsections
Theoretical framework, conceptual framework, or both	In "Literature Review" section (combined) or in separate sections titled "Theoretic Framework" and "Conceptual Framework"; or each concept or definition used in theoretical or conceptual framework may appear as title of separate section or subsection
Hypothesis/research questions	Stated or implied near end of "Introduction" section, which may be labelled; in separate sections or subsection titled "Hypothesis" or "Research Questions"; or, for first time, in "Results" section
Research design	In abstract or introduction (stated or implied) or in section titled "Methods" or "Methodology"
Sample: type and size	Size: may be stated in abstract, in "Methods" section, or in separate "Methods" subsection as "Sample," "Sample/Subjects," or "Participants"
	Type: may be implied or stated in any of previous headings described under size
Legal–ethical issues	In section titled "Methods," "Procedures," "Sample," "Subjects," or "Participants" (in all cases, stated or implied)
Instruments (measurement tools)	In section titled "Methods," "Instruments," or "Measures"
Validity and reliability	In section titled "Methods," "Instruments," "Measures," or "Procedures" (specifically stated or implied)
Data-collection procedure	In "Methods" subsection titled "Procedure" or "Data Collection" or in separate section titled "Procedure"
Data analysis	In "Methods" subsection under subheading "Procedure" or "Data Analysis"
Results	In separate section titled "Results"
Discussion of findings and new findings	Combined with results or in separate section titled "Discussion"
Implications, limitations, and recommendations	Combined with discussion or presented in separate or combined major sections
References	At end of article
Communicating research results	In research articles, poster, and paper presentations

As you read articles, you may notice the difference in style or format between research articles and theoretical or clinical articles. The terms in a research article may be new to you. Reading research articles is a new skill that gets easier with practice. As a student, you are not expected to completely understand a research article; nor are you expected to develop critiquing skills on your own. A primary objective of this book is to help you acquire the skills needed for critical appraisal. No perfect critique exists; your interpretation will be based on your current knowledge, experience, and understanding. Remember that becoming a competent critical thinker and research user takes time, patience, and experience.

The best way to become a knowledgeable research user is to use critical thinking skills when you read research articles. Critical thinking is the rational examination of ideas, inferences, assumptions, principles, arguments, conclusions, issues, statements, beliefs, and actions (Paul & Elder, 2008). As applied to reading research, this means that you are engaged in the following:

- Systematic understanding of the research process
- Thinking that displays a mastery of the criteria for critiquing research and evidence-informed practice
- The art of being able to make your thinking better (i.e., clearer, more accurate, or more defensible) by clarifying what you understand and what you do not know

Being a critical thinker means that you are consciously thinking about your own thoughts and what you say, write, read, or do, as well as what other people say, write, or do. While thinking about all of this, you are also questioning the appropriateness of the content, applying standards or criteria, and seeing how the information measures up. Take the time to reflect so that you more thoroughly consider your own thoughts and feelings and how they impact the decisions you make—your decisions affect not only you but the patients and clients you are caring for (Aveyard et al., 2015). As you read research articles, there are some key critical thinking questions, presented in Box 3.1, to keep in mind.

BOX 3.1	
CRITICAL THINKING QUESTIONS	
Who	Benefits? Is harmed? Makes decisions? Is most affected? Deserves recognition?
What	Is another perspective? Another alternative? A counter-argument? Is most/least important?
Where	Are there similar concepts/situations? In the world is this a problem? Can we get more information?
When	Is this acceptable/unacceptable? Would this benefit society? Cause problems? Has this played a part in our history?
Why	Is this a problem/challenge? Is this relevant? Should people know about this? Have we allowed this to happen?
How	Is this similar to _____? Does this disrupt things? Do we know the truth? Does this benefit/harm us/others? Can we change this?

Source: From Wabisabi Learning. https://wabisabilearning.com/.

Critical reading is "an active, intellectually engaging process in which the reader participates in an inner dialogue with the writer" (Paul & Elder, 2008, p. 461). A critical reader actively looks for assumptions (accepted truths), key concepts and ideas, reasons and justifications, supporting examples, parallel experiences, implications and consequences, and any other structured features of the text so as to interpret and assess the text accurately and fairly (Paul & Elder, 2008).

You will find that critical thinking and critical reading skills used in the nursing process can be transferred to understanding the research process and reading research articles. You will gradually be able to read an entire research article and reflect on it by identifying and challenging assumptions, identifying key concepts, questioning methods, and determining whether the conclusions are soundly based on the study's findings. Once you have obtained this competency in critiquing research, you will be ready to synthesize the findings of multiple research studies to use in developing evidence-informed practice.

STRATEGIES FOR READING AND CRITIQUING RESEARCH STUDIES

Critiquing a research study may require several readings, especially as you are developing critical reading skills. As you begin, you may need to read an article three or four times; this will get faster as you practice. Critical reading is a process that involves the following levels of understanding and allows you to critically assess a study's validity:

- Preliminary: familiarizing yourself with the content (skimming the article)
- Comprehensive: understanding the researcher's purpose or intent
- Analytical: understanding the parts of the study and developing a critique
- Synthesized: understanding the whole article and understanding how it fits with the cumulative body of knowledge

Preliminary Reading

In this first step, keep your research textbook at your side so you can clarify unfamiliar terms and concepts as you read. The goal of a preliminary reading is to ensure the article is relevant for your purposes. Wakefield (2014) suggests a filtering process during this initial reading where you read through the title, then abstract, and then full article (Box 3.2). In addition, you may want to highlight the purpose statement or research question, as well as the identified steps of the research process.

You should also identify the type of article you are reading in this stage. The articles that you read may be broadly divided into research and non-research literature. Research literature includes quantitative studies, qualitative studies, mixed methods studies, and systematic reviews; non-research literature includes theoretical or methodological articles, review articles, dissertations and theses, as well as others (American Psychological Association, 2019). Definitions

---

BOX **3.2**

PRELIMINARY LITERATURE FILTERING PROCESS

TITLE

Look at the title to decide whether it addresses the subject matter you are interested in.

ABSTRACT

Read the abstract in full to compare its content with the topic and your inclusion and exclusion criteria to see if the article addresses these.

FULL TEXT

Read the full text to compare the content with the topic, purpose of the study, and your inclusion and exclusion criteria to see if the article meets all your requirements.

TYPE OF ARTICLE

In this final stage, you will need to decide if the article is what you want. For example, if you want to use only empirical research data in your review.

Source: Wakefield, A. (2014). Searching and critiquing the research literature. *Nursing Standard, 28*(39), 49-57. https//:doi.10.7748/ns.28.39.49.e8867

---

and explanations of the various types of articles are presented in Table 3.3.

Comprehensive Reading

The purpose of this next reading is to understand the aim or intent of the article.

You should be able to identify the main theme of the article in your own words, as well as identify the main steps of the research process, including the phenomenon under study or variables included in the research question (see Chapter 4). Continue to clarify terms and concepts that you are not familiar with. A list of questions is provided in Table 3.4 to help you with this comprehensive reading.

Analytical Reading

As you continue to read an article, you are ready to begin the appraisal process that will help determine a study's value. Critique is the process of

TABLE **3.3**

TYPES OF SCHOLARLY ARTICLES

BROAD CATEGORY	SPECIFIC TYPE OF ARTICLE	DISTINGUISHING FEATURES
Research	Quantitative	Look for explicit use of the words research or study; evidence of ethics approval if it involves human or animal participants; format reflects Introduction, Methods, Results, Discussion; methods of research stated.
	Qualitative	
	Mixed-methods	
	Systematic review	
Non-research	Theoretical	Furthers a theory or theoretical argument.
	Methodological	Present new approaches to research processes or propose modifications to existing processes. These types of articles may discuss research but are not presenting results of research.
	Literature reviews	Not as rigorous or restrictive as a systematic review; may present numerous articles in a table format; offers a summary of previous literature as well as gaps, inconsistencies and relationships between the articles reviewed.
	Other	Often shorter articles such as letters to the editor, editorials, book reviews, comments or responses.

Source: Based on American Psychological Association (2019). Scholarly writing and publishing principles. In *Publication Manual of the American Psychological Association* (7th ed., pp. 3–26). American Psychological Association.

critical appraisal in which a person critically evaluates the content of a research report for scientific validity or merit and applicability to practice. It requires some knowledge of the subject matter, as well as knowledge of how to read critically and use critiquing criteria.

Research Hint

People often think that "being critical" is the same thing as "being negative." When offering a critique, it really means reading with a questioning mindset. While no research study is perfect, many articles will still be useful, and some will be great.

Critiquing criteria are the standards, appraisal guides, or questions used to judge (assess) an article. Guidelines for conducting a critique are presented in several of the following chapters of this book. In addition, there are many critical appraisal tools available, some of which are listed in

Table 3.5. While these are helpful tools to provide structure and consistency in reviewing research articles, you still need to develop further understanding of the research process for them to be useful.

It is important to note that using a critical appraisal tool will not help you if you do not understand the fundamental principles of the research design of the study you are critiquing. It is therefore important to become familiar with the basic research methods of the research papers you have identified. If you do not understand the research methods used by the authors of the studies incorporated in your literature review, you will not be able to critique the studies with any confidence. (Aveyard, 2014, p.111)

In analyzing a research report, you must evaluate each step of the research process and ask whether the author's description of each step of the process meets the criteria. For instance, the

TABLE **3.4**

QUESTIONS FOR COMPREHENSIVE READING

DESCRIPTIVE QUESTIONS	ANALYTICAL QUESTIONS
What is the question I want to address?	Does this article address my question in full or in part, and is it based on empirical research?
What is the quality of the source?	Is the journal and, therefore, the article credible? How do I know and on what am I basing my decision?
Who has written the article?	Is the author a subject expert or novice, and does this matter? How do I know if the author is credible?
In what type of setting has the study taken place?	Is it possible to transfer the findings from this study to my own setting? Is the setting equivalent to my own setting and does this matter? If so, why? If not, why not and can I articulate this?
What was the sample and how was it generated?	Who are the participants? Are they the same or similar to those I want to include? Does this matter and, if so, why? If not, why not and does this matter? Am I able to articulate my rationale for including this study in my review?
What study method was used?	Was the method appropriate and fit for purpose? Was it robust? How do I know? What am I basing my decision on? Has it helped me clarify what methods I want to use as part of my own study?
What were the findings?	Are the findings relevant to what took place in the study and are they relevant to my own needs? Do I understand what the researchers have deduced from the findings? Is it clear how the findings have been generated? Is there a clear trail outlining how, where, when and why the data have been managed?
How were the data analysed?	Were the correct statistical tests used as and where appropriate? How do I know and what am I basing my decision on? Were any themes generated from the qualitative data? How was this done? Is it clear that the ideas expressed came from the data? Was the process of analysing such data robust? How do I know this?
How have the researchers reported or discussed their findings?	Are the findings and modes of analysis transparent, or are they so brief I do not understand what took place? Can I trust the findings and how do I know this?
What are the conclusions?	How realistic and how appropriately derived are the study conclusions? Are they based on the data or do they appear tangential to the study? How applicable are they to my own setting or proposed study?
Is this article worth including and if so, in what context?	Will it form one of the themes of the literature review or will it only be worth using as background information?

Source: Wakefield, A. (2014). Searching and critiquing the research literature. *Nursing Standard, 28*(39), 49-57. https//:doi.10.7748/ns.28.39.49.e8867.

critiquing criteria for assessing a literature review, discussed in Chapter 5, include whether the literature review identifies gaps and inconsistencies in the literature about a subject, concept, or problem, and whether all of the concepts and variables are included in the review. These two criteria relate to critiquing the research question and the literature review. Remember when you are doing a critique you are pointing out strengths as well as weaknesses.

TABLE 3.5

QUALITY APPRAISAL CHECKLISTS

ORGANIZATION	TYPES OF APPRAISAL CHECKLISTS AVAILABLE
British Medical Journal (BMJ, 2021) https://bestpractice.bmj.com/info/toolkit/ebm-toolbox/critical-appraisal-checklists/	• Two-armed Randomized Controlled Trials • Multiple-Armed Randomized Controlled Trials • Diagnostic Test studies • Systematic Reviews
Centre for Evidence-Based Medicine, University of Oxford (2021) https://www.cebm.ox.ac.uk/resources/ebm-tools/critical-appraisal-tools	• Systematic Reviews • Diagnostics • Prognosis • Randomized Controlled Trials • Qualitative studies • Individual Patient Data Review
Critical Appraisal Skills Programme (CASP UK, 2020) https://casp-uk.net/casp-tools-checklists/	• Randomized Controlled Trials • Systematic reviews • Qualitative studies • Cohort study • Diagnostic study • Case Control study • Economic Evaluation • Clinical Prediction
Joanna Briggs Institute (JBI, n.d.) https://jbi.global/critical-appraisal-tools	• Analytical Cross Sectional studies • Case Control studies • Case Reports • Case Series • Cohort studies • Diagnostic Test Accuracy • Economic Evaluation • Prevalence studies • Qualitative Research • Quasi-Experimental studies • Randomized Controlled Studies • Systematic Reviews • Text and Opinion

Research Hint

If you still have difficulty understanding a research study after using the steps related to skimming and comprehensive reading, make another copy of your marked-up research article, include your specific questions or area of difficulty, and ask your professor to read this copy. Comprehensive understanding and synthesis are necessary for analyzing a research article. Understanding the author's purpose and methods for the study reflects critical thinking and facilitates evaluation of the study.

Another useful tool when analysing and critiquing research studies is to determine the level of evidence (Levin & Chang, 2014). Figure 3.1 depicts a model for determining the levels of evidence associated with the design of a study, ranging from systematic reviews of randomized clinical trials to expert opinions. This reflects the relative strength of different research designs to *testing hypotheses,* which is only one reason for doing research. As suggested in Chapter 2, different research methods provide different types of evidence and answer different research questions. Although the hierarchy suggests that evidence provided by qualitative studies ranks lower (i.e., levels V and VI), it is important to remember that qualitative methods are *not* used to test hypotheses and thus would not provide appropriate evidence for hypothesis-testing research or research about intervention effectiveness. However, qualitative research makes equally important contributions to the overall body of knowledge for nursing and

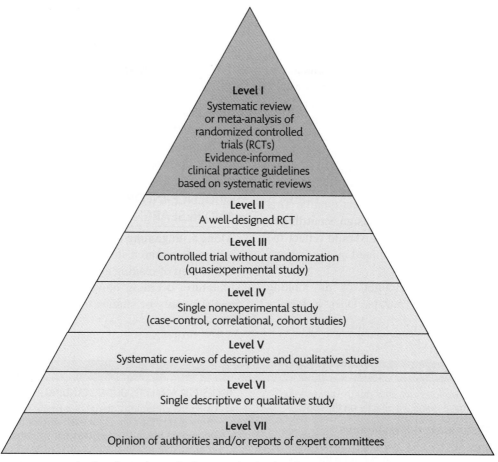

Level I
Systematic review
or meta-analysis of
randomized controlled
trials (RCTs)
Evidence-informed
clinical practice guidelines
based on systematic reviews

Level II
A well-designed RCT

Level III
Controlled trial without randomization
(quasiexperimental study)

Level IV
Single nonexperimental study
(case-control, correlational, cohort studies)

Level V
Systematic reviews of descriptive and qualitative studies

Level VI
Single descriptive or qualitative study

Level VII
Opinion of authorities and/or reports of expert committees

FIG. 3.1   Levels of evidence: hierarchy for rating levels of evidence, associated with a study's design. Evidence is assessed at a level according to its source.
(Based on Melynk, B. M., & Finoult-Overholt, E. (2011). *Evidence-based practice in nursing & literature: A guide to best practice* (2nd ed.). Philadelphia: Lippincott, Williams and Wilkins.)

health care and plays a different role than randomized controlled trials (i.e., level II). Qualitative research can be used to capture experiences of interventions, understand complex causal pathways, generate new theory, explain quantitative findings, or generate hypotheses (Moore et al., 2015).

The importance of an evidence rating system will become clearer to you as you read the chapters on quantitative research. For example, the Jackson and Dennis study (2017; Appendix B) is level II because it is a randomized controlled trial, whereas the study by Pesut et al. (2020; Appendix A) is level VI because of its qualitative design. The level

of evidence, by itself, does not reveal the full worth of a study but is another tool that helps you think about the strengths and weaknesses of research designs for particular purposes and the nature of the evidence provided in the findings and conclusions.

Even though a study may be ranked as a level I or II study, it still needs thorough appraisal to determine its quality and credibility; even a randomized controlled trail can be biased (Djulbegovic & Guyatt, 2017). Assessing the strength of scientific evidence or potential research bias provides a vehicle to guide nurses in evaluating research studies for their applicability in clinical decision-making.

Synthesis of Understanding

After you have completed a critique of the article, compose a one-page summary of the study you have reviewed. Try to use your own words to explain the study, as well as the strengths and weaknesses that you discovered during your critique. If you are critiquing several articles on the same topic, consider using an extraction tool or evidence summary table to make it easier to compare and contrast the findings from different studies. It may also be important to rank the studies you read from highest quality to lowest quality. This ranking can include the study design according to the levels of evidence but also should reflect the quality of the study as determined by the critique that you completed.

Critiquing can be thought of as looking at a completed jigsaw puzzle. Does it form a comprehensive picture, or is a piece out of place? Are all the pieces connected logically together? Are there holes or gaps in the picture that is presented? In the case of reading several studies for synthesis, you need to consider how interrelated each of the studies are and determine the overall strength and quality of evidence and its applicability to practice. Reading for synthesis is essential in critiquing research studies. Box 3.3 summarizes tips for these levels of critical reading.

EVIDENCE-INFORMED PRACTICE AND RESEARCH

Along with gaining confidence while reading and critiquing research studies, you need to undertake a final step of reading and appraising the research literature: deciding how, when, and whether to apply a study or studies to your practice so that

---

BOX 3.3

TIPS FOR CRITICAL READING STRATEGIES

Photocopy or download and print out the article to be critiqued and make notations directly on the copy.

TIPS FOR PRELIMINARY UNDERSTANDING

- Keep a research textbook and a dictionary by your side.
- Review the chapters in the textbook on the various steps of the research process.
- Highlight or underline on your copy of the article any new terms, unfamiliar terms, and significant sentences.
- Look up the definitions of new terms and write them on your copy of the article.
- Highlight or underline identified steps of the research process.
- Find and highlight the purpose statement or research question.
- Determine the type of article.

TIPS FOR COMPREHENSIVE UNDERSTANDING

- Identify the main idea or theme of the article; state it in your own words in one or two sentences.
- Identify the components of the research question.
- Continue to clarify terms that may be unclear on subsequent readings.
- Before critiquing the article, make sure you understand the main points of each reported step of the research process that you identified.

TOOLS FOR ANALYSIS UNDERSTANDING

- Using the critiquing criteria, determine how well the study meets the criteria for each step of the process.
- Determine the level of evidence if you are interested in research about interventions or hypothesis testing.
- Make notes about cues, relationships of concepts, and questions on your copy of the article.
- Ask fellow students to analyze the same study, using the same criteria, and then compare their results with yours.
- Consult faculty members about your evaluation of the study.

TOOLS FOR SYNTHESIS UNDERSTANDING

- Review your notes on the article and determine how each step discussed in the article compares with the critiquing criteria.
- In your own words, compose a one-page summary of the reviewed study.
- Cite article references at the top according to the American Psychological Association (2010) style manual or another reference style.
- In your own words, and using the critiquing criteria, briefly summarize each reported research step.
- In your own words, briefly describe the study's strengths and weaknesses.

your practice is evidence informed. Evidence-informed practice allows you to systematically use the best available evidence with the integration of individual clinical expertise, as well as the patient's values and preferences, in making clinical decisions (Sackett et al., 2000). It is important not to draw hasty conclusions, recognizing that knowledge and science are cumulative (Djulbegovic & Guyatt, 2017). Evidence-informed practice has processes and steps that are followed, as does the research process. Following these steps helps you to decide whether a body of research is of high enough quality and relevance to make a change to practice. Chapter 21 provides further details on evidence-informed practice and introduces you to the steps and strategies associated with developing an evidence-informed practice.

RESEARCH ARTICLES: FORMAT AND STYLE

When you use evidence-informed practice strategies, the first step is to be able to read a research article and understand how each section is linked to each step of the research process. The following section introduces you to the steps of the research process as presented in published articles. When reading research articles, it is important to have a sense of their organization and format. Many journals publish either only research articles or research in addition to clinical or theoretical articles. Although many journals have some common features, they also have unique characteristics. All journals have guidelines for manuscript preparation and submission; these guidelines are published by each journal. A review of these guidelines will give you an idea of the format of articles that appear in specific journals.

A refereed (peer-reviewed) journal has a panel of internal and external reviewers who review submitted manuscripts for possible publication. The external reviewers are drawn from a pool of international and, often interdisciplinary, scholars who are experts in various content areas. In most cases, the reviews are "blind"—that is, the reviewers do not know who the authors of

manuscripts are and vice versa. The reviewers use a set of scholarly criteria to judge whether a manuscript meets the publication standards of the journal. These criteria are similar to those that you use when you are critically appraising the strengths and weaknesses of a study. The credibility of a published theoretical or research article is strengthened by the peer review process.

It is important to remember that even though each step of the research process is discussed at length in this text, you may find only a short paragraph or a sentence in the research article that gives the details of the step in a specific study. However, because of the journal's publishing guidelines, the published study that appears in a journal is a shortened version of the complete work carried out by the researcher or researchers. You will also find that some researchers devote more space in an article to the results, whereas others present a longer discussion of the methods and procedures. Since the 1990s, most authors have given more emphasis to the method, results, and discussion of implications than to the details of assumptions, hypotheses, or definitions of terms. Decisions about the amount of material presented for each step of the research process are constrained by the following:

- A journal's space limitations
- A journal's author guidelines
- The type or nature of the study
- An individual researcher's evaluation of what is the most important component of the study

The following discussion provides a brief overview of each step of the research process and how it might appear in an article (refer to Tables 3.1 and 3.2). It is important to remember that the format of a quantitative research article may differ from that of a qualitative research article.

Abstract

An abstract is a short, comprehensive synopsis or summary of a study at the beginning of an article. An abstract quickly focuses the reader on the main points of a study. A well-presented abstract is accurate, self-contained, concise, specific, nonevaluative, coherent, and readable. In addition to the title of the research study, the abstract will help you to quickly determine if the article is relevant to a topic you are exploring. Keep in mind that abstracts may be misleading, though, so attention still needs to be given to reading the article.

Abstracts vary in length from 50 to 250 words. The length and format of an abstract are dictated by the journal's requirements. Both quantitative and qualitative research studies have abstracts that provide a succinct overview of the study. An example of an abstract can be found at the beginning of the study by Goldsworthy et al. (2019; Appendix D). That abstract follows a structured format that highlights the major steps of the study—background, method, results, and conclusions. Pesut et al. (2020; Appendix A) also follows a structured format. A narrative form of abstract can be seen in Appendix B (Jackson & Denis, 2017) and Appendix C (Bearskin et al., 2016).

Research Hint

A journal abstract is usually a single paragraph that provides a general reference to the research purpose, research questions, or hypothesis, or a combination of these aspects, and highlights the methodology and results, as well as the implications for future practice or research.

Introduction

Early in a research article, in a section that may or may not be titled "Introduction," the researcher presents a background picture of the area researched and its significance to practice. This beginning section should also include a review of the literature and key concepts, building up to the purpose of the study. In the study by Jackson and Dennis (2017; Appendix B) on lanolin use for nipple pain and damage, you can find the basis of the research question early in the report, at the end of the third paragraph:

The purpose of this trial was to evaluate the effect of lanolin on nipple pain among breastfeeding women with damaged nipples. (p. 2)

Jackson and Dennis (2017) use the introduction to set the background of their study that then leads to the purpose statement. They covered why nipple pain is a problem, the previous research done on the topic, and how it could affect breastfeeding.

Another example is found in the first line of the introduction in the study by Bearskin et al. (2016; Appendix C):

The aim of this research was to draw on Cree/Metis understanding through Indigenous research methodologies (IRM), in order to explore how Indigenous knowledge systems are embedded with the nursing practices of four Indigenous nurse scholars.

Bearskin et al. (2016) began with identifying the aim of the study and then continued to explain and situate her research in a larger context. This explanation helps you to understand the context and relevance of the research. Importantly, with Indigenous research you will often see explanations that situate the authors' own personal experience and background. More will be learned on this aspect of the introduction in Chapter 7.

Definition of the Purpose

The purpose of the study is defined either at the end of the researcher's initial introduction or at the end of the "Literature Review" or "Conceptual Framework" section, often immediately preceding the "Methods" section. After reviewing the title and abstract, finding the purpose statement is often a quick way to see if the study is relevant for the topic you are searching. The study's purpose may or may not be labelled as such, or it may be referred to as the study's aim or objective. Pesut et al. (2020; Appendix A) described the goal of the study in the last paragraph of the background section, immediately preceding the methods section:

In this paper, we report on findings from the qualitative phase of the study that revealed the impact of Canada's legislated approach to assisted death on nurses' experiences, and on nursing practice, in Canada. (p. 3)

Goldsworthy et al. (2019; Appendix D) described the purpose of their study in the first sentence of their "Methods" section:

This study used a quasi-experimental design to test the effects of a 16-hour simulation intervention on third-year undergraduate nursing students' confidence and competence in the recognition and response to the rapidly deteriorating adult and paediatric patient. (p. 27)

Literature Review and Theoretical Framework

The literature review section should identify gaps in knowledge that will provide rationale for the purpose of the study. Authors of studies and journal articles present the literature review and theoretical framework in different ways. In many research articles, the literature review is merged with the discussion of the theoretical framework. The resulting section includes the main concepts investigated and may be titled "Review of the Literature," "Literature Review," "Theoretical Framework," "Related Literature," "Background," or "Conceptual Framework"; or it may not be a separate section at all. In reviewing Appendices A through E, you will find differences in the headings used. For example, Jackson et al. (2017) have a general introduction that includes a brief literature review and a review of the literature for previous interventions (Appendix A). Alternately, Pesut et al. (2020) reviewed the history of medical assistance in dying, offered a model for framing the legislation in the section on "Implications of a legislated approach to MAiD," and reviewed literature and policy documents related to nurses in the section "The nursing role in MAiD" (Appendix A). One style is not better than another, as it may be dependent on the

journal guidelines; all of the studies in the appendices contain all of the critical elements but present the elements differently.

Research Hint

Often the background or literature review section of a research study has several citations to other studies. If you use the ideas presented in this section in a scholarly paper, it is important that you locate the original source that was cited and not erroneously attribute the ideas to the author of the article you are reading.

Hypothesis or Research Question

A study's research questions or hypotheses can also be presented in different ways. Research reports in journals often do not have separate headings for reporting the hypotheses or research question. They are often embedded in the "Introduction" or "Background" section or not labelled at all (e.g., as in the studies in the appendices). Quantitative research studies have hypotheses or research questions. If a researcher uses hypotheses in a study, the researcher may report whether the hypotheses were or were not supported; such reporting occurs toward the end of the article, in the "Results" or "Findings" section. Jackson and Dennis (2017) (Appendix B) imbed their hypothesis in the purpose statement, found at the end of the introduction section, as does Goldsworthy et al. (2019) (Appendix D). Qualitative research studies do not have hypotheses but do have research questions and purposes. Pesut et al. (2020) (Appendix A) and Bearskin et al. (2016) (Appendix C) both pose their research questions in the introduction.

Research Design

The type of research design can be found in the abstract, within the purpose statement, and in the introduction to the "Procedures" or "Methods" section. For example, the studies in Appendices A, B, C, and D all identify the design type in both the abstract and the body of the study report.

One of your first objectives is to determine whether the study is qualitative or quantitative, so that the appropriate criteria are used. Although the rigour of the critiquing criteria addressed does not substantially change, some of the terminology of the questions differs for qualitative and quantitative studies. For instance, in the study by Goldsworthy et al. (2019; Appendix D), you might ask whether the hypotheses were generated from the theoretical framework or the literature review and whether the design chosen was appropriate and consistent with the study's questions and purpose. With a qualitative study such as that by Bearskin et al. (2016; Appendix C), however, you might be asking whether the researchers conducted the study in a manner consistent with the principles of qualitative research and specifically an Indigenous research methods, which is described extensively in the "Research Framework" section.

Do not get discouraged if you cannot easily determine the design. More often than not, the specific design is not stated, or, if an advanced design is used, the details are not spelled out. One of the best strategies is to review the chapters in this text that address designs and to ask your professors for assistance. The following tips will help you determine whether the study you are reading employs a quantitative design:

- Hypotheses are stated or implied.
- The terms *control* and *treatment group* appear.
- The term *survey, correlational,* or *ex post facto* is used.
- The term *random* or *convenience* is mentioned in relation to the sample.
- Variables are measured by instruments or scales.
- Reliability and validity of instruments are discussed.
- Statistical analyses are used.

In contrast, qualitative studies do not usually focus on numbers, and you will often see participant quotes in qualitative research reports. Qualitative researchers typically use the terms *informants* or *participants,* rather than *subjects.* Deciding on the type of qualitative design can be confusing; one of the best tools is to review this text's chapters on qualitative design, as well as to critique qualitative studies. The specific qualitative method that is used will often be reported in the "Methods" section of a research report.

Sampling

The population from which the sample was drawn is discussed in the section titled "Methods" or "Methodology" under the subheadings of "Subjects," "Participants," or "Sample." For example, Pesut et al. (2020) discuss the sample in a section titled "Participants" under the larger heading of "Methods" (Appendix A). Bearskin (2016; Appendix C) includes her participants as co-researchers and lists them as authors on her paper—this is consistent with the Indigenous paradigm underpinning the study. Goldsworthy et al. (2019; Appendix D) described their sample in the section titled "Sample." Researchers should describe both the population from which the sample was chosen and the number of participants who took part in the study. They should also mention how participants were recruited, whether participants dropped out of the study, and if they did, how many. For quantitative studies, the process of randomization should be explained, if applicable. The authors of all of the studies in the appendices discuss their samples in enough detail so that who the participants were and how they were selected is clear.

Reliability and Validity

The discussion related to instruments used to measure the variables of a quantitative study is usually included in a "Methods" subsection titled "Instruments" or "Measures." The researcher usually describes the particular measure (i.e., instrument or scale) used by discussing its reliability and validity. Reliability refers to the consistency or constancy of the measuring tool, whereas validity describes whether the measuring tool actually measures the correct phenomenon. Jackson et al. (2017; Appendix B) describe two pain rating instruments used to assess nipple pain and measures for breastfeeding duration, exclusivity, and self-efficacy, along with comments on reliability and validity of these tools. This can be found in the "Methods" section in a subsection titled "Outcome Measures."

Research Hint

Remember that not all research articles include headings related to each step or component of the research process, but each step is presented at some point in the article.

In some cases, researchers do not report the reliability and validity of commonly used, established instruments in an article, and may refer you to other references. Ask for assistance from your instructor if you are in doubt about the validity or reliability of a study's instruments. Qualitative researchers typically report on the trustworthiness of the findings and on how the researcher is positioned in relation to the study (see Chapter 8). A key component of quality in qualitative research is attending to the process of the research, which should be described. For example, Bearskin et al. (2016) described how she attended to the practical values of respect, responsibility, reciprocity, and relevance described by Kirkness and Barnhardt (as cited by Bearskin et al.) in the "Research Framework" section, adding to the trustworthiness of the research.

Procedures and Data Collection Methods

The procedures used to collect data or the step-by-step way in which the researcher used the measures (instruments or scales) is generally described in the "Procedures" section. In each of the studies in Appendices A through D, the researchers indicated how they conducted the study in detail in sections and subsections as follows:

Appendix A: "Methods" with subsection of "Data Collection and Analysis"

Appendix B: "Methods" with subsection of "Outcome Measures"

Appendix C: "Research Framework" with subsection "Data Gathering"

Appendix D: "Methods" with subsection of "Data Collection" with quantitative data in "Statistical Data Collection" and qualitative data in "Qualitative Evaluation"

Notice that the researchers in each study in Appendices A, B, and D also state that the studies were approved by a research ethics board (see Chapter 6), thereby ensuring that each met ethical standards. Appendix C explicitly states that "research ethics were based on IRM principles, thus going beyond the minimum standards outlined" (Bearskin et al., 2016, p. 23).

Data Analysis/Results

The data analysis procedures (i.e., the statistical tests used and the results of descriptive and inferential tests applied in quantitative studies) are presented in the section titled "Results" or "Findings." Often in quantitative research, results are presented in a table format, with a brief narrative description. Qualitative studies may provide descriptive statistics for socio-demographic information for participants. The procedures for analyzing the themes, concepts, and observational or print data in qualitative studies are usually described in the "Methods" or "Data Collection" section and reported in the "Results," "Findings," or "Data Analysis" section. The article by Pesut et al. (2020; Appendix A) describes the process of their qualitative analysis in the "Methods" section, in a subsection titled "Data Collection and Analysis." Goldsworthy et al. (2019) reported both descriptive and inferential statistics used in their analysis in the "Data Analysis" section.

Discussion

The last part of an article about a research study is the "Discussion" section. In this section, the researchers explain how all the parts of the study are related and analyse the study as a whole. The researchers refer to the literature reviewed and discuss how their study is similar to, or different from, other studies. You will often find further literature in the "Discussion" section. This helps readers to understand how the new findings fit in with what is currently known about the topic. Researchers may report the results and discussion in one section but usually report them in separate "Results" and "Discussion" sections (Appendices A, B, C, and D). One way is not better than the other. Journal and space limitations determine how these sections are handled. Any new findings or unexpected findings are usually described in the "Discussion" section.

Recommendations and Implications

In some articles, a separate section titled "Conclusions" describes the implications of the findings for practice and education, as well as related limitations based on the findings, and future studies may be recommended. For example Jackson et al. (2017; Appendix B) include recommendations for practice and for future research in their "Conclusion," stating: "the recommendation of lanolin by health professionals to treat breastfeeding-related nipple pain is questionable and warrants further investigation to ensure the provision of evidence-based care" (p. 561). In other articles, recommendations for research and practice may appear in several sections with titles such as "Discussion," "Limitations," "Nursing Implications," "Implications for Research and Practice," and "Summary." In Appendix D, Goldsworthy et al. (2019) have a section titled "Implications," as well as a "Strengths and Limitations" section. Some authors may include the "Limitations" and other sections discussed above in the section "Discussion."

References

All of the references cited in a research article are included at the end of the article. The main purpose of the reference list is to support the material presented by identifying the sources in a manner that allows for easy retrieval by the reader. Journals have various referencing styles to organize references. American Psychological Association (APA) style is commonly used in the health sciences, although other manuscript and referencing styles are also used in health research, such as Chicago, Vancouver, and Modern Language Association (MLA).

Communicating Results

Communicating the results of a study can take the form of a research article, poster, or paper presentation. All are valid ways of providing nurses with the data and the ability to provide high-quality patient care that is based on research findings. Evidence-informed nursing care plans and practice protocols, guidelines, or standards are outcome measures that effectively indicate communicated research.

As you develop critical thinking and reading skills by using the strategies presented in this chapter, you will become more familiar with the research and appraisal processes. You will be well on your way to becoming a knowledgeable user of research from nursing and other scientific disciplines for application in nursing practice.

Research Hint _____
When writing a paper on a specific concept or topic that requires you to critique and synthesize the findings from several studies, you might find it useful to create an evidence table of the data. Include the following information: author, date, type of study, design, sample, data analysis, findings, and implications.

SYSTEMATIC REVIEWS: META-ANALYSES, INTEGRATIVE REVIEWS, SCOPING REVIEWS, AND META-SYNTHESES

Another variety of articles that is appearing more frequently in the literature and is very important for understanding evidence-informed practice are systematic reviews. "The systematic review is essentially an analysis of the available literature (that is, evidence) and a judgment of the effectiveness or otherwise of a practice, involving a series of complex steps" (Joanna Briggs Institute, 2016, n.p.). Systematic reviews include meta-analyses, integrative reviews, scoping reviews, and meta-syntheses, reflecting a summary of quantitative studies, qualitative studies, or both. Further details on types of systematic reviews can be found in Chapter 21. A systematic review, or meta-analysis of randomized controlled trials is considered Level I evidence for determining the effectiveness of an intervention. The authors of these articles investigate a number of studies related to a specific clinical question and, using a specific set of criteria and methods, evaluate those articles as a whole. An example of a systematic review is included in Appendix E. Chapter 8 has further detail about qualitative approaches to systematic reviews, and Chapter 11 has more detail regarding quantitative systematic reviews.

Systematic reviews are formatted similarly to other research studies but have the purpose of summarizing a body of literature or data. The components of these types of articles may be presented as follows:

- Background: The introduction covers content related to the background of the clinical question and clarifies the specific question that the review answers. The article's authors clarify the definitions of the concepts in the question so that the reader understands the concepts that were used in assessment.
- Methods: The methods used for searching the literature are detailed. The exact electronic databases, the dates, and the keywords used to conduct the search are provided. In addition, the article details the inclusion and exclusion criteria by which the literature was chosen to review and critique. If any articles were found and not used, the authors detail why articles were excluded from the review. This is often presented in a graphic format, such as a PRISMA flow diagram (Moher et al., 2009).
- Appraisal of the literature: The articles that are included in the literature review are discussed in the body of the article, and a data extraction table is used to present the highlights of each article. The author uses the evidence table to compare the articles, critique them for scientific validity, and discuss how well they answer the clinical question. If the author uses a meta-analysis format, a summary of the data is presented.
- Conclusions/summary: In the conclusions or summary, the strength, quality, and consistency of the data are described as they apply to practice. This section contains recommendations about which aspects of practice are supported by the data in the articles and for which aspects further research is needed to more fully answer the question posed in the review.

CLINICAL GUIDELINES

Clinical guidelines are systematically developed statements or recommendations that serve as a guide for practitioners. Guidelines have been developed to assist in bridging practice and research. Guidelines are developed by professional organizations, government agencies, institutions, and convened expert panels. Guidelines provide clinicians with an algorithm for clinical management or for decision making about specific diseases (e.g., colon cancer) or treatments (e.g., pain management). For example, Diabetes Canada has posted clinical practice guidelines on its website that are intended to "guide practice; inform general patterns of care; enhance diabetes prevention efforts in Canada; and reduce the burden of diabetes complications" (Houlden, 2018, p. S1).

Not all guidelines are well developed and, like research, must be assessed before implementation. Clinical guidelines, although they are systematically developed and make explicit recommendations for practice, may be formatted differently. Guidelines should clearly present scope and purpose of the practice, detail who contributed to the development of the guidelines, demonstrate scientific rigour, demonstrate clinical applicability, and demonstrate editorial independence. While improving efficiency in application of evidence into practice, the clinical practice guidelines are only as strong as the research they are based on. Often guidelines will include a summary of the levels of evidence that were available to draw conclusions from. A common appraisal tool is GRADES (Atkins et al., 2004). This will be further described in Chapter 21, along with criteria to use when evaluating clinical practice guidelines.

As you venture through this textbook, you will be challenged to think about not only reading and understanding research studies but also applying the findings to your practice. Nursing has a rich legacy of research that has grown in depth and breadth. Producers of research and clinicians must engage in a joint effort to translate findings into practice that will make a difference in the care of patients and families.

CRITICAL THINKING CHALLENGES

- The critical reading of research articles may require a minimum of three or four readings. Is this always the case? What assumptions underlie this claim?
- Why is it necessary to reach an analysis stage of critical reading before you can critique a study?
- To synthesize a research article, what questions must you first be able to answer?
- Discuss several strategies that might motivate practising nurses to critically appraise research articles.

CRITICAL JUDGEMENT QUESTIONS

1. What level of evidence is presented in the article that appears in Appendix B?
   a. Level I
   b. Level II
   c. Level III
   d. Level IV

2. What are the key features that improve the quality of this study?
   a. Evaluated mechanisms of treatment
   b. Registered as a clinical trial
   c. Researchers are nurses
   d. Randomization and blinding

3. Based on these findings, what would you recommend in practice?
   a. There is insufficient evidence to make recommendations for practice
   b. Lanolin should be used routinely for women who are breastfeeding
   c. Lanolin should not be used routinely for women who are breastfeeding
   d. Lanolin can be used to improve maternal satisfaction but is not effective at reducing nipple pain

KEY POINTS

- Critical thinking and critical reading skills will enable you to question the appropriateness of the content of a research article, apply standards or critiquing criteria to assess the study's scientific merit for use in practice, and consider alternative ways of handling the same topic.
- Critical reading involves active assessment of an article, searching for, interpreting, and evaluating key concepts, ideas, and justifications.
- Critical reading requires four stages of understanding: preliminary (skimming), comprehensive, analysis, and synthesis. Each stage is characterized by specific strategies to increase your critical reading skills.
- Critical reading for preliminary understanding is accomplished by skimming or quickly and lightly reading an article in order to familiarize yourself with its content and to provide you with a general sense of the material.
- Critical reading for a comprehensive understanding is designed to increase your

understanding of both concepts and research terms in relation to the context and of the parts of the study in relation to the whole study, as presented in the article.

- Critical reading for analytical understanding is designed to divide the content into parts so that each part of the study is understood. The critiquing process begins at this stage.
- Critical reading to reach the goal of synthesis understanding combines the parts of a research study into a whole. During this final stage, the reader determines how each step of the research process relates to all the other steps, how well the study meets the critiquing criteria, and the usefulness of the study for practice.
- Critical appraisal is the process of critically evaluating the strengths and weaknesses of a research article for scientific merit and application to practice, theory, and education. The need for more research on the topic or clinical problem is also addressed at this stage.
- Research articles have different formats and styles, depending on journal manuscript requirements and whether they are quantitative or qualitative studies.
- The basic steps of the research process are presented in journal articles in various ways. Detailed examples of such variations can be found in chapters throughout this text.
- Evidence-informed practice begins with the careful reading and understanding of research articles.

🛜 FOR FURTHER STUDY

Go to Evolve at http://evolve.elsevier.com/Canada/ LoBiondo/Research for the Audio Glossary.

REFERENCES

American Psychological Association. (2010). *Publication manual of the American Psychological Association* (6th ed.). Washington, DC: American Psychological Association.

Atkins, D., Best, D., Briss, P. A., et al. (2004). Grading quality of evidence and strength of recommendations. *BMJ, 328*(7454), 1490. https://doi.org/10.1136/bmj.328.7454.1490.

Aveyard, H. (2014). *Doing a literature review in health and social care: A practical guide.* New York: McGraw-Hill Education.

Aveyard, H., Sharp, P., & Woolliams, M. (2015). *A beginner's guide to critical thinking and writing in health and social care* (2nd ed.). Maidenhead, Berkshire, UK: Open University Press.

Bearskin, R. L. B., Cameron, B. L., King, M., & Pillwax, C. W (2016). Mâmawoh Kamâtowin, "Coming together to help each other in wellness": Honouring Indigenous nursing knowledge. *International Journal of Indigenous Health, 11*(1), 18–33. https://doi.org/10.18357/ijih111201615024.

British Medical Journal (2021). *Critical Appraisal Checklists.* https://bestpractice.bmj.com/info/toolkit/ebm-toolbox/critical-appraisal-checklists/.

Centre for Evidence-Based Medicine. (2021). *Critical Appraisal Tools.* University of Oxford. https://www.cebm.ox.ac.uk/resources/ebm-tools/critical-appraisal-tools.

Critical Appraisal Skills Programme (2020). *CASP Checklists.* https://casp-uk.net/casp-tools-checklists/.

Djulbegovic, B., & Guyatt, G. H. (2017). Progress in evidence-based medicine: A quarter century on. *The Lancet, 390*(10092), 415-423. https://doi.org/10.1016/S0140-6736(16)31592-6.

Goldsworthy, S., Patterson, J. D., Dobbs, M., Afzal, A., & Deboer, S. (2019). How does simulation impact building competency and confidence in recognition and response to the adult and paediatric deteriorating patient among undergraduate nursing students? *Clinical Simulation in Nursing, 28*, 25–32. https://doi.org/10.1016/j.ecns.2018.12.001.

Houlden, R. L. (2018). 2018 Clinical practice guidelines: Introduction. *Canadian Journal of Diabetes, 42*, S1–S5. https://doi.org/10.1016/j.jcjd.2017.10.001.

Jackson, K. T., & Dennis, C. L. (2017). Lanolin for the treatment of nipple pain in breastfeeding women: a randomized controlled trial. *Maternal & Child Nutrition, 13*(3), e12357. https://doi.org/10.1111/mcn.12357.

Joanna Briggs Institute (n.d.). *Critical Appraisal Tools.* https://jbi.global/critical-appraisal-tools.

Joanna Briggs Institute. (2016). Critical appraisal tools. http://www.joannabriggs.org/research/critical-appraisal-tools.html.

Levin, R. F., & Chang, A. (2014). Tactics for teaching evidenced-based practice: Determining the level of evidence of a study. *Worldviews on Evidence-Based Nursing, 11*(1), 75–78. https://doi.org/10.1111/wvn.12023.

Moher, D., Liberati, A., Tetzlaff, J., & Altman, D. G. (2009). Preferred reporting items for systematic reviews and meta-analyses: The PRISMA statement. *Annals of Internal Medicine, 151*(4), 264–269. https://doi.org/10.1136/bmj.b2535.

Moore, G. F., Audrey, S., Barker, M., Bond, L., Bonell, C., Hardeman W., ... & Baird, J. (2015). Process evaluation of complex interventions: Medical Research Council guidance. BMJ, 350. https://doi.org/10.1136/bmj.h1258.

Paul, R., & Elder, L. (2008). *The miniature guide to critical thinking concepts and tools*. Dillon Beach, CA: Foundation for Critical Thinking Press.

Pesut, B., Thorne, S., Schiller, C. J., Greig, M., & Roussel, J. (2020). The rocks and hard places of MAiD: A qualitative study of nursing practice in the context of legislated assisted death. *BMC Nursing, 19*(1), 1–14. https://doi.org/10.1186/s12912-020-0404-5.

Sackett, D. L., Straus, S. E., Richardson, W. S., et al. (2000). *Evidence-based medicine: How to practise and teach EBM*. London: Churchill Livingstone.

University of Toronto Libraries (2019). Evidence-based practice: tools and checklists. https://www.guides.library.utoronto.ca/c.php?g=250646&p=5010384.

CHAPTER 4

Developing Research Questions, Hypotheses, and Clinical Questions

Mina D. Singh | Ramesh Venkatesa Perumal

LEARNING OUTCOMES

After reading this chapter, you will be able to do the following:

- Discuss the purpose of developing a research question.
- Describe how the research question and hypothesis are related to the other components of the research process.
- Describe the process of identifying and refining a research question.
- Identify the criteria for determining the significance of a research question.
- Discuss the appropriate use of the purpose, aim, or objective of a research study.
- Discuss how the purpose, research question, and hypothesis suggest which level of evidence is to be obtained from the findings of a research study.
- Identify the characteristics of research questions and hypotheses.
- Describe the advantages and disadvantages of directional and nondirectional hypotheses.
- Compare the use of statistical hypotheses with that of research hypotheses.
- Discuss the appropriate use of research questions versus hypotheses in a research study.
- Discuss the differences between a research question and a clinical question in relation to evidence-informed practice.
- Identify the criteria used for critiquing a research question and a hypothesis.
- Apply the critiquing criteria to the evaluation of a research question and a hypothesis in a research report.

KEY TERMS

clinical question	nondirectional hypothesis	research question
dependent variable	population	statistical hypothesis
directional hypothesis	problem statement	testability
hypothesis	purpose	testable
independent variable	research hypothesis	variable

STUDY RESOURCES

 Go to Evolve at http://evolve.elsevier.com/Canada/LoBiondo/Research for the Audio Glossary.

AS YOU READ EACH CHAPTER, REMEMBER that each step of the research process is defined and discussed as to how that particular step relates to evidence-informed practice. At the beginning of this chapter, you will learn how to generate your own clinical questions that you will use to guide the development of evidence-informed practice projects. Then you will learn about research questions and hypotheses from the perspective of the researcher. From a clinician's perspective, you must understand how the research question and hypothesis align with the rest of the study.

The first step in developing evidence-informed practice is also to ask a question, referred to as a *clinical question*. After posing the clinical question, a quest begins to find the best evidence to answer the question and to apply it to clinical practice. For a clinician making an evidence-informed decision about a patient care issue, a clinical question would guide the nurse in searching for and retrieving the best available evidence. For example, is chlorhexidine or povidone-iodine more effective in preventing infections in central catheters? Finding the evidence, combined with clinical expertise and patient preferences, would provide an answer on which to base the most effective decision about which antiseptic is most effective.

If there is no clear satisfactory answer to the clinical question, a specific research question or hypothesis may be developed to lead a study. All research studies begin with questions and/or hypotheses.

When nurses ask certain questions, they are often well on their way to developing a research question or hypothesis. Such questions include "What is happening in this situation?"; "What are the patient's experiences?"; "Why are things being done this way?"; "I wonder what would happen if . . . ?"; "What characteristics are associated with . . . ?"; and "What is the effect of . . . on patient outcomes?" Research questions are usually generated from situations or problems that emerge from practice. These are often articulated in a **problem statement** such as the following, posed by Jackson and Dennis (2017): "Nipple pain and damage is a common occurrence for breastfeeding women in the early postpartum period" (p. 1). (See Appendix B.)

For an investigator conducting a study, the research question or the hypothesis is a key preliminary step in the research process. The **research question** presents the idea that is to be examined in the study and is the foundation of the research study. Once the research question is clear, the researcher selects the most appropriate research design. If the research question is primarily explorative, descriptive, or theory generating, the researcher opts for qualitative methods. In these studies, a hypothesis is not formulated. For studies in which the researcher is seeking a specific answer to a research question, however, a hypothesis is generated and tested.

Hypotheses can be considered intelligent hunches, guesses, or predictions that help researchers seek the solution or answer to the research question. Hypotheses are a vehicle for testing the validity of the theoretical framework assumptions and provide a bridge between theory and actuality. In the scientific world, researchers derive hypotheses from theories and subject them to empirical testing. A theory's validity is not directly examined. Instead, through testing hypotheses, researchers can evaluate the merit of a theory.

Research questions or hypotheses often appear at the beginning of research articles. However, because of space constraints or stylistic considerations in journal publications, the research question or hypothesis may be embedded in the purpose, aims, goals, or even the results section of the research report. Both the consumer and the producer of research need to understand the importance of research questions and hypotheses as the foundational elements of a research study.

DEVELOPING AND REFINING A CLINICAL QUESTION

Practising nurses, as well as students, are challenged to keep their practice up to date by searching for, retrieving, and critiquing research articles that apply to practice issues that they encounter in their clinical setting to yield positive patient outcomes. As Melnyk and Fineout-Overholt (2019) commented,

> evidenced-based practice (EBP) is a life-long problem-solving approach to clinical practice that integrates the following: a systematic search and critical appraisal of the most relevant and best research (i.e., internal evidence); one's own clinical expertise generated from outcomes management or evidenced-based quality improvement projects, a thorough patient assessment, and evaluation and use of available resources necessary to achieve desired patient outcomes; patient/family preferences and values. (p. 8)

Practitioners strive to use the current best evidence from research in making clinical and health care decisions. Although they may not be conducting research studies, their search for information from practice is also converted into focused, structured clinical questions that are the foundation of evidence-informed practice. Clinical questions often arise from clinical situations for which there are no ready answers. You have probably had the experience of asking, "What is the most effective treatment for . . . ?" or "Why do we still do it this way?"

Focused clinical questions are used as a basis for searching the literature to identify supporting evidence from research. A **clinical question** has five components (Melnyk & Fineout-Overholt, 2019, p. 16):

1. Patient Population
2. Intervention or Issue of Interest
3. Comparison Intervention or Group
4. Outcome
5. Time Frame

These five components, known as PICOT, constitute a format that is effective in helping nurses develop searchable clinical questions (Melnyk & Fineout-Overholt, 2019). Box 4.1 presents each component of the clinical question; in addition, Table 4.1 offers clinical questions based on the PICOT tool.

BOX **4.1**

PICOT COMPONENTS OF A CLINICAL QUESTION

Population: The individual patient or group of patients with a particular condition or health care problem (e.g., adolescents aged 13 to 18 with type 1 insulin-dependent diabetes)

Intervention: The particular aspect of health care that is of interest to the nurse or the health team—for example, a therapeutic intervention (inhaler or nebulizer for treatment of asthma), a preventive intervention (pneumonia vaccine), a diagnostic intervention (measurement of blood pressure), or an organizational intervention (implementation of a bar coding system to reduce medication errors)

Comparison intervention: Standard care or no intervention (e.g., antibiotic or ibuprofen for children with otitis media); a comparison of two treatment settings (e.g., rehabilitation centre or home care)

Outcome: Improved outcome (e.g., improved glycemic control, decreased hospitalizations, decreased medication errors)

Time: Time involved to demonstrate an outcome (e.g., weight loss maintained over a period of 2 years)

Sample Questions using the PICOT Tool:

Intervention: In health care workers (P), how does using N95 masks (I) compared to other masks (C) affect transmission of airborne infections (O)?

Prognosis/Prediction:

1. For patients 65 years and older (P), how does self-isolation (I) compared to no self-isolation (C) influence the risk of developing COVID-19 (O) during the pandemic (T)?

2. In patients who have experienced an acute myocardial infarction (P), how does weekly exercise (3–5 times a week) (I) compared to no exercise (C) influence death and infarction rates (O) during the first 5 years after the myocardial infarction (T)?

Diagnosis: In patients at high risk for gallbladder dysfunction (P), is a HIDA scan (I) compared to an ultrasound (C) more accurate in diagnosing eminent gallbladder function (O)?

Etiology: Are fair-skinned women who have prolonged unprotected UV ray exposure (>1 hour) at increased risk of melanoma compared to darker-skinned women without prolonged unprotected UV ray exposure?

TABLE **4.1**

TEMPLATE FOR ASKING PICOT QUESTIONS

INTERVENTION/TREATMENT: Questions addressing the treatment of an illness or disability.

In _____(P), how does _____ (I) compared to _____
(C) affect _____(O) within _____(T)?

PROGNOSIS/PREDICTION: Questions addressing the act or process of identifying or determining the nature and cause of a disease or injury through assessment/evaluation.

In _____(P), how does _____ (I) compared to _____
(C) influence/affect the risk of/predict _____ (O) over _____ (T)?

DIAGNOSIS/DIAGNOSTIC TEST/ASSESSING: Questions addressing the prediction of the course of a disease.

In _____(P) are/is _____(I) compared to _____
(C) more accurate in diagnosing/assessing _____(O)?

ETIOLOGY/HARM: Questions addressing the causes or origins of disease (i.e., factors that produce or predispose toward a certain disease or disorder).

Are _____ (P), who have _____ (I) compared to those
without _____ (C) at _____ risk for/of _____
(O) over _____ (T)?

MEANING/PROCESS: Questions addressing how one experiences a phenomenon.

How do _____ (P) with _____ (I) perceive/cope
with/adapt to/live with/experience _____ (O) during _____(T)?

Adapted from the PICOT Questions Template; Melnyk and Fineout-Overholt (2019, pp. 45–50).

Meaning: How do young males (P) with a diagnosis of paraplegia (I) perceive their interactions with their romantic significant others (O) during the first year after their diagnosis (T)?

(See also the Practical Application box in Chapter 5 for examples of PICOT and SPIDER.) The SPIDER tool (Cooke et al., 2012) was developed by adapting the PICOT tool and is most suitable to qualitative and mixed method research. It also has five components, as follows:

(S) Sample: suitable for smaller samples used in qualitative research.

(PI) Phenomenon of Interest: qualitative research examines how and why certain experiences, behaviours and decisions are occurring rather than the effectiveness of an intervention or treatment).

(D) Design: the study design influences the trust-worthiness of the study analysis and findings.

(E) Evaluation: include more subjective outcomes (such as meanings, attitudes, experiences etc.).

(R) Research type: qualitative, quantitative and mixed methods research could be searched for. (Figure 4.1):

An example of a SPIDER question is: What are the experiences of first-time mothers using the doula method of childbirth?

The significance of the clinical question becomes obvious as the research evidence from the literature is critiqued. The research evidence is used side by side with clinical expertise and the patient's perspective to develop or revise nursing standards, protocols, and policies that are used to plan and implement patient care

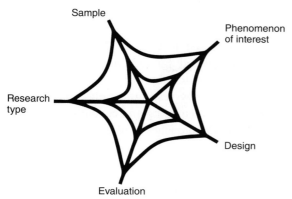

FIG. 4.1 Elements of the SPIDER research tool.
(From Cooke, A., Smith, S., & Booth, A. (2012). Beyond PICO: The SPIDER tool for qualitative evidence synthesis. *Qualitative Health Research, 22*(10), 1435–1443.) SAGE Publications Inc.

(Melnyk & Fineout-Overholt, 2019). Issues or questions can arise from multiple clinical and managerial situations (see the Practical Application box).

Practical Application

With regard to the example of pain, a nurse working in a palliative care setting wondered whether completing pain diaries was useful for patients with advanced cancer who were receiving palliative care. She wondered whether they were spending time developing something that had previously been shown to be useless or even harmful—it is conceivable that monitoring one's pain in a diary actually heightens one's awareness and experience of pain. To focus her search of the literature, the nurse developed the following question: "Does the use of pain diaries in the palliative care of patients with cancer lead to improved pain control?"

Sometimes it is helpful for nurses who develop clinical questions from a consumer's perspective to consider three elements—(1) the situation, (2) the intervention, and (3) the outcome—as they frame their focused question:

- The situation is the patient or problem being addressed. This can be a single patient or a group of patients with a particular health problem (palliative care of patients with cancer).

- The intervention is the dimension of health care interest, and the question is often about whether a particular intervention (in this case, pain diaries) is a useful treatment.

- The outcome encompasses the effect of the treatment (intervention) for this patient or the patient population in terms of quality (e.g., decreased pain perception) and cost (low cost). It essentially answers whether the intervention makes a difference for the patient population.

The individual parts of the question are vital pieces of information to remember when you search for evidence in the literature. One of the easiest ways to do this is to use a table, such as Table 4.1. Examples of clinical questions are highlighted in Box 4.2. Chapter 5 provides examples of how to effectively search the literature to find answers to questions posed by researchers and research consumers.

BOX **4.2**

EXAMPLES OF RESEARCH QUESTIONS

- What is the mother's level of confidence in caring for her late preterm infant (Premji et al., 2018)?
- Does hand massage have sustained effects on pain intensity and pain-related interference in cardiac surgery critically ill patients (Boitor et al., 2019)?
- How do first-time mothers access support and information (online and offline) during the first 6 months of their postpartum period (Price et al., 2018)? What are adolescents' mothers' perceptions of a mobile phone-based peer support (MPPS) intervention designed to prevent postpartum depression (Chyzzy et al., 2020)?
- What are palliative care nurses' attitudes toward medical assistance in dying (Freeman et al., 2020)? What is the relationship between coping strategies and psychological well-being of Bhutanese refugees resettled in Ottawa (Subedi et al., 2019)?
- What is the experience of managing chronic conditions in the community from the perspectives of older adults, family caregivers, and health care providers working in a variety of settings (Ploeg et al., 2017)?

DEVELOPING AND REFINING A RESEARCH QUESTION

A researcher spends a great deal of time refining a research idea or problem into a research question. Unfortunately, the evaluator of a research study is not privy to this creative process because it occurs during the study's conceptualization. The final research question usually does not appear in the research article unless the study is qualitative rather than quantitative. Although this section does not teach you how to formulate a research question, it does provide an important glimpse into the researcher's process of developing a research question.

Research questions or topics do not arise spontaneously. As shown in Table 4.2, research questions should indicate that practical experience, critical appraisal of the scientific literature, or interest in an untested theory was the basis for the generation of a research idea. The research question should reflect a refinement of the researcher's initial thinking. The evaluator of a nursing research study should be able to discern that the researcher has done the following:

1. Defined a specific topic area
2. Reviewed the relevant scientific literature
3. Examined the question's potential significance in nursing
4. Pragmatically examined the feasibility of studying the research question

When conducting research with Indigenous people in Canada, it must be noted that the researcher acknowledges that the topic and/or research question originated in the community itself and is defined, analyzed, and solved with the community. Thus, the community actively participates in developing the research question(s), which differs from the Western/mainstream research. This is also discussed in Chapter 7. The researcher should be invited by Indigenous communities to conduct research that they have identified as a priority, thereby respecting self-determination in research and ensuring and encouraging active, participatory approaches to research.

Defining the Research Question

Brainstorming with teachers, advisers, or colleagues may provide valuable feedback to help the researcher focus on a specific question area. For example, suppose a researcher told a colleague that an area of interest was whether men and women recovered differently after cardiac surgery. The colleague may have said, "What is it about the topic that specifically interests you?" Such a conversation may have initiated a train of thought that resulted in a decision to explore the recovery processes and gender differences. Box 4.3 illustrates how a broad area of interest was narrowed to a specific research topic.

Beginning the Literature Review

The literature review should reveal a collection of relevant individual studies and systematic reviews that have been critically examined (see Chapter 5). Concluding sections in such articles—that is, the recommendations and implications for practice—often identify remaining gaps in the literature, the need for replication, the need for extension of the knowledge base about a particular research focus, or to understand the phenomenon of interest.

The literature review also helps researchers determine whether their study can contribute to the field of nursing.

TABLE **4.2**

HOW PRACTICAL EXPERIENCE, SCIENTIFIC LITERATURE, AND UNTESTED THEORY INFLUENCE DEVELOPMENT OF A RESEARCH IDEA

AREA	INFLUENCE	EXAMPLE
Practical experience	Clinical practice provides a wealth of experience from which research problems can be derived. The nurse may observe the occurrence of a particular event or pattern and become curious about why it occurs, as well as its relationship to other factors in the patient's environment.	Critically ill patients commonly require artificial airways and mechanical ventilation that prohibits verbal communication. Difficulties in communication can result in unmet needs. Santiago et al. (2019) explored the feasibility and usefulness of using a tablet equipped with communication app in the intensive care unit with patients who are unable to communicate using verbal speech.
Critical appraisal of the scientific literature	The critical appraisal of research studies that appear in journals may indirectly suggest a problem area by stimulating the reader's thinking. Nurses may observe the outcome data from a single study or a group of related studies that provide the basis for developing a pilot study or quality improvement project to determine the effectiveness of this intervention in their own practice.	Adults 65 years of age and older represent a small proportion of the population yet account for roughly half of the hospitalizations in Canada. Health care practices that restrict older adults' functioning contribute to functional decline and related complications in this patient population. Research that advances understanding of the mechanisms by which geriatric care environment (GPE) is associated with the overall quality of care for hospitalized older adults and their families is needed to help decision-makers identify key areas for quality improvement. Thus, Fox et al. (2018) tested the relationships between GPE, geriatric nursing practice, and overall quality of care for older adults and their families as reported by nurses working in hospitals, while controlling for nurse and hospital characteristics.
	A research idea may also be suggested by a critical appraisal of the literature that identifies gaps and suggests areas for future study. Research ideas also can be generated by research reports that suggest the value of replicating a particular study to extend or refine the existing body of scientific knowledge.	The use of multiple-choice questions (MCQs) is widely used as a testing format in nursing education. There is widespread adoption of four-option and five-option MCQs. According to Hartigan-Rodgers et al. (2019), there is nearly a century of educational research that has demonstrated that three-option MCQs are as valid and reliable as the four- or five-option one. Thus, they replicated a 2012 study to address this knowledge within nursing.
	Verification of an untested nursing theory provides relatively uncharted territory from which research questions can be derived. Inasmuch as theories themselves are not tested, a researcher may think about investigating a particular concept or set of concepts related to a particular nursing theory. The deductive process would be used to generate the research question. The researcher would pose questions such as "If this theory is correct, what kind of behaviour will I expect to observe in particular patients and under which conditions?" or "If this theory is valid, what kind of supporting evidence will I find?"	The concepts of nursing competence and confidence have been used to describe nurses' preparedness for, and level of performance in, nursing practice. There is considerable work supporting the premise that health professionals' scope of competence should be explored within a lens relevant to the context of their work environment. Thus, Penz et al. (2019) conducted a study to test their model of rural and remote RN/NP confidence and competence.

The databases that researchers use for the literature review—for example, Cumulative Index to Nursing and Allied Health Literature (CINAHL), PsycINFO, MEDLINE, and PubMed—contain relevant articles that have been critically examined and gray literature, which are reports based on a specific topic from organizations. Concluding sections in such articles and reports (i.e., the recommendations and implications for practice) often identify remaining gaps in the literature, the need for replication, or the need for extension of the knowledge gleaned on a particular research focus.

In the example in Appendix D on the evaluation of evidence-informed changes to an internationally educated nurse (IEN) registration process, (see Box 4.3), the researchers conducted a preliminary review of journals for research studies on evidence-informed regulation for IENs and found that there was no comprehensive, international review of scopes of practice or of nursing education practices for this population.

The search for relevant factors for effective policy and practice changes led to a review of the characteristics of education and employment at critical points in the registration process. The researcher can then use this information to further define the research question, to address a gap in the literature, and to extend the body of knowledge related to making policy and practice changes to IENs in Canada. At this point, the researcher could write the following tentative research question: "How does previous education and currency of practice influence IEN registration success across Canada?" After reading this question, you should be able to envision the interrelatedness of the initial definition of the research question, the literature review, and the refined research question. Readers of research reports examine the end product of this process in the form of a research question, hypothesis, or both. Thus, readers need an appreciation of how the researcher formulates the final research question directing the study.

BOX 4.3

DEVELOPMENT OF A RESEARCH QUESTION

IDEA EMERGES
- Palliative care

BRAINSTORMING
- How does the aging population influence the need for palliative care approaches?
- How do health care workers perceive or know about palliative care?
- How is the palliative approach implemented?

LITERATURE REVIEW
- Characteristics of a palliative approach from a knowledge synthesis iPanel
- Enhancing integration of palliative approach needs self-perceived competence of nurses and care aides
- Elements of a conceptual framework such as Bandura's social cognitive theory to frame perception of competence
- Dimensions of self-perceived competence
- Impact of the work environment

VARIABLES
- Self-perceived competence in a palliative approach
- A measure of application of the approach
- Work environment
- Patients characteristics

RESEARCH QUESTION
- What is the extent to which nurses' and care aides' self-perceived palliative care competence explain variation in the application of a palliative care approach across home, hospital, and residential care settings?

From Sawatzky, R., Roberts, D., Russell, L., Bitschy, A., Ho, S., Desbiens, F-F., Chan, E.K.H., Tayler, C., &Stajduhar, K. (2019). Self-perceived competence of nurses and care aides providing a palliative approach in home, hospital, and residential care settings: A cross-sectional survey. *Canadian Journal of Nursing, 53*(1), 64–77. https://doi.org/10.1177/0844562119881043

Research Hint

Reading the literature review or theoretical framework section of a research article helps you trace the development of the implied research question, hypothesis, or both.

Examining Significance

When considering a research question, it is crucial that the researcher has examined the question's potential significance to nursing. The research question should have the potential to contribute to and extend the scientific body of nursing knowledge. Guidelines for selecting research questions should meet the following criteria:

- Patients, nurses, the medical community in general, and society will potentially benefit from the knowledge derived from the study.
- The results will be applicable for nursing practice, education, or administration.
- The results will be theoretically relevant.
- The findings will lend support to untested theoretical assumptions, extend or challenge an existing theory, or clarify a conflict in the literature.
- The findings could lead to improved patient outcomes.
- The findings will potentially enable professionals to formulate or alter nursing practices or policies.

If the research question has not met any of these criteria, the researcher needs to extensively revise the question or discard it. For example, in the final research question in Kwan et al. (2019), "Did using evidence-based policy increase the efficiency and transparency of the registration process for IENs?" (see Box 4.3), the significance of the question includes the following facts:

- Transparency facilitates the registration process.
- Transparency contributes to efficiency and vice versa.

Evidence-Informed Practice Tip

Without a well-developed research question, the researcher may search for incorrect, irrelevant, or unnecessary information. Such information is a barrier to identifying the potential significance of the study.

Determining Feasibility

The feasibility of a research question must be examined pragmatically. Regardless of how significant or researchable a question may be, pragmatic considerations—such as time; availability of participants, facilities, equipment, and money; experience of the researcher; and any ethical considerations—may render the question inappropriate because it lacks feasibility. One of the most frequent issues is whether a sufficient number of participants can be recruited. If potential issues emerge affecting the feasibility of the study, the researcher may need to reconsider the research question and/or design.

THE FULLY DEVELOPED RESEARCH QUESTION

As discussed previously, qualitative researchers develop and refine a research question that outlines a general topic area. Examples include the following:

- What are parents' perceptions and experiences of support from health and social services communities when living with a child with a rare NDD [neurodevelopmental disorder] (Currie, Currie & Szabo, 2020)?
- What is your experience in caring for LPIs [late preterm infant] as a PHN [Public Health Nurse] (Currie et al., 2018)?
- What are the components of an educational intervention that support the development of clinical nursing leadership in 1st year (Ha & Pepin, 2018)?

As a quantitative researcher finalizes a research question, the following three characteristics should be evident:

1. The *variables* under consideration are clearly identified.
2. The *population* being investigated is specified.
3. The possibility of empirical *testing* is implied.

Because each of these elements is crucial in the formulation of a satisfactory research question, the criteria are discussed in greater detail in the following sections. These elements can often be found in the introduction of the published article; however, they are not always stated in an explicit manner.

Research Hint _____

Remember that research questions are used to guide all types of research studies.

Evidence-Informed Practice Tip _____

The answers to questions generated by qualitative data reflect evidence that may provide the first insights about a phenomenon that has not been studied previously.

Variables

Researchers call the properties that they study *variables*. Such properties take on different values. Thus, a **variable** is, as the name suggests, something that varies. Properties that differ from each other, such as age, weight, height, religion, and ethnicity, are examples of variables. Researchers attempt to understand how and why differences in one variable relate to differences in another variable. For example, a researcher may be concerned about the rate of pneumonia in postoperative patients on ventilators in critical care units. This rate is a variable because not all critically ill postoperative patients on ventilators have pneumonia. A researcher may also be interested in what other factors can be linked to ventilator-acquired pneumonia (VAP). Clinical evidence suggests that elevation of the head of the bed is also associated with VAP. You can see that these factors are also variables that need to be considered in relation to the development of VAP in postoperative patients.

When speaking of variables, the researcher is essentially asking, "Is X related to Y? What is the effect of X on Y? How are X_1 and X_2 related to Y?"* The researcher is asking a question about the relationship between one or more independent variables *(X)* and a dependent variable *(Y)*.

_____
*Note: In cases in which multiple independent or dependent variables are present, subscripts are used to indicate the variable number.

An **independent variable**, usually symbolized by X, is the variable that has the presumed effect on the dependent variable. In experimental research studies, the researcher manipulates the independent variable. For example, a nurse may study how different methods of administering pain medication affect the patient's perception of pain intensity. The researcher may manipulate the independent variable (i.e., the method of administering pain medication) by using nurse- versus patient-controlled administration of analgesics. In nonexperimental research, the independent variable is not manipulated and is assumed to have occurred naturally before or during the study. For example, the researcher may be studying the relationship between gender and the perception of pain intensity. The independent variable—gender—is not manipulated; it is presumed to exist and is observed and measured in relation to pain intensity.

The **dependent variable**, represented by Y, is often referred to as the consequence or the presumed effect that varies with a change in the independent variable. The dependent variable is not manipulated. It is observed and assumed to vary with changes in the independent variable. Predictions are based on how changes to the independent variable will affect the dependent variable. The researcher is interested in understanding, explaining, or predicting the response of the dependent variable. For example, a researcher might assume that the perception of pain (i.e., the dependent variable) will vary according to the person's gender (i.e., the independent variable). In this case, the researcher is trying to explain the perception of pain in relation to gender: that is, male or female. Although variability in the dependent variable is assumed to depend on changes in the independent variable, this assumption does not imply that a causal relationship exists between X and Y or that changes in X cause Y to change.

In a hypothetical study about nurses' attitudes toward patients with hepatitis C, the researcher may discover that older nurses had a more negative attitude about such patients than did younger nurses. The researcher cannot conclude that the nurses' attitudes toward patients with hepatitis C were negative because of their age; however, it is apparent that there was a directional relationship between age and negative attitudes about patients with hepatitis C—that is, the older the nurses were, the more negative their attitudes about patients with hepatitis C. This example highlights the fact that causal relationships are not necessarily implied by the independent and dependent variables; rather, only a relational statement with possible directionality is proposed.

Table 4.3 presents a number of examples to help you learn how to write research questions. Practise substituting other variables for the examples in the table. You will be surprised at the skill you develop in writing and critiquing research questions.

Although one independent variable and one dependent variable were used in the examples just given, there is no restriction on the number of variables that can be included in a research question. Remember, however, that questions should not be unnecessarily complex or unwieldy, particularly in beginning research efforts. Research questions that include more than one independent or dependent variable may be divided into more concise subquestions.

Finally, note that variables are not inherently independent or dependent. A variable that is classified as independent in one study may be considered dependent in another study. For example, a nurse may review an article about sexual behaviours that are predictive of the risk for HIV infection or AIDS. In this case, HIV/AIDS is the dependent variable. In another article in which the relationship between HIV/AIDS and maternal parenting practices is considered, HIV/AIDS

TABLE **4.3**

RESEARCH QUESTION FORMAT

TYPE	FORMAT	EXAMPLE
QUANTITATIVE		
Correlational	Is there a relationship between X (independent variable) and Y (dependent variable) in the specified population?	Is there a relationship between the effectiveness of pain management strategies and quality of life?
Comparative	Is there a difference in Y (dependent variable) between people who have characteristic X (independent variable) and those who do not have characteristic X?	Is there a difference in prevention of osteoporosis in at-risk survivors of breast cancer who receive a combination of long-term progressive strength training exercises, alendronate, calcium, and vitamin D, in comparison with those who do not receive this treatment?
Experimental	Is there a difference in Y (dependent variable) between Group A, which received X (independent variable), and Group B, which did not receive X?	What is the difference in physical, social, and emotional adjustment in women with breast cancer (and their partners) who have received phase-specific standardized education by video versus phase-specific telephone counselling?
QUALITATIVE		
Phenomenological	What is or was it like to have X?	What is the experience of self in Canadian youth living with anxiety (Woodgate et al., 2020)?
Ethnographic	What is the experience of a select culture group with a specific phenomenon?	What are the experiences of frail, older adults undergoing a transcatheter aortic valve implantation (Baumbausch et al., 2018)?

status is the independent variable. Whether a variable is independent or dependent depends on the role it plays in a particular study.

Population

The **population** (a well-defined set that has certain properties) is either specified or implied in the research question. If the scope of the question has been narrowed to a specific focus and the variables have been clearly identified, the nature of the population is evident to the reader of the research report. For example, a research question may be "Is there a relationship in outcomes between a partnership model of discharge planning model for older adults hospitalized with heart failure and their caregivers compared to other older adults who received the usual discharge planning?" This question suggests that the population under consideration includes older adults hospitalized for heart failure and their caregivers. The question also implies that some of the older adults and their caregivers were involved in a provider–patient partnership model of discharge planning, in contrast to other older adults who received the usual discharge planning. The researcher or reader will have an initial idea of the composition of the study population from the outset.

Evidence-Informed Practice Tip

Make sure that the population of interest and the setting have been clearly described so that if you plan to replicate the study, you will know exactly who the study population needs to be.

Testability

The research question must be phrased in such a way that there is a specific issue that needs to be answered. In many cases, the question is **testable**—that is, measurable by quantitative methods. For example, the research question "Should postoperative patients control how much pain medication they receive?" is stated incorrectly, for a variety of reasons. One reason is that the question is not

testable; it represents a value statement rather than a relational problem statement. A scientific or relational question must propose a relationship between an independent variable and a dependent variable in such a way that the variables can be measured. Many interesting and important questions are not valid research questions because they are not amenable to testing.

The question "Should postoperative patients control how much pain medication they receive?" could be revised from a philosophical question to a research question that implies testability. Examples of the revised research question are as follows:

- Is there a relationship between patient-controlled analgesia versus nurse-administered analgesia and the perception of postoperative pain?
- What is the effect of patient-controlled analgesia on pain ratings provided by postoperative patients?

These examples illustrate the relationship between the variables, identify the independent and dependent variables, and imply the testability of the research question.

Table 4.4 lists the components of the research question regarding variance in the perception of pain in relation to a person's age and gender.

TABLE 4.4	
COMPONENTS OF THE RESEARCH QUESTION AND RELATED CRITERIA	
Testability	Differential effect of pain intensity and number of painful sites on functional disability (physical and social functioning)
Population	Adolescent males and females
Variables	**Independent Variables:** Pain intensity, Pain sites, Gender, Health (number of limiting diagnoses) **Dependent Variables:** Management effectiveness, Functional status

Research Hint

Remember that research questions are often not explicitly stated. The reader must infer the research question from the report's title, the abstract, the introduction, or the purpose.

STUDY PURPOSE, AIMS, OR OBJECTIVES

Once the research question is developed and the literature review is critiqued in terms of the level, strength, and quality of evidence available for the particular research question, the purpose, aims, or objectives of the study become focused. In all paradigms of research, quantitative, qualitative, and mixed methods, researchers clearly articulate the purpose of the study. In quantitative studies, the researcher can then decide whether a hypothesis should be tested or answering the research question is sufficient.

The **purpose** of the study encompasses the aims or objectives the investigator hopes to achieve with the research, not the question to be answered. For example, a nurse working with patients with bladder dysfunction who are in rehabilitation may be disturbed by the high incidence of urinary tract infections. The nurse may propose the following research question: "What is the optimum frequency of changing urinary drainage bags in patients with bladder dysfunction to reduce the incidence of urinary tract infection?" If this nurse were to design a study, its purpose might be to determine the differential effect of 1-week and 4-week schedules of changing urinary drainage bags on the incidence of urinary tract infections in patients with bladder dysfunction.

The purpose communicates more than just the nature of the question. Through the researcher's selection of verbs, the purpose statement suggests the manner in which the researcher sought to study the question. Verbs such as *discover, explore,* or *describe* suggest an investigation of a relatively underresearched topic that might be more appropriately guided by research questions than by hypotheses. In contrast, verbs such as *test* (testing the effectiveness of an intervention) or *compare* (comparing two alternative nursing strategies) suggest a study with a better-established body of knowledge that is hypothesis testing in nature. Box 4.4 provides other examples of purpose statements.

Evidence-Informed Practice Tip

The purpose, aims, or objectives often provide the most information about the intent of the research question and hypotheses and suggest the level of evidence to be obtained from the findings of the study.

DEVELOPING THE RESEARCH HYPOTHESIS

Like the research question, hypotheses are often not stated explicitly in a research article. The hypotheses are often embedded in the data analysis, results, or discussion section of the research

---

BOX **4.4**

EXAMPLES OF PURPOSE STATEMENTS

"The aim of this study was to explore nurse leaders' perceptions of the impact of their participation in the reflective practice program (Lavoie-Tremblay et al., 2018).

"The purpose of the Parachute**TM** Concussion Awareness for Players (PCAP) Program was to deliver standardized concussion education to youth and adolescent soccer players during summer camps and measure its effectiveness in knowledge and attitude (Macartney et al., 2019).

"The aim of this research was to draw on Cree/Métis understanding through Indigenous research methodologies (IRM), in order to explore how Indigenous knowledge systems and identity are embedded in the nursing practices of four Indigenous nurse scholars (Bourque-Bearskin et al., 2016, p. 20) .

"The objective of this study was to examine the process that South Asians undergo when managing their hypertension (HTN) (King-Shier et al., 2019, p. 321)

report. You then need to discern the nature of the hypotheses being tested. Similarly, the population may not be explicitly described but is identified in the background, significance, and literature review. It is then up to you to discern the nature of the hypotheses and population being tested.

Hypotheses flow from the research question, literature review, and theoretical framework. Figure 4.2 illustrates this flow. A **hypothesis** is a statement about the relationship between two or more variables that suggests an answer to the research question. A hypothesis converts the question posed by the research question into a declarative statement that predicts an expected outcome. It explains or predicts the relationship or differences between two or more variables in terms of the expected results or outcomes of a study. Hypotheses are formulated before the study is actually conducted; they provide direction for the collection, analysis, and interpretation of data.

Research Hint

When hypotheses are not explicitly stated by the author at the end of the "Introduction" section or before the "Methods" section, they are embedded or implied in the "Results" or "Discussion" section of a research article.

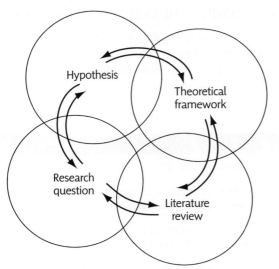

FIG. 4.2 Interrelationship of the research question, literature review, theoretical framework, and hypothesis.

Characteristics

Nurses who are conducting research or critiquing published research studies must have a working knowledge of what constitutes a "good" hypothesis. Such knowledge provides a standard for evaluating their own work and the work of others. The following discussion about the characteristics of hypotheses presents criteria to be used when a hypothesis is formulated or evaluated.

Relationship Statement

The first characteristic of a hypothesis is that it is a declarative statement identifying the predicted relationship between two or more variables. This implies a systematic relationship between an independent variable (X) and a dependent variable (Y). The direction of the predicted relationship is also specified in this statement. Phrases such as "greater than"; "less than"; "positively related," "negatively related," or "curvilinearly related"; and "difference in" connote the directionality that is proposed in the hypothesis. The following is an example of a directional hypothesis: "The rate of continuous smoking abstinence [dependent variable] at 6 months postpartum, according to self-report and biochemical validation, will be significantly higher in the treatment group [receiving postpartum counselling intervention] than in the control group [independent variable]." The dependent and independent variables are explicitly identified, and the relational aspect of the prediction in the hypothesis is contained in the phrase "significantly higher than."

The nature of the relationship, either causal or associative, is also implied by the hypothesis. A causal relationship is one in which the researcher can predict that the independent variable (X) causes a change in the dependent variable (Y). In research, it is rare that a definitive stand can be assumed about a cause-and-effect relationship. For example, a researcher might hypothesize that relaxation training would have a significant effect on the physical and psychological health status of patients who have suffered myocardial infarction.

The researcher would have difficulty predicting a strong cause-and-effect relationship, however, because the multiple intervening variables (e.g., age, medication, and lifestyle changes) might also influence the participant's health status.

Variables are more commonly related in non-causal ways; that is, the variables are related but in an associative way. This means that variables change in relation to each other. For example, because strong evidence exists that asbestos exposure is related to lung cancer, a researcher may be tempted to state a causal relationship between asbestos exposure and lung cancer. However, not all individuals exposed to asbestos develop lung cancer and, conversely, not all individuals who have lung cancer have been exposed to asbestos. Thus, a position advocating a causal relationship between these two variables would be scientifically unsound. Instead, only an associative relationship exists between the variables of asbestos exposure and lung cancer, with a strong systematic association between the two phenomena.

Testability

The second characteristic of a hypothesis is its **testability**. The variables of the study must lend themselves to observation, measurement, and analysis. The hypothesis is either supported or not supported after the data have been collected and analyzed. The predicted outcome proposed by the hypothesis is or is not congruent with the actual outcome when the hypothesis is tested. Hypotheses advance scientific knowledge by confirming or refuting theories.

A hypothesis may fail to meet the criteria of testability because the researcher has not made a prediction about the anticipated outcome, because the variables are not observable or measurable, or because the hypothesis is couched in terms that are value laden.

Research Hint

When a hypothesis is complex (i.e., contains more than one independent or dependent variable), it is difficult for the findings to indicate unequivocally that the hypothesis is supported or not supported. In such cases, the reader must infer which relationships are significant from the "Findings" or "Discussion" section.

Theory Base

A sound hypothesis is consistent with an existing body of theory and research findings. Whether a researcher arrives at a hypothesis inductively or deductively, the hypothesis must be based on a sound scientific rationale. Readers should be able to identify the flow of ideas from the research question to the literature review, to the theoretical framework, and to the hypotheses.

Wording the Hypothesis

As you become more familiar with the scientific literature, you will observe that a hypothesis can be worded in various ways. Regardless of the specific format used to state the hypothesis, the statement should be worded in clear, simple, and concise terms. If this criterion is met, the reader will understand the following:

- The variables of the hypothesis
- The population being studied
- The predicted outcome of the hypothesis

Information about hypotheses may be further clarified in the "Instruments," "Sample," or "Methods" section of a research report.

Statistical Versus Research Hypotheses

Readers of research reports may observe that a hypothesis is further categorized as either a research or statistical hypothesis. A **research hypothesis**, also known as a *scientific hypothesis*, consists of a statement about the expected relationship of the variables. A research hypothesis indicates what the outcome of the study is expected to be. A research hypothesis is also either directional or nondirectional. If the researcher obtains statistically significant findings for a research hypothesis, the hypothesis is supported. The examples in Table 4.5 represent research hypotheses.

TABLE **4.5**

EXAMPLES OF HOW TO WORD A HYPOTHESIS

VARIABLES	HYPOTHESIS	TYPE OF DESIGN; LEVEL OF EVIDENCE SUGGESTED

1. There are significant differences in self-reported cancer pain, symptoms accompanying pain, and functional status according to gender.

Independent Gender	Nondirectional, research	Nonexperimental; level IV
Dependent Self-reported cancer pain Symptoms accompanying pain Functional status		

2. Individuals who participate in usual care plus blood pressure telemonitoring will have a greater reduction in blood pressure from baseline to 12-month follow-up than will individuals who receive only usual care.

Independent Telemonitoring Usual care	Directional, research	Experimental; level II
Dependent Blood pressure		

3. There will be a greater decrease in state anxiety scores for patients receiving structured informational videos before abdominal or chest tube removal than for patients receiving standard information.

Independent Preprocedure structured video information Standard information	Directional, research	Experimental; level II
Dependent State anxiety		

4. The incidence and degree of severity of participants' discomfort will be lower after administration of medications by the Z-track intramuscular injection technique than after administration of medications by the standard intramuscular injection technique.

Independent Z-track intramuscular injection technique Standard intramuscular injection technique	Directional, research	Experimental; level II
Dependent Participant discomfort		

5. Nurses with high levels of social support from co-workers have low perceived job stress.

Independent Social support	Directional, research	Nonexperimental; level IV
Dependent Perceived job stress		

6. There will be no difference in rates of complications from anaesthetics between hospitals in which anaesthetics are administered primarily by certified registered nurse anaesthetists (CRNAs) and hospitals in which anaesthetics are administered primarily by anaesthesiologists (MDs).

Independent Type of anaesthesia provider (CRNA or MD)	Nondirectional; null	Nonexperimental; level IV
Dependent Anaesthesia complication rate		

7. There will be no significant difference in the duration of patency of a 24-gauge intravenous lock in a neonatal patient when flushed with 0.5 mL of heparinized saline (2 U/mL), standard practice, in comparison with 0.5 mL of 0.9% normal saline.

Independent Heparinized saline Normal saline	Nondirectional; null	Experimental; level II
Dependent Duration of patency of intravenous lock		

TABLE **4.6**		
EXAMPLES OF STATISTICAL (NULL) HYPOTHESES		
HYPOTHESIS	**VARIABLES**	**TYPE OF DESIGN SUGGESTED**
Oxygen inhalation by nasal cannula of up to 6 L/min does not affect oral temperature measurement taken with an electronic thermometer.	Independent: Oxygen inhalation by nasal cannula Dependent: Oral temperature	Experimental
There will be no difference in performance accuracy between adult nurse practitioners (ANPs) and family nurse practitioners (FNPs) in formulating accurate diagnoses and acceptable interventions for suspected cases of domestic violence.	Independent: Nurse practitioner (ANP or FNP) category Dependent: Diagnosis and intervention performance accuracy	Nonexperimental

According to a **statistical hypothesis** (also known as a *null hypothesis*), there is no relationship between the independent and dependent variables. The examples in Table 4.6 illustrate statistical hypotheses. If, in the data analysis, a statistically significant relationship emerges between the variables at a specified level of significance, the statistical hypothesis is rejected. Rejection of the statistical hypothesis is equivalent to acceptance of the research hypothesis. For example, Bilik et al. (2020) sought to identify differences in Critical Thinking Motivational scores on the five domains of expectancy, attainment, utility, value and cost between students receiving web-based concept mapping education and those who did not receive such education. The statistical hypothesis is that there would be no differences in Critical Thinking Motivational scores. This statistical hypothesis was partially supported for value and cost. Because the difference in outcomes was not greater than that expected by chance, the statistical hypothesis was accepted. To further differentiate between a statistical hypothesis and a research hypothesis, consider the following hypotheses:

Research hypothesis: Hospitals with higher nurse-to-patient ratios will have fewer adverse patient events.

Statistical (null) hypothesis: There is no difference in the number of adverse patient events in hospitals with higher nurse-to-patient ratios.

You will note that research hypotheses are generally used more often than statistical hypotheses because they are more desirable for stating the researcher's expectation. In all studies, the statistical hypothesis is typically what is tested using statistics, as we want to reject the null hypothesis by demonstrating that any effect/relationship was unlikely to be due to chance alone.

Directional Versus Nondirectional Hypotheses

Hypotheses can be formulated directionally or nondirectionally. A **directional hypothesis** specifies the expected direction of the relationship between the independent and dependent variables. The reader of a directional hypothesis may observe not only that a relationship is proposed but also the nature or direction of that relationship. The following is an example of a directional hypothesis: "Exercise and the use of mindfulness will reduce stress levels." Examples of directional hypotheses can also be found in examples 2 to 7 of Table 4.5.

Whereas a **nondirectional hypothesis** indicates the existence of a relationship between the variables, it does not specify the anticipated direction of the relationship. The following is an example of a nondirectional hypothesis: "The addition of warm shower and perineal exercise interventions during childbirth will result in significant group differences regarding pain, anxiety, and stress-related hormonal levels" (Henrique et al., 2018, p. 2).

Nurses who are learning to critique research studies should be aware that both the directional and nondirectional forms of hypothesis statements are acceptable. There are definite advantages and disadvantages that pertain to each form.

Proponents of the directional hypothesis argue that researchers naturally have hunches, guesses, or expectations about the outcome of their research. It is the hunch, the curiosity, or the guess that initially leads them to speculate about the question. The literature review and the conceptual framework provide the theoretical foundation for deriving the hypothesis. For example, the theory (e.g., self-efficacy theory) provides a critical rationale for proposing that relationships between variables have particular outcomes. When there is no theory or related research on which to base a rationale, or when findings in previous research studies are ambivalent, a nondirectional hypothesis may be appropriate. As you read research articles, you will note that directional hypotheses are much more commonly used than nondirectional hypotheses.

In summary, when you evaluate a hypothesis, note that directional hypotheses have several advantages that make them appropriate for use in most studies:

- Directional hypotheses indicate that a theory base was used to derive the hypotheses and that the phenomena under investigation have been critically examined and interrelated. You should note that nondirectional hypotheses may also be deduced from a theory base. Because of the exploratory nature of many studies for which the hypotheses are nondirectional, in contrast, the theory base may not be as developed.
- Directional hypotheses provide a specific theoretical frame of reference within which the study is being conducted.
- They suggest that the researcher believes that the evidence is indicative of a particular outcome, and as a result, the analyses of data can be accomplished in a statistically more sensitive way.

The important point about the directionality of the hypotheses is whether the rationale for the choice the researcher has proposed is sound.

RELATIONSHIP AMONG THE HYPOTHESIS, THE RESEARCH QUESTION, AND THE RESEARCH DESIGN

Regardless of whether the researcher uses a statistical or research hypothesis, there is a suggested relationship among the hypothesis, the research question, the research design of the study, and the level of evidence provided by the results of the study. The type of design, experimental or nonexperimental, influences the wording of the hypothesis. For example, when an experimental design is used, the research consumer would expect to see hypotheses that reflect relationship statements, such as the following:

- X_1 is more effective than X_2 on Y.
- The effect of X_1 on Y is greater than that of X_2 on Y.
- The incidence of Y will not differ in participants receiving X_1 and X_2 treatments.
- The incidence of Y will be greater in participants after X_1 than after X_2.

Such hypotheses indicate that an experimental treatment (i.e., independent variable X) will be used and that two groups of participants, experimental and control groups, are being used to test whether the difference in the outcome (i.e., dependent variable Y) predicted by the hypothesis exists. Hypotheses reflecting experimental designs also concern the effect of the experimental treatment (i.e., independent variable X) on the outcome (i.e., dependent variable Y).

In contrast, hypotheses related to nonexperimental designs reflect associative relationship statements such as the following:

- X will be negatively related to Y.
- A positive relationship will exist between X and Y.

Thus, in a study in which the hypotheses were associative relationship statements, the evidence provided by the results of that investigation have level IV strength (nonexperimental design).

The Critical Thinking Decision Path will help you determine both the type of hypothesis presented in a study and the study's readiness for a hypothesis-testing design.

Evidence-Informed Practice Tip ___

Think about the relationship between the wording of the hypothesis, the type of research design suggested, and the level of evidence provided by the findings of a study with each kind of hypothesis. The research consumer may want to consider which type of hypothesis potentially will yield the strongest results applicable to practice.

CRITIQUING THE RESEARCH QUESTION

The Critiquing Criteria box on p. 78 provides several criteria for evaluating this initial phase of the research process: the research question. Because the research question represents the basis for the study, it is usually introduced at the beginning of the research report to indicate the focus and direction of the study. Readers are then in a position to evaluate whether the rest of the study logically pertains to this basis. The author often begins by identifying the background and significance of the issue that led to crystallizing development of the unanswered question. The clinical and scientific background, significance, or both are summarized, and the purpose, aim, or objective of the study is identified. Finally, the research question and any related subquestions are proposed before or after the literature review.

The purpose of the introductory summary of the theoretical and scientific background is to provide the reader with a contextual glimpse of how the author critically thought about the development of the research question. The introduction to the research question places the study within an appropriate theoretical framework and begins the description of the study. This introductory section should also include the significance of the study (i.e., why the investigator is conducting the study). For example, the significance may be to answer a question encountered in the clinical area and thereby improve patient care, to resolve a conflict in the literature regarding a clinical issue, or to provide data supporting an innovative form of nursing intervention that is more effective and is also cost-effective.

Sometimes readers find that the research question is not clearly stated at the conclusion of the introduction. In some cases, the author only hints at the research question, and the reader is challenged to identify it. In other cases, the author embeds the research question in the introductory text or purpose statement. To some extent, where or whether the author states the research question depends on the style of the journal. Nevertheless, the evaluator must remember that the main research question should be implied if it is not clearly identified in the introductory section—even if the subquestions are not stated or implied.

When critiquing the research question, the reader looks for the presence of the three key elements, described on p. 78:

- Does the research question express a relationship between two or more variables or, at least, between an independent variable and a dependent variable?
- Does the research question specify the nature of the population being studied?
- Does the research question imply the possibility of empirical testing?

You will use these three elements as criteria for judging the soundness of a stated research question. If the variables, the population, and the implications for testability are unclear, then the remainder of the study will probably falter. For example, a research study on anxiety during the perioperative period contained introductory material on anxiety in general, anxiety as it relates to the perioperative period, and the potentially beneficial influence of nursing care in relation to anxiety reduction. The author concluded that the purpose of the study was to determine whether selected measures of patient anxiety could be shown to vary when different approaches to nursing care were used during the perioperative period. The author did not state the research questions.

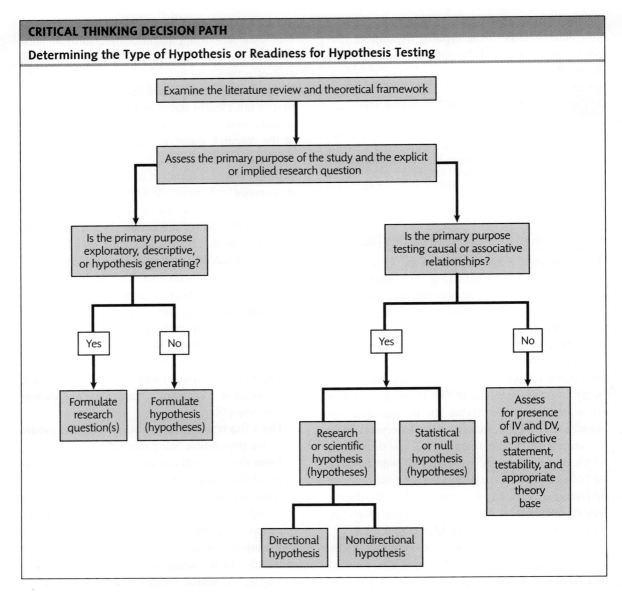

CRITICAL THINKING DECISION PATH

Determining the Type of Hypothesis or Readiness for Hypothesis Testing

A restatement of the problem in question form might be as follows:

What is the difference in patient anxiety level in relation to different approaches to nursing care during the perioperative period?

If this process of developing a research question is clarified at the outset of a research study, the report that follows can develop logically. Readers will have a clear idea of what the report should convey and can knowledgeably evaluate the material that is presented. When you critically appraise clinical questions, remember that they should be focused and specify the patient or problem being addressed, the intervention, and the outcome for a particular patient population. The author should provide evidence that the clinical question guided the literature search and that the question suggests the design and level of evidence to be obtained from the study findings.

CRITIQUING THE HYPOTHESES

As illustrated in the Critiquing Criteria box, several criteria for critiquing the hypotheses should be used as a standard for evaluating the strengths and weaknesses of the hypotheses in a research report:

1. When reading a research study, you may find the hypotheses clearly delineated in a separate hypothesis section of the research article (i.e., after the literature review or theoretical framework section or sections). In many cases, the hypotheses are not explicitly stated and are only implied in the results or discussion section of the article. In such cases, you must infer the hypotheses from the purpose statement and the type of analysis used. You should not assume that if hypotheses do not appear at the beginning of the article, they do not exist in the particular study. Even when hypotheses are stated at the beginning of an article, they are re-examined in the results or discussion section as the findings are presented and discussed.

2. If a hypothesis or set of hypotheses is presented, the data analysis should answer the hypotheses directly. Because the hypothesis should reflect the culmination and expression of this conceptual process, its placement in the research report logically follows the literature review and the theoretical framework discussion. It should be consistent with both the literature review and the theoretical framework.

3. Although a hypothesis can legitimately be nondirectional, it is preferable and more common for the researcher to indicate the direction of the relationship between the variables in the hypothesis. You will find that when data for the literature review are unavailable (i.e., the researcher has chosen to study a relatively undefined area of interest), a nondirectional hypothesis may be appropriate. Enough information simply may not be available for making a sound judgement about the direction of the proposed relationship. All that can be proposed is that there will be a relationship

between two variables. Essentially, you will want to determine the appropriateness of the researcher's choice regarding directionality of the hypothesis.

4. The notion of testability is central to the soundness of a hypothesis. One criterion related to testability is that the hypothesis should be stated in such a way that it can be clearly supported or dismissed. Although this criterion is very important to keep in mind, you should also understand that, ultimately, theories or hypotheses are never proved beyond a doubt through hypothesis testing. Claims that certain data have "proved" the validity of their hypothesis should be regarded with grave reservation. At best, findings that support a hypothesis are considered tentative. If repeated replication of a study yields the same results, more confidence can be placed in the conclusions advanced by the researchers. It is important to remember about testability that although hypotheses are more likely to be accepted with increasing evidence, they are ultimately never proved.

5. Another point about testability to consider is that the hypothesis should be objectively stated and devoid of any value-laden words. Value-laden hypotheses are not empirically testable. Quantifiable phrases—such as "greater than"; "less than"; "decrease"; "increase"; "positively related"; "negatively related"; and "related"—convey the idea of objectivity and testability. You should immediately be suspicious of hypotheses that are not stated objectively.

6. You should recognize that how the proposed relationship of the hypothesis is phrased suggests the type of research design that is appropriate for the study, as well as the level of evidence to be derived from the findings. For example, if a hypothesis proposes that treatment X_1 will have a greater effect on Y than treatment X_2, an experimental (level II evidence) or quasiexperimental design (level III evidence) is suggested. If a hypothesis

proposes that there will be a positive relationship between variables X and Y, a non-experimental design (level IV evidence) is suggested. Table 4.5 contains additional examples of hypotheses, the type of research design, and the level of evidence that is suggested by each hypothesis. The design and level of evidence have important implications for the remainder of the study in terms of the appropriateness of sample selection, data collection, data analysis, interpretation of findings, and—ultimately—the conclusions advanced by the researcher.

7. If the research report contains research questions rather than hypotheses, you will want to evaluate whether this is appropriate for the study. One criterion for making this decision, as presented earlier in this chapter, is whether the study is of an exploratory, a descriptive, or a qualitative nature. If it is, then it is appropriate to have research questions rather than hypotheses.

APPRAISING THE EVIDENCE

The Research Question and Hypotheses

The care taken by a researcher when developing the research question or hypothesis is often representative of the overall conceptualization and design of the study. A methodically formulated research question provides the basis for hypothesis development. In a quantitative research study, the remainder of the study revolves around testing the hypothesis or, in some cases, the research question. In a qualitative research study, the objective is to answer the research question. This task may be a time-consuming, sometimes frustrating, endeavour for the researcher, but in the final analysis, the outcome, as evaluated by the consumer, is most often worth the struggle. Because this text focuses on the nurse as a critical consumer of research, the sections in this chapter pertain primarily to the evaluation of research questions and hypotheses in published research reports.

CRITIQUING CRITERIA

THE RESEARCH QUESTION

1. Was the research question introduced promptly?
2. Is the question stated clearly and unambiguously in declarative or question form?
3. Does the research question express a relationship between two or more variables or at least between an independent variable and a dependent variable, thereby implying its empirical testability?
4. Does the research question specify the nature of the population being studied?
5. Has the research question been substantiated by adequate experiential and scientific background material?

6. Has the research question been placed within the context of an appropriate theoretical framework?
7. Has the significance of the research question been identified?
8. Have pragmatic issues, such as feasibility, been addressed?
9. Have the purpose, aims, or goals of the study been identified?
10. Are research questions appropriately used (i.e., for an exploratory, descriptive, or qualitative study or in relation to ancillary data analyses)?

THE HYPOTHESES

1. Is the hypothesis related directly to the research question?
2. Is the hypothesis stated concisely in a declarative form?

3. Are the independent and dependent variables identified in the statement of the hypothesis?
4. Are the variables measurable or potentially measurable?
5. Is each of the hypotheses specific to one relationship so that each hypothesis can be either supported or not supported?
6. Is the hypothesis stated in such a way that it is testable?
7. Is the hypothesis stated objectively, without value-laden words?
8. Is the direction of the relationship in each hypothesis clearly stated?
9. Is each hypothesis consistent with the literature review?
10. Is the theoretical rationale for the hypothesis explicit?

CRITICAL THINKING CHALLENGES

- Drawing from your nursing experience, develop some research questions using both the PICOT and SPIDER tools. How do the questions differ?

- Discuss how the wording of a research question or hypothesis suggests the type of research design and level of evidence that will be provided.

- A nurse is caring for patients in a clinical situation that produces a clinical question that has no ready answer. The nurse wants to develop and refine this clinical question by using the PICOT approach so that it becomes the basis for an evidence-informed practice project. How can the nurse accomplish that objective?

CRITICAL JUDGEMENT QUESTIONS

1. Which of the following is the purpose of a hypothesis for any study?
   a. To provide the objective of the research by identifying the expected outcome
   b. To identify dependent and independent variables in a study
   c. To define the appropriate measures needed to test the research question
   d. To provide a means to know whether or not the study of the research problem is feasible

2. Which of the following identified research problems has enough significance to warrant further development?
   a. Children between 6 and 10 years do not eat the broccoli in their school lunches.
   b. Women above 100 years old are at moderate risk for development of breast cancer.
   c. Obese males are at risk for heart attacks.
   d. The rate of sunscreen use among Aboriginal people is less than 10%.

3. Which part of the following research question is the dependent variable? "How does maternal employment among nurses affect infant health during the first 6 months of life?"
   a. "Infant health"
   b. "Maternal employment"
   c. "First 6 months of life"
   d. "Nurses"

KEY POINTS

- Focused clinical questions arise from clinical practice and guide the literature search for the best available evidence to answer the clinical question.
- Formulation of the research question and stating the hypothesis are key preliminary steps in the research process.
- The research question is refined through a process that proceeds from the identification of a general idea of interest to the definition of a more specific and circumscribed topic.
- A preliminary literature review reveals related factors that appear to be critical for the research topic of interest and helps further define the research questions.
- The significance of the research question must be identified in terms of its potential contribution to patients, nurses, the medical community in general, and society. The applicability of the question for nursing practice and its theoretical relevance must be established. The findings should also have the potential for formulating or altering nursing practices or policies.
- The feasibility of a research question must be examined in light of pragmatic considerations: for example, time; the availability of participants, money, facilities, and equipment; the nurse's experience; and ethical issues.
- The final research question consists of a statement about the relationship of two or more variables. The question clearly identifies the relationship between the independent variables and dependent variables, specifies the nature of the population being studied, and implies the possibility of empirical testing.
- A hypothesis is an attempt to answer the research question. When the validity of the assumptions of the theoretical framework is tested, the hypothesis connects the theory and reality.
- A hypothesis is a declarative statement about the relationship between two or more variables in which an expected outcome is

predicted. The characteristics of a hypothesis include a relationship statement, implications regarding testability, and consistency with a defined theory base.

- Hypotheses can be formulated directionally or nondirectionally. Hypotheses can be further categorized as either research or statistical (null) hypotheses.
- Research questions may be used instead of hypotheses in exploratory, descriptive, or qualitative research studies. Research questions may also be formulated in addition to hypotheses to answer questions related to ancillary data.
- The purpose, research question, or hypothesis provides information about the intent of the research question and hypothesis and suggests the level of evidence to be obtained from the study findings.
- The critiquing criteria are a set of guidelines for evaluating the strengths and weaknesses of the research question and hypotheses as they appear in a research report.
- In critiquing, the reader assesses the clarity of the research question and the related subquestions, the specificity of the population, and the implications for testability.
- The interrelatedness of the research question, the literature review, the theoretical framework, and the hypotheses should be apparent.
- The appropriateness of the research design suggested by the research question is also evaluated.
- The purpose of the study (i.e., why the researcher is conducting the study) should be differentiated from the research question.
- The reader evaluates the wording of the hypothesis in terms of the clarity of the relational statement, its implications for testability, and its congruence with theory. The appropriateness of the hypothesis in relation to the type of research design is also examined. In addition, the appropriate use of research questions is evaluated in relation to the type of study conducted.

🛜 FOR FURTHER STUDY

Go to Evolve at http://evolve.elsevier.com/Canada/LoBiondo/Research for the Audio Glossary.

REFERENCES

Bilik, Ö., Kankaya, E. A., & Deveci, Z. (2020). Effects of web-based concept mapping education on students' concept mapping and critical thinking skills: A double blind, randomized, controlled study. *Nurse Education Today, 86*, Article 104312. https://doi.org/10.1016/j.nedt.2019.104312.

Boitor, M., Martorella, G., Maheu, C., Laizner, A. M., & Gélinas, C. (2019). Does hand massage have sustained effects on pain intensity and pain-related interference in the cardiac surgery critically ill? A randomized controlled trial. *Pain Management Nursing, 20*(6), 572–579. https://doi.org/10.1016/j.pmn.2019.02.011.

Bourque-Bearskin, R. L., Cameron, B., King, M., & Pillwax, C. (2016). Mâmawoh Kamâtowin, "Coming together to help each other in wellness": Honouring Indigenous Nursing Knowledge. *International Journal of Indigenous Health, 11*(1), 18. https://doi.org/10.18357/ijih111201615024.

Chyzzy, B., Nelson, L. E., Stinson, J., Vigod, S., & Dennis, C.-L. (2020). Adolescent mothers' perceptions of a mobile phone-based peer support intervention. *Canadian Journal of Nursing Research, 52*(2), 129–138. https://doi.org/10.1177/0844562120904591.

Cooke, A., Smith, S., & Booth, A. (2012). Beyond PICO: The SPIDER tool for qualitative evidence synthesis. *Qualitative Health Research, 22*(10), 1435–1443. https://doi.org/10.1177/1049732312452938.

Currie, G., & Szabo, J. (2020). Social isolation and exclusion: the parents' experience of caring for children with rare neurodevelopmental disorders. *International Journal of Qualitative Studies on Health and Well-Being, 15*(1), Article 1725362. https://doi.org/10.1080/17482631.2020.1725362.

Currie, G., Dosani, A., Premji, S., Riley, S., Lodha, A., & Young, M. (2018). Caring for late preterm infants: Public health nurses' experiences. *BMC Nursing, 17*(1), 16. http://dx.doi.org/10.1186/s12912-018-0286-y.

Fox, M., McCague, H., Sidani, S., & Butler, J. (2018). The relationships between the geriatric practice environment, nursing practice, and the quality of hospitalized older adults' care. *Journal of Nursing Scholarship, 50*(5), 513–521. https://doi.org/10.1111/jnu.12414.

Freeman, L. A., Pfaff, K. A., Kopchek, L., & Liebman, J. (2020). Investigating palliative care nurse attitudes towards medical assistance in dying: An exploratory cross-sectional study. *Journal of Advanced Nursing, 76*, 535–545. https://doi.org/10.1111/jan.14252.

Ha, L., & Pepin, J. (2018). Clinical nursing leadership educational intervention for first-year nursing students: A qualitative evaluation. *Nurse Education in Practice, 32*, 37–43. https://doi.org/10.1016/j.nepr.2018.07.005.

Hartigan-Rogers, J. A., Redmond, S., Cobbett, S., et al. A, B, or C? (2019). A quasi-experimental multi-site study investigating three option multiple choice questions. *International Journal of Nursing Education Scholarship, 16*(1). https://doi.org/10.1515/ijnes-2019-0061.

Henrique, A. J., Gabrielloni, M. C., Rodney, P., & Barbieri, M. (2018). Non-pharmacological interventions during childbirth for pain relief, anxiety, and neuroendocrine stress parameters: A randomized controlled trial. *International Journal of Nursing Practice, 24*, e12642. https://doi.org/10.1111/ijn.12642.

Jackson, K. T., & Dennis, C. L. (2017). Lanolin for the treatment of nipple pain in breastfeeding women: A randomized controlled trial. *Maternal and Child Nutrition, 13*(3), 1–10. https://doi.org/10.1111/mcn.12357.

King-Shier, K. M., Dhaliwal, K. K., Puri, R., LeBlanc, P., & Johal, J. (2019). South Asians' experience of managing hypertension: A grounded theory study. *Patient Preference andAadherence, 13*, 321–329. https://doi.org/10.2147/PPA.S196224.

Kwan, J. A., Wang, M., Cummings, G. G., Lemermeyer, G., Nordstrom, P., Blumer, L., Horne, N., & Giblin, C. (2019). The evaluation of evidence-informed changes to an internationally educated nurse registration process. *International Nursing Review, 66*, 309–319.

Lavoie-Tremblay, M., Cyr, G., Primeau, G., & Aube, T. (2018). Nurse leaders' perceptions of the impact of their participation in a reflective practice program. *Journal of Nursing Education and Practice, 9*(4). https://doi.org/10.5430/jnep.v9n4p38.

Macartney, G., Vassilyadi, V., Zemek, R., Chen, W., Aglipay, M., Macartney, A., & Goulet, K. (2019). The effect of the ParachuteTM concussion awareness for players program on the acquisition of concussion knowledge and attitude in children who play soccer. *Canadian Journal of Neuroscience Nursing, 9*(1), 14–22.

Melnyk, B. M., & Fineout-Overholt, E. (2019). *Evidence-based practice in nursing and healthcare: A guide to best practice* (4th ed). New York: Wolters Kluwer.

Penz, K. L., Stewart, N. J., Karunanayake, C. P., Kosteniuk, J. G., & MacLeod, M. L. P. (2019). Competence and confidence in rural and remote nursing practice: A structural equation modelling analysis of national data. *Journal of Clinical Nursing, 28*, 1664–1679. https://doi.org/10.1111/jocn.14772.

Ploeg, J., Matthew-Maich, N., Fraser, K., et al. (2017). Managing multiple chronic conditions in the community: A Canadian qualitative study of the experiences of older adults, family caregivers and healthcare providers. (Report). *BMC Geriatrics, 17*(1), 40. https://doi.org/10.1186/s12877-017-0431-6.

Premji, S. S., Pana, G., Currie, G., Dosani, A., Reilly, S., Young, M., Hall, M., Williamson, T., & Lodha, A. K. (2018). Mother's level of confidence in caring for her late preterm infant: A mixed method study. *Journal of Clinical Nursing, 27*(5-6), e1120–e1133.

Price, S. L., Aston, M., Monaghan, J., et al. (2018). Maternal knowing and social networks: Understanding first-time mothers' search for information and support through online and offline social networks. *Qualitative Health Research, 28*(10), 1552–1563. https://doi.org/10.1177/1049732317748314.

Santiago, C., Roza, D., Porretta, K., & Smith, O. (2019). The use of tablet and communication app for patients with endotracheal or tracheostomy tubes in the medical surgical intensive care unit: A pilot, feasibility study. *Canadian Journal of Critical Care Nursing, 30*(1), 17–23. https://doi.org/10.13140/RG.2.2.19835.57125.

Sawatzky, R., Roberts, D., Russell, L., Bitschy, A., Ho, S., Desbiens, F-F., Chan, E. K. H., Tayler, C., & Stajduhar, K. (2019). Self-perceived competence of nurses and care aides providing a palliative approach in home, hospital, and residential care settings: A cross-sectional survey. *Canadian Journal of Nursing, 53*(1), 64–77. https://doi.org/10.1177/0844562119881043.

Subedi, A., Edge, D. S., Goldie, C. L., & Sawhney, M. (2019). Resettled Bhutanese refugees in Ottawa: What coping strategies promote psychological well-being? *Canadian Journal of Nursing Research, 51*(3), 168–178. https://doi.org/10.1177/0844562119828905.

Woodgate, R. L., Tailor, K., Tennent, P., Wener, P., & Altman, G. (2020). The experience of the self in Canadian youth living with anxiety: A qualitative study. *PLoS ONE, 15*(1), Article e0228193. https://doi.org/10.1371/journal.pone.0228193.

CHAPTER 5

Finding and Appraising the Literature

Lorraine Thirsk

LEARNING OUTCOMES

After reading this chapter, you will be able to do the following:

- Explain the relationship of the literature review to nursing theory, research, education, and practice.
- Outline the purposes of the literature review for research projects and for evidence-informed practice projects.
- Identify the differences between primary and secondary sources.
- Compare the advantages and disadvantages of commonly used online databases for conducting a literature review.
- Develop strategies for an effective electronic search of the literature.
- Outline the steps to effectively retrieve and select articles appropriate for an evidence-informed practice project.
- Apply critiquing criteria to the evaluation of literature reviews in selected research studies.

KEY TERMS

Boolean operator
citation management
   software
controlled vocabulary

literature review
online database
primary sources
print indexes

refereed (peer-reviewed)
journal
secondary sources

STUDY RESOURCES

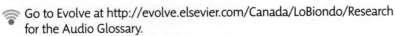 Go to Evolve at http://evolve.elsevier.com/Canada/LoBiondo/Research for the Audio Glossary.

THE PURPOSE OF THIS CHAPTER IS to introduce you to the **literature review** as it is used in both research and evidence-informed practice projects. Searching for, retrieving, critically appraising and synthesizing the literature is a key step in the process for researchers and for nurses implementing evidence-informed practice. Your ability to locate and retrieve research studies, critically appraise them, and decide that you have the best available evidence to inform your practice decision making is a skill essential for your current role as a student and your future role as a nurse who is a competent research user.

This chapter provides you with the tools to (1) conduct an appropriate, comprehensive literature search for research studies, systematic reviews, documents, and statistical reports; (2) critically appraise the literature to determine which resources are useful for your topic; (3) differentiate between different types of articles and sources; and (4) understand the relevance of literature review section of a research report. This set of tools will help you develop your competencies as a research user and apply them to your academic papers and evidence-informed practice projects.

While Chapter 3 gave an overview of critically appraising an individual article, it is also important that you develop skills to search, retrieve, critique, and synthesize several articles related to your topic of interest. This will help you in determining the breadth and depth of evidence, which is important when considering evidence-informed practice projects.

REVIEW OF THE LITERATURE

The Literature Review: Evidence-Informed Project

With an evidence-informed practice approach, you search the literature widely and gather multiple resources to answer a clinical question or to solve a clinical problem. This process includes (1) asking clinical questions; (2) identifying and gathering the evidence; (3) critically appraising and synthesizing the evidence or literature; (4) acting to change practice by using the best available evidence, coupled with your clinical experience and patient preferences (values, setting, and resources); and (5) evaluating the use of the research evidence found to assess applicability of the research findings to the practice change. In Box 5.1, objectives 1 through 3 reflect the purposes of a literature review for nurses involved in evidence-informed practice projects.

BOX 5.1
OVERALL PURPOSES OF A LITERATURE REVIEW

MAJOR GOAL

To develop a strong knowledge base to carry out a research study or an evidence-informed practice project

OBJECTIVES

A review of the literature helps you do the following:
1. Uncover one or more new practice interventions or obtain supporting or contrary evidence for revising, maintaining, or stopping current interventions, protocols, and policies
2. Promote evidence-informed revision and development of new practice protocols, policies, and projects or activities related to nursing practice
3. Generate clinical questions that guide development of evidence-informed practice projects
4. Determine what is known and unknown about a subject, concept, or problem
5. Determine gaps, consistencies, and inconsistencies in the literature about a subject, concept, or problem
6. Discover conceptual traditions used to examine problems
7. Generate useful research questions and hypotheses
8. Determine an appropriate research design, methodology, and analysis for answering the research questions or hypotheses on the basis of an assessment of the strengths and weaknesses of earlier works
9. Determine the need for replication of a study or refinement of a study
10. Synthesize the strengths and weaknesses and findings of available studies on a topic or problem

As a student or practising nurse, you may be asked to generate a clinical question for an evidence-informed practice project. For this you need to search for, retrieve, review, and critically appraise the literature to identify the "best available evidence" that provides the answer to a clinical question. As described in Chapter 4, a clear and precise articulation of a question is crucial for finding the best evidence. Evidence-informed questions may sound like research questions, but they are questions used to search the existing literature for answers. As a practising nurse, you may be called on to revise or continue current evidence-informed practice protocols, practice standards, or policies in your health care organization or to develop new ones. This requires that you know how to retrieve and critically appraise research articles, systematic reviews, and practice guidelines to determine the degree of support or lack of support found in the literature. A critical appraisal of the literature related to a specific clinical question uncovers data that contribute evidence to support current practice and clinical decision making, as well as for making changes in practice.

The Literature Review: Research Study

Research producers also systematically find and appraise literature. As a researcher user, you are most likely looking for recent research articles that will help you in making decisions about how you practice; researcher producers will look more broadly at the literature on a particular topic to account for the historical development of knowledge and different theoretical viewpoints (Spurlock, 2019). The research process requires that researchers position their study in the context of the larger knowledge base. The section of a published research study titled "Literature Review" generally appears near the beginning of a research article. It provides an abbreviated version of the complete literature review conducted by a researcher and represents the foundation for the study. Therefore, the literature review, a systematic and critical appraisal of the most important literature on a topic, is a key step in the research process that provides the basis of a research study.

The conceptual framework, or theoretical framework, of a research report is a structure of concepts or theories pulled together as a map for the study; this map provides rationale for the development of research questions or hypotheses. This section of a research report is often a titled subsection of the literature review and may be accompanied by a diagram illustrating the proposed relationships between and among the concepts. Alternatively, the conceptual/theoretical framework may not be separately identified; it may be embedded in the literature review section of an article or simply not included. As described in Chapter 2, it is important to understand the conceptual/theoretical framework as this will help you with the links between theory, research, education, and practice.

The overall purpose of the literature review in a research study is to present a strong knowledge base for the conduct of the research study. Objectives 4 through 10 listed in Box 5.1 reflect the purposes of a literature review for conducting research. It is important to understand when you read a research article that the researcher's main goal when developing the literature review was to develop the knowledge foundation for a sound study, generate research questions and hypotheses, and determine how to best design a particular study.

An extensive literature review is essential for all types of quantitative research and for most qualitative studies, with occasional exceptions. From this perspective, the review is broad and systematic, as well as in-depth. It is a critical collection and evaluation of the important published literature in journals, monographs, books, and book chapters, as well as unpublished research print and online materials (e.g., doctoral dissertations and masters' theses), audiovisual materials (e.g., audio and video recordings), and sometimes personal communications (e.g., conference presentations).

The following brief overview about the use of the literature review in relation to the steps of the research process will help you to understand how literature is used throughout a research article (Figure 5.1). A critical review of relevant literature affects the steps of the research process as follows:

- Theoretical or conceptual framework: A literature review reveals conceptual traditions, concepts, theories, or conceptual models from nursing and other related disciplines that can be used to examine problems. This framework presents the context for studying the problem and can be viewed as a map for understanding the phenomenon being studied. In quantitative research, the literature review provides rationale for the variables and explains concepts, definitions, and relationships between or among the independent and dependent

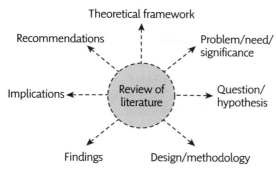

FIG. 5.1 Relationship of the review of the literature to the steps of the research process.

variables used in the study. In qualitative research, the literature review may provide an overview of similar studies, support for using a particular method, and a theoretical or conceptual frame for the research. In many research articles the literature review may be labelled "Background" and is usually at the beginning of the article. The authors of the study will usually provide several citations in this section.

- Research question and hypothesis: The literature review helps you determine what is known and not known; uncover gaps, consistencies, or inconsistencies; or to disclose unanswered questions in the literature about a subject, concept, theory, or problem that generate or allow for refinement of research questions, hypotheses, or both.
- Design and method: The literature review exposes the strengths and weaknesses of previous studies in terms of designs and methods and helps the researcher choose an appropriate new, replicated, or refined design, including data-collection method, sampling strategy and size, valid and reliable measurement instruments, an effective data analysis method, and appropriate informed consent forms. Literature may also be used to support decisions made regarding ethical process in the research. Often, because of journal space limitations, researchers only include abbreviated information about these aspects in their journal article.

- Outcome of the analysis (i.e., findings, discussion, implications, and recommendations): The literature review is used to help the researcher accurately interpret and discuss the results or findings of a study. In the discussion section of a research article, the researcher refers to the research studies and theoretical articles or books described earlier in the article in the literature review and uses this conceptual and research literature to interpret and explain the study's findings. Further literature may be examined to help explain the new findings of the research project.
- Systematic reviews are another type of literature review but follow a rigorous, in-depth research methodology and are considered research studies. More information about systematic reviews can be found in Chapter 8 (qualitative systematic reviews), Chapter 12 (quantitative systematic reviews) and Chapter 21 (comparison of systematic reviews).

Research Hint

If you are new to a topic, finding a recent systematic review, or integrated literature review, can help to give you an overview or summary of what is known on the topic. This will give you a sense of how nurse researchers have examined the topic previously and should also identify gaps in current knowledge.

Differences and Similarities in Literature Reviews for Evidence-Informed Projects and Research Studies

How does the literature review differ whether it is used for evidenced-informed practice purposes or for a research study? The literature review in a research study is used to develop a sound research proposal for a research study that will generate knowledge. From a broader perspective, the major focus of reviewing the literature for an evidence-informed project is to uncover multiple sources of evidence on a given topic that have been generated by researchers in their research studies that can potentially be used to improve clinical practice and patient outcomes.

Research Hint _____

Remember that the findings of one study on a topic do not usually provide enough evidence to support a change in practice; be cautious when anyone suggests that you change your practice on the basis of the results of one study.

From a student perspective, the ability to critically appraise the literature is essential to acquiring a skill set for successfully completing scholarly papers, presentations, debates, and evidence-informed practice projects. Both types of literature reviews are similar in that both should be framed in the context of previous research and theoretical literature and pertinent to the objectives presented in Box 5.1.

Although reviewing the literature for research purposes and practice questions requires the same critical thinking and reading skills, a literature review for a research proposal is usually much more extensive and comprehensive, and the critiquing process is more in-depth. From an academic standpoint, requirements for a literature review for a class assignment differ depending on the level and type of course, as well as the specific objective of the assignment. These factors determine whether a student's literature search requires a limited, selective review or a major/extensive review. Regardless of extent, discovering knowledge is the goal of any search; therefore, you must know how to search the literature.

Evidence-Informed Practice Tip _____

For a research user, formulating a clinical question provides a focus that guides the literature review.

SEARCHING FOR EVIDENCE

There is currently a wealth of information that is readily available, and it can be overwhelming to determine accurate and reliable sources of information for your practice (Aveyard et al., 2015). Developing a solid search strategy, the skills to conduct and refine a literature search, and critically

appraise and synthesize research, is a key tool for your practice. It is important in searching for literature that you move beyond "finding some articles" to systematically retrieving, sorting, reading, and appraising quality evidence. It is also important to avoid confirmation bias—where you look for and use only those articles that confirm what you already believe.

In your student role, when you are preparing an academic paper, you read the required course materials, as well as additional literature retrieved from the library. You search the literature to uncover research and conceptual information to prepare an academic term paper on a certain topic. You search for **primary sources**, which are articles, books, or other documents written by the person who conducted the study, developed the theory, or prepared the scholarly discussion on a concept, topic, problem, or issue of interest.

The literature review, or background section, of a research article will likely refer to other sources. The authors of the study likely read these sources directly. If you want to use this information, it is important that you find the original, or primary, source unless the primary source is unavailable (American Psychological Association, 2019). If it is a historical document, or written in another language, it may not be available to you, and you may need to cite it as a secondary source. Relying on **secondary sources** can eventually lead to misinterpretations and misrepresentations of the original study or theory (Aveyard, 2014).

Research Hint _____

There are several references used throughout this textbook—when you read this textbook, it is a secondary source of these materials. For example, if you wanted to use the information by Aveyard (2014) about the consequences of using secondary sources, you should retrieve that handbook and read the primary source directly, rather than relying on our interpretation.

Reference librarians and technicians can provide excellent help in searching for various sources of scholarly literature and are excellent resources for both research producers and research users. Table 5.1 provides you with an overview of the steps and strategies for conducting a literature search.

Research Hint

Librarians are experts at searching literature and finding information. Research courses often include a session with a librarian, and the library at your institution may have tutorials and guides to help students navigate online databases and conduct successful searches. If you are unfamiliar with the process of conducting a scholarly database search, your reference librarian is an invaluable resource.

Step 1: Determine the Topic and Generate Keywords

The first step in your search strategy is to define your question or topic. The PICOT or SPIDER (Cooke et al., 2012) questions should be refined prior to starting your search (see Chapter 4). These are mnemonics that structure the elements of a practice question. These questions will become the source for your keywords. An example of a clinical question is provided in the following Practical Application box.

When conducting a search, you should use a rigorous focusing process; otherwise, you may end up with hundreds or thousands of citations. Retrieving too many citations is usually a sign that there was something wrong with your search technique or that you may have not sufficiently narrowed your clinical question. Retrieving too few citations may be a sign that your search is too narrow, you need to change your keywords, or there is limited research on the topic. Finding the right keywords for a computer search is an important aspect of conducting a search. Once you have the keywords from your question, generate as many synonyms as you can, and use the thesaurus function in your academic database (Wakefield, 2014).

When it is possible, you want to match the words that you use to describe your question with

TABLE **5.1**	
STEPS AND STRATEGIES FOR CONDUCTING A LITERATURE SEARCH	
STEPS OF LITERATURE REVIEW	**STRATEGY**
Step 1: Determine the topic and generate keywords.	Form your PICOT or SPIDER question and spend some time refining it so it is focused. Generate keywords related to the terms used in your question and explore the controlled vocabulary in key databases to check for other search terms.
Step 2: Choose databases to search	Choose at least two databases to search. If your library has a unified database, remember that it may not link all indexed articles (e.g., EBSCO's Discover search does not include ProQuest indexed articles).
Step 3: Conduct your search	Get help from a librarian if you can when conducting the search. Remember Boolean operators, wild cards, and filters that can limit your search results.
Step 4: Refine search results	Scan through your search, read the abstracts provided, and make a note of only those that fit your topic; select "references," as well as "search history" and "full-text articles" if available, before printing, saving, or emailing your search.
Step 5: Select relevant sources	Review the full articles and discard those that are not relevant. Download or print the relevant resources. Consider using reference management software.
Step 6: Critically read, summarize, and synthesize	Review the critical appraisal strategies described in chapter 3. Consider making an extraction table to keep track of the key findings from each of the articles and make further comparison and synthesis easier.
Step 7: Present the findings	Decide how you will present your synthesis of overall strengths and weaknesses of the reviewed articles (e.g., chronologically or according to type: research or conceptual) and type up the synthesized material and a reference list.

Practical Application

One group of students was interested in whether regular exercise prevented osteoporosis for postmenopausal women who had osteopenia. The PICOT format for the clinical question that guided their search was as follows:

P: Postmenopausal women with osteopenia
I: Regular exercise program
C: No regular exercise program
O: Prevention of osteoporosis
T: After 1 year

Another set of students was interested in whether regular exercise improved the quality of life for post-menopausal women who had osteopenia. The SPIDER format that guided their search was as follows:

S: Postmenopausal women with osteopenia
PI: Quality of life of postmenopausal women with osteopenia who regularly exercised
D: Exploratory studies, lived experience, survey, focus group, case study
E: Quality of life, well-being, attitude, experience
R: Qualitative, mixed-research, quantitative

Their assignment required that the students do the following:

- Search the literature by using electronic databases (e.g., Cumulative Index to Nursing and Allied Health Literature [CINAHL] via EBSCO; MEDLINE; Scopus; and Cochrane Database of Systematic Reviews) for the background information that enabled them to identify the significance of osteopenia and osteoporosis as a health problem in women.
- Identify systematic reviews, practice guidelines, and individual research studies that provided the "best available evidence" related to the effectiveness and experiences of regular exercise programs on prevention of osteoporosis.
- Critically appraise systematic reviews, practice guidelines, and research studies in accordance with standardized critical appraisal criteria (see Chapter 21).
- Synthesize the overall strengths and weaknesses of the evidence provided by the literature.
- Establish a conclusion about the strength, quality, and consistency of the evidence.
- Make recommendations on the applicability of the evidence to clinical nursing practice that guides development of a health promotion project about osteoporosis risk reduction for postmenopausal women with osteopenia.

the terms that indexers have assigned to the articles. In many **online databases**, you can browse the controlled vocabulary terms and search. Used to conduct searches in databases, controlled vocabulary terms are carefully selected words and phrases that are applied to similar pieces of information units. While most databases can be searched with keywords you generate, it can be helpful to explore the controlled vocabulary to ensure your search is comprehensive, and you are not inadvertently missing important terms. If you are still having difficulty, ask your reference librarian for help.

Consider the example in the Practical Application box. Some keywords that might be helpful for the search might be: women, female, aging, menopause, menopausal, postmenopausal, exercise, fitness, physical activity, bone loss, osteoporosis, osteopenia, joints, arthritis. Searching the controlled vocabulary Subject Headings in CINAHL reveals that Menopause, Postmenopausal Disorders and Osteoporosis are Subject Headings. In other words, these are the official, controlled keywords associated with the articles that might be relevant for your search.

Step 2: Choosing Online, Academic Databases

Why use an academic database? You are likely very familiar with search engines such as Google or Yahoo. You may have even used these search tools and found some relevant information for your paper or project. These search engines are not the most appropriate and efficient way to find the latest and strongest research on a topic that affects nursing practice decisions. Academic databases are designed for advanced searching, are discipline specific, and often have direct access to academic journals and books, giving you more relevant resources (Aveyard, 2014). They allow you to specifically search peer-reviewed research that will be higher quality than what Google searches find. If you take the time to learn how to perform a sound database search, building your information literacy skills, you will have the essential competency needed for nursing in an increasingly information-intensive environment (Purnell et al., 2020). Following the strategies and hints provided in this chapter will help you gain the essential competencies needed for your course assignments and career in nursing. The Critical Thinking Decision Path illustrates a method for locating evidence to support your research or clinical question.

An online, academic database is used to find journal sources (periodicals) of research and conceptual articles on a variety of topics (e.g., doctoral dissertations), as well as the publications of professional organizations and various governmental agencies. These databases contain bibliographic citation information such as the author, title, journal, date, and indexed terms (controlled keywords) for each record. Some also include the abstract. Box 5.2 lists examples of the more commonly used online databases.

Your college or university probably enables you to access such databases online. It is a good idea to conduct your search in at least two databases; however, many libraries now have unified database search engines that allow you to search multiple databases (Spurlock, 2019). The most relevant and frequently used source for nursing literature remains CINAHL (Cumulative Index to Nursing and Allied Health Literature). Another premier resource is MEDLINE, which is produced by the National Library of Medicine in the United States. MEDLINE focuses on the life sciences, and its sources date back to the early 1950s.

Most college and university libraries also have an online catalogue to find print and online books, journals (titles only), videos and other media items, scripts, monographs, conference proceedings, masters' theses, dissertations, archival materials, and more. Before the 1980s, a search was usually done manually with print indexes, which were listings of published material. This was a tedious and time-consuming process. The print indexes are useful today for finding sources that have not been entered into electronic (online) databases. The print index started in 1956 but is no longer produced.

Other Types of Search Engines and Databases

Some databases contain more than just journal article information. These online resources contain either summaries or synopses of studies, overviews of diseases or conditions, or a summary of the most recent evidence to support a treatment. For example, the Cochrane Library is an online resource that consists of six databases, including the Cochrane Database of Systematic Reviews. Table 5.2 lists sources of *free* online information. Review the table carefully to determine whether it is a good source of primary research studies. Note that some sites are sources of health information and others are clinical guidelines based on systematic reviews of the literature, but most websites are not a primary source of research studies.

Prioritizing the Search for Evidence

In Chapter 3, an evidence hierarchy is presented for grading the strength and quality of evidence provided by individual studies or resources located during a search. In this chapter, an evidence-informed model, called the "6S" pyramid, is used to help you identify the highest-level information resource to facilitate your search for the best evidence about your clinical question or problem (DiCenso et al., 2009). This model, as illustrated in Figure 5.2, suggests that when searching the literature, consider prioritizing your search strategy and begin by looking for the highest-level information resource available. For example, individual original studies such as those found in MEDLINE or CINAHL (e.g., a randomized clinical trial) are at the lowest level of the information resource pyramid. The next information resource levels of the 6S pyramid are synopses of studies (e.g., a brief summary of a high-quality study), then syntheses (e.g., Cochrane Library), followed by synopses

BOX **5.2**

ONLINE DATABASES

COCHRANE LIBRARY

- Collection of databases that contain high-quality evidence
- Includes the Cochrane Database of Systematic Reviews
- Full Cochrane Library available from Wiley Online Library; other databases that make up the Cochrane Library available from other vendors, including Ovid Technologies
- Cochrane systematic reviews are indexed and searchable in both CINAHL and MEDLINE

CUMULATIVE INDEX TO NURSING AND ALLIED HEALTH LITERATURE (CINAHL)

- Initially called Cumulative Index to Nursing Literature
- Produced by CINAHL
- Electronic version available as part of the EBSCO online service
- Over 1,800 journals indexed for inclusion in database
- Citations in CINAHL are assigned index terms from a controlled vocabulary

EDUCATION RESOURCE INFORMATION CENTER (ERIC)

- Sponsored by the Institute of Education and the U.S. Department of Education
- Focuses on education research and information
- Currently indexes more than 600 journals and includes references to books, conference papers, and technical reports
- References date from 1966
- Available from the ERIC website and by subscription from EBSCO, OCLC, and Ovid Technologies

EXCERPTA MEDICA

- Biomedical database
- More than 24 million indexed records
- Approximately 7,500 current, mostly peer-reviewed journals

MEDLINE (MEDICAL LITERATURE ANALYSIS AND RETRIEVAL SYSTEM ONLINE)

- Produced by the National Library of Medicine
- Premier bibliographic database for journal articles in life sciences
- References date from 1950, and approximately 5,200 worldwide journals are indexed
- Indexed with MeSH (Medical Subject Headings)
- MEDLINE is available for free through PubMed (tutorial available; National Library of Medicine, 2016) and by subscription from EBSCO, OCLC, and Ovid Technologies

PROQUEST DISSERTATIONS AND THESES

- Produced by ProQuest
- PDF downloads available for over 1 million dissertations
- Available from ProQuest (n.d.)

PSYCINFO

- Produced by the American Psychological Association (APA, n.d.)
- An abstract database of the psychosocial literature beginning with citations dating back to 1800
- Covers more than 2,150 journals
- Of the journals covered, 98% are peer reviewed
- Also includes book chapters and dissertations
- Indexed with the Thesaurus of Psychological Index Terms
- Available through APA PsycNET, EBSCO, Ovid Technologies, and ProQuest

SCOPUS

- Largest abstract and citation database of peer-reviewed science literature and quality Web sources
- Provides 100% MEDLINE coverage
- Offers sophisticated tools to track, analyze, and visualize research

OCLC (ONLINE COMPUTER LIBRARY CENTER)

- A global library network representing 100 countries
- Provides shared technology services and original research
- Provides an comprehensive database of information about library collections
- OCLC also conducts research

THE JOANNA BRIGGS INSTITUTE

A not-for-profit research and development centre within the Faculty of Health Sciences at the University of Adelaide, South Australia that promotes and supports the synthesis, transfer, and utilization of evidence through identifying feasible, appropriate, meaningful, and effective health care practices to assist in the improvement of health care outcomes globally.

The free JBI COnNECT+ provides easy access to evidence-based resources such as the following:

- JBI databases (including the JBI Library of Systematic Reviews, Best Practice Information Sheets, Evidence Summaries, and Evidence Based Recommended Practices)
- JBI Library of Systematic Reviews
- External databases (including the Cochrane Library, PubMed)

TABLE 5.2

SELECTED EXAMPLES OF FREE WEBSITES FOR LITERATURE SEARCHES

WEBSITE	SCOPE	NOTES
Canadian Institute for Health Information: www.cihi.ca	CIHI gathers and organizes health data from a variety of sources. Their goal is to improve health care and health systems by supporting databases, measurement, and standards.	An independent, non-profit organization. Access to some reports and primary data is free.
Canadian Nurses Association (CNA): http://www.nurseone.ca	This site gives CNA members access to online libraries including electronic books, full-text journals, and evidence-informed resources in EBSCO databases (including CINAHL and MEDLINE), Cochrane Collaboration, e-CPS (Electronic drug manual), e-Therapeutics, STAT!Ref Electronic Health Library, and much more.	This site is managed by the CNA and can only be accessed by members.
Canadian Patient Safety Institute (and provincial patient safety organizations): https://www.canada.ca/en/health-canada/services/quality-care/patient-safety/current-patient-safety-organizations-canada.html	These organizations are involved in a range of activities related to patient safety and quality care.	Numerous sources of primary data related to health care quality and patient safety.
Cochrane Collaboration: http://www.cochrane.org	Provides free access to abstracts from the Cochrane Database of Systematic Reviews. Full text of reviews and access to the databases that are part of the Cochrane Library—Database of Abstracts of Reviews of Effectiveness, Cochrane Controlled Trials Register, Cochrane Methodology Register, Health Technology Assessment database (HTA), and National Health Service (NHS) Economic Evaluation Database (EED)—are accessible through Wiley Online library.	Abstracts of Cochrane Reviews are available without charge and can be browsed or searched; many databases are used in its reviews, including CINAHL via EBSCO and MEDLINE; some are primary sources (e.g. systematic reviews/meta-analyses); others (if commentaries of single studies) are a secondary source. Important source for clinical evidence but limited as a provider of primary documents for literature reviews.
National Guideline Clearinghouse: https://www.guideline.gov	Public resource for evidence-informed clinical practice guidelines. It contains more than 1,900 guidelines, including non-U.S. publications.	Offers a useful online feature of side-by-side comparison of guidelines.

Continued

TABLE 5.2

SELECTED EXAMPLES OF FREE WEBSITES FOR LITERATURE SEARCHES—cont'd

WEBSITE	SCOPE	NOTES
National Institute of Nursing Research: https://www.ninr.nih.gov	Promotes science for nursing practice, funding for nursing and interdisciplinary research, and nurse scientist training programs. Provides links to many nursing organizations and search sites. Excellent site for graduate students.	Able to link to Computer Retrieval of Information on Scientific Projects (CRISP) and PubMed (search service of the National Library of Medicine), which accesses literature via MEDLINE and PreMEDLINE and other related material from online journals; however, this site has limited utility for the beginning consumer of research for conducting scholarly review of nursing research literature because MEDLINE alone does not include all nursing literature; searching CINAHL and MEDLINE on your own would be your first choice. Useful site for graduate students in addition to CINAHL and MEDLINE and as third database related to topic.
Statistics Canada: http://www.statcan.gc.ca	Collects data on the Canadian population that are related to demographic trends, labour, health, trade, and education. Data on health trends are useful in identifying populations at risk and suggest associations among health determinants, health status, and population characteristics. Research papers on a variety of topics are also published.	Free source of primary data essential for comprehensive demographic data and socioeconomic trends; updated daily.
Turning Research into Practice (Trip): http://www.tripdatabase.com	Content from a wide variety of free online resources, including synopses, guidelines, medical images, electronic textbooks, and systematic reviews; accessed together by the Trip search engine (Trip, 2016).	Provides a wide sampling of available evidence.
Virginia Henderson Global Nursing e-Repository: https://www.nursinglibrary.org/vhl/	Open access to the Registry of Nursing Research database, which contains nearly 30,000 abstracts of research studies and conference papers.	Service offered without charge; locate conference abstracts and research study abstracts. This library is supported by Sigma Theta Tau International, honour society of nursing.

CRITICAL THINKING DECISION PATH

Search for Evidence Thought Flow

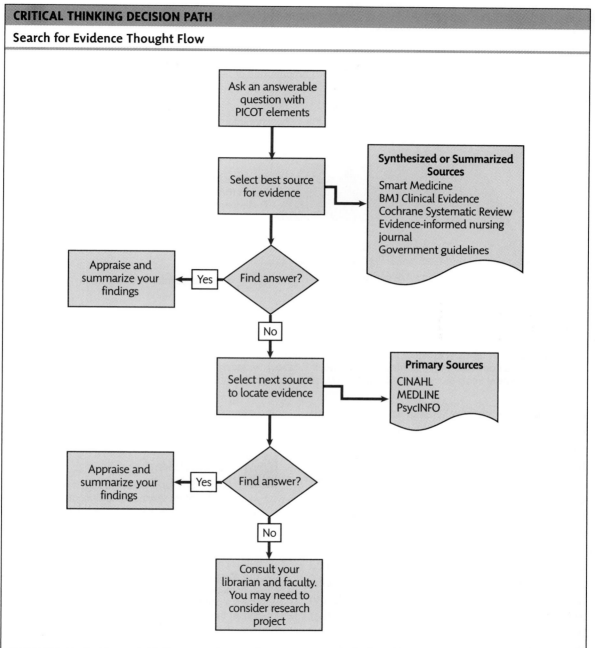

BMJ, British Medical Journal; CINAHL, Cumulative Index to Nursing and Allied Health Literature; PICOT, population, intervention, comparison, outcome, time. Based on Kendall, S. American College of Physicians (ACP). (2008). Evidence-based resources simplified. Canadian Family Physician, 54(2), 241–243. ©2001,2003, 2004 Sandra Kendall (Mount Sinai Hospital), reprinted with permission.

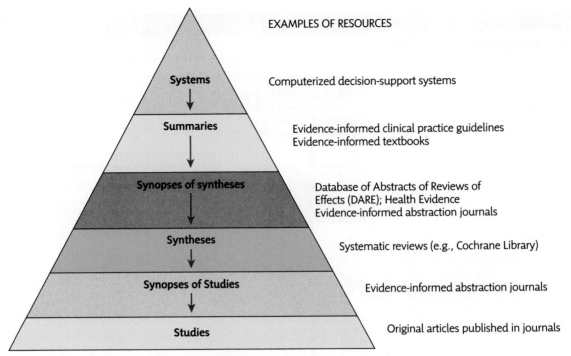

EXAMPLES OF RESOURCES

Systems — Computerized decision-support systems

Summaries — Evidence-informed clinical practice guidelines
Evidence-informed textbooks

Synopses of syntheses — Database of Abstracts of Reviews of Effects (DARE); Health Evidence
Evidence-informed abstraction journals

Syntheses — Systematic reviews (e.g., Cochrane Library)

Synopses of Studies — Evidence-informed abstraction journals

Studies — Original articles published in journals

FIG. 5.2   *6S levels of evidence from health care research.*
(Adapted from: DiCenso, A., Bayley, L., & Haynes, R.B. (2009). Accessing pre-appraised evidence: Fine-tuning the 5S model into a 6S model. *Evidence Based Nursing, 12*(4), 99–101. http://dx.doi.org/10.1136/ebn.12.4.99-b.)

of syntheses (a comprehensive summary of all the research related to a clinical question), and summaries (e.g., evidence-informed clinical practice guidelines and textbooks).

The highest information resource level portrayed in the 6S levels of organization (see Figure 5.2) pertains to computerized decision support systems, a resource built into an electronic medical record that links your patient's distinctive needs with current evidence-informed practice guidelines. These computerized systems help to synthesize large volumes of research into a format that is accessible to nurses and other health care providers and presents it in a format that aids in decision-making at the point of care (Djulbegovic & Guyatt, 2017). The 6S model is a tool that can help guide your search for the strongest and most relevant evidence-informed information; however, it does not replace the importance of critically reading each piece of evidence

and assessing its quality and applicability for current practice.

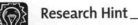 **Research Hint** _____

Google Scholar should generally not be used for your initial literature searches as it is not discipline specific and does not have the advanced filtering functions of academic databases like CINAHL. It can be useful for other purposes. If you have one particularly good article on your topic, you can see if that article has been "cited by" other authors more recently. This is called descendant searching and, along with ancestry searching, is a method to find literature that might have been missed in your original search. This is a particularly important strategy if you are trying to find all the literature on a topic and helps to position the research chronologically within a body of knowledge.

Step 3: Conduct your Search

The goal of this step is to acquire several resources to answer your question using the databases and the keywords that you generated previously. You

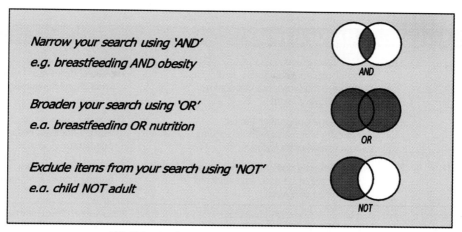

Narrow your search using 'AND'
e.g. breastfeeding AND obesity

AND

Broaden your search using 'OR'
e.g. breastfeeding OR nutrition

OR

Exclude items from your search using 'NOT'
e.g. child NOT adult

NOT

FIG. 5.3   Boolean operators: Combining keywords

can do this yourself, or with the help of a librarian. You want your search to be broad enough to ensure you do not overlook relevant sources, but it also needs to be specific enough that you are not too overwhelmed with articles that are not relevant. There are several tools available in the databases that will help you to refine your search and focus on the most relevant articles. These are Boolean operators, wild cards, and filters.

Boolean operators dictate the relationship between words and concepts; "AND," "OR," "NOT" are Boolean operators. "AND" requires that both concepts be located within the results that are returned; "OR" allows you to group together like terms or synonyms; and "NOT" eliminates terms from your search (see Figure 5.3). As noted, you have the option of a search using the controlled vocabulary of CINAHL or a keyword search. If you wanted to locate articles about maternal–fetal attachment as they relate to the health practices or health behaviours of low-income mothers, you would first want to construct your PICOT:

P: Maternal–fetal attachment in low-income mothers (specifically defined group)
I: Health behaviours or health practices (event to be studied)
C: None (comparison intervention)

O: Neonatal outcomes (outcome)
T: 2010–2020

In this example, the two main concepts are maternal–fetal attachment and health practices and how these impact neonatal outcomes. Many times when conducting a search, you only enter in keywords or controlled vocabulary for the first two elements of your PICOT—in this case, maternal–fetal attachment and health practices or behaviours. The other elements can be added if your list of results is overwhelming, but often you can pick from the results you have by just combining the first two.

Maternal–fetal attachment should be part of your search as a keyword search, but "prenatal bonding" is the appropriate CINAHL subject heading. To be comprehensive, you should use "OR" to link these terms together. The second concept, health practices OR health behaviours, is accomplished in a similar manner. The subject heading or controlled vocabulary assigned by the indexers could be added in for completeness.

Note that these two concepts are connected with the Boolean operator, which defines the relationships between words or groups of words in your literature search. To restrict our retrieval to research, the "Research Article" limit has been applied. Searching is an iterative process and takes some

TABLE **5.3**		
WILD CARD SYMBOLS FOR DATABASE SEARCHES		
SYMBOL	**FUNCTION**	**EXAMPLE**
Asterisk (*)	Matches multiple characters, usually at the end of a word, but can also be used within a word.	The search term *nurs** will include findings: *nurse, nursing, nurses*
Hash (#)	Matches one optional character, typically when an alternate spelling contains an extra letter.	The search term *p#ediatric* will include findings: *pediatric* and *paediatric*
Question mark (?)	Matches exactly one character within a word, cannot be used as a wildcard at the end of a word.	The search term *ne?t* will include findings: *next, nest, neat*.

Source: Adapted from EBSCO Connect (June 26, 2019). *Searching with Wildcards in EDS and EBSCOhost.* https://connect.ebsco.com/s/article/Searching-with-Wildcards-in-EDS-and-EBSCOhost?language=en_US

trial and error to use the correct terms to locate the articles you will find useful for your search question.

Wild cards are another important search tool. These symbols indicate specific search instructions to the database. See Table 5.3 for descriptions and examples of wild cards. Keep in mind both Boolean operators and wild cards may work differently in different databases, so be sure to check how they function in the database you are using.

A final important tool to help with searching are **filters** or limiters. These filters include or exclude based on certain features. Check with your librarian to see how these filters may affect your search. If you have too many articles these can be helpful; if you have too few you will have to remove some of these search filters. Some common filters include:

- *Year of publication.* For an evidence-informed practice project, you may want to limit the search to the last 5 years. For a class assignment, your instructor may set parameters on how recent the literature is.
- *Language.* It can be helpful to restrict the articles to those that you can read, so select languages that you are fluent in. English is the dominant language in scientific publication, allowing for a common language for communication (Di Bitetti & Ferreras, 2017) although there are nursing articles published in other languages as well.

- *Full text.* This is not a recommended filter and needs to be used cautiously. While it may seem efficient to limit your search to full text articles, it may result in you missing important and easily accessible resources. This filter limits findings to those directly housed in the database and may not reflect all the full-text resources that your library has (Spurlock, 2019).
- *Age.* This filter will restrict findings based on age of the participants in the study. This does not always filter perfectly but can be helpful when you are looking specifically at an age-related topic such as with pediatric or geriatric populations.
- *Scholarly (Peer Reviewed) Journals.* This can be useful if it is a requirement of your assignment, but the articles retrieved still need to be assessed to determine if they were peer-reviewed and if they are of good quality.

Research Hint

Look for useful tools within the search interfaces of online databases to make your searching more efficient. For example, when you search for a particular age group, use the built-in limits of the database instead of relying on a keyword search. Other shortcuts include the "Clinical Queries" in CINAHL and MEDLINE that retrieve articles about therapy or diagnosis.

Each online database explains each feature; it is worth your time to click on each icon and explore the explanations offered because this will increase your confidence. Also keep in mind the types of articles you are retrieving. Many online resources allow you to limit your search to randomized controlled trials or systematic reviews. In CINAHL, there is a limit for "Research" that will restrict the number of citations you retrieve to research articles.

A general timeline for most academic or evidence-informed practice papers and projects is to go back in the literature at least 3 years, but preferably 5 years, although some research projects may warrant going back 10 years or more until the researcher is satisfied that he or she has found literature that accurately represents the body of knowledge. In some cases, influential or ground-breaking research in the field should be reviewed regardless of publication date. This is particularly relevant if you are trying to locate the primary source of an idea. For example, conducting a literature review on the effects of stress would not be complete without reading Hans Selye's (1955) pioneering work on stress.

Research Hint
Reading systematic reviews, if they are available, on your clinical question or topic will enhance your ability to implement evidence-informed nursing practice because they generally offer the strongest and most consistent level of evidence. If you come across a systematic review on your specific clinical topic, scan it to see what years the review covers; then begin your search from the last year to the present.

Step 4: Refine Search Results

Most searches with electronic databases include not only citation information but also the abstract of the article and options for obtaining the full text. Reading the abstract is critical for determining whether you need to retrieve the full text of an article. Keep your initial question handy as you review the abstracts, to ensure you stay focused on your topic.

As you scroll through and mark the citations you wish to include, make sure you include all relevant fields when you save or print the publications. If you are writing a paper and need to produce a

bibliography, you can export your citations to citation management software, which is a software program that formats and stores your citations so that they are available for electronic retrieval when they must be inserted in a paper you are writing. Quite a few of these programs are available; some, such as Zotero and Mendeley are free, and others, including EndNote and RefWorks, must be purchased, by either you or your institution. Microsoft Word also has a reference tab that allows you to manage your citations and references. It may also be worthwhile to create an account in CINAHL so that you can save your searches and organize the articles you wish to keep.

Do not be discouraged if not all the retrieved articles are as useful as you first thought; this happens with the most experienced reviewers of literature. If most of the articles are not useful, be prepared to perform another search, but discuss your keyword selection and your database selection with your instructor or the reference librarian first. You may want to add a third database. In the previous example of a search to locate articles on maternal–fetal attachment, the third database of choice may be PsycINFO (see Box 5.2).

Research Hint
- Take the time to set up your computer for electronic library access.
- If the full text of an article is unavailable through your electronic search, read the abstract to determine whether you want to order the article through interlibrary loan.
- Sign up for a free reference manager software program, such as Zotero or Mendeley, to help you track, organize, and manage your literature searches.
- Keep track of the search terms that you use. Some search engines have options for you to save your searches, including the terms used.

Step 5: Select Literature

Once you have reviewed the abstracts and selected the articles you wish to keep, you need to retrieve the full text and either print or download the full articles. Now the truly important aspect of your searching begins: your critical reading of the retrieved materials. Critically reading scholarly material, especially research articles, requires several readings and the use of critiquing criteria (as discussed in Chapter 3). A preliminary reading of the full article may result in further discarding articles that are not relevant for your topic.

Research Hint_____

Read the abstract carefully to determine whether the article is about research. Next, you may want to locate the research question or purpose, as this will help to clarify what the article is about. It is also a good idea to review the references of the articles; if any seem relevant, you can retrieve them.

A major portion of most literature reviews—whether for evidence-informed practice projects, class assignments, or research articles—consists of journal articles. In contrast to books and textbooks, which take much longer to publish, journals are a ready source of up-to-date information on almost any subject. Therefore, journals are the preferred mode of communicating the most recent theory or results of a research study. For you as a beginning research user, **refereed journals** should be your first choice when looking for theoretical, clinical, or research articles. Most refereed journals are available in print and accessible electronically through your library's online resources.

Evidence-Informed Practice Tip _____

You may wish to sort the research articles you retrieve according to the model of levels of evidence in Chapter 3. For questions about treatment effectiveness, the hierarchy of evidence is a helpful tool. More broadly, Aveyard (2014) suggests sorting the literature you find according to your levels of evidence—in other words, which evidence is most suited to answer your clinical practice question? You can then decide on including only those articles that provide the best evidence for your question.

Step 6: Critically Read, Summarize, and Synthesize

Once you have your materials down to only relevant articles, you will need to review each article and assess it for quality. The studies selected for the literature review for your practice project, or for your class assignment, should offer the best and most appropriate evidence available on the topic. You will likely read the articles several times during this process, as described in the steps of critical appraisal in Chapter 3. A table or extraction tool can help you to organize the information you read in each article and ensure you are looking for the same details across the articles (Wakefield, 2014). You may choose to extract information such as location of the research, participants, type of intervention, measurement tools/instruments used, themes found, outcomes, and a general summary. You may also wish to include the major critiques of the article—whether these are strengths or limitations. See Table 5.4 for an example extraction tool.

Extraction tools also help you to notice similarities and differences across the studies you have included—this is helpful in moving from describing and summarizing individual articles to synthesizing the findings from several articles (Wakefield, 2014). Wakefield offered several tips for moving from summarizing individual articles to synthesizing several articles:

- Search for patterns, words or phrases that occur across multiple articles.
- Consider what the collective group of authors have written about from a variety of viewpoints.
- Highlight areas of agreements between the articles—this gives you support for evidence-based conclusions.
- Think critically about differences between articles: Do newer articles represent different ideas and a shift in thinking? Are differences the result of flawed study design, or misinterpreted evidence?

Research Hint_____

- Use standardized critical appraisal criteria to evaluate your research articles.
- Make a table to represent the components of your topic and fill in your evaluation to help you see the "big picture" of your analysis.
- Synthesize the results of your analysis to try to determine what was similar or different among and between these studies in relation to your topic or clinical question, and then draw a conclusion.

TABLE **5.4**					
SAMPLE EXTRACTION TABLE					
Full reference for article, including publication date	Population targeted and number of participants	Intervention or area of interest	Study method used by author/ authors	Summary of the findings	Similarities and differences between other studies

Source: Wakefield (2014). Searching and critiquing the research literature. *Nursing Standard, 28*(39), 49–57. https:// doi.10.7748/ns.28.39.49.e8867.

Step 7: Formatting the Literature Review

Familiarity with the format and process of the literature review will help you to critically appraise the literature used in a research report. Literature reviews should be written in a logical and organized manner. Typically the findings of a literature review are presented chronologically, thematically, or methodologically (Wakefield, 2014) and will be influenced by the following:

- The research or clinical question or topic
- The number of retrieved sources reviewed
- The number and type of research materials versus conceptual materials

Some reviews are written according to the variables being studied and presented chronologically in the discussion of each variable. In others, the entire material is presented chronologically, and subcategories or variables are discussed within each time period. In still others, the variables are presented, and the subcategories are related to the study's type or designs or related variables. Review the literature reviews in Appendices A–D to appreciate the different styles.

An example of how literature is incorporated into a research article (Figure 5.1) is seen in Appendix D. Goldsworthy et al. (2019) provide a section at the beginning of their article titled "Literature Review." They also provide a review of how knowledge and skills of students are assessed, particularly in relation to simulation in a section titled "Knowledge and Skills Measurement." They have listed several studies together that have consistent findings:

The investigators found significant increases in student nurses' knowledge, skills performance, confidence, and perception of team work following simulation experiences (Buckley & Gordon, 2011; Cooper et al., 2015a, b; Davies, Nathan, & Clarke, 2012; Goldsworthy et al., 2019, p. 26; Kelly et al., 2014; Liaw, Zhou, Lau, Siau, & Chan, 2014). (p. 26)

In the "Theoretical Framework" section, they have not only reviewed literature related to self-efficacy but also cited other articles that used this theory for simulation studies with nursing students. Lastly, in the "Discussion" section, Goldsworthy et al. (2019) refer back to literature that they cited at the beginning of the paper indicating that their study conforms with previous research.

Researchers always compare the literature review with their findings. In some cases, the reviewed literature is used during the analysis process as well. In a study on medical assistance in dying, Pesut et al. (2020; Appendix A) discovered wide variation in practices across Canada. After the analysis, Pesut et al. looked at literature that would help to explain and discuss their findings—for example, the design of health authorities allows for flexibility in providing services to a specific population but also allows for variance across populations.

Research Hint _____

If you are writing a literature review for an assignment, include enough information so that your professor or fellow students could re-create your search path and come up with the same results. This means specifying the databases searched, the date you searched, years of coverage, terms used, and any limits or restrictions that you used.

APPRAISING THE EVIDENCE

Review of the Literature

Whether you are a researcher writing the literature review for the research study you are planning to conduct or a nurse writing a literature review for an evidence-informed practice project, you need to critically appraise individual research reports by using appropriate criteria. If you are appraising an individual research study that is to be included in a literature review, it must be evaluated in terms of critical appraisal criteria that are related to each step of the research process so that the strengths and weaknesses of each study can be identified. Standardized critical appraisal tools (e.g., Critical Appraisal Skills Programme [CASP] Tools and Appraisal of Guidelines for Research and Evaluation [AGREE] Guidelines) available for specific types of research designs (e.g., clinical trials, cohort studies, systematic reviews) can also be used to critically appraise an individual research study.

Critiquing the literature review of research or conceptual reports is a challenging task for seasoned consumers of research, so do not be surprised if you feel a little intimidated by the prospect of critiquing the published research. The important issue is to determine the overall value of the literature review, including both the research and theoretical materials. The purposes of a literature review (see Box 5.1) and the characteristics of a well-written literature review (Box 5.3) provide the framework for developing the evaluation criteria for a literature review.

The literature review should be presented in an organized manner. The theoretical and research literature can be presented chronologically from earliest studies to most recent; sometimes the theoretical literature that provided the foundation for the existing research is presented first, followed by the research studies that were derived from this theoretical base. Other times, the literature can be clustered by concept, grouped according to supportive or nonsupportive positions, or categorized by evidence that highlights differences in theoretical and/or research findings. The overall question to be answered is "Does the review of the literature develop and present a knowledge base that builds on previous research, identifies a conflict or gap in the literature, or proposes to extend the current knowledge base?" (see Box 5.1).

Regardless of how the literature review is organized, it should provide a strong knowledge base for carrying out the research, educational, or clinical practice project.

Questions related to the logical organization and presentation of the reviewed studies are somewhat more challenging for beginning research consumers. The more you read research studies, the more competent you will become at differentiating a well-organized literature review from one that has no organizing framework.

Whenever possible, read both qualitative (metasyntheses) and quantitative (meta-analyses) systematic reviews that pertain to a clinical question. Systematic reviews represent a synthesis of studies and they often represent the best available evidence on a particular clinical issue. An example of a systematic review is provided in Appendix E. In another example, Singh et al. (2017) conducted a quantitative systematic review in which they critically appraised and synthesized the evidence from research studies related to the psychological impact of rapid diagnostic centres for women related to breast cancer. After retrieving 846 studies, screening, and subsequently synthesizing 6 studies, Singh et al. concluded that "all of the studies in the review, regardless of measures used, found significantly lower anxiety levels in women who received their results on the same day in the short-term." (p. 353). In the article "Factors Associated with Pain Assessment for Nursing Home Residents: A Systematic Review and Meta-Synthesis" Knopp-Sihota et al. (2019) gathered 31 primary qualitative studies on barriers and facilitators to pain assessment in nursing home residents. After synthesizing the studies, Knopp-Sihota et al. reported "that cognitive impairment was the most common barrier to pain assessment at the nursing home resident level" (p. 890).

The Critiquing Criteria box summarizes general critiquing criteria for a review of the literature. Two broad questions to start with are: "Does the literature search seem accurate?" and "Does the report demonstrate scholarly writing?" The first place to begin is to determine whether the source is a refereed journal. It is reasonable to assume that the manuscripts published in a scholarly refereed journal are adequately referenced, are based mainly on primary sources, and are written in a scholarly manner. This does not mean, however, that every study reported in a refereed journal meets all the critiquing criteria for a literature review and other components of the study in an equal manner. Because of style differences and space constraints,

APPRAISING THE EVIDENCE—*cont'd*

Review of the Literature

each citation summarized is often very brief, or related citations may be summarized as a group and lack a critique.

The key to a strong literature review is a careful search of the published and unpublished literature. Whether you write or critically appraise a literature review written for a published research study, it should reflect a synthesis or compilation of the main points or value of all of the sources reviewed in relation to the study's research question or hypothesis (see Box 5.1). The relationship between and among these studies must be explained. The synthesis of a written review of the literature usually appears at the end of the review section before the section about the research question or hypothesis.

Searching the literature, like critiquing the literature, is an acquired skill. Practising your search and critical appraisal skills on a regular basis will make a huge difference. Seeking guidance from faculty is essential for developing critical appraisal skills. Synthesizing the body of literature you have critiqued is even more challenging but will help you apply new knowledge to practice.

CRITIQUING CRITERIA

1. Are all the relevant concepts and variables included in the review?
2. Does the search strategy include an appropriate and adequate number of databases and other resources to identify key published and unpublished research and theoretical sources?
3. Are both theoretical literature and research literature included?
4. Does an appropriate theoretical or conceptual framework guide the development of the research study?
5. Are mainly primary sources used?
6. What gaps or inconsistencies in knowledge does the literature review uncover?
7. Does the literature review build on the findings of earlier studies?
8. Does the summary of each reviewed study reflect the essential components of the study design (e.g., type and size of sample, reliability and validity of instruments, consistency of data-collection procedures, appropriate data analysis, identification of limitations)?
9. Does the critique of each reviewed study mention strengths, weaknesses, or limitations of the design; conflicts; and gaps in information related to the area of interest?
10. Does the synthesis summary follow a logical sequence in which the overall strengths and weaknesses of the reviewed studies are presented and a logical conclusion is established?
11. Is the literature review presented in an organized format that flows logically (e.g., chronologically, clustered by concept or variables), enhancing the reader's ability to evaluate the need for the particular research study or evidence-informed practice project?
12. Does the literature review follow the proposed purpose of the research study or evidence-informed practice project?
13. Does the literature review generate research questions or hypotheses or answer a clinical question?

BOX 5.3

CHARACTERISTICS OF A WELL-WRITTEN REVIEW OF THE LITERATURE

Each reviewed source of information reflects critical thinking and scholarly writing and is relevant to the study, topic, or project, and the content satisfies the following criteria:

- The literature review is organized in a systematic approach.
- Each research or conceptual article is summarized succinctly and with appropriate references.
- Established critical appraisal criteria are used for specific study designs to evaluate the study for strengths, weaknesses, or limitations, as well as for conflicts or gaps in information that relate directly or indirectly to the area of interest.

- Evidence of a synthesis of the critiques is provided to highlight the overall strengths and weaknesses of the studies reviewed.
- The review consists of mainly primary sources; there are a sufficient number of research sources.
- The review concludes with a synthesis of the reviewed material that reflects why the study or project should be implemented.
- Research questions and hypotheses are identified, or clinical questions are answered.

CRITICAL THINKING CHALLENGES

■ Using the PICOT format, generate a clinical question related to health promotion for children in elementary school.

■ How does a research article's theoretical or conceptual framework interrelate concepts, theories, conceptual definitions, and operational definitions?

■ A general guideline for a literature search is to use a timeline of 3 to 5 years. When would a nurse researcher need to search beyond this timeline?

■ What is the relationship of the research article's literature review to the theoretical or conceptual framework?

CRITICAL JUDGEMENT QUESTIONS

1. What is an appropriate reason to use a secondary source?

   a. The original article is not freely available
   b. The primary source is written in a language you do not know
   c. The source was originally published in a print journal
   d. The primary article is older than 5 years

2. When retrieving evidence to answer a clinical practice question, what is the most useful resource?

   a. A high-quality single study
   b. A systematic review
   c. A series of single studies
   d. Computerized decision support tools

3. Which of the following sections in a research article can help you quickly decide if a research article is relevant for your purposes?

   a. The abstract and the conclusion
   b. The title and the method
   c. The abstract and the purpose statement
   d. The title and the findings

KEY POINTS

• The review of the literature is defined as a broad, comprehensive, in-depth, systematic critique and synthesis of scholarly publications, unpublished scholarly print and online materials, audiovisual materials, and personal communications.

• The review of the literature is used for development of research studies, as well as other activities for consumers of research, such as development of evidence-informed practice projects.

• With regard to conducting and writing a literature review, the main objectives for the consumer of research are to acquire the abilities to accomplish the following: (1) conduct an appropriate search of electronic or print research on a topic; (2) efficiently retrieve a sufficient amount of materials for a literature review in relation to the topic and scope of project; (3) critically appraise (i.e., critique) research and theoretical material in accordance with accepted critiquing criteria; (4) critically evaluate published reviews of the literature in accordance with accepted standardized critiquing criteria; (5) synthesize the findings of the critiqued materials for relevance to the purpose of the selected scholarly project; and (6) determine applicability of the findings to practice.

• Primary research and theoretical resources are essential for literature reviews.

• The use of secondary sources, such as commentaries on research articles from peer-reviewed journals, is part of a learning strategy for developing critical critiquing skills.

• It is more efficient to use electronic rather than print databases for retrieving scholarly materials.

• Strategies for efficiently retrieving scholarly nursing literature include consulting the reference librarian and using at least two online sources (e.g., CINAHL and MEDLINE).

• Literature reviews are usually organized according to variables, as well as chronologically.

- Critiquing and synthesizing a number of research articles, including systematic reviews, are essential for implementing evidence-informed nursing practice.

FOR FURTHER STUDY

Go to Evolve at http://evolve.elsevier.com/Canada/LoBiondo/Research for the Audio Glossary.

REFERENCES

American Psychological Association. (n.d.). PsycINFO. Retrieved from http://www.apa.org/pubs/databases/psycinfo/index.aspx.

American Psychological Association. (2019). *Publication Manual of the American Psychological Association.* Washington, DC: American Psychological Association.

Aveyard, H. (2014). *Doing a literature review in health and social care: A practical guide.* New York: McGraw-Hill Education.

Averyard, H., Sharp, P., & Woolliams, M. (2015). *A beginner's guide to critical thinking and writing in health and social care* (2nd ed.). Maidenhead, Berkshire, UK: Open University Press.

Cooke, A., Smith, D., & Booth, A. (2012). Beyond PICO: The SPIDER tool for qualitative evidence synthesis. *Qualitative Health Research, 22*(10), 1435–1443.

Di Bitetti, M. S., & Ferreras, J. A. (2017). Publish (in English) or perish: The effect on citation rate of using languages other than English in scientific publications. *Ambio, 46*(1), 121–127. https://doi.org/10.1007/s13280-016-0820-7.

DiCenso, A., Bayley, L., & Haynes, R. B. (2009). Accessing pre-appraised evidence: Fine-tuning the 5S model into a 6S model. *Evidence Based Nursing, 12*(4), 99–101. http://dx.doi.org/10.1136/ebn.12.4.99-b.

Djulbegovic, B., & Guyatt, G. H. (2017). Progress in evidence-based medicine: A quarter century on. *The Lancet, 390*(10092), 415–423. https://doi.org/10.1016/S0140-6736(16)31592-6.

EBSCO Connect (June 26, 2019). Searching with Wildcards in EDS and EBSCOhost. https://connect.ebsco.com/s/article/Searching-with-Wildcards-in-EDS-and-EBSCOhost?language=en_US.

Goldsworthy, S., Patterson, J. D., Dobbs, M., Afzal, A., & Deboer, S. (2019). How does simulation impact building competency and confidence in recognition and response to the adult and paediatric deteriorating patient among undergraduate nursing students? *Clinical Simulation in Nursing, 28*, 25–32. https://doi.org/10.1016/j.ecns.2018.12.001.

Knopp-Sihota, J. A., Dirk, K. L., & Rachor, G. S. (2019). Factors associated with pain assessment for nursing home residents: A systematic review and meta-synthesis. *Journal of the American Medical Directors Association, 20*(7), 884–892. https://0-doi-org.aupac.lib.athabasPcau.ca/10.1016/j.jamda.2019.01.156.

Pesut, B., Thorne, S., Schiller, C. J., Greig, M., & Roussel, J. (2020). The rocks and hard places of MAiD: A qualitative study of nursing practice in the context of legislated assisted death. *BMC Nursing, 19*(1), 1–14. https://doi.org/10.1186/s12912-020-0404-5.

ProQuest. (n.d.). ProQuest dissertations and theses global: Fast facts. Retrieved from http://www.proquest.com/products-services/pqdtglobal.html.

Purnell, M., Royal, B., & Warton, L. (2020). Supporting the development of information literacy skills and knowledge in undergraduate nursing students: An integrative review. *Nurse Education Today, 95*, Article 104585. https://doi.org/10.1016/j.nedt.2020.104585.

Selye, H. (1955). Stress and disease. *Science, 122*, 625–631.

Singh, M., Maheu, C., Brady, T., & Farah, R. (2017). The psychological impact of the rapid diagnostic centres in cancer screening: A systematic review. *Canadian Oncology Nursing Journal, 27*(4), 348–364. https://0-doi-org.aupac.lib.athabascau.ca/10.5737/23688076274348355.

Spurlock, D. (2019). Searching the literature in preparation for research: Strategies that matter. *Journal of Nursing Education, 58*(8), 441–443. https://doi.org/10.3928/01484834-20190719-02.

Turning Research into Practice [Trip]. (2016). What is Trip? Retrieved from http://www.tripdatabase.com/about.

Wakefield, A. (2014). Searching and critiquing the research literature. *Nursing Standard, 28*(39), 49–57. https://doi.10.7748/ns.28.39.49.e8867.

CHAPTER 6

Legal and Ethical Issues

Mina D. Singh | Ramesh Venkatesa Perumal

LEARNING OUTCOMES

After reading this chapter, you will be able to do the following:

- Describe the historical background that led to the development of ethical guidelines for the use of human participants in research.
- Identify the essential elements of an informed consent form.
- Evaluate the adequacy of an informed consent form.
- Describe the role of the research ethics board in the research review process.
- Identify populations of participants who require special legal and ethical research considerations.
- Appreciate the nurse researcher's obligations to conduct and report research in an ethical manner.
- Describe the nurse's role as patient advocate in research situations.
- Discuss the nurse's role in ensuring that Health Canada guidelines for testing of medical devices are followed.
- Discuss animal rights in research situations.
- Critique the ethical aspects of a research study.

KEY TERMS

animal rights
anonymity
assent
beneficence
benefits
confidentiality

consent
ethics
informed consent
justice
process consent
product testing

research ethics board (REB)
respect for persons
risk–benefit ratio
risks

STUDY RESOURCES

 Go to Evolve at http://evolve.elsevier.com/Canada/LoBiondo/Research for the Audio Glossary.

NURSES ARE IN AN IDEAL POSITION to promote the public's awareness of the role played by research in the advancement of science and improvement in patient care. In Canada, the professional code of ethics (Canadian Nurses Association [CNA], 2017) outlines the ethical standards for practice, which can include research and patients' rights with regard to research. Not only do the standards represent rules and regulations regarding practice, but when research becomes the domain of a nurse, these standards can be applied to the participation of human research participants to ensure that nursing research is conducted legally and ethically. The Code states that nurses must strive to uphold human rights and call attention to any violations of these rights. The Code of Ethics for Registered Nurses, originally published in 1985, was revised in 2008 and 2017. The revised 2017 CNA code includes new content addressing medical assistance in dying and advocating for quality work environments that support the delivery of safe, compassionate, competent and ethical care. There are seven primary values within this Code. Under the first value of Providing Safe, Compassionate, Competent and Ethical Care, there are ethical responsibilities related to research (p. 8) These responsibilities also translate to patients' or participants' rights in research around "informed consent, the risk-benefit balance, the privacy and confidentiality of data and the monitoring of research" (p. 9). Nurses need to be advocates in this context to ensure that ethical concepts in nursing research are upheld.

Researchers and caregivers of patients who are research participants must be fully committed to the tenets of informed consent and patients' rights. The principle "the ends justify the means" must never be tolerated. Researchers and caregivers of research participants must take every precaution to protect the people being studied from physical or mental harm or discomfort (although it is not always clear what constitutes harm or discomfort).

The focus of this chapter is on the legal and ethical considerations that need to be addressed before, during, and after the conducting of research to ensure that the research does not harm the patient. Informed consent, research ethics boards (REBs), and research involving vulnerable populations—older adults, pregnant women, children, prisoners, Indigenous people, and persons with acquired immune deficiency syndrome (AIDS) or other serious illnesses, as well as animals—are discussed. The nurse's role as patient advocate, whether functioning as researcher, caregiver, or research consumer, is addressed.

ETHICAL AND LEGAL CONSIDERATIONS IN RESEARCH: A HISTORICAL PERSPECTIVE

Past Ethical Dilemmas in Research

Ethical and legal considerations regarding medical research first arose in the United States and received focused attention after World War II. Lawyers defending war criminals intended to justify the atrocities committed by Nazi physicians by claiming their actions were in the name of "medical research." On learning of this defense, the U.S. Secretary of State and the Secretary of War asked the American Medical Association to appoint a group to develop a code of ethics for research to serve as a standard for judging the medical experiments committed by physicians on concentration camp prisoners.

The Code of Ethics, developed as 10 rules, became known as the Nuremberg Code (Box 6.1). The Nuremberg Code's definitions of the terms voluntary, legal capacity, sufficient understanding, and enlightened decision have been the subject of numerous court cases and U.S. presidential commissions involved in setting ethical standards in research (Amdur & Bankert, 2011). The Code that was developed requires informed consent in all cases but makes no provisions for any special treatment of children, older adults, or people who are mentally incompetent. Several other international standards have followed; the most notable is the Declaration of Helsinki, adopted in 1964 by the World Medical Assembly and revised in 1975 (Levine, 1979).

The research heritage in the United States and Canada is well documented and is used here to illustrate the human consequences of not adhering to ethical standards when conducting research. Some examples are highlighted in Table 6.1 and incorporated into Table 6.2 to show the violation of human rights that occurred in these studies.

ARTICLES OF THE NUREMBERG CODE

1. The voluntary consent of the human subject is absolutely essential.
2. The study should be conducted so as to yield fruitful results for the good of society, unprocurable by other means of study, and not random and unnecessary in nature.
3. The experiment should be so designed and based on the results of animal experimentation and knowledge of the natural history of the disease or other problems under study that the anticipated results will justify the performance of the experiment.
4. The experiment should be conducted to avoid all unnecessary physical and mental suffering and injury.
5. No experiment should be conducted where there is an a priori reason to believe that death or disabling injury will occur.
6. The degree of risk to be taken should never exceed that determined by the humanitarian importance of the problem to be solved by the experiment.

7. Proper preparations should be made and adequate facilities provided to protect the subject against even remote possibilities of injury, disability, or death.
8. The experiment should be conducted only by scientifically qualified persons.
9. The human subject should be at liberty to bring the experiment to an end.
10. During the course of the experiment the scientist in charge must be prepared to terminate the experiment at any stage, if he [or she] has probable cause to believe . . . that a continuation of the experiment is likely to result in injury, disability, or death to the experimental subject.

From United States Government Printing Office. (2008). The medical case. In *Trials of war criminals before the Nuremberg Military Tribunals under Control Council Law No. 10* (Vol. 2, pp. 3–31). Washington, DC: Author, 1949. Retrieved from http://www.loc.gov /rr/frd/Military_Law/pdf/NT_war-criminals_Vol-II.pdf.

In the United States, under the National Research Act of 1974 (Public Law 93-348), the National Commission for the Protection of Human Subjects of Biomedical and Behavioral Research was created. A major charge of the commission was to identify the basic principles that should underlie the conduct of biomedical and behavioural research involving human participants and to develop guidelines to ensure that research is conducted in accordance with those principles (Levine, 1986). Three ethical principles (Box 6.2) were identified as relevant to the conduct of research involving human participants:

- **respect for persons** (the idea that people have the freedom to participate or not participate in research),
- **beneficence** (the obligation to do no harm and maximize possible benefits), and
- **justice** (the principle that human subjects should be treated fairly).

These three principles have formed the basis of many ethical guidelines in Canada.

In Canada, for the protection of human participants in all types of research, Health Canada has adopted the Good Clinical Practice: Consolidated Guidelines (Health Canada, 2019). There are also guideline documents related to "Drugs for Clinical Trials involving Human Subjects" (https://www. canada.ca/en/health-canada/services/drugs-health-products/compliance-enforcement/good-clinical-practices/guidance-documents.html).

The collaboration of the three major funding agencies—the Canadian Institutes of Health Research (CIHR), the Natural Sciences and Engineering Research Council of Canada (NSERC), and the Social Sciences and Humanities Research Council of Canada (SSHRC)—has led to a joint statement for the protection of human participants. The revision of this document, the Tri-Council Policy Statement: Ethical Conduct for Research Involving Humans (CIHR et al., 2018), offers a more inclusive approach to delineating current trends in ethical issues. This revised document, sometimes called the Tri-Council Policy Statement-2, is henceforth referred to as TCPS 2.

Respect for human dignity is articulated through the three core principles "Respect for Persons," "Concern for Welfare," and "Justice" (CIHR et al., 2018, p.6). Respect for Persons "incorporates the dual moral obligations to respect

TABLE **6.1**

HIGHLIGHTS OF UNETHICAL RESEARCH STUDIES CONDUCTED IN THE UNITED STATES AND CANADA

RESEARCH STUDY	DATE OF STUDY	FOCUS OF STUDY	ETHICAL PRINCIPLE VIOLATED
Series of nutrition studies on First Nations communities in northern Manitoba and residential schools across Canada. (See Mosby, 2013.)	1942–1952	Experiments with vitamin supplements/fortified foods and food policy in malnourished populations. All participants in control and intervention groups were fed diets known to be nutritionally inadequate.	There was no informed consent or likely even knowledge of being involved in a study. The prevailing belief at the time was that "Indians" would not understand the research and it should not be explained to them (Mosby, 2013). A 5 year experiment included use of children at residential schools, as wards of the state, without consent or assent. Children were denied access to usual care (i.e., dental services) so researchers could better study the effects of malnutrition. The study continued despite worsening levels of anemia.
Tuskegee syphilis study, Tuskegee, Alabama	1932–1973	For 40 years, the U.S. Public Health Service conducted a study using two groups of poor Black male sharecroppers. One group consisted of men with untreated syphilis; the other group was judged to be free of the disease. Treatment was withheld from the group with syphilis even after penicillin became generally available and accepted as effective treatment for syphilis in the 1950s. Steps were even taken to prevent the research participants from obtaining penicillin. The researcher wanted to study the untreated disease.	Many of the research participants who consented to participate in the study were not informed about the purpose and procedures of the research. Others were unaware that they were participants. The degree of risk outweighed the potential benefit. Withholding of known effective treatment violates the participants' right to fair treatment and protection from harm (Levine, 1986).
Sterilization experiments in Auschwitz concentration camp, Germany	1940–1944	Sterilization experiments	Basic human rights and rights to fair and ethical treatment were violated, and the research participants did not give informed consent. Nurses who were prisoners were forced to participate in the experiments, which was against their prima facie duty to protect (Benedict & Georges, 2006).

Continued

TABLE **6.1**

HIGHLIGHTS OF UNETHICAL RESEARCH STUDIES CONDUCTED IN THE UNITED STATES AND CANADA—cont'd			
RESEARCH STUDY	**DATE OF STUDY**	**FOCUS OF STUDY**	**ETHICAL PRINCIPLE VIOLATED**
Dr. Ewen Cameron's psychiatric experiments, Allan Memorial Psychiatric Institute, Montreal, Quebec	1950s–1960s	The U.S. Central Intelligence Agency (CIA) funded psychic driving, or brain-washing, experiments on patients with psychiatric illnesses (Collins, 1988, as cited in Charron, 2000). Psychic driving is a psychiatric procedure pioneered by Dr. Cameron in which electroconvulsive therapy (ECT) and psychedelic drugs, such as lysergic acid (LSD), are used in an attempt at mind control. To develop the psychic driving, increasingly higher levels of ECT were applied to patients as often as three times a day. This treatment would continue for 30 days. Considerable damage was done to patients after such severe treatment. Patients were unable to walk or feed themselves and were incontinent (Gillmor, 1987, as cited in Charron, 2000).	The ethical principles of respect for persons and beneficence were severely violated. Dr. Cameron used patients with diminished autonomy (patients with psychiatric illnesses), even though, as a physician, he was obliged to protect them. The ECT treatments did more harm than good.
Hyman v. Jewish Chronic Disease Hospital, Jewish Chronic Disease study, New York City	1965	Doctors injected aged, senile patients with cancer cells to study the patients' response to injection of the cells.	Informed consent was not obtained, and no indication was given that the study had been reviewed and approved by an ethics committee. The two physicians involved claimed that they did not wish to evoke emotional reactions or New York City refusals to participate by informing the research participants of the nature of the study (Hershey & Miller, 1976).
Milledgeville, Georgia study	1969	Researchers administered investigational drugs to mentally disabled children without first obtaining the opinion of a psychiatrist.	The study protocol or institutional approval of the program was not reviewed before implementation (Levine, 1986).
San Antonio contraceptive study, San Antonio, Texas	1969	In a study of the adverse effects of oral contraceptives, 76 impoverished Mexican American women were randomly assigned to an experimental group receiving birth control pills or a control group receiving placebos. Research participants were not informed about the placebo and the attendant risk of pregnancy. Of the participants, 11 became pregnant; 10 of these women were in the placebo control group.	Principles of informed consent were violated; full disclosure of the potential risk, harm, results, and adverse effects was not evident in the informed consent document. The potential risk outweighed the benefits of the study. The participants' right to fair treatment and protection from harm was violated (Levine, 1986).

TABLE **6.1**			
HIGHLIGHTS OF UNETHICAL RESEARCH STUDIES CONDUCTED IN THE UNITED STATES AND CANADA—cont'd			
RESEARCH STUDY	**DATE OF STUDY**	**FOCUS OF STUDY**	**ETHICAL PRINCIPLE VIOLATED**
Willowbrook Hospital study, New York State	1972	Children with mental incompetence (N = 350) were not admitted to Willowbrook Hospital, a residential treatment facility, unless parents consented to their children's being research participants in a study of the natural history of infectious hepatitis and the effect of γ-globulin. The children were deliberately infected with the hepatitis virus under various conditions; some received γ-globulin, whereas others did not.	The principle of voluntary consent was violated. Parents were coerced into consenting to their children's participation for the research. Participants or their guardians have a right to self-determination; in other words, they should be free of constraint, coercion, and undue influence of any kind. Many participants feel pressured to participate in studies if they are in powerless, dependent positions (Rothman, 1982).
Schizophrenia medication study, University of California, Los Angeles	1983	In a study of the effects of withdrawing psychotropic medications in 50 patients receiving treatment for schizophrenia, 23 research participants suffered severe relapses after their medication was stopped. The goal of the study was to determine whether some patients with schizophrenia might do better without medications that had deleterious adverse effects.	Although all participants signed informed consent documents, they were not informed about how severe their relapses might be or that they could suffer worsening symptoms with each recurrence. Principles of informed consent were violated; full disclosure of the potential risk, harm, results, and adverse effects was not evident in the informed consent document. The potential risk outweighed the benefits of the study. The participants' right to fair treatment and protection from harm was violated (Hilts, 1995).
Côte d'Ivoire, Africa, AIDS/AZT case	1994	In research supported by the U.S. government and conducted in the Côte d'Ivoire, Dominican Republic, and Thailand, some pregnant women infected with HIV were given placebo pills rather than AZT, a drug known to prevent passing of the virus from mothers to their babies. Babies born to these mothers were in danger of contracting a fatal disease.	Research participants who consented to participate and who were randomly assigned to the control group were denied access to a medication regimen with a known benefit. This denial violates the participants' right to fair treatment and protection (French, 1997; Wheeler, 1997).

AIDS, acquired immune deficiency syndrome; *AZT*, azidothymidine; *HIV*, human immunodeficiency virus.

autonomy and to protect those with developing, impaired or diminished autonomy" (p. 6). An important aspect of enacting respect for persons is the requirement to seek their free, informed, and ongoing consent. Concern for Welfare includes balancing harm and benefits, such that the researcher maximizes benefit and minimizes harm. If the research on individuals affects the welfare

TABLE **6.2**

PROTECTION OF HUMAN RIGHTS

BASIC HUMAN RIGHT	DEFINITION
Right to self-determination	This right is based on the ethical principle of respect for persons; people should be treated as autonomous agents who have the freedom to choose without external controls. An autonomous agent is one who is informed about a proposed study and is allowed to choose to participate or not to participate (Brink, 1992). Moreover, research participants have the right to withdraw from a study without penalty.
Right to privacy and dignity	This right is based on the ethical principle of respect for persons; privacy is the freedom of a person to determine the time, extent, and circumstances under which private information is shared or withheld from other people.
Right to anonymity and confidentiality	This right is based on the ethical principle of respect for persons; anonymity exists when the participant's identity cannot be discerned, even by the researcher, from his or her individual responses (American Nurses Association, 1985).
	Confidentiality means that the individual identities of participants will not be linked to the information they provide and will not be publicly divulged.

VIOLATION OF BASIC HUMAN RIGHT	EXAMPLE
A participant's right to self-determination is violated through the use of coercion, deception, and covert data collection • In coercion, an overt threat of harm or excessive reward is presented to ensure participants' compliance. • In deception, participants are misinformed about the purpose of the research. • In covert data collection, people become research participants and are exposed to research treatments without knowing it. • The potential for violation of the right to self-determination is greater for research participants with diminished autonomy, who have decreased ability to give informed consent and are vulnerable.	Participants may believe that their care will be adversely affected if they refuse to participate in research. The Willowbrook Hospital Study (see Table 6.1) is an example of how coercion was used to obtain the consent of parents of vulnerable children with mental retardation, who would not be admitted to the institution unless they participated in a study in which they were deliberately injected with the hepatitis virus. The Jewish Chronic Disease Hospital Study (see Table 6.1) is an example of a study in which patients and their personal physicians did not know that cancer cells were being injected. In Milgram's (1963) study, research participants were deceived when asked to administer electric shocks to another person, who was an actor pretending to suffer from the shocks. Participants administering the shocks were very distressed by participating in this study, although they were not administering shocks at all. This study is an example of deception.
The U.S. Privacy Act of 1974 was instituted to protect participants from privacy violations. These violations occur most frequently during data collection, when responses to invasive questions might result in the loss of a job, friendships, or dignity or might create embarrassment and mental distress. These violations also may occur when participants are unaware that information is being shared with other people.	Research participants may be asked personal questions such as "Were you sexually abused as a child?"; "Do you use drugs?"; and "What are your sexual preferences?" When questions are asked in the presence of hidden microphones or hidden recording devices, the participants' privacy is invaded because they have no knowledge that the data are being shared with other people. Participants' right to control access of other people to their records is also violated.
Anonymity is violated when the participants' responses can be linked to their identity.	Researchers who choose to identify data by using the participant's name are breaching the basic human right of anonymity. Instead, researchers should assign participants a code number that is used for identification purposes. Research participants' names are never used in the reporting of findings.

TABLE **6.2**

PROTECTION OF HUMAN RIGHTS—cont'd

BASIC HUMAN RIGHT	DEFINITION
Confidentiality is breached when a researcher, by accident or direct action, allows an unauthorized person to gain access to study data that contain information about the participant's identity or responses, which creates a potentially harmful situation for the participant.	Breaches of confidentiality with regard to sexual preference, income, drug use, prejudice, or personality variables can be harmful to research participants. Data should be analyzed as group data so that participants cannot be identified by their responses.
Right to fair treatment	This right is based on the ethical principle of justice; people should be treated fairly and should receive what they are due or owed. "Fair treatment" refers to the equitable selection of research participants and their treatment during the research study. This treatment includes selection of participants for reasons directly related to the problem studied, as opposed to selection of participants because of convenience, the compromised position of the participants, or their vulnerability. Fair treatment also extends to the treatment of participants during the study, including fair distribution of risks and benefits of the research regardless of age, race, or socioeconomic status.
Right to protection from discomfort and harm	This right is based on the ethical principle of beneficence; people must take an active role in promoting good and preventing harm both in the world around them and in research studies. Discomfort and harm can be physical, psychological, social, or economic in nature. The five levels of harm and discomfort are as follows: 1. No anticipated effects 2. Temporary discomfort 3. Unusual level of temporary discomfort 4. Risk of permanent damage 5. Certainty of permanent damage Participants with diminished autonomy are entitled to protection. They are more vulnerable because of age, legal or mental incompetence, terminal illness, or confinement to an institution. A justification for the use of vulnerable participants must be provided.
VIOLATION OF BASIC HUMAN RIGHT	EXAMPLE
Injustices with regard to participant selection have occurred as a result of social, cultural, racial, and gender biases in society.	The Tuskegee Syphilis Study that ended in 1973 (Levine, 1986), the Jewish Chronic Disease Study of 1965 (Hershey & Miller, 1976), the San Antonio Contraceptive Study of 1969 (Levine, 1986), and the Willowbrook Hospital Study of 1972 (Rothman, 1982) (see Table 6.1) all are examples of unfair participant selection and the use of vulnerable populations.
Historically, research participants were often recruited from groups of people who were regarded as having less "social value," such as people living in poverty, prisoners, slaves, people who are mentally incompetent, and people who are dying. Participants were often treated carelessly, without consideration of physical or psychological harm.	Investigators should not be late for data-collection appointments, should terminate data collection on time, should not change agreed-upon procedures or activities without consent, and should provide agreed-upon benefits, such as a copy of the study findings or a participation fee.

Continued

TABLE **6.2**

PROTECTION OF HUMAN RIGHTS—cont'd

BASIC HUMAN RIGHT	DEFINITION
Research participants' right to be protected is violated when discomfort or disabling injury will occur and, thus, the benefits do not outweigh the risks.	Temporary physical discomfort involving minimal risk includes fatigue or headache; emotional discomfort includes the expense involved in travelling to and from the data-collection site. Studies of sensitive issues (such as rape, incest, or spouse abuse) might cause unusual levels of temporary discomfort by increasing participants' awareness of current or past traumatic experiences. In these situations, researchers assess distress levels and provide debriefing sessions, during which the participant may express feelings and ask questions. The researcher has the opportunity to make referrals for professional intervention. Studies with the potential to cause permanent damage are more likely to be medical in nature rather than nursing in nature, inasmuch as physiological damage may be permanent. One clinical trial of a new drug, a recombinant activated protein C (Zovan) for treatment of sepsis, was halted when interim findings from the phase III clinical trials revealed that the rate of mortality among the patients receiving treatment was lower than that among those receiving the placebo. Evaluation of the data led to termination of the trial to make a known beneficial treatment available more quickly to all patients. In some research, such as the Tuskegee Syphilis Study or Nazi medical experiments, participants experienced permanent damage or died. In Dr. Cameron's study (see Table 6.1), the continued electroconvulsive therapy increased the damage.

BOX **6.2**

BASIC ETHICAL PRINCIPLES RELEVANT TO THE CONDUCTING OF RESEARCH

RESPECT FOR PERSONS

People have the right to self-determination and to treatment as autonomous agents. Thus they have the freedom to participate or not participate in research. Persons with diminished autonomy are entitled to protection.

BENEFICENCE

Beneficence is an obligation to do no harm and maximize possible benefits. Persons are treated in an ethical manner when their decisions are respected, they are protected from harm, and efforts are made to secure their well-being.

JUSTICE

Human subjects should be treated fairly. An injustice occurs when benefit to which a person is entitled is denied without good reason or when a burden is imposed unduly.

From Elder, G. (1981). Social history & life experience. In D. H. Eichorn, J. A. Clausen, N. Haan, et al. (Eds.), *Present and past in middle life* (pp. 3–31). New York: Academic Press.

of a group, "the weight given to the group's welfare will depend on the nature of the research being undertaken, and the individuals or group in question" (p. 8). Justice implies fairness and equitable treatment; there should not be an imbalance of power between the researcher and participant or an inequity with vulnerable groups.

 Research Hint _____

The qualitative researcher must be especially diligent in protecting the privacy and confidentiality of participants. When the participants' verbatim quotations are used in the "Results" or "Findings" section of the research report to highlight the findings, the smallness of the sample size may make it easy to identify an individual participant. Moreover, when researchers and REBs are engaging in naturalistic observation, the TCPS 2 indicates that these boards "and researchers need to consider the methodological requirements of the proposed research project and the ethical implications associated with observational approaches, such as the possible infringement of privacy. They should pay close attention to the ethical implications of such factors as the nature of the activities to be observed, the environment in which the activities are to be observed, whether the activities are staged for the purpose of the research, the expectations of privacy that prospective participants might have, the means of recording the observations, whether the research records or published reports involve identification of the participants, and any means by which those participants may give permission to be identified" (CIHR et al., 2018, p. 139).

The Evolution of Ethics in Nursing Research

The evolution of ethics in nursing research can be traced back to 1897 and the constitution of the Nurses' Associated Alumnae Organization in the United States. One of the first purposes of this organization was to establish a code of ethics for the nursing profession. In 1900, Isabel Hampton Robb wrote Nursing Ethics: For Hospital and Private Use. In describing the moral laws by which people must abide, she stated the following:

Etiquette, speaking broadly, means a form of behavior or manners expressly or tacitly required on particular occasions. It makes up the code of polite life and includes forms of ceremony to be observed, so that we invariably find in societies that certain etiquette is required and observed either tacitly or by expressed agreement.

Although Robb's comments reflect the norms of Victorian society, they also highlight a historical concern for ethical actions by nurses as health care providers (Robb, 1900). In 1953, the International Council of Nurses (ICN) adopted the Code of Ethics for Nurses, and it is used as the standard for nurses worldwide.

The Code is regularly reviewed and revised, most recently in 2017, in response to the changing trends and realities in nursing. The Code guides nurses and nursing to demonstrate respect for human rights, the right to life and to dignity, and the right to be treated with respect. The ICN code of ethics also supports a nurse's right to refuse to participate in activities that conflict with caring and healing (ICN, 2012).

In Canada, most disciplines have developed their own code of ethics with guidelines for research. The CNA's first document on ethical principles related to nursing research, Ethical Guidelines for Nurses in Research Involving Human Participants, was released in 1983. It was revised in 1994 and 2002 and is now titled Ethical Research Guidelines for Registered Nurses (CNA, 2002).

Clearly, ignorance and naïveté regarding ethical and legal guidelines for conducting research are never an excuse for a nurse's failure to be familiar with such guidelines and to act on behalf of patients, whose human rights must be safeguarded at all times. Nurse researchers are often among the most responsible and conscientious investigators in respecting the rights of human participants. All nurses should be aware that, in addition to the ethical research guidelines of the CNA, universities and hospitals may also have supplemental sets of ethical guidelines to follow.

Current and Future Ethical Dilemmas in Research

Ethics is the theory or discipline dealing with principles of moral values and moral conduct. The ethical dilemmas in research for the twenty-first century concern biotechnology, the use of animals for research, and the creation of an organizational culture that values and nurtures research ethics and the rights of people who engage in research either as investigators or as participants. For example, in only 12 years, the Human Genome Project, an international research project launched in 1988 by investigators in the United States, provided a vast amount of data on DNA, including the molecular details about the DNA of more than 26 organisms. To engage in genome research, genetic engineering and genetic information are required (Carroll & Ciaffa, 2003), which can raise ethical concerns about the purpose of the engineering. If the purpose is to treat a disease, then the research is ethically acceptable, but the existence of germline intervention raises "more significant ethical concerns, because risks will extend across generations, magnifying the impact of unforeseen consequences" (Carroll & Ciaffa, 2003). Ethical concerns also arise with regard to the privacy of genetic information, mandatory testing of newborns, and mandatory genetic screening.

Other areas of research that engender much discussion and controversy are fetal tissue research and the use of women who are of child-bearing potential as participants in drug or therapeutic studies. The Tri-Council (i.e., the CIHR, the NSERC, and the SSHRC) worked over a period of several years to make stem cell research a reality in Canada, with the appropriate ethical guidelines for the use of embryos, fetuses, gametes, and pluripotent stems cells. These guidelines are detailed in the TCPS 2 (CIHR et al., 2018).

Of note is the following information:

Researchers conducting genetic research shall:

(a) in their research proposal, develop a plan for managing information that may be revealed through their genetic research;
(b) submit their plan to the REB; and
(c) advise prospective participants of the plan for managing information revealed through the research. (CIHR et al., 2018, p. 184, Article 13.2)

In the past, women of child-bearing potential were denied participation in studies of a drug or potential therapy because of the unknown, potentially teratogenic effects of drugs and other therapies that were in various stages of testing. Guidelines related to the inclusion of pregnant women as research participants have been even more stringent than previous guidelines; as a result, women have been excluded from many important drug and research studies over the years.

Given the history of injustices, including unethical research, with Indigenous peoples in Canada, the TCPS 2 also has a well-articulated policy on the ethical guidelines for research with Indigenous populations to ensure protection of the rights of those communities (CIHR et al., 2018). Further information on the history of research with Indigenous communities, as well as the particular ethical requirements for research, are detailed in Chapter 9.

PROTECTION OF HUMAN RIGHTS

Human rights are the claims and demands that have been justified according to an individual or by a group of individuals. The term *human rights* is applied to the following five rights outlined in the CNA's (2002) guidelines and linked to the Tri-Council's principles of respect for research participants:

1. Right to self-determination
2. Right to privacy and dignity
3. Right to anonymity and confidentiality
4. Right to fair treatment
5. Right to protection from discomfort and harm

These rights apply to everyone involved in a research project, including research team members involved in data collection, practising nurses involved in the research setting, and people participating in the study. As consumers of research read a research article, they must realize that any issues highlighted in Table 6.2 should have been addressed and resolved before a research study is approved for implementation.

Procedures for Protecting Basic Human Rights

Informed Consent

Informed consent, illustrated by the ethical principles of respect and the related right to self-determination, is outlined in Box 6.3. Nurses need to understand the elements of informed consent to be knowledgeable participants when either obtaining informed consent from patients or critiquing this process as it is presented in research articles.

Informed consent is the legal principle that requires a researcher to inform individuals about the potential benefits and risks of a study before the individuals can participate voluntarily. In theory, this principle governs the patient's ability to accept or reject individual medical interventions designed to diagnose or treat an illness. According to the TCPS 2 (CIHR et al., 2018), free and informed consent is at the heart of ethical research

BOX **6.3**

ELEMENTS OF INFORMED CONSENT

1. A statement that the study involves research
2. An explanation of the purposes of the research, delineating the expected duration of the subject's participation
3. A description of the procedures to be followed and identification of any procedures that are experimental
4. A description of any reasonably foreseeable risks or discomforts to the subject
5. A description of any benefits to the subject or to others that may reasonably be expected from the research
6. A disclosure of appropriate alternative procedures or course of treatment, if any, that might be advantageous to the subject
7. A statement describing the extent to which the anonymity and confidentiality of the records identifying the subject will be maintained
8. For research involving more than minimal risk, an explanation as to whether any medical treatments are available if injury occurs and, if so, what they consist of or where further information may be obtained
9. An explanation about whom to contact for answers to questions about the research and researcher subjects' rights and whom to contact in the event of a research-related injury to the subject
10. A statement that participation is voluntary, that refusal to participate will not involve any penalty or less benefit to which the subject is otherwise entitled, and that the subject may discontinue participation at any time without penalty or loss of otherwise entitled benefits

From Code of Federal Regulations: Protection of human subjects, 45 CFR 46, *OPRR Reports*, revised March 8, 1983.

and is a process of dialogue and information sharing to allow participants the choice to participate in research. Free and informed consent must be given without manipulation, undue influence, or coercion.

For example, Benbow et al. (2019) examined the multidimensional nature of social exclusion in the lives of mothers experiencing homelessness. Approval for the use of human participants was obtained from appropriate ethics review boards before the data collection. Another example involves a study with nursing students on exploring how simulation impacts competence and confidence in recognizing and responding to the adult and pediatric deteriorating patient; therefore, Goldsworthy et al. (2019) (Appendix D) obtained ethical approval from the university's ethics board, then recruited nursing students in their third year of study.

No investigator may involve a human being as a research participant until the legally effective informed consent has been obtained from either the participant or a legally authorized representative of the participant, and prospective participants must have time to decide whether to take part in a study. The researcher must not coerce the participant into taking part in the study, nor may researchers collect data on participants who have explicitly refused to take part in a study.

An ethical violation of this principle is illustrated by the case of Halushka v. University of Saskatchewan et al. (1965). In this landmark case, a university student volunteered for a study testing a new anaesthetic, for which he would be paid $50. He consented to be in the study, based on the following information disclosed to him: the test would last a few hours, the test was safe and had been conducted many times before, and the student had nothing to worry about. He was informed that the procedure would include placement of electrodes on his arms, legs, and head and insertion of a catheter into a vein in his arm. He signed a consent form releasing the physicians and the university from liability for any untoward effects or accidents, which were explained to him as "falling down the stairs at home after the test and then trying to sue the University hospital as a result" (McLean, 1996, p. 49). The test proceeded with administration of an untested anaesthetic, and the student suffered a cardiac arrest. He was unconscious for 4 days in the hospital and left with a residual inability to concentrate. The physicians and the university were found negligent for failing to disclose that there was risk involved with the use of an anaesthetic and that this particular drug had not been previously tested by them.

When composing an informed consent form, researchers must ensure that the language is understandable. For example, the level of language used should be appropriate to the age and comprehension/reading level of the participant population, generally at approximately a grade 6–8 reading level (Health Canada, 2019b). The elements that need to be contained in an informed consent form are listed in Box 6.3. Note that many institutions require additional elements. Figure 6.1 is an example of an informed consent form for a quantitative study; Figure 6.2 is an example of an informed consent form for a qualitative study. Note that in each consent form, the elements of participation, risk and benefits, withdrawal, confidentiality, and whom to contact for further queries are clearly outlined.

Research Hint

Remember that research reports rarely provide readers with detailed information regarding the degree to which the researcher adhered to ethical principles, such as informed consent; this is because of space limitations in journals, which make it impossible to describe all aspects of a study. Failure to mention procedures to safeguard participants' rights does not necessarily mean that such precautions were not taken.

Most investigators obtain **consent** (agreement to participate in a study) through personal discussion with potential participants. This process allows the person who is the potential participant to obtain immediate answers to questions. Consent forms, written in narrative or outline form, highlight elements that both inform and remind participants of the nature of the study and their participation When one participant is scheduled to participate in many interviews, the participant must give **process consent** (voluntary continued participation in a study, which can be verbal) for each data-collection point.

Assurance of anonymity and confidentiality (defined in Table 6.2), which is conveyed in writing, is sometimes difficult in unique research situations that capture the public's attention. For example, when physicians at Loma Linda University Hospital in California transplanted a baboon's heart into a 2-week-old infant, her identity was hidden (**anonymity**)—she was known only as Baby Fae—and **confidentiality** was ensured in that the reports could not be linked to her and her family. Maintaining anonymity and confidentiality is particularly important for qualitative researchers because the researcher often functions as the data-collection "instrument" and meets the participant. The consent form must be signed and dated by the participant. The presence of witnesses is not always necessary but does constitute evidence that the participant concerned actually signed the form. In cases in which the participant is a minor or is physically or mentally incapable of signing the consent, the signature must be obtained from a legal guardian or representative. The investigator also signs the form to indicate commitment to the agreement of anonymity and confidentiality.

In studies in which the researcher suspected child abuse or neglect, the participants need to be clearly informed that the researcher has a legal responsibility to report any suspicions to the child welfare agency, even though the participants' anonymity and confidentiality were guaranteed. Another strategy that can be used to ensure confidentiality is to ask the transcribers, who are not part of the research team, in a qualitative study to sign a confidentiality agreement.

In general, the signed informed consent form is given to the participant. The researcher should also keep a copy. Some research, such as a retrospective chart audit, may require only institutional approval, not informed consent. In some cases, when minimal risk is involved, the investigator may have to provide the participant only with an information sheet and a verbal explanation. In other cases, such as a volunteer convenience sample, completion and return of research instruments constitute evidence of consent. The REB advises on exceptions to these guidelines, as in cases in which the REB might grant waivers or amend its guidelines in other ways. The REB

CONSENT TO PARTICIPATE IN A RESEARCH STUDY

Title
VISUAL DIFFERENTIATION IN LOOK-ALIKE MEDICATION NAMES

University Health Network Principal Investigator
Tasmine Halevy, Clinical Director of Pharmacy, UHN, 416-XXX-XXXX

Study Principal Investigator
Monica Blum, Associate Professor, Reed University, 416-XXX-XXXX

Co-Investigators
Joyce Davis, Vice President, ISMP Canada
Dr. Mina D. Singh, Associate Professor, York University, Faculty of Health, School of Nursing
Ravinder Sharma, Human Factors Engineer, Red Forest Consulting
Dr. Irmgard Mirren, Psychiatrist, Child and Parent Resource Institute
Evan Ross, Chief Pharmacist, Child and Parent Resource Institute

Collaborator
Jude Hartman

Sponsors
Canadian Patient Safety Institute, ISMP Canada; Red Forest Consulting; Child and Parent Resource Institute; York University Faculty of Graduate Studies, Department of Design and Faculty of Health

Introduction
You are being asked to take part in a research study. Please read this explanation about the study and its risks and benefits before you decide if you would like to take part. You should take as much time as you need to make your decision. You should ask the Principal Investigator or Research Assistants to explain anything that you do not understand and make sure that all of your questions have been answered before signing this consent form. Before you make your decision, feel free to talk about this study with anyone you wish. Participation in this study is voluntary.

Background and Purpose
This study will look at the visual display of look-alike medication names. It is hoped that this research will contribute to the design of shelf labelling, packaging, and computer displays to help reduce instances of medication errors due to look-alike medication names. The results from this research are intended to support health care workers in the safe delivery of health care. You have been asked to take part in this research study because you have or may come into contact with look-alike medications. A total of 130 to 135 nursing staff and 10 pharmacy staff from Princess Margaret Hospital, Toronto General Hospital and Toronto Western Hospital will participate in this study.

Study Design
You will help us evaluate the best ways to display look-alike names for ease and accuracy in recognition and selection of medications. If you choose to participate in this study, you will be asked to answer a short questionnaire to establish your demographic information and to ask you your opinion of current practices related to the display of look-alike medication names. You will participate in three experiments that emulate the selection of medications. The first two experiments are screen based, and you will be asked to identify look-alike names on a laptop display. For the third experiment, you will be asked to select medications from a series of baskets. The tasks will be explained thoroughly before each experiment. Your commitment for this study will be one session lasting approximately 45 to 60 minutes.

FIG. 6.1 Example of an informed consent form for a quantitative study. *ISMP*, Institute for Safe Medication Practices; *UHN*, University Health Network.

Continued

CONSENT TO PARTICIPATE IN A RESEARCH STUDY—cont'd

Risks Related to Being in the Study

There are no known risks if you take part in this study, but you may refuse to answer questions or stop the experiments at any time if there is any discomfort. Your responses to the questionnaires will not have an impact on your employment, nor will they be shared with your supervisors or managers.

Benefits to Being in the Study

You will not receive any direct benefit from being in this study. Information learned from this study may help in the safe delivery of health care.

Voluntary Participation

Your participation in this study is voluntary. You may decide not to be in this study, or to be in the study now and then change your mind later. You may leave the study at any time without affecting your employment status. You may refuse to answer any question you do not want to answer on the questionnaire by writing "pass," or stop participating in the experiment at any time.

Confidentiality

The information that is collected for the study will be kept in a locked and secure area at York University by the study Principal Investigator for 10 years. Only the study team and the people or groups listed below will be allowed to look at the data. All information collected during this study will be kept confidential and will not be shared with anyone outside the study unless required by law. Any information about you that is collected for the study will have a code and will not show your name or address, or any information that directly identifies you. You will not be named in any reports, publications, or presentations that may come from this study. If you decide to leave the study, the information about you that was collected before you left the study will still be used. No new information will be collected without your permission. Representatives of the University Health Network Research Ethics Board may look at the study records to check that the information collected for the study is correct and to make sure the study followed proper laws and guidelines.

Questions about the Study

If you have any questions or concerns, or would like to speak to the study team for any reason, please call: Tasmine Halevy, University Health Network, at **416-XXX- XXXX** or Monica Blum, Reed University, **416-XXX-XXXX.**

The research has been reviewed and approved by the University Health Network Research Ethics Board (REB) and the Human Participants Review Committee (HPRC) at Reed University for compliance with senate ethics policy. If you have any questions about your rights as a research participant or have concerns about this study, call the Chair of the UHN (REB) or the Research Ethics office number at 416-XXX-XXXX or Manager, Research Ethics—Alicia Collins-Walker: 309 Elsevier Lanes, Reed University, 416-XXX-XXXX. The HPRC and REB are groups of people who oversee the ethical conduct of research studies. These people are not part of the study team. Everything that you discuss will be kept confidential.

Consent

This study has been explained to me and any questions I had have been answered. I know that I may leave the study at any time. I agree to take part in this study.

---   --   ----------------------

Print Study Participant's Name   Signature   Date

(You will be given a signed copy of this consent form.)

My signature means that I have explained the study to the participant named above. I have answered all questions.

---   --   ----------------------

Print Name of Person Obtaining Consent   Signature   Date

FIG. 6.1   cont'd

INFORMATION AND INFORMED CONSENT STATEMENT: INTERVIEW

Title
BETTER UNDERSTANDING HOW COUPLES COPE WITH A CHILD'S LIFE-THREATENING ILLNESS

Principal Investigator
Dr. Susan Cadell, Associate Professor; Director, Manulife Centre for Healthy Living; Lyle S. Hallman Faculty of Social Work, Wilfrid Laurier University, 519-XXX-XXXX

Co-Investigators
Dr. Rosemary Stiles, School of Nursing, York University
Dr. Anna DeLaurentis, The Centre for Health and Coping Studies, University of British Columbia

Research Assistants
Matilde Negrini, Faculty of Social Work, Wilfrid Laurier University
Julian Millman, Faculty of Social Work, Wilfrid Laurier University
Nella Leone, Faculty of Social Work, Wilfrid Laurier University

Contact Person
Matthew Philips, Research Coordinator: 1-800-XXX-XXXX

We are inviting couples to participate in the next phase of this research study. The purpose of this study is to discover the experience of spouses/partners who are together caring for a child with a life-limiting illness. This study is being conducted by Dr. Susan Cadell, Associate Professor and Director of the Manulife Centre for Healthy Living at Wilfrid Laurier University, and Co-Investigator on the Canadian Institutes for Health Research's New Emerging Team (NET): *Transitions in Pediatric Palliative and End-of-Life Care.*

Information
During the interview, you and your spouse/partner will be interviewed together. You will be asked questions about your personal experience of caring for a child with a life-limiting condition, as well as questions about the role that each spouse/partner plays in the coping of the other. The interview will take approximately 1.5 to 2 hours. The interview will be conducted by a trained, sensitive interviewer and will take place at a location convenient to you. In order to make sure that we have an accurate record of what you have shared during the interview, your interview will be recorded and transcribed. All identifying information will be removed from the transcripts and only the investigators and research staff will have access to them. The recordings and transcripts will be identified only by code number and stored in a locked filing cabinet or secured information system. They will be stored for 5 years after the publication of the results from this study. After 5 years, the recordings and the transcripts will be destroyed. The recordings will not be used for any other purposes without your additional permission.

Phase Two of this study will involve the participation of approximately 15 to 20 couples who are together caring for their child. Due to the nature of this study, it is possible that quotes from your interview may be used in publication. To maintain confidentiality, all identifying information will be removed from the quotations. If a specific family or disease characteristic is rare and could potentially be identifying, the information will be changed in the quote. Please indicate your preference below regarding the use of your quotations.

Name: _____   Name: _____
☐ Yes – I can be quoted with no identifying information.   ☐ Yes – I can be quoted with no identifying information.
☐ No – Please do not use quotes.   ☐ No – Please do not use quotes.

FIG. 6.2   Example of an informed consent form for a qualitative study.

Continued

INFORMATION AND INFORMED CONSENT STATEMENT: INTERVIEW—cont'd

Risk
This research project deals with a sensitive topic. The interviewer will monitor your distress level and will stop the interviewing process if you become upset. The interviewer will then ensure that you are aware of your right not to answer any questions asked and your right to terminate the interview at any time. If necessary, the interviewer will refer you to appropriate services and resources to ensure your support needs are met.

Benefits
You may benefit from the ability to communicate your experiences of pediatric palliative care in a safe, nonjudgemental setting. In addition, your participation may benefit other families, researchers, and policy makers in pediatric palliative care by providing a better understanding of the caregiver experience.

Confidentiality
Confidentiality will be provided to the fullest extent possible by law. Your identity and the identity of all family members will be kept strictly confidential. All identifying information will be removed from the data. All documents and recordings will be identified only by code number and the information will be retained in a secured information system and locked filing cabinet. All identifying information will be kept separate from the data. All documents that are kept on a computer will be password protected. Identifying information will not be emailed to anyone at any time. You will not be identified by name in any reports of the completed study. Only study personnel will have access to the study data.

Compensation
For participating in this study, you and your spouse/partner will each receive $30 at the beginning of the interview. If you withdraw from the study after this point, you will still receive the full amount.

Participation
Your participation in this study is voluntary; you may decline to participate without penalty. If you decide to participate, you may withdraw from the study at any time without penalty and without loss of benefits to which you are otherwise entitled. If you withdraw from the study before data collection is completed, your data will be destroyed. You have the right to omit any question(s)/procedure(s) you choose.

Feedback and Publication
It is expected that the results of this study will be presented and published as a journal article. If you would like to be notified of the results of the study, please indicate below.

Name: _____   Name: _____
☐ Yes – I would like to be notified of results.   ☐ Yes – I would like to be notified of results.

Contact
If you have questions at any time about the study or the procedures, or if you experience adverse effects as a result of participating in this study, you may contact the Research Coordinator, Matthew Philips, at 1-800-XXX- XXXX. This project has been reviewed and approved by the University Research Ethics Board at Wilfrid Laurier University. If you feel you have not been treated according to the descriptions in this form, or your rights as a participant in research have been violated during the course of this project, you may contact Dr. Mark Billingsley, Chair, University Research Ethics Board, Wilfrid Laurier University, 519-XXX-XXXX.

Consent
I have read and understand the above information. I have received a copy of this form. I agree to participate in this study.

_____   _____
Participant's signature   Date

_____   _____
Participant's signature   Date

_____   _____
Investigator's signature   Date

FIG. 6.2   cont'd

makes the final determination regarding the most appropriate documentation format. Research consumers should note whether and what kind of evidence of informed consent has been provided in a research article.

💡 Research Hint

Note that researchers often do not obtain written informed consent when the major means of data collection is through self-administered questionnaires. Implied consent is usually assumed in such cases; in other words, the return of the completed questionnaire reflects the respondent's voluntary consent to participate.

Research Ethics Boards

Research ethics boards (REBs) are panels that review research projects to assess whether ethical standards are met in relation to the protection of the rights of human participants. Such boards are established in agencies to review biomedical and behavioural research involving human subjects within the agency or in programs sponsored by the agency. Universities, hospitals, and other health agencies applying for a grant or contract for any project or program that involves the conduct of biomedical or behavioural research with human participants are required by the Tri-Council and most funding agencies to submit with their application assurances that they have established an REB that reviews the research projects and protects the rights of the human participants (CIHR et al., 2018). The Panel on Research Ethics has an online applied course with 10 modules for researchers and members of REBs, which can be found at http://www.pre.ethics.gc.ca/eng/education/tutorial-didacticiel/. Students engaged in research are encouraged to complete this tutorial.

The Tri-Council also requires that the REB have at least five members, including both men and women. Membership must include at least two professionals who have expertise in relevant research disciplines, fields, and methodologies covered by the REB; at least one who is knowledgeable in ethics; at least one who is knowledgeable in the relevant law (but that member should not be the institution's legal counsel or risk manager); and at least one who is a community member and has no affiliation with the institution but is recruited from the community served by the institution (CIHR et al., 2018).

The REB is responsible for protecting participants from undue risk and loss of personal rights and dignity. For a research proposal to be eligible for consideration by an REB, it must already have been approved by a departmental review group, such as a nursing research committee, that attests to the proposal's scientific merit and congruence with institutional policies, procedures, and mission. The REB reviews the study's protocol to ensure that it meets the requirements of ethical research. Most boards provide guidelines or instructions for researchers that include steps to be taken to receive REB approval. For example, guidelines for writing a standard consent form or criteria for qualifying for an expedited rather than a full REB review may be available. The REB has the authority to approve research, require modifications, or disapprove a research study, on the basis of the guidelines outlined in Box 6.4. A researcher must receive REB approval

---

BOX **6.4**

PARTIAL GUIDELINES FOR RESEARCH ETHICS BOARD APPROVAL OF RESEARCH STUDIES

To approve research, the REB must determine that the following guidelines have been satisfied:
1. There is an analysis of balance and distribution of harms and benefits.
2. There is a proportionate approach based on the general principle that the level of review is determined by the level of risk presented by the research: the lower the level of risk, the lower the level of scrutiny (delegated review); the higher the level of risk, the higher the level of scrutiny (full board review).
3. There is a formal informed consent process.

REB, research ethics board.
From Canadian Institutes of Health Research, Natural Sciences and Engineering Research Council of Canada, & Social Sciences and Humanities Research Council of Canada. (2014, December). *Tri-Council policy statement: Ethical conduct for research involving humans.* Retrieved from https://ethics.gc.ca/eng/policy-politique_tcps2-eptc2_2018.html

before beginning to conduct research. Subedi et al. (2019) assess the relationship between coping strategies and psychological well-being of Bhutanese refugees. After REB approval, written consent was obtained from each participant and confidentiality maintained throughout data collection and analysis. Two counsellors were available if participants became emotionally upset or distressed. REBs have the authority to suspend or terminate approval of research that is not conducted in accordance with REB requirements or that has been associated with unexpected serious harm to participants.

REBs in Canada also provide for reviewing research in an expedited manner when the risk to research participants is minimal. An expedited review usually shortens the length of the review process but does not automatically exempt the researcher from obtaining informed consent.

Not all research requires an ethical review. To follow protocol, researchers can submit a proposal to their own REB; however, according to the TCPS 2 (CIHR et al., 2018), this step is not necessary when the research relies exclusively on information that is publicly available through a mechanism set out by legislation or regulation and that is protected by law. Legally accessible information includes registries of deaths, court judgements, and public archives and publicly available statistics (e.g., Statistics Canada public use files).

REB review is also not required when researchers use information exclusively in the public domain and the individuals to whom the information refers have no reasonable expectation of privacy. For example, identifiable information may be disseminated in the public domain through print or electronic publications; film, audio, or digital recordings; press accounts; official publications of private or public institutions; artistic installations, exhibitions, or literary events freely open to the public; or publications accessible in public libraries. Research that is nonintrusive and does not involve direct interaction between the researcher and individuals through the Internet also does not require REB review. Online material such as documents, records, performances, online archival materials, or published third-party interviews to which the public is given uncontrolled access on the Internet and for which there is no expectation of privacy is considered to be publicly available information.[1]

The TCPS 2 exempts quality assurance studies, quality improvement studies, performance reviews, or testing within normal educational requirements from REB reviews. However, performance reviews or studies that contain an element of research in addition to assessment may need ethics review (CIHR et al., 2018, Article 2.5).

The Critical Thinking Decision Path illustrates the ethical decision-making process an REB might use in evaluating the risk–benefit ratio of a research study.

Protecting the Basic Human Rights of Vulnerable Groups

Researchers are advised to consult their agency's REB for the most recent guidelines when considering research involving vulnerable groups such as older adults, children, pregnant women, unborn children, persons who are emotionally or physically disabled, prisoners, deceased persons, students, and persons with AIDS or other serious illnesses.

In addition, researchers should consult the REB before planning research that potentially involves an oversubscribed research population, such as patients who have undergone organ transplantation, patients with AIDS, or "captive" and convenient research populations, such as prisoners. The use of special populations does not preclude undertaking research; safeguards must be undertaken,

[1]Adapted from Canadian Institutes of Health Research, Natural Sciences and Engineering Research Council of Canada, & Social Sciences and Humanities Research Council of Canada. (2018). *Tri-Council policy statement: Ethical conduct for research involving humans.* Chapter 2, "Scope and approach." Retrieved from https://ethics.gc.ca/eng/policy-politique_tcps2-eptc2_2018.html.

CRITICAL THINKING DECISION PATH

Evaluating the Risk–Benefit Ratio of a Research Study

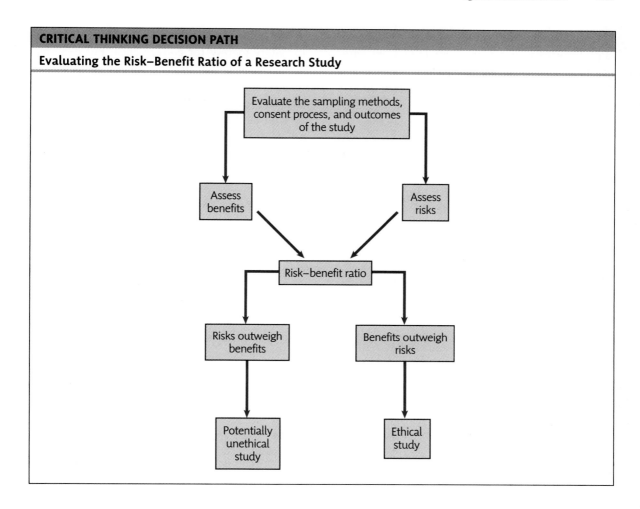

however, to protect the rights of these participants (CIHR et al., 2018). Individuals or groups whose circumstances may make them vulnerable in the context of research should not be inappropriately included or automatically excluded from participation in research on the basis of their circumstances. Researchers and REBs shall carefully examine the relationship between the circumstances of the individuals and groups and the proposed research question. Individuals should not be considered vulnerable simply because of assumptions made about the vulnerability of the group to which they belong (CIHR et al., 2018, Article 4.7).

Pediatric research can be particularly problematic. **Assent**—an aspect of informed consent that pertains to protecting the rights of children as research subjects—is composed of the following three fundamental elements:

1. A basic understanding by the child of what the child will be expected to do and what will be done to the child
2. A comprehension by the child of the basic purpose of the research
3. An ability of the child to express a preference regarding participation

An example of research in a pediatric group in which assent was used is the study of Stewart and colleagues (2019). These researchers examined the use of interactive distraction versus oral midazolam to reduce pediatric preoperative anxiety, emergence delirium, and postanesthesia length of stay. Informed consent was attained from caregivers or legally authorized representatives, and verbal assent was attained from children aged 8 to 12 years.

In contrast to assent, consent requires a relatively advanced level of cognitive ability. Informed consent reflects competency standards requiring abstract appreciation of and reasoning about the information provided. According to Health Canada (2019b), "a child under 16 years of age should provide his/her assent and may refuse to participate even if the parent has provided their consent. The age of consent to participate in research in Quebec is 18 years of age, and the assent form for the involvement of minors in research should be used for any individuals under the age of 18" (p. 1).

If the research involves more than minimal risk and does not offer a direct benefit to the individual child, then both parents must grant permission. When children reach maturity, usually at 18 years of age in the case of research, they may render their own consent. They may do so at a younger age if they have been legally declared emancipated minors. Questions regarding assent, consent, and the age of the individual should be addressed by the REB or research administration office and not left to the discretion of the researcher to answer.

Special ethical considerations also exist when research is conducted with older adults. The issue of the legal competence of older adults is often raised, but no issue exists if the potential participant can supply legally effective informed consent. Competence is not clearly measurable. The complexity of the study may affect an individual's ability to consent to participate. The capacity to give informed consent should be assessed in each individual for each research protocol being considered. For example, an older person may be able to consent to participate in a simple observation study but not in a clinical drug trial.

No vulnerable population may be singled out for study merely for convenience. For example, neither people with mental illness nor prisoners may be studied simply because they are available and their presence is convenient. Prisoners may be studied if the study pertains to them—for example, studies concerning the effects and processes of incarceration. Similarly, people with mental illness may participate in studies that focus on expanding knowledge about psychiatric disorders and treatments. Students also are often a conveniently available group. They must not, however, be singled out as research participants because of convenience; the research questions must have some bearing on their status as students.

Researchers and patient caregivers involved in research with vulnerable people are well advised to seek advice from appropriate REBs, clinicians, lawyers, ethicists, and other professionals. In all cases, the burden should be on the investigator to show the REB that it is appropriate to involve vulnerable participants in research.

Research Hint

Keep in mind that researchers rarely mention explicitly that the study participants were vulnerable participants or that special precautions were taken to appropriately safeguard the human rights of this vulnerable group. Research consumers need to be attentive to the special needs of individuals who may be unable to act as their own advocates or are unable to adequately assess the risk–benefit ratio of a research study.

SCIENTIFIC FRAUD AND MISCONDUCT

Fraud

Periodically, articles reporting the unethical actions of researchers appear in the professional and lay literature. Data may have been falsified or fabricated, or participants may have been coerced into participating in a research study (Gupta, 2013). In a climate of "publish or perish" in academic and scientific settings and declining research dollars, academics and scientists are under increasing pressure to produce significant research findings. Job security and professional recognition are coveted, essential, and often predicated on being a productive scientist and a prolific writer. These pressures have been known to overpower some people, who then take shortcuts, fabricate data, and falsify findings to advance their positions.

The risks of engaging in fraudulent research are many, including harming research participants or basing clinical practice on false data. As advocates of patient welfare and professional practice, nurses should be aware that sometimes they might observe or suspect a researcher's misconduct. In such cases, nurses must contact the appropriate group, such as the REB, to ensure that this matter receives appropriate attention and review.

Misconduct

Of equal importance is the issue of basing nursing practice on reports that appear in journals when subsequent research and reports on those participants change the scientific basis for practice. Corrections or further research in follow-up reports may be buried, obscure, or underreported. As patient advocates and research consumers, nurses must keep up to date on scientific reports related to nursing practice and must adjust their practice as directed by ever-evolving, evidence-informed research findings. In addition, researchers have a responsibility to keep current with federal compliance regulations on prevention, detection, investigation, and adjudication of scientific misconduct.

Unauthorized Research

At times, ad hoc or informal and unauthorized research is conducted, including **product testing** (the testing of medical devices). Although the testing may seem harmless, it is, again, not the purview of the investigator to make that determination. Nurses must carefully avoid being involved in unauthorized research, for a number of reasons, including the following:

- These treatments or methods of care are usually not monitored as closely for untoward

effects; hence, the patient may be exposed to unwarranted risk.
- Patients' rights to informed consent in clinical trials are not protected.
- The success or failure of these unrecorded trials contributes nothing to the organized scientific knowledge of the efficacy or complications of the treatment.
- The lack of independent quality supervision allows deviations from the adopted experimental program that may eliminate the program's effectiveness.

Product Testing

Nurses are often approached by manufacturers to test products on patients. Often, nurses assume the role of research coordinator in clinical drug or product trials. Consequently, nurses should be aware of the Health Products and Food Branch Inspectorate guidelines (see Health Canada, 2019a; 2020) and regulations for testing of medical devices before they initiate any form of clinical testing. Medical devices are classified according to the extent of control necessary to ensure the safety and effectiveness of each device.

LEGAL AND ETHICAL ASPECTS OF ANIMAL EXPERIMENTATION

The laws that have been written regarding **animal rights**—guidelines used to protect the rights of animals in the conduct of research—in research emanate from an interesting history of attitudes toward animals and the value that people place on them. In 1963, the Medical Research Council of Canada (now CIHR) requested that a committee be established to investigate the care and use of experimental animals. The Canadian Council on Animal Care (CCAC) was formed and became a nonprofit, autonomous, and independent body in 1982 (CCAC, 2021). It is the oversight body for scientific animal use and is described on the CCAC website. It is now funded by the CIHR and the NSERC and conducts assessment visits to each institution every 3 years, often unannounced. The CCAC requires that institutions conducting animal-based research, teaching, or testing establish an animal care committee and that this committee be functionally active. Assessments of institutional animal ethics and care programs are based on CCAC guidelines (animal care; types of animals; procedures; and program management) and assessment policies, as well as other relevant documents. Compliance with CCAC guidelines and policies is a requirement to receive a CCAC Certificate of GAP – Good Animal Practice®, as determined by CCAC assessment panels (https://www.ccac.ca/en/standards /guidelines/).

The CIHR scrutinized the proposed amendments to the Cruelty to Animal Provisions of the Criminal Code of Canada, Bill-C15. The objective of these changes is to strengthen but simplify the existing penal code and "to enhance the effectiveness of the offence provisions for clearly abusive, brutal and cruel treatment of animals." The CIHR supported this objective in principle and, with the NSERC, prepared a joint submission to the House of Commons Standing Committee on Justice and Human Rights in the fall of 2001, recommending amendments to clarify certain provisions of the bill with regard to their application to health research.

This section serves only as an introduction to the concept of legal and ethical issues related to animal experimentation. Principles of protection of animal rights in research have evolved over time. Animals, unlike humans, cannot give informed consent, but other conditions related to their welfare must not be ignored. Nurses who encounter the use of animals in research should be alert to their rights.

RESEARCH INVOLVING HUMAN GAMETES, EMBRYOS, OR FETUSES

Research on the human genome and other reproductive issues have caused much ethical debate and concern; thus, the Tri-Council (CIHR

et al., 2018) developed pertinent guidelines, as demonstrated by these examples:

- Materials related to human reproduction for research use shall not be obtained through commercial transaction, including exchange for services (Article 12.6).
- Research on in vitro embryos already created and intended for implantation to achieve pregnancy is acceptable if:
  - The research is intended to benefit the embryo
  - Research interventions will not compromise the care of the woman or the subsequent fetus
  - Researchers closely monitor the safety and comfort of the woman and the safety of the embryo
  - Consent was provided by the gamete donors (Article 12.7)
- Research involving embryos that have been created for reproductive or other purposes permitted in Canada under the Assisted Human Reproduction Act (CIHR et al., 2018, Article 12.8), but are no longer required for these purposes, may be ethically acceptable if:
  - The ova and sperm from which they are formed were obtained in accordance with Article 12.7
  - Consent was provided by the gamete donors
  - Embryos exposed to manipulations not directed specifically to their ongoing normal development will not be transferred for continuing pregnancy
  - Research involving embryos will take place only during the first 14 days after their formation by combination of the gametes, excluding any time during which embryonic development has been suspended (Article 12.8)
- Research involving a fetus or fetal tissue (CIHR et al., 2018, Article 12.9):
  - Requires the consent of the woman
  - Should not compromise the woman's ability to decide whether to continue her pregnancy

Nurses working in labour rooms, especially those being required to assist with embryonic research, should be aware of these ethical issues.

APPRAISING THE EVIDENCE

The Legal and Ethical Aspects of a Research Study

Research articles and reports often do not contain detailed information regarding either the degree to which or all of the ways in which the investigator adhered to the legal and ethical principles presented in this chapter. Space considerations in articles preclude extensive documentation of all legal and ethical aspects of a research study. Lack of written evidence regarding the protection of human rights does not imply that appropriate steps were not taken.

The Critiquing Criteria box provides guidelines for evaluating the legal and ethical aspects of a research report. Although research consumers reading a research report will not see all areas explicitly addressed in the research article, they should be aware of them and should determine that the researcher has addressed them before gaining REB approval to conduct the study. A nurse who is asked to serve as a member of an REB will find the critiquing criteria useful in evaluating the legal and ethical aspects of the research proposal.

Information about the legal and ethical considerations of a study is usually presented in the "Methods" section of a research report, probably in the subsection on the sample or data-collection methods. The author most often indicates in a few sentences that informed consent was obtained and that approval from an REB or similar committee was granted. A manuscript without such a discussion will probably not be accepted for publication; thus, it is almost impossible for unauthorized research to be published. Therefore, when a research article provides evidence of having been approved by an external review committee, the reader can feel confident that the ethical issues raised by the study have been thoroughly reviewed and resolved.

CRITIQUING CRITERIA

1. Was the study approved by an REB or other agency committee members?
2. Is there evidence that informed consent was obtained from all participants or their representatives? How was it obtained?
3. Were the participants protected from physical or emotional harm?

4. Were the participants or their representatives informed about the purpose and nature of the study?
5. Were the participants or their representatives informed about any potential risks that might result from participation in the study?
6. Was the research study designed to maximize the benefit or benefits and to minimize the risks to human participants?

7. Were participants coerced or unduly influenced to participate in this study? Did they have the right to refuse to participate or withdraw without penalty? Were vulnerable participants used?
8. Were appropriate steps taken to safeguard the privacy of participants? How have data been kept anonymous or confidential?

To protect participant and institutional privacy, the locale of the study frequently is described in general terms in the report's subsection on the sample. For example, the article might state that data were collected at a 500-bed tertiary care centre in Ontario, without mentioning the centre's name. Protection of participant privacy may be explicitly addressed by statements indicating that the anonymity or confidentiality of the data was maintained or that grouped data were used in the data analysis.

Determining whether participants were subjected to physical or emotional risk is often accomplished indirectly by evaluating the study's "Methods" section. The reader evaluates the **risk–benefit ratio**: that is, the extent to which the **benefits** of the study—the potential positive outcomes of participation in a research study—are maximized and the **risks**—the potential negative outcomes of participation in a research study—are minimized, so that participants are protected from harm during the study. The Practical Application boxes list examples of how researchers attempt to protect study participants from harm.

> ### Practical Application
> Dahlke et al. (2019) conducted a study to examine how the learning processes inherent in a pre-licensure nursing program are socializing students to work with older people. After university ethics approval, the Associate Dean of the pre-licensure nursing program forwarded an email invitation to all 963 nursing students to participate in an online survey about their perceptions of older people. The email guaranteed students that completing or not completing the survey would have no bearing on their status as a student in the nursing program. They were also assured of confidentiality and anonymity in completing the survey and that completing the survey implied consent.

> ### Practical Application
> Currie and Szabo (2020) conducted a study to co-construct new meanings and interpretations of parenting a child with complex disabilities by having an increased understanding of the struggles and barriers for parents. Prior to commencing the semi-structured interviews, human research ethics approval was received. Due to the sensitive nature of the narratives, the researcher worked closely with participants to attend vulnerability with disclosure.

The obligation to balance the risks and benefits of a study is the responsibility of the researcher. However, the research consumer reading a research report also should be confident that participants have been protected from harm.

When considering the special needs of vulnerable participants, research consumers should be sensitive to whether the investigators have addressed the special needs of individuals who are unable to act on their own behalf. For example, has the right of self-determination been addressed by the informed consent protocol identified in the research report? Woodgate et al. (2020) explored the experience of the self in Canadian youth living with anxiety. After ethical approval was obtained, those participants over the age of 18 years of age gave written informed consent. For those under the age of 18 years of age, assent and written consent from youth and parents respectively were obtained.

When qualitative studies are reported, verbatim quotations from informants often are incorporated into the "Findings" section of the article. In such cases, the reader can evaluate how effectively the author protected the informant's identity, either by using a fictitious name or by withholding information such as age, gender, occupation, or other potentially identifying data.

Although the need for guidelines for the use of human and animal participants in research is evident and the principles themselves are clear, many instances arise in which nurses must use their best judgement, as both patient advocates and researchers, when evaluating the ethical nature of a research project. In any research situation, the basic guiding principle of protecting the patient's human rights must always apply. When conflicts arise, nurses must feel free to raise suitable questions with appropriate resources and personnel. In an institution, raising questions may include contacting the researcher first; then, if there is no resolution, the matter must be raised with the director of nursing research and the chairperson of the REB. In cases in which ethical considerations in a research article are in question, clarification from a colleague, agency, or the researcher's REB is indicated. Nurses should pursue their concerns until they are satisfied that the patient's rights and their rights as professionals are protected.

CRITICAL THINKING CHALLENGES

- As part of a needs assessment for future health care delivery planning, the Ministry of Health is interested in determining the number of babies infected with the human immunodeficiency virus (HIV). A province-wide study is funded that will include the testing of all newborns for HIV, but the mothers will not be told that the test is being done, nor will they be told the results. Using the basic ethical principles found in Box 6.2, defend or refute this practice.

- The REB of your health care agency does not include a nurse, and you think it should. You discuss this matter with your supervisor, who states that including a nurse is not necessary because the REB uses strict guidelines. What essential arguments and explanations should your proposal address for including a nurse on your institution's REB?

- A qualitative researcher intends to conduct a phenomenological study on caring and to recruit informants who are severely and persistently mentally ill and attend an outpatient clinic. The REB denies the study, indicating that informed consent cannot be obtained and that these patients will not be able to tolerate an interview. What assumptions have the members of this REB made? If you were the researcher and you were given the opportunity to address their concerns, what would you say? Include information from Table 6.2.

- How do you see electronic databases and websites assisting researchers in conducting ethical studies? Do you think that REBs can use this technology to assist them in their goals?

CRITICAL JUDGEMENT QUESTIONS

1. You are a staff nurse, and you observe a health care professional coercing a client to agree to participate in a research study. What should you do in this situation?
   a. Contact the hospital's REB
   b. Confront the researcher with your concerns
   c. Document your suspicions in the client's medical record
   d. Secretly tape-record the researcher's interaction with the client

2. A woman newly diagnosed with breast cancer is asked to participate in a clinical trial for a new chemotherapy agent. Which of her human rights is protected by her freedom to choose whether or not to participate in the study?
   a. Right to fair treatment
   b. Right to self-determination
   c. Right to privacy and confidentiality
   d. Right to anonymity

3. Which of the following ethical principles is violated when a potential subject refuses to participate in a clinical study and, in response, the physician takes less time to answer this patient's questions than he does with other patients?
   a. Promoting Justice
   b. Promoting Health and Well-Being
   c. Maintaining Privacy and Confidentiality
   d. Preserving Dignity

KEY POINTS

- Ethical and legal considerations in research first received attention after World War II, during the Nuremberg trials, which resulted in the development of the Nuremberg Code. This code became the standard for research guidelines protecting the human rights of research participants.
- The U.S. National Research Act, passed in 1974, created the National Commission for the Protection of Human Subjects of Biomedical and Behavioral Research. The findings, contained in the Belmont Report (National Commission for the Protection of Human Subjects of Biomedical and Behavioral Research, 1978), are discussed with regard to the three basic ethical principles of respect for persons, beneficence, and justice that underlie the conduct of research involving human participants. U.S. federal regulations developed in response to the Commission's report provide guidelines for informed consent and REB protocols.

- Protection of human rights includes the rights to (1) self-determination, (2) privacy and dignity, (3) anonymity and confidentiality, (4) fair treatment, and (5) protection from discomfort and harm.
- Procedures for protecting basic human rights include obtaining informed consent, which illustrates the ethical principle of respect, and obtaining REB approval, which illustrates the ethical principles of respect, beneficence, and justice.
- Special consideration of ethics should be addressed in studies involving vulnerable populations, such as children, older adults, prisoners, and those who are mentally or physically disabled.
- Scientific fraud or misconduct represents unethical conduct, and professional responsibility must include monitoring for such conduct. Informal, ad hoc, or unauthorized research may expose patients to unwarranted risk and may not protect participants' rights adequately.
- Nurses who are asked to be involved in product testing should be aware of Health Canada guidelines and regulations for testing medical devices before becoming involved in product testing and, perhaps, violating guidelines for ethical research.
- Animal rights need to be protected, and regulations for animal research have evolved over time. Nurses who encounter the use of animals in research should be alert to their rights.
- As consumers of research, nurses must be knowledgeable about the legal and ethical components of a research study so that they can evaluate whether a researcher has ensured appropriate protection of human or animal rights.

📶 FOR FURTHER STUDY

Go to Evolve at http://evolve.elsevier.com/Canada/LoBiondo/Research for the Audio Glossary.

REFERENCES

Amdur, R., & Bankert, E. A. (2011). *Institutional review board: Member handbook* (3rd ed.). Boston: Jones & Bartlett.

American Nurses Association. (1985). *Code for nurses with interpretive statements*. Kansas City, MO: Author.

Benbow, S., Forchuk, C., Berman, H., Gorlick, C., & Ward-Griffin, C. (2019). Spaces of exclusion: Safety, stigma, and surveillance of mothers experiencing homelessness. *Canadian Journal of Nursing Research, 51*(3), 202–213. https://doi.org/10.1177/0844562119859138.

Benedict, S., & Georges, J. M. (2006). Nurses and the sterilization experiments of Auschwitz: A postmodernist perspective. *Nursing Inquiry, 13*, 277–288.

Brink, P. J. (1992). Autonomy versus do no harm. *Western Journal of Nursing Research, 14*, 264–266.

Canadian Council on Animal Care (CCAC) (2021). *About CCAC*. Retrieved from https://ccac.ca/en/standards/guidelines/.

Canadian Institutes of Health Research, Natural Sciences and Engineering Research Council of Canada, & Social Sciences and Humanities Research Council of Canada. (2018). Tri-Council policy statement: Ethical conduct for research involving humans - TCPS 2 (2018). Retrieved from https://ethics.gc.ca/eng/policy-politique_tcps2-eptc2_2018.html.

Canadian Nurses Association. (2002). Ethical research guidelines for registered nurses. Ottawa: Author.

Canadian Nurses Association. (2017). Code of ethics for registered nurses: 2017 edition. Ottawa: Author. Retrieved from https://www.cna-aiic.ca/~/media/cna/page-content/pdf-en/code-of-ethics-2017-edition-secure-interactive.

Carroll, M. L., & Ciaffa, J. (2003). The human genome project: A scientific and ethical overview. Retrieved from http://www.actionbioscience.org/genomics/carroll_ciaffa.html.

Charron, M. (2000). Ewen Cameron and the Allan Memorial Psychiatric Institute: A study in research and treatment ethics. Retrieved from http://www.illuminati-news.com/ewen-cameron.htm.

Collins, A. (1988). *In the sleep room: The story of the CIA brainwashing experiments in Canada*. Toronto: Lester & Orpen Dennys.

Currie, G., & Szabo, J. (2020). Social isolation and exclusion: the parents' experience of caring for children with rare neurodevelopmental disorders. *International Journal of Qualitative Studies on Health and Well-Being, 15*(1), Article 1725362. https://doi.org/10.1080/17482631.2020.1725362.

Dahlke, S., Davidson, S., Duarte Wisnesky, U., Kalogirou, M. R., Salyers, V., Pollard, C., Fox, M. T., Hunter, K. F., & Baumbusch, J. (2019). Student nurses' perceptions about older people. *International Journal of Nursing Education Scholarship* (1), Article 20190051. https://doi.org/10.1515/ijnes-2019-0051.

French, H. W. (1997, October 9). AIDS research in Africa: Juggling risks and hopes. *New York Times,* pp. A1, A12.

Gillmor, D. (1987). *I swear by Apollo: Dr. Ewen Cameron and the CIA-brainwashing experiments.* Montreal: Eden Press.

Goldsworthy, S., Patterson, J. D., Dobbs, M., Afzal, A., & Deboerin, S. (2019). How does simulation impact building competency and confidence in recognition and response to the adult and paediatric deteriorating patient among undergraduate nursing students? *Clinical Simulation in Nursing, 28*, 25–32, https://doi.org/10.1016/j.ecns.2018.12.001.

Gupta, A. (2013). Fraud and misconduct in clinical research: A concern. *Perspectives in Clinical Research, 4*(2), 144–147. https://doi .org/10.4103/2229 -3485.111800.

Halushka, V. University of Saskatchewan. (1965). 53 D.L.R. (2nd) 436, 52 W.W.R. 608 (Sask. CA).

Health Canada. (2019). ICH Guidance E6: Good clinical practice: Consolidated guideline. Ottawa: Health Products and Food Branch. Retrieved from https://www.canada.ca/en/health-canada/services /drugs-health-products/drug-products/applications -submissions/guidance-documents/international -conference-harmonisation/efficacy/good-clinical -practice-consolidated-guideline-topic.html.

Health Canada. (2019b). Requirements for informed consent documents. Retrieved from https://www.canada .ca/en/health-canada/services/science-research /science-advice-decision-making/research-ethics -board/requirements-informed-consent-documents .html.

Health Canada. (2020). Drugs and health products: Medical devices. Retrieved from https://www.canada .ca/en/health-canada/services/drugs-health-products /medical-devices.html.

Hershey, N., & Miller, R. D. (1976). *Human experimentation and the law.* Wheat Ridge, CO: Aspen Systems.

Hilts, P. J. (1995, March 9). Agency faults a UCLA study for suffering of mental patients. *New York Times,* pp. A1, A11.

International Council of Nurses (ICN). (2012). ICN Code of Ethics for Nurses. Retrieved from https://www.icn .ch/sites/default/files/inline-files/2012_ICN _Codeofethicsfornurses_%20eng.pdf.

Levine, R. J. (1979). Clarifying the concepts of research ethics. *Hastings Center Report, 93*(3), 21–26.

Levine, R. J. (1986). *Ethics and regulation of clinical research* (2nd ed.). Baltimore: Urban and Schwartzenberg.

McLean, P. (1996, November). Biomedical research and the law of informed consent. *Canadian Nurse, 92,* 49–50.

Milgram, S. (1963). Behavioral study of obedience. *Journal of Abnormal and Social Psychology, 67,* 371–378.

Mosby, I. (2013). Administering colonial science: Nutrition research and human biomedical experimentation in Aboriginal communities and residential schools, 1942–1952. *Histoire Sociale/Social History, 46*(1), 145–172. https://www.muse.jhu.edu /article/512043.

National Commission for the Protection of Human Subjects of Biomedical and Behavioral Research. (1978). *Belmont report: Ethical principles and guidelines for research involving human subjects* (DHEW Pub. No. [OS] 78-0012). Washington, DC: U.S. Government Printing Office.

Robb, I. H. (1900). *Nursing ethics: For hospital and private use.* Milwaukee, WI: GN Gaspar.

Rothman, D. J. (1982). Were Tuskegee and Willowbrook studies in nature? *Hastings Centre Report, 12*(2), 5–7.

Stewart, B., Cazzell, M. A., & Pearcy, T. (2019). Single-blinded randomized controlled study on use of interactive distraction versus oral Midazolam to reduce pediatric preoperative anxiety, emergence delirium, and postanesthesia length of stay. *Journal of PeriAnesthesia Nursing, 34*(3), 567–575.

Subedi, A., Edge, D. S., Goldie, C. L., & Sawhney, M. (2019). Resettled Bhutanese refugees in Ottawa: What coping strategies promote psychological well-being? *Canadian Journal of Nursing Research, 51*(3), 168–178. https://doi.org/10.1177/0844562119828905.

Wheeler, D. L. (1997). Three medical organizations embroiled in controversy over use of placebos in AIDS studies abroad. *Chronicle of Higher Education,* A15–A16.

Woodgate, R. L., Tailor, K., Tennent, P., Wener, P., & Altman, G. (2020). The experience of the self in Canadian youth living with anxiety: A qualitative study. *PLoS ONE, 15*(1): Article e0228193. https://doi.org/10.1371/journal.pone.0228193.

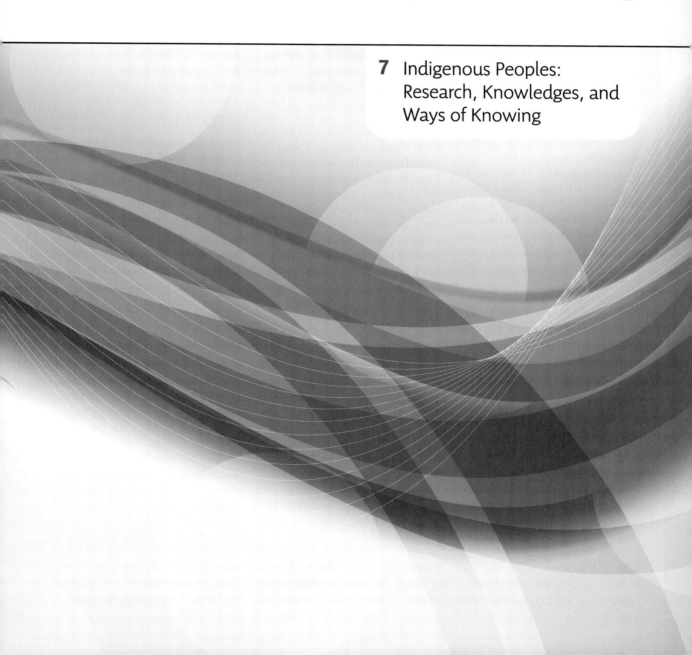

PART TWO

Indigenous Peoples: Research, Knowledges, and Ways of Knowing

RESEARCH **VIGNETTE**

An Interview With Dr. Evelyn Voyageur

Caroline Foster-Boucher & Evelyn Voyageur
Assistant Professor
Department Nursing Science
MacEwan University
Calgary, Alberta

WHAT IS YOUR BACKGROUND? HOW DID YOU BECOME INTERESTED IN NURSING?

I started my education late in life because I was in the Residential School (RS). We were not encouraged to stay in school then. Once we were in grade 8, or reached 16 years old, we were told to leave. We were taught the very basics, no academic subjects. So many of us never went beyond grade 8, and some did not even reach that grade if they reached 16 years old before that grade.

Something in my life happened that made me want to go further in school. So, I started doing correspondence. I studied at home for my grade 9 and 10. By this time, the government gave Indians permission to go further in school. I went to Victoria, B.C. to complete my grade 10, then took up practical nursing. I did very well in my studies, received a reward for top grades in grade 10, then another one when I graduated in LPN training for top bedside manner.

I faced some challenges while studying in BCIT (British Columbia Institute of Technology). The principal took me aside and said to me, "Evelyn, you have 2 strikes against you. One is that you have

to prove you can do this course to complete it and the other is your race. I have 2 great teachers, but they are racist." Luckily for me, there was a black lady in our class. The teachers picked on her and made her cry many times. I felt so sorry for her. We stuck together.

After working as an LPN, I knew I wanted to work with our people but needed to upgrade to be eligible to go do the RN training. I was convinced to do the RN training because I saw the need to be more vocal for the inequality for other races I now saw in the healthcare system. I had seen this inequality in the treatment of First Nations people when doctors and nurses visited our villages, but I did not think I had the right to say anything because I was not trained as a healthcare person. Now, I want to say more to help. Once more, I entered school to do my grades 11 and 12. I was accepted in Langara School of Nursing in 1975. I did well, never failed any exams, but was failed by a racist teacher. She failed me in my bedside manner, where I had been awarded for that in the LPN program.

A few months later, I saw an ad in a newspaper from Douglas College, challenging all LPNs to take a test to see if they qualify to take a year's training to become a RN. I took it and passed the test—one of the top 10. I graduated in 1978. I am ever so grateful to Douglas College for the opportunity to reach my goal—now I could work

towards getting into the First Nations Communities. I am so grateful for good, non-racist teachers at Douglas College.

I went to work in Northern Alberta. While working, I studied for my BScN, distance learning from the University of Victoria (UVIC). When I returned to B.C. to work in Native communities, I decided to go to school in UVIC. I had done three semesters by distance but was finding it took too long to complete my studies. So I took three semesters in UVIC to finish. I will explain the reason for continuing on with my education later.

WHAT ARE THE MOST IMPORTANT THINGS NURSING STUDENTS NEED TO KNOW ABOUT INDIGENOUS KNOWLEDGE AND RESEARCH WITH INDIGENOUS PEOPLES?

The students must know and understand that Indigenous knowledge is the way of being. These teachings are embedded in their lives since time immemorial. These knowledges are handed down, generation after generation, orally. For there was no written language in those days. These Indigenous knowledges are our laws and guide us to be a good person. They are our policies in our lives, but not like the western policies; these were to guide the people in their daily lives.

To do research with Indigenous people, researchers must come with respect, honesty, and patience. A demanding and controlling researcher will not be welcomed. Too many non-natives have come into our communities with disrespectful attitudes. In my own research with my people, I always say, "You will be helping me to be a better nurse by telling me what I can do for the community." This is a journey for the researcher and the researched to walk hand in hand.

When our team of researchers (students and faculty) is wanting to go to a community, we first of all meet to ask permission to come visit. Then we plan with the community what we should do while there, who to talk with, where to go visit. All these plans must be agreed upon with the community. No one should make the community, or a person, feel that they are not important in these interviews. We are all equal. Researchers are welcomed and treated with respect everywhere we have visited. Everyone participates in the journey, as stories are being heard.

WHAT DOES RESEARCH LOOK LIKE FOR YOU?

In the beginning, I did not like research, as a lot of First Nations people (FNP) did too. It was because FNP have been studied to death. So much studies are done on our people, but not often the truth. I have read many books about us, the Indigenous peoples, and have had many disappointments, because of the full story not being told. These books should be critiqued by a First Nations scholar before being published, to make sure it is the truth. On the other hand, there are more First Nation scholars doing research, using a cultural way as the methodology. It has taken a long time for these papers to come, but it is sad that they are not used in education. Research must be done by a researcher who truly knows themselves, their background, and their

history. In the Indigenous worldview, these were very important— the stories, beliefs, values, ceremonies, and philosophies. All are spiritual to the Indigenous people and must be respected.

As I do my research, I honour all that I hear and honour the interviewed person, and I openly ask questions when I am not sure about something. I am grateful that I have dealt with my own personal challenges, so I am able to work with all people I encounter. I know who I am, where I come from, my family history, my community, tribe, and clan. These are a must in our lives, so that we are connected to our inner selves. When I was doing my Master's in John Bastyr University in Seattle, one of my teachers said, "One of the 10 signs of a healthy person is knowing your history 4 generations back." Wow, I thought to myself, this is what our ancestors taught us, "always know who you are." So to me research is listening to the stories of the knowledge keepers of the Indigenous people. These knowledge keepers are not all old people either. Some knowledge keepers are very young, who have been schooled in the culture early in their lives. So to me research is a very basic level to establish, to maintain, and to nurture a respectful relationship amongst all involved persons.

WHAT ARE YOUR THOUGHTS ON THE EVIDENCE-INFORMED PRACTICE MOVEMENT?

I believe this looks good, but if all the research is based on written work, it's not acceptable. I was working in a community where TB testing was being done. One

older man tested positive. He refused prophylactic meds. He said, "I know what TB is. I've seen my sister and brother very sick with it, I don't have a cough and I am not sick. I drink our traditional herbs too. Evelyn, if I did feel ill, I would gladly take meds, to prevent my grandchildren from getting TB. But I know I am not sick." I relayed this to the doctor; his answer was: "But the drinks have not being scientifically proven." I argued with him that my people have used it for years and that no one died from TB until the Europeans came with their meds.

I've seen my mother, father, grandparents, and all older people use our herbs and they were healthy. Yes, our stories of how health was treated should be listened to, and be believed as evidence, proof of good use. To the western worldview, the traditional medicines are not accepted as evidence based, but to the Indigenous people, it is evidenced informed. My ancestors have informed many of us on the use of our traditional herbs.

WHAT ARE THE OPPORTUNITIES AND CHALLENGES FACED BY INDIGENOUS SCHOLARS?

The Indigenous scholar may be, or could be, the highest educated in an organization or institution, but overlooked in being hired over a non-native person who may be less qualified. There are not many Indigenous in top jobs. There is much discrimination in the world.

When doing their theses or dissertations, the institution readers of paper keep wanting them to change what they are writing about. I know some writers who have had to do their papers over and over again.

There are workshops done in educational institutions now to help the students understand what happened to Indigenous people during contact, such as Building Bridges, or Blanket exercises.

Some students now go to Indigenous villages to do some first hand learning—very beneficial for their studying. Having Indigenous instructors in the classes has helped too. I have been asked to read three (thesis) papers by universities to help them grade when it has been a paper on Indigenous topics, so that is an opportunity.

WHAT ARE THE THREE MOST IMPORTANT TOPICS FOR US TO COVER IN THIS CHAPTER?

This is where I will explain why I kept returning to school and why it is important to bring this to the attention of everyone who is working with people.

I was so elated, for I reached my goal, working with my own people, First Nations. I was very happy. I loved the work, but as time went on, I soon learned that I did not fully know the people I was serving. I began to ask many questions. Why are these people not prepared for emergencies, why don't they have bandages, why don't they have aspirins? You see, I had parents and grandparents who taught me all this. I was so puzzled. Then, one day a man said to me, "You know, Evelyn, we had no role models, positive that is, in the school. Yes, we all were in the RS, as our parents and grandparents. We had never seen our parents raise our younger brothers or sisters. That is why

we don't know to look after each other." It made me think, I need to take more classes in how to understand the why's of the many lacks. I asked my boss, Medical Services, to send me to workshops on relationships, how to work with addicts. That is what most of the people were addicted to, drugs, alcohol, or gambling. I went to Nechi, a 25-day training, to understand addicts. The first 10 days was basic counselling, the next 10 days was advanced counselling, and last 5 days was personal growth. This was healing of our own pain. I had denied being abused in the RS because I was not sexually or physically abused. But it surfaced that I was emotionally and spiritually abused. For I was snatched from the safe haven of my parents' home into a place that did not nurture us at all. I shed many tears and let go of my pain. I returned to work a better person, a more empathetic, good listener, non-judgemental nurse, a better person. All that I learned about the traumas of the clients, I now understood where it all originated from: the loss of identity, voice, and choice in the schools.

Their behaviours now are the defense mechanism to their traumas. I know the reasons why there were differences from my family. None of my family went to RS, whereas these people have been affected for five to seven generations. Now they have systemic behaviours. It was my own openness to my healing that helped to understand and do a better job. So knowing self and being healed are the key to fully understanding clients. I continued on to do my PhD. Even though I have learned a lot about

understanding FNP, I was hungry to learn more. While researching my dissertation, "*Loss of Identity Through Colonization, Christianity, Oppression; Who Am I?*" (Voyageur, 2020), I interviewed many people and learned more. I now understand them more, give them choices, and how to help themselves. That is why I continued to study, to learn more about working with the clients more effectively.

This leads to cultural safety—knowing self. Cultural safety *must be learned experientially*, not just from books or online. When you are culturally safe, you will feel you belong, no matter where you work. When doing cultural safety, let yourself really hear, see, and feel; let yourself be a human being. Only when you are real with yourself can you begin to find the right path to be successful in relationship with the people who need help. If this is not done experientially, only your head talks or hears; the heart and mind are not going to do the walk.

Despite going to St. Michael's Residential School at age 10, Dr. Evelyn Voyageur is a fluent speaker of Kwak'wala and an active matriarch in the Kwakwaka'wakw culture and traditions. She has dedicated her life to improving the health of Indigenous peoples through her more than five decades in the nursing profession.

A leader in the transformation of Indigenous healthcare, Elder Voyageur is bringing back the holistic way of looking at health in First Nations communities by integrating spiritual, emotional, physical, and mental health in her work. She has co-authored a number of publications on cultural safety and nursing, sharing her knowledge with generations of nurses to come. She was instrumental in the development of A'eka-lixl, a community-led health initiative where culture is the foundation of wellness in Wuikinuxv First Nation and D'zawada'enuxv First Nation.

From 1999 to 2003, Elder Voyageur worked with the Indian Residential School Society, where she supported survivors healing from the trauma they experienced.

At North Island College, Dr. Voyageur has worked to make changes to the nursing curriculum and help bring cultural awareness to the program. (Indspire, 2020, Dr. Evelyn Voyageur) ▨

REFERENCES

Indspire (2020). Dr. Evelyn Voyageur. *https://indspire.ca/laureate/dr-evelyn-voyageur/*.

Voyageur, E. (2002). *Loss of Identity Through Colonization, Christianity, Oppression; Who Am I?* (dissertation): University of Stratford.

CHAPTER 7

Indigenous Peoples: Research, Knowledges, and Ways of Knowing

Caroline Foster-Boucher | Lorraine Thirsk

LEARNING OUTCOMES

After reading this chapter, you will be able to do the following:

- Develop a beginning understanding of the history of First Nations, Inuit, and Métis peoples.
- Identify the effects of Canadian government policies that led to systemic racism and cultural genocide.
- Understand the history of colonization in research related to Indigenous peoples in Canada.
- Understand the application of the Royal Commission on Aboriginal Peoples and the Truth and Reconciliation Commission's recommendations for research with Indigenous peoples.
- Recognize the influence of privileging a Western research paradigm.
- Recognize the validity and history of Indigenous ways of knowing.
- Identify ways in which Indigenous and Western knowledge can be integrated.
- Understand ethical principles of research with Indigenous peoples.
- Understand the importance of Indigenous research paradigms.
- Identify key aspects of Indigenous research methodologies.
- Identify further resources and practical tips for research with First Nations, Inuit, and Métis peoples.

KEY TERMS

Assimilation
Colonization
Decolonization
First Nations
Inuit

Indigenous peoples
Indigenous research
   paradigm
Indigenous methodologies
Indigenous knowledge

Métis
Sixties scoop
Systemic racism
Truth and Reconciliation
   Commission (TRC)

STUDY RESOURCES

Go to Evolve at http://evolve.elsevier.com/Canada/LoBiondo/Research for the Audio Glossary.

THE VERY ACTIVITY OF WRITING THIS chapter in a textbook reflects a knowledge tradition based on a Western, institutionalized, academic paradigm. It places a value on the written word over oral traditions (Kirkness & Barnhardt, 1991), a domination of European knowledge development, history, and the power of "experts" who are granted the privilege of writing this chapter to convey this knowledge to students. Yet in a spirit of reconciliation, this is our opportunity to explore and share the history, context, and relationships of Indigenous and Western knowledge in a format that recognizes the problems with privileging only a Western paradigm, as well as the potential for integration of two worldviews.

This chapter will provide you with an important opportunity to learn more about Indigenous knowledge and research by/ with **Indigenous peoples**. A brief history of **First Nations, Inuit, and Métis** peoples is provided; however, it is imperative that your understanding of the history, context, and outcomes of **colonization** go beyond what is covered in this chapter. We have included a list of additional recommended readings and resources at the end of the chapter (Box 7.1). The main focus of this chapter will be to increase understanding of Indigenous knowledge and worldviews; to understand the privileging of Western knowledge in research and academic institutions; and to gain awareness of how research has perpetuated inequality and racism, inaccurately representing Indigenous peoples and cultures while very often not benefitting Indigenous peoples. In understanding this context, it is then possible to appreciate **Indigenous research paradigms and methodologies**, be aware of ethical principles and values in research with Indigenous communities, and understand the role of research in reconciliation. Lastly, we provide you with some practical strategies to consider when beginning to work with Indigenous peoples

BOX 7.1

SEMINAL AND SUGGESTED READINGS/ RESOURCES

Brown, L. A., & Strega, S. (Eds.). (2005). *Research as resistance: Critical, indigenous and anti-oppressive approaches*. Toronto, ON: Canadian Scholars' Press.

Canadian Institutes of Health Research, Natural Sciences and Engineering Research Council of Canada, & Social Sciences and Humanities Research Council of Canada. (2018). *Tri-Council Policy Statement: Ethical Conduct for Research Involving Humans*. www.pre .ethics.gc.ca.

Kirkness, V. J., & Barnhardt, R. (1991). First Nations and Higher Education: The Four R's–Respect, Relevance, Reciprocity, Responsibility. *Journal of American Indian Education, 30*(3), 1–15.

Kovach, M. (2009). *Indigenous methodologies: Characteristics, conversations, and contexts*. Toronto, ON: University of Toronto Press, Scholarly Publishing Division.

MacDonald, C., & Steenbeek, A. (2015). The Impact of colonization and Western assimilation on health and wellbeing of Canadian Aboriginal people. *International Journal of Regional and Local History, 10*(1), 32–48.

Tuhiwai Smith, L. (2012). *Decolonizing methodologies: Research and indigenous peoples* (2nd ed). London: Zed Books Ltd.

United Nations. (2007). *United Nations declaration on the rights of Indigenous peoples*. Https://www .un.org/development/desa/indigenouspeoples/wp -content/uploads/sites/19/2018/11/UNDRIP_E_web.pdf.

University of Alberta. (2020). *Indigenous Canada* [Open Online Course]. https://www.ualberta.ca/ admissions-programs/online-courses/indigenous-canada/index.html.

Wilson, S. (2001). What is an Indigenous research methodology? *Canadian Journal Of Native Education, 25*(2), 175–179.

and tools for critical appraisal that are specific to research with Indigenous peoples and communities.

Evidence-Informed Practice Tip

One of the foundational concepts to keep in mind when learning about Indigenous peoples is that this term represents numerous cultures, and not a single population. While there are some similarities amongst Indigenous peoples, there are also many differences. This will be reflected in worldviews, values, ceremonies, and knowledge.

Practical Application

Establishing oneself in relationship to research, knowledge, the land, and its inhabitants is fundamental to an Indigenous worldview (Kovach, 2009). "Knowing the researcher's location allows others to assess the researchers' credibility, and thus the validity of the research" (Johnston et al., 2018, p. 11). As authors of this chapter, we believed it was important and congruent with the spirit of reconciliation to present our location to people and lands.

I (CFB) was born in Edmonton, Alberta on Treaty Six Territory, to a Dene woman from Fort Chipewyan Alberta. My birth father was from a settler family of Norwegian, Scottish, and Irish heritage. My mother was also a residential school survivor and disappeared shortly after my birth, becoming one of the Missing and Murdered Indigenous Women in Canada. I was adopted by a British family who had recently moved to Canada and was raised in Edmonton generally in a British household. I am therefore a **Sixties Scoop** survivor as I did not have my Dene language, or culture. I started to learn about Cree culture in my twenties, attending ceremonies and other gatherings, found my birth family when I was in my thirties, and began to get to know Fort Chipewyan and surrounding area. I live in Edmonton currently and recognize that I am a settler on these lands, as well as an Indigenous traveller. My birth family's traditional homelands are in northeastern Alberta in Treaty Eight territory. I am grateful for the opportunities I have had in living in Treaty Six territory in many aspects of my life including education, housing, recreation, and the relationships I have with Indigenous peoples in this area who have shared their cultural teachings and practices with me. My main interest in nursing is in Indigenous health and the relationship between Indigenous peoples and non-Indigenous peoples in Canada, as well as post-colonialism and decolonization.

I (LT) was born in a rural area in Alberta, on Treaty 6 territory, traditional lands for First Nations and Métis. My father's family were English and Swiss immigrants who moved, four generations ago, to the Battle River area to farm and operate a store in the late 19th century. My great-great-grandfathers would likely have known two nearby Métis settlements/wintering sites near Dried Meat Hill/Lake and Buffalo Lake. On my mother's side, I am a third-generation immigrant with a grandfather that was born in Scotland and a grandmother born in Wales. Both immigrated to Calgary/Treaty 7 territory as children in the 1910s. They lived in the growing city of Calgary, where my mother was also born. I grew up within a Western European, Christian, rural, agricultural community and culture. Both of my parents completed university degrees, and I am grateful for the opportunities that education has provided me. I married a first-generation immigrant from Norway, and we are currently living and working in Edmonton/Treaty 6 territory. Over my nursing career I have seen firsthand the health inequities that are faced by Indigenous peoples including increased disease burden and lack of equitable access to health services. I have also met several Indigenous scholars and learned about their lives and work. I felt compelled to contribute towards reconciliation by advocating for the inclusion of an Indigenous chapter in this textbook and supporting the writing of this section of the book. It has been a significant learning opportunity that will shape my nursing practice.

HISTORY AND CONTEXT OF INDIGENOUS PEOPLES[1]

The three Indigenous groups—First Nations, Métis, and Inuit—have their own unique languages, heritages, cultural practices, and spiritual beliefs (Indigenous and Northern Affairs Canada, [INAC], 2016a). These groups contain many subgroups, each with its own unique culture. In the last census, 1,673,785 people self-identified as Indigenous, accounting for 4.9% of the total population of Canada (Statistics Canada, 2016a).

Between 2006 and 2016, the Indigenous population grew by 42.5%—more than four times faster than the increase for the non-Indigenous population (Statistics Canada, 2016a). In 2016, 55.8% of Indigenous peoples lived in urban areas; this proportion increased from 49% in 1996 (National Collaborating Centre of Aboriginal Health [NCCAH], 2013; Statistics Canada, 2016a). Furthermore, the Indigenous population is, on average, younger than the non-Indigenous population. About one-third of First Nations and Inuit people are aged 14 and younger, in comparison to 16.4% of the non-Indigenous population (Statistics Canada, 2016a). For Métis, 22.3% of the population is aged 14 or younger.

---

[1]This section is adapted from Barton, S., & Foster-Boucher, C. (2019). Indigenous health. In Fundamentals of nursing (6th ed., pp. 133–153). Elsevier.

Definitions and Identities

The legal term *Indian* describes all the Indigenous peoples in Canada who are not Inuit. This includes the nations or groups of people who were originally living in Canada before the European explorers began to arrive in the 1600s (pre-contact), and the Métis, who are a specific cultural entity formed after contact with Europeans (post-contact) and before colonization. Legal definitions used to describe Indians in Canada include Status, non-Status, and Treaty Indians. Status Indians are registered under the Indian Act (INAC, 2013a), which regulates the management of reserves and sets out certain federal obligations. A Treaty Indian is a Status Indian who belongs to a First Nation that signed a treaty with the Crown (INAC, 2013a). The term *First Nation/s* refers to a person or a group of First Nations people legally known as an Indian band (INAC, 2013a). Currently there are 634 First Nations or Indian bands in Canada.

Until recently, non-Status Indians and Métis peoples were not included as Indians under Section 91(24) of the Constitution Act. However, in 1999, four claimants brought legal action against the Canadian federal government, seeking a declaration that Métis and non-Status Indians fall within federal jurisdiction. This would mean that Métis and non-Status Indians have the right to be consulted by, and to negotiate with, the federal government over needs, rights, and interests as Indigenous peoples. In 2016, the Supreme Court of Canada, in what is now known as the "Daniels Decision" (Daniels v. Canada [Indian Affairs and Northern Development]), sided in favour of non-Status Indians and Métis as being "Indian" under S.91(24) of the Constitution Act. Currently, the federal government is closely examining this ruling to determine its meaning in terms of legislative authority (INAC, 2017; Supreme Court of Canada, 2016).

The Inuit have inhabited northern Canada for over 5,000 years. In 2016, there were 62,025 Inuit, which comprise 3.9% of the Indigenous population and 0.2% of the Canadian population (Statistics Canada, 2016b). Almost three-quarters of Inuit live in the northern part of Canada, in four territories (Inuit Nunangat) that were negotiated in land claim agreements with the federal government (Penny et al., 2012; Statistics Canada, 2013). The four areas of Inuit Nunangat include Nunatsiavut (Northern Labrador), Nunavik (Northern Quebec), the Territory of Nunavut, and the Inuvialuit Settlement Region (Northwest Territories) (Penny et al., 2012). Each of the four regions has its own flag and history, as well as distinct geography and regional experiences of the people (Inuit Tapiriit Kanatami, 2018).

The Inuit were traditionally hunters and gatherers who, for more than four centuries, experienced regular appearances from outsiders such as traders, whalers, explorers, and scientists (Inuit Tapiriit Kanatami, 2004; Wright, 2014). The Inuit have used oral storytelling to ensure continuity of information about their history from generation to generation (Inuit Tapiriit Kanatami, 2004). Inuit ancestors, the Sivullirmiut and the Thule people, moved from the Bering Strait eastward and south across northern Canada over a period of about 1,000 years, hunting, fishing, and making tools that are found today by archeologists. Arctic exploration by Europeans started in the 1500s, and by the 1800s, Inuit culture was being affected by European whalers. Missionaries started schools in the early 1900s, and the Royal Canadian Mounted Police (RCMP) soon followed to 'protect' (p. 13) northern biological resources and examine territorial sovereignty (Inuit Tapiriit Kanatami, 2004). Since the 1950s, several other events have impacted Inuit culture, including relocations of groups into completely different regions, the mass killing of sled dogs by the Canadian Government, the removal of Inuit children from families, and the separation of families for medical care in the south (Qikiqtani Inuit Association, 2014; Wright, 2014).Currently climate change is a crisis that is impacting severely the way of life for Inuit peoples (Wright, 2014).

The Métis have been noted as a distinct Indigenous group in Canada, born from the union of Indigenous women and European men during the fur trade era, post-contact but precolonially (Métis National Council, 2020). There was a gradual establishment of Métis communities, the ancestral Métis homelands, distinct from either Indigenous or settler communities. These communities gradually formed a culture of their own, with cultural aspects including the language Michif, the red river cart, the Métis sash, fiddler music and a specific dance style known as jigging (Métis Nation British Columbia, n.d.; Métis Nation of Alberta, n.d.; Métis Nation of Saskatchewan, n.d.; Métis Nation of Manitoba, n.d.; Métis Nation of Ontario, n.d.; Métis National Council, 2020). According to a number of scholars and the main Métis political groups in Ontario, British Columbia and the Canadian prairie provinces, the Métis are a distinct people; in order to be identified as Métis, one must self-identify as such; be descended from the historic Métis who lived in ancestral Métis homelands; and be accepted by the Métis Nation (Métis National Council, 2020). Métis homelands include "the three prairie provinces, and extend[ing] into Ontario, British Columbia, the Northwest Territories and the Northern United States" (Métis National Council, 2020) used and occupied by the Métis (Métis Nation of Alberta, 2017; Province of Alberta, 2015).

Métis understand themselves to be descended from families who lived in the historic homelands of the Métis and who received land scrip or land grants under the Manitoba Act of Dominion Lands Act in 1876. Currently 5,054 Métis live on eight provincial constitutionally protected settlements in Alberta, which are the only lands set aside for the Métis (Government of Alberta, 2020; Métis Settlements General Council, n.d.). In 2016, The Manitoba Métis Federation signed an agreement with the federal government to negotiate a land claim based on the 1870 Manitoba Act in which the Métis were promised land never received (Malone, 2016). The Métis have suffered great inequity and social exclusion from Canadian society, in part due to land dispossession through scrip and unresolved land claims. Currently, accurate statistics about the health of the Métis are minimal, owing to issues related to identity and misunderstood identity, interpretation of statistics, and other political pressures that influence defining who is Métis and how the data are gathered and interpreted (Andersen, 2016; Leroux & Gaudry, 2017).

More than 70 Indigenous languages in 12 different language families are still spoken in Canada, with Algonquian being the largest and most widespread language family (Statistics Canada, 2016a). Many Indigenous languages have identifiable dialects; however, some are in decline, and many are endangered, owing to the history of **assimilation** policies carried out by the Canadian government, such as residential schooling. Language shapes the way people think about and interact with the world around them. Much cultural knowledge and history is contained within language and therefore it is an important aspect of Indigenous knowledges (Tuhiwai Smith, 2012).

The Indigenous peoples of Canada are exceptionally diverse—culturally, linguistically, socially, economically, and historically—as well as in many other ways. There are distinct cultural differences between the Indigenous groups, derived from history and geographic influences on day-to-day life. The diversity of Indigenous peoples exists within Indian bands or First Nations across Canada (Assembly of First Nations, n.d.), among the Métis, and where differences emanate from particular historical experiences and geographic locations of the Inuit (Pauktuutit Inuit Women of Canada, 2006).

Indigenous people vary in what they prefer to be called. Common terms include *Indigenous*, *Aboriginal*, *First Nations/Inuit/Métis*, or a specific term in their own language, such as *Nehiyawak* for Cree people. Inuit means "the people," and the singular term is *Inuk* (preferred term when describing a group; Inuk refers to a single person [Wilson, 2018]). It is best to ask each person how they would like to be referred to. For the purposes of this chapter, we use the term *Indigenous peoples* to include First Nations, Inuit, and Métis of Canada. We may also use the term *Aboriginal peoples* if that was the term presented in the original reference documents.

Indigenous History in Canada and Colonization

Working with Indigenous peoples in research requires a deep understanding of the historical, social, and economic contexts in which Indigenous families and communities are situated. An appreciation of Indigenous history requires a knowledge of the history of colonization that includes pre-European and post-European contact. Pre-European contact refers to the history of Indigenous peoples before exploration and settlement of the Americas by Europeans. During that period, Indigenous peoples were composed of distinct cultures from the Arctic, Western Subarctic, Eastern Subarctic, Northeastern Woodlands, Plains, Plateau, and Northwest Coast.

The Indian Act was first passed in 1876 and has been amended a number of times since. Its main purpose was to assimilate First Nations people into Canadian society. It sets out federal obligations toward "Indians" and regulates the management of reserves, money, and other resources for "Indians."

Colonialism is a theoretical framework for understanding the complexities of the relationship that evolved between Indigenous peoples and Europeans as they came into contact and as they later sustained those initial relationships in building a new reality in North America. Specifically, colonialism is the development of institutions and policies by European imperial and Euro-American settler governments toward Indigenous peoples (Truth and Reconciliation Commission [TRC], 2015b, p. 43-50). There

are several categories of colonialism including **settler colonialism**, as experienced in the Americas, New Zealand, and Australia. Settler colonialism occurs when the colonizers become the dominant society—the colonizers' intent is to displace the original population with a new society (LeFevre, 2015).

In Canada, as well as elsewhere in the world, experiences of colonialism resulted in much **historical trauma** (the nature of trauma as experienced over many years) and **systemic racism** for Indigenous people. European contact began in the Eastern Arctic, where Norse made contact initially with Inuit starting in 1000 BC and continuing throughout the centuries. French explorers and fur traders settled on the lower east coast and introduced diseases such as smallpox, tuberculosis (TB), and measles, which killed tens (and perhaps hundreds) of thousands of Indigenous people. Scarce resources diminished Indigenous livelihoods, and malnutrition, starvation, and alcohol consumption made circumstances worse (Dickason & Newbigging, 2015; Waldram et al., 2006).

During post-European contact, Europeans established relationships with Indigenous people and colonization influenced Indigenous systems of government, trade, and health care. Over the years, the Canadian government displaced Indigenous people from their traditional lands and developed policies to isolate and assimilate them into Canadian society, which resulted in the destruction of Indigenous cultures. These oppressive and suppressive policies and the acts that followed had extensive negative effects on Indigenous cultural identities and governance structures (TRC, 2015c, p. 3-4). The Indian residential school system, for example, which no longer exists in Canada, left a legacy over several generations resulting in physical and psychological abuse that "is reflected in the significant educational, income, health and social disparities between Aboriginal people and other Canadians" (TRC, 2015b, p. 135).

Residential Schools

Residential schools and associated policies were a central element in colonial practices in Canada, wherein Indigenous children as young as 5 years old were separated from their parents, in many cases forcibly. The children were sent to residential schools to board year-round, in order to sever the link between identity and culture. This was part of a policy to eliminate Indigenous people as a distinct group and to assimilate them into mainstream Canadian society. The ulterior motive was to avoid the legal and financial obligations that the federal government had with Indigenous people, as well as to gain control over their lands and resources, thereby eliminating treaties, reserves, and Indigenous rights (TRC, 2015b, p. 3).

The government of Canada funded churches that included Roman Catholic, Anglican, United, Methodist, and Presbyterian to operate at least 139 residential schools beginning in the 1880s, the last one closing in 1996 (TRC, 2015b, p. 3) At least 150,000 Indigenous children attended these schools over approximately 130 years, in poorly built and maintained buildings, with limited numbers of inadequately trained staff. There was minimal and weakly enforced regulation. The children were harshly disciplined and were forbidden to speak their language or practise any part of their own culture, including spirituality. They received a rudimentary education and were often forced to engage in chores to maintain the schools' operations. At least 3,200 children are estimated to have died from malnourishment, diseases such as TB, and abuse, as well as those who ran away and died from accidents or freezing to death. The number of children who died could be 5 to 10 times higher; however, given poor record-keeping, the full number may never be known (Mas, 2015; TRC, 2015a). In many cases, the schools did not record the name or gender of the children who died and generally did not send the child's body back to their home community to be buried (TRC, 2016a, p. 118; TRC, 2015b, p. 100). Physical and sexual abuse were rampant throughout the schools (TRC, 2015b, p. 105-110) and usually went unreported. If abuse was reported, little was done other than moving the perpetrator to another school or having the person resign. Few police investigations occurred, and prosecutions were rare.

The legacy of residential schools, one of the longest-lasting effects of colonialism, has had devastating consequences for Indigenous communities across Canada. Students who stayed at residential schools became institutionalized, disconnected from their language and culture, and had no experience of being parented. Because of their institutional upbringing, they were unable to learn how to parent; no such lessons were taught, and no such family interactions existed. The children and grandchildren of residential school survivors tell of growing up in abusive homes, with minimal affection and severe strictness and discipline—experiences similar to what the survivors experienced in residential school (Elias et al., 2012; TRC, 2015c, p. 11-12, 32-33). This is now understood as intergenerational trauma. **Intergenerational trauma** is defined as the pathways by which the nature of trauma is understood and experienced by "Aboriginal survivors of the residential school system and their descendants" as well as "the pathways by which this trauma is transmitted from one generation to the next" (Aguiar & Halseth, 2015, p. 23). Suicide rates are much higher among children and grandchildren of survivors than for survivors themselves. Some survivors turned to alcohol and other substances to cope with post-traumatic stress disorder; the effects of addiction have had a stronghold on some families and communities for decades (Ross et al., 2015; TRC, 2015c). Diets have been poor as a result of minimal knowledge of nutrition and of food pattern issues derived from residential schools. Sexual abuse is rampant in some communities, as evidenced by recent reports (Elias et al., 2012; Kirkup & Ubelacker, 2016; TRC, 2015c, p. 70).

The government of Canada has failed in its assimilation goal, with Indigenous people surviving the atrocities of residential schools. However, the legacy of residential schools is still reflected in the significant health, educational, and income disparities between Indigenous people and other Canadians (TRC, 2015d). Furthermore, intergenerational trauma is rampant, with some children who were abused becoming abusers, developing addictions as a way of coping, and being unable to parent their own children because of lack of experience of being parented (Menzies, 2008; Barker et al., 2019).

Truth and Reconciliation

In the 1960s, with the onset of the assertion of Indigenous rights globally, the Civil Rights Movement in the United States, and the Catholic social justice movement that came to be known as liberation theology, churches began to examine their relationship with Indigenous peoples in Canada (TRC, 2015d). A number of churches apologized in the 1970s, 1980s, and 1990s for their treatment of, and the impact of their work on, Indigenous peoples in Canada (TRC, 2015d).

From the 1970s through the 1990s, residential school survivors wrote memoirs, accounts, and histories of their experiences. During this time, the Royal Commission on Aboriginal Peoples (RCAP, 1996) was established to study the evolution of the relationship among Aboriginal peoples, the government of Canada, and Canadian society as a whole. The final report was released in 1996, in which a full chapter was dedicated to residential schools. In response to RCAP, the federal government issued an action plan that included an apology and a healing fund entitled the *Aboriginal Healing Foundation* (AHF) (TRC, 2015d, p. 551-579).

Residential school survivors, however, organized into associations and by 2005, more than 18,000 residential school survivors had filed lawsuits against the churches, the federal government, and other organizations involved as well as individuals who had committed the abuses. As a result of the staggering number of civil court cases and complex litigation, increasing costs, and the crippling effect on churches, the federal government created the Office of Indian Residential Schools Resolution (OIRSR) who after negotiations, launched the National Resolution Framework, which was ineffective. In the early 2000s, over 20 class action lawsuits were filed against the federal government. Eventually Indigenous organizations, church organizations, and the federal government began talks that would lead to the Indian Residential Schools Settlement Agreement (TRC, 2015d).

There were five main components of Truth and Reconciliation, of which the **Truth and Reconciliation Commission (TRC)** was one. These included the Common Experience Payment (CEP), in which all who had resided at a residential school would be eligible for financial compensation (TRC, 2015d). There was also an independent assessment process available for those who had suffered abuse or neglect who would be eligible for more financial compensation; $20 million was set aside for commemoration initiatives and $125 million was set aside for the AHF to address the healing needs of Aboriginal people affected. The Anglican, Presbyterian, United, and Catholic churches all contributed funds (TRC, 2015d).

This agreement only covered Aboriginal people within the series of lawsuits, and the list of schools was limited to those with a residential component. It did not address the claims of Métis students, or a number of other situations and places, such as day schools (TRC, 2015d). There continue to be issues still being dealt with today.

In 2008, Prime Minister Stephen Harper issued a national apology in Parliament to Indigenous peoples in Canada. Then, government opposition party leaders issued their own apologies and Indigenous leaders such as Assembly of First Nations National Chief Phil Fontaine, Mary Simon, President of the Inuit Tapiriit Kanatami, and various others responded to the apologies (TRC, 2015d).

The TRC issued its final report in 2015. It comprises 10 books, or volumes, of information covering the full history, from early European imperialism to the year 2000; the final report includes survivors' stories and documentation of Inuit and Métis experiences, missing children and unmarked burials, and the legacy of residential schools. The TRC found that many of the 150,000 children who attended residential school were abused sexually, physically, emotionally, and spiritually. The TRC also stated that Canada was guilty of **cultural genocide** with respect to Indigenous people in Canada, which is the "destruction of those structures and practices that allow the group to continue as a group" (TRC, 2015a, p. 3). Instances of destruction of practices and structures included occupying and seizing land; forcing relocation of Indigenous peoples; confining them to reserves; disempowering them through replacement of existing forms of Indigenous government; and denying them basic rights, such as the right to practise their faith, the right to assemble, and the right to legal counsel.

The TRC released 94 Calls to Action to address the ongoing legacy of residential schools in Canada for Indigenous peoples. These Calls to Action address policy as well as institutional and governmental structures within Canada, such as child welfare, justice, education, language rights, government Indigenous funding programs, and health care. To help enact such actions, the TRC encourages citizens to become settler allies—teachers and learners who question how non-Indigenous people can change, as opposed to just Indigenous people changing. In addition, Calls to Action were directed at the government to take steps to improve its policies and funding practices for a variety of aspects within the Indigenous realm, such as commencement of the inquiry into missing and murdered Indigenous women in Canada and adoption of the United Nations *Declaration on the Rights of Indigenous Peoples* (TRC, 2015c). There are several Calls to Action from the TRC that are important and relevant to health, nursing, and research (Box 7.2).

IMPLICATIONS FOR RECONCILIATION AND RESEARCH

The overview of Canada's history with Indigenous peoples is the basis for your appreciation of research with Indigenous peoples and Indigenous ways of knowing. Moreover, it provides a background to consider the implications for research ethics and research processes. In this section we focus on how colonization has led to Indigenous people's general skepticism of research as well as the work towards reconciliation. Around the world, research has been used by Europeans for colonization purposes (Tuhiwai Smith, 1999). The historical privileging of Western European knowledge systematically discounted Indigenous knowledge, which relied on oral traditions (Kirkness & Branhardt, 1991). This resulted in research that was not only unhelpful to Indigenous peoples but moreover was often unethical and harmful (Tuhiwai Smith, 2012). Indigenous communities and peoples have been "researched to death" (Brant-Castellano, 2004) with methods and outcomes that perpetuated racism and inequity and benefited mostly non-Indigenous people and institutions (Tuhiwai Smith, 2012). The current Tri-Council Policy Statement explains (Canadian Institute of Health Research [CIHR] et al., 2018):

> Research involving Indigenous peoples in Canada has been defined and carried out primarily by non-Indigenous researchers. The approaches used have not generally reflected Indigenous worldviews, and the research has not necessarily benefited Indigenous peoples or communities. As a result, Indigenous peoples continue to regard research, particularly research originating outside their communities, with a certain apprehension or mistrust. (p. 107)

Research has a poor reputation among Indigenous peoples in Canada with a widespread lack of trust and resistance to research (Assembly of First Nations [AFN], 2009). For decades, research involving Indigenous peoples was executed in ways that were harmful, disrespectful, and destructive to lives and communities (Tuhiwai Smith,

BOX **7.2**

TRUTH AND RECONCILIATION COMMISSION RECOMMENDATIONS

CALLS TO ACTION REGARDING HEALTH:

18. We call upon the federal, provincial, territorial, and Aboriginal governments to acknowledge that the current state of Aboriginal health in Canada is a direct result of previous Canadian government policies, including residential schools, and to recognize and implement the health-care rights of Aboriginal people as identified in international law, constitutional law, and under the Treaties.

19. We call upon the federal government, in consultation with Aboriginal peoples, to establish measurable goals to identify and close the gaps in health outcomes between Aboriginal and non-Aboriginal communities, and to publish annual progress reports and assess long term trends. Such efforts would focus on indicators such as: infant mortality, maternal health, suicide, mental health, addictions, life expectancy, birth rates, infant and child health issues, chronic diseases, illness and injury incidence, and the availability of appropriate health services.

20. In order to address the jurisdictional disputes concerning Aboriginal people who do not reside on reserves, we call upon the federal government to recognize, respect, and address the distinct health needs of the Métis, Inuit, and off-reserve Aboriginal peoples.

21. We call upon the federal government to provide sustainable funding for existing and new Aboriginal healing centres to address the physical, mental, emotional, and spiritual harms caused by residential schools, and to ensure that the funding of healing centres in Nunavut and the Northwest Territories is a priority.

22. We call upon those who can effect change within the Canadian health-care system to recognize the value of Aboriginal healing practices and use them in the treatment of Aboriginal patients in collaboration with Aboriginal healers and Elders where requested by Aboriginal patients.

23. We call upon all levels of government to: i. Increase the number of Aboriginal professionals working in the health-care field. ii. Ensure the retention of Aboriginal health-care providers in Aboriginal communities. iii. Provide cultural competency training for all healthcare professionals.

24. We call upon medical and nursing schools in Canada to require all students to take a course dealing with Aboriginal health issues, including the history and legacy of residential schools, the United Nations Declaration on the Rights of Indigenous Peoples, Treaties and Aboriginal rights, and Indigenous teachings and practices. This will require skills-based training in intercultural competency, conflict resolution, human rights, and anti-racism.

CALLS TO ACTION REGARDING RESEARCH:

65. We call upon the federal government, through the Social Sciences and Humanities Research Council, and in collaboration with Aboriginal peoples, post-secondary institutions and educators, and the National Centre for Truth and Reconciliation and its partner institutions, to establish a national research program with multi-year funding to advance understanding of reconciliation.

78. We call upon the Government of Canada to commit to making a funding contribution of $10 million over seven years to the National Centre for Truth and Reconciliation, plus an additional amount to assist communities to research and produce histories of their own residential school experience and their involvement in truth, healing, and reconciliation.

From: Truth and Reconciliation Commission of Canada. (2015e). *Truth and reconciliation commission of Canada: Calls to action.* Retrieved from http://trc.ca /assets/pdf/Calls_to_Action_English2.pdf.

2012). Indigenous peoples were used as "subjects" often without their consent or knowledge (see, for example, Mosby, 2013). There was a lack of cultural safety for Indigenous peoples, a paucity of respectful relationships made with Indigenous peoples, and a disregard of research concerns and needs of Indigenous peoples (AFN, 2009). There are numerous examples to draw from to illustrate the challenges Indigenous peoples have had with research and researchers in their communities.

In the 1940s, medical experiments were carried out on Cree communities in northern Manitoba without knowledge or consent from the research subjects (Mosby, 2013). The experiments—which involved vitamin supplementation while neglecting adequate caloric intake—were prompted by the state of poor health of the First Nations people at the time in Norway House, Cross Lake, God's Lake Mine, Ross Lake, and The Pas Manitoba. There had been widespread hunger and malnutrition in the area for years due to the decline of the fur trade, and for the economic toll of World War II as well as insufficient unemployment relief from the Government of Canada (Mosby, 2013). It is now well documented that poor nutrition was also commonplace at Indian Residential schools across Canada and in this instance, there were more nutrition experiments carried out at six Indian Residential schools (Mosby, 2013; TRC, 2015d). These research studies did little to help Indigenous peoples in their time of starvation and poor health (Mosby 2013).

There is also evidence that much of the tuberculosis treatment provided to Aboriginal people in the 1940s and 1950s was experimental, as "Indian" bodies were seen as disposable (Lux, 2016). The Charles Camsell Hospital in Edmonton, associated with the University of Alberta medical school, experimented with tuberculosis treatments such as painful surgeries to remove ribs and parts of lungs, under local anaesthetic (Lux, 2016).

As Indigenous peoples were increasingly able to gain access to academia, sufficient capacity was built to influence the conduct of research with Indigenous peoples and communities. In Canada, a shift began with the Royal Commission on Aboriginal People and the research committee co-led by Denise Brant-Castellano (Brant-Castellano, 2004). While Indigenous peoples are increasingly accessing university education, there is still insufficient capacity. New researchers, Indigenous and non-Indigenous, need to be specifically trained to understand the respectful way to do research *with*

and *for* rather than *to* Indigenous peoples. With a focus on self-determination in research, the benefits must be for the communities, not for non-Indigenous academics and institutions.

Education

Calls to reform university education (see Kirkness & Barnhardt, 1991) to make it more accessible and useful to Indigenous students extends to nursing and nurse researchers. While there is a significant increase in the numbers of Indigenous people attaining a university degree (9.8% in 2011, compared with 22% in 2016), there is still a persistent gap in university level attainment for First Nations people compared to non-Indigenous Canadians, with only 22% of First Nations people completing university while 45% of non-Indigenous people have completed university (Assembly of First Nations, 2018; Statistics Canada, 2013). In 2016, only 3% of registered nurses in Canada identified as Indigenous, while forming 4.5% of the population in Canada (Canadian Indigenous Nurses Association (CINA), 2018). Of all Indigenous people who are health professionals, the majority (74.5%) are registered nurses; of the overall health workforce, only 1.2% are Indigenous (CINA, 2018).

Although our communities have a critical perspective of universities and what they represent, at the same time these same communities want their members to gain Western educations and high-level qualifications. But they do not want this to be achieved at the cost of destroying people's indigenous identities, their languages, values, and practices...For many students it [attending university] can be an alienating and destructive experience. (Tuhiwai Smith, 2012, p. 135)

There are an increasing number of First Nations, Inuit, and Métis scholars in both academic and community research settings (CIHR et al., 2018). "We need a critical mass of Aboriginal researchers who are educated in the ethics of their own traditions and also open to seeing the common ground that they share with other traditions, including settler society" (Brant-Castellano in Gentelet et al., 2018, p. 835). Being a researcher in an academic institution is not without challenges for Indigenous researchers, who are often faced with navigating universities and communities as an insider and an outsider (Tuhiwai Smith, 1999). Creating partnerships and negotiating requirements across the university and Indigenous communities can be difficult and time-consuming for health researchers, even those who are Indigenous (Anderson & Cidro, 2019; Kovach, 2009).

The National Collaborating Center for Indigenous Health (2020) maintains a database of researchers who publish in the area of Indigenous health. In searching for researchers associated with a nursing faculty in Canada, 31 people are listed, with only 3 of those identifying as Indigenous. Indigenous nurse scholars report numerous barriers to obtaining graduate education that would lead to work in universities and/or community research positions: they may be living with their own effects of colonization, such as intergenerational trauma, helping their own families and communities to live well as Indigenous peoples, and often receive and respond to many requests on their time (C. Foster-Boucher, personal communication, February 2020). In addition there are funding barriers, a lack of Indigenous content in courses, a lack of Indigenous faculty members who can be role models for Indigenous students, faculty lacking knowledge about Indigenous—settler history and relations, and institutional racism that comes across in acts of everyday microaggressions (Indspire, 2018).

Kirkness and Barnhardt's (1991) seminal article outlined the four "Rs" of education that would transform higher education for First Nations' peoples: respect, relevance, reciprocity, and responsibility (Table 7.1). Kirkness and Barnhardt called for a shift in perspectives around the issue of university completion rates for First Nations students—rather than focusing on the attrition and drop-out rates, the focus should be on creating a more hospitable and valuable experience for First Nations people that recognizes and incorporates knowledge, culture, values, and communities that differ from Western-oriented institutions and worldviews. These have been adopted and adapted to apply broadly to Indigenous research (Pidgeon, 2019). These "Rs" happen in the context of relationships and are the actions in the relationships (Johnston et al., 2018). Engaging in authentic relationships in research is foundational to conducting ethical research with Indigenous peoples (Bull, 2010; Pidgeon, 2019).

INDIGENOUS KNOWLEDGE AND RESEARCH

Indigenous peoples had their own knowledge systems that were interrupted and dominated by colonization (Tuhiwai Smith, 2012). Indigenous knowledge (IK), also sometimes referred to as Aboriginal Traditional Knowledge (ATK), reflects numerous ways of knowing and knowledge systems embedded in communities, traditions, and history (Native Women's Association of Canada [NWAC], 2015; Smylie et al., 2004; Tuhiwai Smith, 2012). It is important to keep in mind that *these knowledge systems exist outside the academic realm.* Systems for knowledge accumulation and dissemination in Indigenous communities existed prior to contact with Europeans and have historically been invalidated by colonizing policies and the privileging of Western knowledge. "Aboriginal knowledge has always been informed by research, the purposeful gathering of information and the thoughtful distillation of meaning" (Brant Castellano, 2004, p. 98). Accumulating and transferring knowledge continues to happen in Indigenous communities, through oral traditions, and outside the structure of universities (AFN, 2009; Lightbourn, 2017).

Cultural longevity depends on the ability to sustain cultural knowledges. At the heart of a cultural renaissance, Indigenous or otherwise, is a restoration and respectful use of that culture's knowledge systems. Colonial history has

TABLE 7.1			
THE "Rs" OF HIGHER EDUCATION			
THE FOUR RS	**DESCRIPTION**	**IMPLICATIONS FOR HIGHER EDUCATION**	**IMPLICATIONS FOR RESEARCH**
Respect	Respect FNs people as individuals and people who have knowledge, value, and culture.	Institutional respect for Indigenous knowledge that is bound to cultural context and acquired through real-world experiences.	Respect means egalitarian relationships where researchers adapt to participants, express humility and honour. and acknowledge contributions.
Relevance	Legitimize Indigenous knowledge; incorporate and build on customary ways of knowing.	Institutes of higher education need to be more relevant, accepting, and responsive to needs of students.	Research should be relevant to the community, ideally initiated by the community.
Reciprocity	Recognize Western hierarchies of producers vs consumers of knowledge.	Make teaching and learning a two-way process; teachers make an effort to learn the cultural background of students; students learn the culture of the institution.	Research should serve a purpose to the community, ideally improve the community; the community chooses the researcher.
Responsibility	Commitment to culturally appropriate, accessible, quality education.	Institutions created and controlled by FNs; recognize incentives and purposes for FN students (i.e., community rather than personal gain).	Responsibility as a human being in relationship with others; network of family and community to ensure research is done in a good way; ensure research is not misused or used in a way that causes harm.
Relationships	Fundamental to Indigenous ways of knowing; relationships to knowledge, the land, others (living and non-living)		Foundation of research; relationship with knowledge, researcher, participants, land, ancestors, future generations.

Source: Adapted from Kirkness, V. J., & Barnhardt, R. (1991). First Nations and higher education: The four R's—Respect, relevance, reciprocity, responsibility. *Journal of American Indian Education, 30*(3), 1–15; MacGregor et al. (2018). *Indigenous Research: Theories, Practices, and Relationships.* Toronto, ON: Canadian Scholars' Press.

disrupted the ability of Indigenous peoples to uphold knowledges by cultural methodologies." (Kovach, 2009, p. 12).

The process of decolonizing means looking at, acknowledging, and giving voice to these systems of knowledge—whether or not they are documented in written forms and part of university/academic research endeavours. Decolonizing means decentering from non-Indigenous aims to an Indigenous agenda by "adopting Indigenous perspectives, knowledge and methodologies" (Asselin & Basile, 2018, p. 644).

Indigenous Research Paradigms and Methodologies

As described in Chapter 2, paradigms or worldviews shape how we understand the world and what we consider knowledge, and thus influence research methodology—the types of research questions asked, as well as how research is conducted. Kovach (2009) argued that because policy and practices are based on research, and methodology influences the outcomes of the research, that Indigenous methodologies have the potential to improve policies and practices in the

Indigenous context (p. 13). Indigenous methodologies "in the plural, describe the theory and method of conducting research that flows from an Indigenous epistemology" (Kovach, 2009, p. 20). Indigenous paradigms influence all aspects of research; "it is holistic, relational, and characterized by particular protocols and culturally sanctioned ways of living" (Fellner, 2018, p. 37).

Research should draw on Indigenous worldviews and knowledge as part of a movement towards reconciliation (MacGregor et al., 2018).

Science is the pursuit of knowledge. Approaches to gathering that knowledge are culturally relative. Indigenous science incorporates traditional knowledge and Indigenous perspectives, while non-Indigenous scientific approaches are commonly recognized as Western science. Together, they contribute substantially to modern science.

Although the value of integrating Indigenous science with Western science has been recognized, we have only begun to scratch the surface of its benefits…Both Western and Indigenous science approaches and perspectives have their strengths and can greatly complement one another." (Popp, 2018, para. 2, 3, 4)

Western paradigms begin in the assertion that knowledge is individually earned, gained, and owned and that humans have knowledge. Indigenous paradigms begin with the understanding that knowledge cannot be owned but is shared among all entities (Wilson, 2001; Yantz, 2005). Indigenous worldview sees humans as one small aspect in a universe that includes animals, plants, minerals, space, water, and other entities all sharing the space and all interconnected; as such, research is seen as something that is shared with all of creation (Wilson, 2001). One's reality is connected to the idea of the relationship one has with all that is in one's life. A chair is not just an object but is an item with which we have a relationship in which we use the chair to sit in. Everything around us is in relationship with us. This is where Indigenous methodologies are born. Indigenous

research methodologies therefore are about relationships first and foremost (Wilson, 2001).

When using Indigenous research methodologies, it is vital that one recognizes and respects the great diversity in Indigenous communities. "Indigenous research offers a clear commitment to recognize and support diversity and nationhood—intellectual self-determination" (Johnston et al., 2018, p. 2). In order to conduct research, appropriate protocols must be followed according to the community in which the research will be conducted (Johnston et al., 2018). One must also have an understanding of the history of the community in relation to land, the traditions, impacts of colonialism such as residential school, and who the current leadership is (Johnston et al., 2018). By having these understandings, following protocol is better understood.

Indigenous methodologies hold space for recognizing traditional and contemporary Indigenous knowledge (Johnston et al., 2018). Indigenous knowledge is a constantly changing and evolving entity, and therefore contemporary knowledge is as important as traditional. Furthermore, Indigenous research values the community leadership and communal ownership of knowledge. Indigenous knowledges are both individual and collective from experiences in relation to a specific place (Fellner, 2018). As such it is necessary to recognize and value the ownership of the knowledge—that it may be a community that owns the knowledge rather than just one individual. This has implications for how consent is obtained, particularly considering the protocols and traditions of the community (Baydala et al., 2013). Indigenous research respects the voice of the community leadership as they know and live with the community and have been chosen to lead the community.

"Indigenous research holds the potential to regenerate and revitalize the life of Indigenous peoples and communities along with the 'knowing' that sustains their ongoing vitality" (Johnston et al., 2018, p. 2). Indigenous peoples and communities have been devastated by colonialism, losing much in terms of vital traditional knowledge and practices through forced movement onto reserves, forced attendance at residential schools, and the banning of ceremonies and spiritual practices over the past century (TRC, 2015e). By having control over what, why, and how research is conducted, Indigenous communities and peoples can regain and revitalize their knowledge, which will support self-determination (Brown, 2018; MacGregor et al., 2018).

Indigenous scholars face a dilemma in that they are viewing themselves through the knowledge systems of others, rather than from an Indigenous perspective, as they have been schooled in Eurocentric universities (Kovach, 2009; Tuhawi Smith, 2012). As such, it is necessary to understand these systems in which they have been educated including how they represent and misrepresent, how knowledge construction works, and how knowledge is made legitimate in the eyes of academia including the embedding of power (MacGregor et al., 2018). By understanding this, Indigenous scholars can then emancipate themselves from these systems by utilizing their own realities, and perspectives to develop practices and methodologies that better reflect the Indigenous viewpoint (Rigney, 2016).

Advancing the Indigenous viewpoint, and making the Indigenous voice heard, does not mean that Indigenous researchers are anti-intellectual or atheoretical, nor is their research meant only for Indigenous peoples (Rigney, 2016). Rather, this research opens the arena to "exploration of frameworks that encourage the possibilities of intellectual, political, social, and economic emancipation" (Rigney, 2016, p. 42). Kovach (2009) further offered that "many non-Indigenous people are attracted to Indigenous approaches as well because, I believe, it has to do with a generation seeking ways to understand the world without harming it." (p. 11).

While recognizing that there are many methodologies, there are some common key tenets:

- Indigenous communities and participants determine the value of the research, not academic experts (Johnston et al., 2018)
- Ethical research in Indigenous communities requires an ongoing investment and commitment in relationships and to the community (Bull et al., 2020; Srigley & Varley, 2018)
- An individual is always in relationship—to family, community, Elders and traditional knowledge keepers, and all beings ("living" and "non-living") (Johnston et al., 2018, p. 13)
- The research must be useful to people (Wilson, 2001)

Indigenous methodologies are not just a response to colonialism (Wilson, 2008); they exist based on worldviews, ontology, and epistemology of diverse Indigenous nations (Johnstone et al., 2018). Indigenous research methodologies vary from community to community as they are based on specific Indigenous teachings and frameworks. Teachings and frameworks may include and/or be influenced by the Medicine Wheel used in a variety of ways: treaty practices and frameworks, oral teachings passed down from generation to generation that differ among communities based on local history, geography and culture, and specific cultural teachings and understandings (Mashford-Pringle, 2018; Bell, 2018; Martin, 2018; Luby et al., 2018; Restoule et al., 2018).

There are some research methods and designs, based on a Western worldview, that have been used with Indigenous communities. For example, there is some acceptance with ecological approaches and participatory action research (Brant Castellano, 2004); critical feminist and critical theory (Tuhiwai Smith, 2012); and some natural alliances with qualitative research and community-based approaches (Kovach, 2009). Kovach (2009) argued that even though some of these are "in alliance with the ethical and community dynamics of research with Indigenous peoples" (p. 13) that distinct methodologies that are wholly Indigenous are needed. It is important that Indigenous research move beyond placing an Indigenous lens on non-Indigenous paradigms (Wilson, 2001). Indigenous researchers, located in Western universities, integrate Indigenous cultural knowledge into their research to manage the tension and conflict they face in upholding cultural knowledge in an academic context (Kovach, 2009).

Contemporary universities are centres where knowledge is created, maintained, and upheld. Research powers this force. By entering these knowledge centres, Indigenous peoples are well positioned to carry out research that upholds cultural knowledges. Indigenous research frameworks are conceptual tools that can assist. (Kovach, 2009, p. 12).

Kovach offered three practices as part of an Indigenous methodology: self-location, cultural grounding, and purpose. Self-locating involves sharing about your group, community, culture, and/or epistemology—this is an introduction, shows respect, and makes the researcher aware of their perspective and power (Kovach, 2009). In addition, reflecting on and knowing one's purpose and motivation for conducting the research is important, as personal motivation for conducting can further help in understanding the perspective and reflects honesty (Kovach, 2009). Purpose can also reflect the obligation for research to have a collective purpose, to be relevant to the community (Kovach, 2009). Lastly, cultural grounding means recognizing that culture permeates the research at many levels; "what matters is that there is room within Indigenous research to acknowledge the meaningful role of culture within our inquiries" (Kovach, 2009, p. 177).

A final consideration for Indigenous research paradigms and methodologies is language.

Fellner (2018) described English language as a "cage" representing Euro-Western ideology. Many Indigenous peoples and communities have lost their language due to assimilation policies, or to protect themselves, children, and grandchildren; this loss of language was part of the policies and practices of the residential schools (TRC, 2015e). Tuhiwai Smith (2012) described the irony of indigenous peoples needing to write and converse in the language of the colonizer. As explorers and colonizers traversed the globe collecting artifacts, stories were told and retold often with mistranslation, a lack of knowledge about cultural context, and often with a cascade of misrepresentations that were then accepted as fact (Tuhiwai-Smith, 2012). As ITK and methodologies are increasingly used in research, it is vital that language translation and cultural translation is carried out correctly and ethically. Johnson (1992) discussed the difficulties associated with translation of cultural knowledge of Dene knowledge keepers:

> Much of the knowledge is transmitted in the form of stories and legends using metaphors and sophisticated Dene terminology that may not be well understood by younger interviewers. One community researcher frequently commented on the elders use of hidden words: North Slavey terms or metaphors, which were indirect references to certain animals or their behaviour, that could not be translated literally into English. Unless the interviewer is familiar with the stories and understands how to extract the ecological data from the narrative, an important source of information may be overlooked. (p. 27)

There are an increasing number of articles and books that detail research methods and designs that align with Indigenous paradigms. In looking at how one can use both western and Indigenous paradigms in research, Two-Eyed Seeing is a methodology that "refers to learning to see from one eye with the strengths of Indigenous knowledges and ways of knowing, and from the other eye with the strengths of Western knowledges and ways of knowing, and to using both these eyes together, for the benefit of all" (Bartlett et al., 2012, p. 335). This methodology was developed by two Mi'kmaw Elders—Albert Marshall and Murdena Marshall—and a biologist—Cheryl Bartlett—at Cape Breton University and has been utilized in numerous research endeavors (Hall et al., 2015; Hovey, Delormier, McComber, Levesque & Martin, 2017; Marsh, Cote-Meek, Toulouse, Najavits, & Young, 2015; Martin, Thompson, Ballard, & Linton, 2017). It was developed as

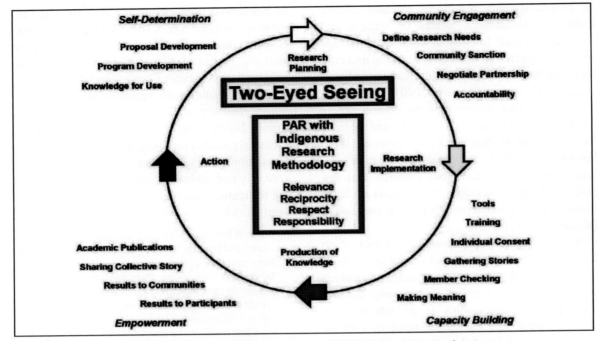

FIG. 7.1 Participatory action research with Indigenous methodologies as Two-Eyed seeing. This model was adapted from the Jacklin and Kinoshameg (2008) *Wikwemikong Community Needs Assessment Research Model.*

part of a program of Integrative Sciences and is noted as "the most profound" (p. 340) of eight of the "Lessons Learned" when the authors were working with how to weave together Western and Indigenous knowledges and ways of knowing (Bartlett et al., 2012). Peltier (2018) used a Two Eyed Seeing approach, combining Indigenous methodologies and participatory action research, to understand the contributions of Indigenous healing to cancer care and *mno-bimaadiziwin* (an understanding of wellness; Peltier, 2018). The process of this research can be seen in Figure 7.1.

ETHICS AND PRINCIPLES OF INDIGENOUS RESEARCH

Over the last few decades there has been considerable work to understand, support, and conduct more ethical research with Indigenous peoples

and communities, both in Canada and around the world. Researchers need to follow several protocols and principles when conducting research including making meaningful relationships with the communities and people, researching what Indigenous people want researched, ensuring appropriate consent is given, researching with involvement of Indigenous peoples and communities, helping to build research capacity, and ensuring that the findings are given back to the community in a way that is helpful for them. Overall, this means not perpetuating colonialism and working towards reconciliation through the bringing together of both Indigenous and Western knowledge. In this section we review standards, policies, and guidelines for the ethical conduct of research with Indigenous peoples and communities and provide examples of recent nursing research that demonstrates these points.

Principles and Guidelines From Indigenous Communities

In 2010, the First Nations Information Governance Center (FNIGC) was officially incorporated and works towards the vision of every First Nation achieving data sovereignty with its distinct worldview (FNIGC, 2018). Among other research, this organization conducts the First Nations Regional Health Survey using both Western and traditional knowledge of health and illness (FNIGC, 2018). The OCAP® principles (see Table 7.2) are the expected standards for data collection, use, and dissemination; "they are the defacto standard for how to conduct research with First Nations" (FNIGC, 2020, What is OCAP®). OCAP® was developed to recognize *community* rights, a concept that was not reflected in Western society, as well as in response to research that was not done by, or for the benefit of, First Nations (FNIGC, 2020).

The Métis National Council represents the Métis Nation and Métis peoples nationally and internationally, comprised of Métis Nations of British Columbia, Alberta, Saskatchewan, Manitoba, and Ontario (Métis National Council [MNC], 2021). While there is no research guidance directly from the MNC, individual Métis Nations may have frameworks and processes for engaging in research with their communities.

In 2018, the National Inuit Strategy on Research (NISR) was launched. The strategy "identifies areas for partnership and action that can strengthen the impact and effectiveness of Inuit Nunangat research for Inuit" (Inuit Tapiriit Kanatami, 2018, News, NISR). A copy of the opening letter from the Inuit Tapiriit Kanatami president is included in the *Practical Application* box.

Principles & Guidelines from Canadian Government Institutions

In response to the Royal Commission on Aboriginal Peoples and the Truth and Reconciliation Commission's Calls to Action, Canadian Government research funding agencies have worked towards improving research with Indigenous

---

TABLE **7.2**

FIRST NATIONS PRINCIPLES OF OCAP®

Principle and Definition

Ownership refers to the relationship of First Nations to their cultural knowledge, data, and information. This principle states that a community or group owns information collectively in the same way that an individual owns his or her personal information.

Control affirms that First Nations, their communities, and representative bodies are within their rights in seeking to control over all aspects of research and information management processes that impact them. First Nations control of research can include all stages of a particular research project-from start to finish. The principle extends to the control of resources and review processes, the planning process, management of the information and so on.

Access refers to the fact that First Nations must have access to information and data about themselves and their communities regardless of where it is held. The principle of access also refers to the right of First Nations' communities and organizations to manage and make decisions regarding access to their collective information. This may be achieved, in practice, through standardized, formal protocols.

Possession While ownership identifies the relationship between a people and their information in principle, possession or stewardship is more concrete: it refers to the physical control of data. Possession is the mechanism by which ownership can be asserted and protected.

OCAP® is a registered trademark of The First Nations Information Governance Centre (FNIGC)
Source: Based on First Nations Information Governance Centre (2020). The First Nations principles of OCAP®. https://fnigc.ca/ocap-training/

Practical Application

The term *research* invokes strong reactions among Inuit because researchers have historically been and continue to be the primary beneficiaries of research involving our people, wildlife, and environment. While we recognize the important role research can play in informing actions that create safer, healthier, and more resilient communities, Inuit from across Inuit Nunangat have long insisted that researchers and research institutions respect Inuit self-determination in research through partnerships that enhance the effcacy, impact, and usefulness of research.

For far too long, researchers have enjoyed great privilege as they have passed through our communities and homeland, using public or academic funding to answer their own questions about our environment, wildlife, and people. Many of these same researchers then ignore Inuit in creating the outcomes of their work for the advancement of their careers, their research institutions, or their governments. This type of exploitative relationship must end.

Inuit, governments, and research institutions can do so by working together to transform research relationships. Inuit and researchers have reaped the benefits of research relationships premised on respect for Inuit self-determination and are seeking coherent and consistent research relationships across Inuit Nunangat. In recent years, a number of researchers, research institutions, and Inuit have developed meaningful partnerships and undertaken research that has created value for our

people and communities. These meaningful partnerships have been developed in a fragmented fashion because they are dependent upon goodwill and respect between individual researchers, institutions, and Inuit.

Achieving Inuit self-determination in research can lead to an evolution of the outdated policies and processes that determine our relationship with research, as well as enhanced capacity for Inuit-led research.

The National Inuit Strategy on Research (NISR) outlines the coordinated actions required to improve the way Inuit Nunangat research is governed, resourced, conducted, and shared. This strategy builds upon the important strides taken by Inuit towards self-determination in research by offering solutions to challenges our people have grappled with for decades. It envisions research being utilized as a building block for strong public policies, programs, and initiatives that support optimal outcomes for Inuit that in turn benefit all Canadians.

Many people have contributed to the creation of the NISR. I would like to acknowledge the guidance of the Inuit Tapiriit Kanatami (ITK) Board of Directors and the expertise and advice of the Inuit Qaujisarvingat National Committee in the writing of this strategy.

Nakummek,
Natan Obed

Source: Inuit Tapiriit Kanatami (2018). *Letter from ITKs president.* National Inuit Strategy on Research. Author.

peoples. Indigenous research has been defined by the Social Sciences and Humanities Research Council (SSHRC; 2019) as

Research in any field or discipline that is conducted by, grounded in or engaged with First Nations, Inuit, Métis or other Indigenous nations, communities, societies or individuals, and their wisdom, cultures, experiences or knowledge systems, as expressed in their dynamic forms, past and present. Indigenous research can embrace the intellectual, physical, emotional and/or spiritual dimensions of knowledge in creative and interconnected relationships with people, places and the natural environment.

Whatever the methodologies or perspectives that apply in a given context, researchers who conduct Indigenous research, whether they are Indigenous or non-Indigenous themselves, commit to respectful relationships with all Indigenous peoples and

communities...Research by and with Indigenous peoples and communities emphasizes and values their existing strengths, assets and knowledge systems. (SSHRC, 2019, definition of terms)

The Canadian Institute for Health Research (CIHR, 2020a) has identified the importance of building respectful relationships with Indigenous communities and improving the health and well-being of Indigenous peoples "through the establishment of research environments that are socially, spiritually, emotionally and physically safe" (CIHR, 2020a, Indigenous Health Research at CIHR). The Institute of Indigenous Peoples Health was established to "improve and promote the health of First Nations, Inuit and Métis peoples in Canada, through research, knowledge translation and capacity building. The Institutes pursuit of research excellence is enhanced by respect for community research priorities and Indigenous knowledge, values and cultures" (CIHR, 2020b, Institute of Indigenous People's Health).

The Tri-Council Policy Statement 2.0 (TCPS) is a joint document from CIHR, SSHRC, and the National Science and Engineering Research Council (CIHR et al., 2018), which outlines requirements for the ethical conduct of research with people. Although researchers in Canada who receive funding from this agency are required to follow this policy, it is widely adopted in Canada as a basis for ethical research, regardless of the funding source (see Chapter 6). Chapter 9 of the TCPS 2.0 is focused on *Research Involving First Nations, Inuit and Métis Peoples of Canada* and how the value of human dignity and the core principles of respect, welfare, and justice apply to research involving Aboriginal peoples (CIHR et al., 2018). While this document is intended to provide guidance to researchers, it recognizes the diversity of First Nations, Inuit, and Métis peoples and that the specific codes of conduct of research will be negotiated with communities on an ongoing basis. In other words, the TCPS 2.0, Chapter 9, does not replace, but rather emphasizes, the need to engage in relationships with Indigenous communities to ensure ethics of the research.

Research Hint

Relationships are fundamental to research with Indigenous peoples. "Taking time to establish a relationship can promote mutual trust and communication, identify mutually beneficial research goals, define appropriate research collaborations or partnerships, and ensure that the conduct of research adheres to the core principles of Respect for Persons, Concern for Welfare... and Justice" (CIHR et al., 2018, p. 110).

The core principle of *Respect for Persons* includes recognizing the importance of community and interrelationships in Aboriginal communities and preserving distinctive knowledge, cultures, and identities (CIHR et al., 2018). *Concern for Welfare* is interpreted in Chapter 9 of the TCPS 2.0 more broadly to acknowledge the collective rights, interests, and

responsibilities of Aboriginal peoples as well as protection of participants in their "physical, social, economic and cultural environment" (p. 109). The core principle of *Justice* attends to the power imbalance that exists between researcher and participants. For Aboriginal peoples, there have been many abuses of this power, including: "misappropriation of sacred songs, stories and artefacts; devaluing of aboriginal peoples' knowledge as primitive or superstitious; violation of community norms regarding the use of human tissue and remains; failure to share data and resulting benefits; and dissemination of information that has misrepresented or stigmatized entire communities" (CIHR et al., 2018, p. 109).

While it may seem that there are two distinct groups presented here (the researcher and the participants), keep in mind that these distinctions are not always clear cut. There are Indigenous researchers who work at research institutions who may or may not be doing research within their own communities. In addition, community-based and institution-based researchers may be using Indigenous methodologies, Western methodologies, or a combination of these to conduct research. First Nations, Inuit, and Métis communities and peoples continue with traditional knowledge practices as well as initiating, leading, and conducting research—sometimes in collaboration with an Indigenous or non-Indigenous researcher located outside their communities. "As the academic landscape shifts with an increasing Indigenous presence, there is a desire among a growing community of non-Indigenous academics to move beyond the binaries found within Indigenous–settler relations to construct new, mutual forms of dialogue, research, theory, and action" (Kovach, 2009, p. 12).

Research Hint

Getting ethical approval from the Ethics board is not the same as getting ethical approval from the Indigenous community (Bull et al., 2020). Obtaining consent with Indigenous communities is complex—it involves building relationships and ensuring both the researcher and the community are clear about the benefits and outcomes (Anderson & Cidro, 2019).

Research Processes

In this section, we review three research reports to provide some specific examples of the process of research with Indigenous peoples/communities.

An example of research led by an Indigenous nurse scholar can be found in Appendix A. Bourque-Bearskin et al. (2016) explored how Indigenous knowledge manifests in the practice of Indigenous nurses. In the introduction, Bourque-Bearskin et al. describes drawing on Cree/Métis understanding through Indigenous research methodologies. In subsequent paragraphs there is a description of the background and context of the research, and the first author locates herself in terms of culture, history, and current practice of nursing. There is a thorough explanation of the Indigenous research methodology as well as more concrete descriptions of how data collection and analysis were conducted. This extensive description is something you may not see in other research reports but is an important part of an Indigenous research paradigm. The four nurses that Bourque-Bearskin et al. (2016) interviewed are named in the results section (without pseudonyms) and are also included as authors on the research report. This reflects the contributions of the participants as co-researchers and respects their knowledge by giving them credit. The findings of the report are focused on how these nurses incorporate Indigenous ways of knowing, being, and doing in their nursing practice.

As part of a program of research on cancer care survivorship, Gifford et al. (2019) provide a detailed protocol for a knowledge translation study. Publishing this protocol sets out the key processes for the research team and helps to set the context for their study. They begin with a background section that presents an argument for why their research is important, reviews the literature and current situation, and ends with three clearly stated research questions. They describe how knowledge will be co-produced, strategies to ensure collaboration, use of Indigenous knowledge translation frameworks, and how they will engage knowledge users and communities throughout the research process:

> Culturally relevant channels of dissemination will be utilized such as kinship networks, talking circles and stories, and participation of community leaders, chiefs, elders, and community members. The continued engagement of community members in our previous study has allowed us to establish partnerships with community leaders, elders, healthcare providers, cancer survivors, and families to plan, design, conduct, and disseminate this study using a participatory, integrated Indigenous KT approach. (Gifford et al., 2019)

This study was the third in a program of research. They write about how this project builds on previous work, as well as the strategies to maintain relationships with the communities including regular meetings, and co-developing analysis that reflects culturally relevant beliefs (Gifford et al., 2019).

Camargo Plazas et al. (2018) used popular theatre to disseminate research findings from a community-based action research project that developed an Indigenous-led intervention to improve access to health care (Cameron et al., 2014). Based on narrative from the intervention research project (Cameron et al., 2014), five skits were developed by high school students in a First Nations community in collaboration with a theater instructor. These skits were then performed at a community symposium attended by community members, health care professionals, and managers. This dissemination strategy was "a powerful tool to strengthen our collaboration with community members and deepen our understanding of access to healthcare services for Indigenous people in a rural setting" (Camargo Plazas et al., 2018, p. 494). Throughout the article, the authors describe the background and relationships with the Indigenous communities, Community Health Representatives (CHRs), Indigenous liaison person, and the research team, as well as how the research team collaborated with the students to develop this dissemination project. The entire research project was conducted under the guidance of an elder (Camargo Plazas et al., 2018). This

APPRAISING THE EVIDENCE

Critiquing Criteria

Appraising research done by and with Indigenous peoples requires attention to ethical processes and relationships. When reading research reports about Indigenous peoples/communities, keep these critical thinking questions in mind:

1. Who are the researchers? What is their relationship to the people and land that they are reporting on?
2. At what stage of the research were relationships developed?
3. Were Indigenous peoples involved in deciding on or directing the research question/project?
4. Is there evidence of commitment to relationships with the people and communities they are working with?
5. How are these relationships initiated, built, and maintained?
6. Is it clear who is benefitting from the research?
7. Is there evidence of developing partnerships and building research capacity within the community?
8. Are the results presented in a manner that is respectful, reflects reciprocity, is relevant and responsible?
9. Does the research primarily reflect a Western worldview or Indigenous worldview?
10. Does the report reflect self-determination of Indigenous peoples/communities in the research process?
11. Does the research perpetuate or challenge stereotypes?
12. From whose perspective is the research question framed?
13. From whose perspective are the implications and recommendations framed?
14. Is the methodology congruent with an Indigenous research paradigm/methodology?

research project was used to lobby the government for increased use of CHRs in hospitals.

SUMMARY

As you read research by and about Indigenous peoples, recall the history of First Nations, Inuit, and Métis peoples in Canada. Consider the effects of historical and intergenerational trauma—this means recognizing and valuing Indigenous knowledge and culture, as well as the risks of privileging Western knowledge that may be continuing to oppress an Indigenous worldview and peoples. Also consider how research by and with Indigenous peoples, as well as that built on Western paradigms, can be brought together in a beneficial way. By creating ethical space (Ermine, 2007) for engagement between Indigenous communities and Western communities, we all work towards reconciliation and decolonization of research and knowledge. "The implications for indigenous research...seem to be clear and straightforward: the survival of peoples, cultures and languages" (Tuhiwai Smith, 2012, p. 143).

CRITICAL THINKING CHALLENGES

- Thinking about the health-related or research-related Calls to Action from the Truth and Reconciliation Commission report, identify an action you could take personally to work towards reconciliation.

- Find a recent research article written on a health topic that involved an Indigenous community and review it using the questions provided in the Appraising Evidence box.

- How might you incorporate Indigenous perspectives and cultural competence in an evidence-informed practice project?

CRITICAL JUDGEMENT QUESTIONS

1. Which of the following should be present in a research report about Indigenous peoples?
   a. Evidence of ethical approval from the council of the First Nations
   b. Evidence of established and ongoing relationships
   c. Evidence of ATK (Aboriginal Traditional Knowledge) and ceremony
   d. Evidence of adherence to the principles of OCAP®

2. What was one of the main effects of residential schools on Indigenous knowledge?

   a. Loss of language and transmission of knowledge
   b. Abuse and neglect, including malnutrition
   c. The difficulty navigating school as an insider–outsider
   d. Loss of parenting role models

3. Why is use of an Indigenous methodology important for research?

   a. It is a requirement of the TCPS 2.0 for ethical research
   b. It is the only paradigm that allows for inclusion of Indigenous cultures
   c. Many viewpoints can be represented in the methodology
   d. Changes in policies and practices will better reflect Indigenous contexts

KEY POINTS

- *Indigenous* is an umbrella term that includes many different cultural groups.
- Indigenous peoples had systems for the accumulation and dissemination of knowledge for thousands of years prior to contact with Europeans. These knowledge systems were primarily based on oral traditions.
- First Nations, Inuit, and Métis peoples in Canada have been subjected to harmful assimilation policies of the Canadian government that have resulted in intergenerational trauma.
- Not only have research practices that have privileged Western knowledge been of little benefit to Indigenous peoples; these practices have often been harmful.
- Research with Indigenous peoples and communities is centred on building and maintaining authentic, ethical relationships.

🔊 FOR FURTHER STUDY

Go to Evolve at http://evolve.elsevier.com/Canada/LoBiondo/Research for the Audio Glossary.

REFERENCES

Aguiar, W., & Halseth, R. (2015). *Aboriginal peoples and historic trauma: The processes of intergenerational transmission.* Centre de collaboration nationale de la santé autochtone: [National Collaborating Centre for Aboriginal Health].

Andersen, C. (2016). The colonialism of Canada's Métis health population dynamics: Caught between bad data and no data at all. *Journal of Population Research, 33,* 67–82. doi:10.1007/s12546-016-9161-4.

Anderson, K., & Cidro, J. (2019). Decades of doing: Indigenous women academics reflect on the practices of community-based health research. *Journal of Empirical Research on Human Research Ethics, 14*(3), 222.

Asselin, H., & Basile, S. (2018). Concrete ways to decolonize research. *ACME: An International E-Journal for Critical Geographies, 17*(3), 643–650.

Assembly of First Nations. (n.d.). First Nations Ethics Guide on research and Aboriginal Traditional Knowledge. Retrieved from https://www.afn.ca/uploads/files/fn_ethics_guide_on_research_and_atk.pdf.

Assembly of First Nations (AFN). (2009). Ethics in First Nations research. Retrieved from https://www.afn.ca/uploads/files/rp-research_ethics_final.pdf.

Assembly of First Nations (AFN). (2018). First Nations Post-secondary Education Fact Sheet. Retrieved from https://www.afn.ca/wp-content/uploads/2018/07/PSE_Fact_Sheet_ENG.pdf.

Barker, B., Sedgemore, K., Tourangeau, M., et al. (2019). Intergenerational trauma: The relationship between residential schools and the child welfare system among young people who use drugs in Vancouver, Canada. *Journal of Adolescent Health, 65*(2), 248–254. doi:10.1016/j.jadohealth.2019.01.022.

Bartlett, C., Marshall, M., & Marshall, M. (2012). Two-eyed seeing and other lessons learned within a co-learning journey of bringing together indigenous and mainstream knowledges and ways of knowing. *Journal of Environmental Studies and Sciences, 2*(4), 331–340. doi:10.1007/s13412-012-0086-8.

Barton, S. S., & Foster-Boucher, C. (2019). Indigenous health. In B. J Astle, W. Duggleby, P. A. Potter, A. G. Perry, P. A. Stockert, & A. M. Hall (Eds.), *Canadian fundamentals of nursing* (6th ed., pp. 133–156). Oxford: Elsevier Canada.

Baydala, L. T., Worrell, S., Fletcher, F., Letendre, S., & Ruttan, L. (2013). "Making a Place of Respect": Lessons learned in carrying out consent protocol with First Nations Elders. *Progress in Community Health Partnerships: Research, Education, and Action, 7*(2), 135–143. https://doi.org/10.1353/cpr.2013.0015.

Bell, N. (2018). Anishnaabe research, theory and methodology as informed by Nanaboozhoo, the Bundle Bag, and the Medicine Wheel. In D. McGregor, J.-P. Restoule, & R. Johnston (Eds.), *Indigenous research: Theories, practices and relationships* (Chapter 10). Toronto, ON: Canadian Scholars Press.

Bourque-Bearskin, R. L., Cameron, B. L, King, M., Weber-Pillwax, C., Stout, M., Voyageur, E., Reid, A., Bill, A., & Martial, R. (2016). Mâmawoh kamâtowin, "coming together to help each other in wellness": Honouring indigenous nursing knowledge. *International Journal of Indigenous Health, 11*(1), 18–33. http://dx.doi.org/10.18357/ijih111201615024.

Brant Castellano, M. B. (2004). Ethics of aboriginal research. *Journal of Aboriginal Health, 1*(1), 98–114. http://www.nvit.ca/docs/ethics%20of%20aboriginal%20research.pdf.

Brown, C. (2018). Self determination and data control vital to Indigenous health research. *Canadian Medical Association Journal, 190*(29), E893. doi:10.1503/cmaj109-5631.

Bull, J. R. (2010). Research with Aboriginal peoples: Authentic relationships as a precursor to ethical research. *Journal of Empirical Research on Human Research Ethics, 5*(4), 13–22. https://doi.org/10.1525/jer.2010.5.4.13.

Bull, J., Beazley, K., Shea, J., et al. (2020). Shifting practise: Recognizing Indigenous rights holders in research ethics review. *Qualitative Research in Organizations & Management, 15*(1), 21.

Camargo Plazas, P., Cameron, B. L., Milford, K., Hunt, L. R., Bourque-Bearskin, L., & Santos-Salas, A. (2018). Engaging Indigenous youth through popular theatre: Knowledge mobilization of Indigenous peoples' perspectives on access to healthcare services. *Action Research, 17*(4), 492–509. doi:10.1177/1476750318789468.

Cameron, B. L., Camargo Plazas, M., del, P., Santos Salas, A., Bourque-Bearskin, L., & Hungler, K (2014). Understanding inequalities in access to healthcare services for Aboriginal people: A call for nursing action. *Advances in Nursing Science, 37*(3), E1–E16.

Canadian Indigenous Nurses Association (CINA). (2018). *Aboriginal nursing in Canada.* Retrieved from https://indigenousnurses.ca/resources/publications/2018-university-saskatchewan-cinas-fact-sheet-aboriginal-nursing-canada.

Canadian Institutes of Health Research (CIHR). (2020a). *Indigenous health research at CIHR.* Retrieved from https://cihr-irsc.gc.ca/e/50339.html.

Canadian Institutes of Health Research (CIHR). (2020b). *Institute of Indigenous people's health.* Retrieved from https://cihr-irsc.gc.ca/e/8668.html.

Canadian Institutes of Health Research, Natural Sciences and Engineering Research Council of Canada, & Social Sciences and Humanities Research Council of Canada. (2013). *Tri-council policy statement: Ethical conduct for research involving humans.* Retrieved from www.pre.ethics.gc.ca.

Dickason, O. P., & Newbigging, W. (2015). *A concise history of Canada's first nations.* Oxford: Oxford University Press.

Elias, B., Mignone, J., Hall, M., Hong, S. P., Hart, L., & Sareen, J. (2012). Trauma and suicide behaviour histories among a Canadian indigenous population: an empirical exploration of the potential role of Canada's residential school system. *Social Science & Medicine, 74*(10), 1560–1569. https://doi.org/10.1016/j.socscimed.2012.01.026.

Ermine, W. (2007). The ethical space of engagement. *Indigenous Law Journal, 6,* 193. https://heinonline.org/HOL/Page?collection=journals&handle=hein.journals/ilj6&id=194&men_tab=srchresults.

Fellner, K. D. (2018). Miyo pimatisiwin: (Re)claiming voice with our original instructions. In D. McGregor, J.-P. Restoule, & R. Johnston (Eds.), *Indigenous research: Theories, practices and relationships* (pp. 25–45). Toronto, ON: Canadian Scholars.

First Nations Information Governance Center (FNIGC). (2018). *Frequently asked questions.* Retrieved from. https://fnigc.ca/about-fnigc/frequently-asked-questions.html.

First Nations Information Governance Center (FNIGC). (2020). *What is OCAP®.* Retrieved from https://fnigc.ca/ocap.

Gentelet, K., Basile, S., & Asselin, H. (2018). We have to start sounding the trumpet for things that are working": An interview with Dr. Marlene Brant-Castellano on concrete ways to decolonize research. *ACME: An International E-Journal for Critical Geographies, 17*(3), 832–839.

Gifford, W., Thomas, R., Barton, G., & Graham, I. D. (2019). Providing culturally safe cancer survivorship care with Indigenous communities: study protocol for an integrated knowledge translation study. *Pilot and Feasibility Studies, 5*(1), 33. https://doi.org/10.1186/s40814-019-0422-9.

Government of Alberta. (2020). Metis settlements and First Nations in Alberta community profiles. Retrieved from https://open.alberta.ca/dataset/d3004449-9668-4d02-bb88-f57d381a6965/resource/17fba338-6b1f-401a-8408-521851b5fba7/download/ir-metis-settlements-and-first-nations-in-alberta-community-profiles-2020-05.pdf.

Hall, L., Dell, C. A., Fornssler, B., Hopkins, C., Mushquash, C., & Rowan, M. (2015). Research as cultural renewal: Applying two-eyed seeing in a research project about cultural interventions in First Nations addictions treatment. *International Indigenous Policy Journal, 6*(2), 1–15. doi:10.18584/iipj.2015.6.2.4.

Hovey, R. B., Delormier, T., McComber, A. M., Levesque, L., & Martin, D. (2017). Enhancing Indigenous health promotion research through two-eyed seeing: A hermeneutic relational process. *Qualitative Health Research, 27*(9), 1278–1287. doi:10.1177/1049732317697948.

Indigenous and Northern Affairs Canada (INAC). (2016). *Common terminology*. Retrieved from https://www.aadnc-aandc.gc.ca/eng/1358879361384/1358879407462.

Indigenous and Northern Affairs Canada (INAC). (2016a). *Indigenous peoples and communities*. Retrieved from https://www.aadnc-aandc.gc.ca/eng/1100100013785/1304467449155.

INAC. (2017). *2017–18 departmental plan - Operating contexts: Conditions affecting our work*. Retrieved from https://www.aadnc-aandc.gc.ca/eng/1483561566667/1483561606216.

Indspire. (2018). *Post-secondary experience of Indigenous students following the Truth and Reconciliation Commission: Summary of survey findings*. Retrieved from https://indspire.ca/wp-content/uploads/2019/10/PSE-Experience-Indigenous-Students-Survey-Summary-Sept2018.pdf.

Inuit Tapiriit Kanatami. (2004). *5000 years of Inuit history and heritage*. Retrieved from https://www.itk.ca/?s=history.

Inuit Tapiriit Kanatami. (2018). *National Inuit strategy on research*. Retrieved from https://www.itk.ca/national-strategy-on-research/.

Johnson, M. (1992). *Lore: Capturing traditional environmental knowledge*. Retrieved from https://idl-bnc-idrc.dspacedirect.org/bitstream/handle/10625/19497/IDL-19497.pdf?sequence=1.

Johnston, R., McGregor, D., & Restoule, J.-P. (2018). Introduction: Relationships, respect, relevance, reciprocity, and responsibility: Taking up Indigenous research approaches. In *Indigenous Research: Theories, Practices, and Relationships* (pp. 1–21). Toronto, ON: Canadian Scholars' Press.

Kirkness, V. J., & Barnhardt, R. (1991). First Nations and higher education: The four R's—Respect, relevance, reciprocity, responsibility. *Journal of American Indian Education, 30*(3), 1–15.

Kirkup, K., & Ubelacker, S. (2016). Open secret: Sexual abuse haunts children in Indigenous communities: *CBC*. Retrieved from http://www.cbc.ca/news/Indigenous/Indigenous-sexual-assault-1.3839141.

Kovach, M. (2009). *Indigenous methodologies: Characteristics, conversations, and contexts*. Toronto: University of Toronto Press, Scholarly Publishing Division.

LeFevre, T. A. (2015). *Settler colonialism*. Oxford: Oxford University Press. https://doi.org/10.1093/obo/9780199766567-0125.

Leroux, D., & Gaudry, A. (2017). Becoming Indigenous: The rise of Eastern Métis in Canada. *The Conversation*. Retrieved from https://theconversation.com/becoming-indigenous-the-rise-of-eastern-Métis-in-canada-80794.

Lightbourn, D. (Dec. 20, 2017). Stories from the bush: Traditional teachings from a lifetime Oskapiyos. *Alberta Native News*. https://www.albertanativenews.com/stories-from-the-bush-traditional-teachings-from-a-lifetime-oskapiyos/.

Luby, B., Arsenault, R., Burke, J., Graham, M., & Valenti, T. (2018). Treaty #3: A tool for empowering diverse scholars to engage in Indigenous research. In D. McGregor, J.-P. Restoule, & R. Johnston (Eds.), *Indigenous research: theories, practices, and relationships* (pp. 200–218). Toronto, ON: Canadian Scholars' Press.

Lux, M. K. (2016). *Separate beds: A history of Indian hospitals in Canada, 1920s–1980s*. Toronto, ON: University of Toronto Press, Scholarly Publishing Division.

MacGregor, D., Restoule, J.-P., & Johnston, R. (2018). *Indigenous research: theories, practices, and relationships*. Toronto, ON: Canadian Scholars' Press.

Malone, K. (2016). Métis Nation 'finding ourselves in Confederation' with land claim negotiations, President of MMF says. *CBC News*. Retrieved from http://www.cbc.ca/news/canada/manitoba/m%C3%A9tis-confederation-land-claim-negotiations-mmf-1.3854022.

Manitoba Metis Federation. (2021). Michif language. https://www.manitobametis.com/michif-language/.

Marsh, T. N., Cote-Meek, S., Toulouse, P., Najavits, L. M., & Young, N. L. (2015). The application of two-eyed seeing decolonizing methodology in qualitative and quantitative research for the treatment of intergenerational trauma and substance use disorders. *International Journal of Qualitative Methods, 14*(5), 1–13. doi:10.1177/1609406915618046.

Martin, D. E., Thompson, S., Ballard, M., & Linton, J. (2017). Two-eyed seeing in research and its absence in policy: Little Saskatchewan First Nation elder's experiences of the 2011 flood and forced displacement. *The International Indigenous Policy Journal, 8*(4), 1–27. doi:10.18584/iipj.2017.8.4.6.

Martin, G. (2018). Storytelling and narrative inquiry: Exploring research methodologies. In D. McGregor, J.-P. Restoule, & R. Johnston (Eds.), *Indigenous research: theories, practices, and relationships* (pp. 1–21). Toronto, ON: Canadian Scholars' Press.

Mas, S. (2015). Truth and reconciliation commission final report points to 'growing crisis' for Indigenous youth. *CBC News*, 14. Retrieved from http://www.cbc.ca/news/politics/truth-and-reconciliation-final-report-1.3361148.

Mashford-Pringle, A. (2018). Aboriginal children in Toronto: Working together to improve services. In D. McGregor, J.-P. Restoule, & R. Johnston (Eds.), *Indigenous research: theories, practices, and relationships* (pp. 142–154). Toronto, ON: Canadian Scholars' Press.

Menzies, P. (2008). Developing an Aboriginal healing model for intergenerational trauma. *International Journal of Health Promotion and Education*, *46*(2), 41–48. doi:10.1080/14635240.2008.10708128.

Métis Nation British Columbia. (n.d.). *Citizenship, ID and registry*. Retrieved from https://www.mnbc.ca/directory/view/301-Métis-citizenship-registry.

Métis Nation of Alberta. (n.d.). *Frequently asked questions*. Retrieved from http://albertaMétis.com/registry/registry-frequently-asked-questions/.

Métis Nation of Alberta. (2021). History. https://alberta-metis.com/metis-in-alberta/history/.

Métis Nation of Ontario. (n.d.). *Citizenship*. Retrieved from http://www.Métisnation.org/registry/citizenship/.

Métis Nation Saskatchewan. (n.d.). *Citizenship*. Retrieved from https://Métisnationsk.com/citizenship/#eligibility.

Métis National Council. (2020). *Who are the Méetis?* Retrieved from https://www2.Métisnation.ca/about/faq.

Métis Settlements General Council. (n.d.). *Our land*. Retrieved from https://msgc.ca/#ourland.

Mosby, I. (2013). Administering colonial science: Nutrition research and human biomedical experimentation in Aboriginal communities and residential schools, 1942-1952. *Histoire sociale/Social History*, *46*(91), 145–172. https://muse.jhu.edu/article/512043/pdf.

National Aboriginal Health Organization. (2018). *Principles of ethical Métis research*. Retrieved from https://achh.ca/wp-content/uploads/2018/07/Guide_Ethics_NAHOMétisCentre.pdf.

National Collaborating Centre for Aboriginal Health. (2013). *An overview of Aboriginal health in Canada*. Retrieved from https://www.nccih.ca/en/publications-view.aspx?sortcode=2.8.10.16&id=101.

National Collaborating Center for Indigenous Health. (2020). *Indigenous health researchers database*. Retrieved from https://www.nccih.ca/512/researchers.aspx?sortcode=2.12.23&search=nursing.

Native Women's Association of Canada. (2015). *Aboriginal women and Aboriginal traditional knowledge (ATK): Input and insight on ATK*. Retrieved from https://www.nwac.ca/wp-content/uploads/2015/05/2014-NWAC-Aborignal-Women-and-A borignal-Traditional-Knowledge-Report1.pdf.

Pauktuutit Inuit Women of Canada. (2006). *The Inuit way: A guide to Inuit culture*. Retrieved from https://www.relations-inuit.chaire.ulaval.ca/sites/relations-inuit.chaire.ulaval.ca/files/InuitWay_e.pdf.

Peltier, C. (2018). An application of two-eyed seeing: Indigenous research methods with participatory action research. *International Journal of Qualitative Methods*, *17*(1), Article 1609406918812346.

Penny, C., O'Sullivan, E., & Senecal, S. (2012). *The community well-being index (CWB): Examining well-being in Inuit communities*. Unpublished report: Aboriginal Affairs and Northern Development Canada. Retrieved from http://assembly.nu.ca/library/Edocs/2012/000818-e.pdf.

Pidgeon, M. (2019). Moving between theory and practice within an Indigenous research paradigm. *Qualitative Research*, *19*(4), 418–436. https://doi.org/10.1177/1468794118781380.

Popp, J. (2018). *How Indigenous knowledge advances modern science and technology*. Retrieved from https://theconversation.com/how-indigenous-knowledge-advances-modern-science-and-technology-89351.

Province of Alberta. (2015). *Metis Settlements Act*. Revised Statutes of Alberta 2000 Chapter M-14. Alberta Queen's Printer. http://www.qp.alberta.ca/1266.cfm?page=m14.cfm&leg_type=Acts&isbncln=9780779786541.

Qikiqtani Inuit Association. (2014). *Thematic reports and special studies 1950-1975. QTC final report - Achieving Saimaqatigiingniq*. Retrieved from https://www.qtcommission.ca/sites/default/files/public/thematic_reports/thematic_reports_english_final_report.pdf.

Restoule, P., Dokis, C., & Kelly, B (2018). Working to protect the water: Stories of connection and transformation. In D. McGregor, J.-P. Restoule, & R. Johnston (Eds.), *Indigenous research: Theories, practices, and relationships* (pp. 219–239). Toronto, ON: Canadian Scholars' Press.

Rigney, L.-I. (2016). Indigenist research and Aboriginal Australia. In J. Kunnie, & N. I. Goduka (Eds.),

Indigenous people's wisdom and power: Affirming our knowledge through narratives (pp. 32–48). Oxford: Routledge.

Ross, A., Dion, J., Cantinotti, M., Collin-Vezina, D., & Paquette, L. (2015). Impact of residential schooling and of child abuse on substance use problem in Indigenous peoples. *Addictive Behaviors, 51,* 184–192. https://doi.org/10.1016/j.addbeh.2015.07.014.

Royal Commision on Aboriginal Peoples (RCAP). (1996). *Report of the Royal Commission on Aboriginal Peoples.* Retrieved from https://www.bac-lac.gc.ca/eng/discover/aboriginal-heritage/royal-commission-aboriginal-peoples/Pages/final-report.aspx.

Smylie, J., Martin, C. M., Kaplan-Myrth, N., Steele, L., Tait, C., & Hogg, W. (2004). Knowledge translation and indigenous knowledge. *International Journal of Circumpolar Health, 63*(supp. 2), 139–143. https://doi.org/10.3402/ijch.v63i0.17877.

Social Sciences and Humanities Research Council of Canada (SSHRC). (2019). *Definitions of terms; Indigenous research.* Retrieved from https://www.sshrc-crsh.gc.ca/funding-financement/programs-programmes/definitions-eng.aspx?pedisable=false&wbdisable=true#a11.

Statistics Canada. (2013). *NHS in brief: The educational attainment of Aboriginal peoples in Canada, National Household Survey 2011.* Retrieved from https://www12.statcan.gc.ca/nhs-enm/2011/as-sa/99-012-x/99-012-x2011003_3-eng.pdf.

Statistics Canada. (2016a). *Aboriginal peoples in Canada: Key results from the 2016 Census.* Retrieved from https://www150.statcan.gc.ca/n1/daily-quotidien/171025/dq171025a-eng.htm?indid=14430-1&indgeo=0.

Statistics Canada. (2016b). *Focus on geography series: Aboriginal peoples.* Retrieved from https://www12.statcan.gc.ca/census-recensement/2016/as-sa/fogs-spg/Facts-CAN-eng.cfm?Lang=Eng&GK=CAN&GC=01&TOPIC=9.

Supreme Court of Canada. (2016). *Daniels v. Canada (Indian Affairs and Northern Development).* Retrieved from https://scc-csc.lexum.com/scc-csc/scc-csc/en/item/15858/index.do.

Truth and Reconciliation Commission of Canada. (2015a). Canada's residential schools: The history, Part 1 Origins to 1939. The final report of the Truth and Reconciliation Commission of Canada. Vol. 1. Montreal, Canada: McGill-Queen's University Press.

Truth and Reconciliation Commission of Canada. (2015b). *Honouring the truth, reconciling for the future. Summary of the final report of the Truth and Reconciliation Commission of Canada.* Retrieved from https://ehprnh2mwo3.exactdn.com/wp-content/uploads/2021/01/Executive_Summary_English_Web.pdf.

Truth and Reconciliation Commission of Canada. (2015c). Canada's residential schools: The legacy. The final report of the Truth and Reconciliation Commission of Canada. Vol. 5. Montreal, Canada: McGill Queen's University Press. Retrieved from https://ehprnh2mwo3.exactdn.com/wp-content/uploads/2021/01/Volume_5_Legacy_English_Web.pdf.

Truth and Reconciliation Commission of Canada. (2015d). *Canada's residential schools: The history part 2, 1939-2000. The final report of the Truth and Reconciliation Commission Of Canada.* Vol. I. Retrieved from https://ehprnh2mwo3.exactdn.com/wp-content/uploads/2021/01/Volume_1_History_Part_2_English_Web.pdf.

Truth and Reconciliation Commission of Canada. (2015e). *Truth and reconciliation commission of Canada: Calls to action.* Retrieved from http://trc.ca/assets/pdf/Calls_to_Action_English2.pdf.

Tuhiwai Smith, L. (1999). *Decolonizing methodologies: Research and indigenous peoples.* London: Zed Books Ltd.

Tuhiwai Smith, L. (2012). *Decolonizing methodologies: Research and indigenous peoples* (2nd ed). London: Zed Books Ltd.

United Nations (2007). *United Nations declaration on the rights of Indigenous peoples.* Retrieved from .Https://www.un.org/development/desa/indigenous-peoples/wp-content/uploads/sites/19/2018/11/UNDRIP_E_web.pdf.

University of Alberta (2020). *Indigenous Canada* [Open Online Course]. Retrieved from https://www.ualberta.ca/admissions-programs/online-courses/indigenous-canada/index.html.

Waldram, J. B., Herring, A., & Young, T. K. (2006). *Aboriginal health in Canada: Historical, cultural, and epidemiological perspectives.* Toronto, ON: University of Toronto Press.

Wilson, S. (2001). What is an Indigenous research methodology? *Canadian Journal of Native Education, 25*(2), 175–179.

Wilson, K. (2018). Pulling together: Foundations guide. Victoria, BC: BCcampus. Retrieved from https://opentextbc.ca/indigenizationfoundations/.

Wright, S. (2014). *Our ice is vanishing/Sikuvut Nunguliqtut: A history of Inuit, newcomers, and climate change.* Montreal: McGill-Queen's University Press.

Yantz, J. (2005). *Indigenous knowledge of the land and protected areas: Fond du Lac Denesuline Nation and the Athabasca Sand Dunes.* [Thesis].

Qualitative Research

RESEARCH **VIGNETTE**

Public Health Nursing and the Social Construction of Mothering

Megan Aston, PhD, RN
Professor
School of Nursing
Dalhousie University
Halifax, Nova Scotia

In 1986, I began my career working as a public health nurse in the community visiting new mothers, elderly clients, and schools. I enjoyed supporting clients where they were at with their health needs and to collaboratively make plans that were meaningful to them. Education was part of what I did, but it was more about building relationships and trust to provide support and ensure people felt empowered to take care of themselves in whatever way they needed. Working with other public health nurses enabled me to learn from them and subsequently develop my own nursing skills of critical assessments, caring, empathy, communication, building therapeutic relationships, advocating, and leadership. Although our practice was very independent as we individually went out on home visits and to schools, we also met daily to support each other.

I then went back to school to obtain my Master's and PhD so that I could teach and conduct research. I also continued to work as a public health nurse during this time and ultimately focused my research in the area of public health nursing and maternal, newborn, and child health because this was my passion. I wanted to understand the challenges that mothers experienced early

postpartum and how public health nurses could best support them. I used qualitative feminist poststructuralism as my research methodology (Aston, 2016) that provided a lens to understand not only personal experiences but also how the social construction of mothering had a significant impact on mothers' daily practices. Not only did I begin to understand how relations of power explained how mothers and public health nurses continued to be socially and personally constructed as invisible, but I also began to understand how both mothers and public health nurses used their agency to challenge everyday practices that might be oppressive or marginalizing.

I will provide examples from two research studies that demonstrate how an understanding of the social construction of mothering and public health nursing can inform healthcare practices to address both the oppression and empowerment of mothers and public health nurses. In our first study, entitled *Listening to the voices of mothers and public health nurses, personal social and institutional aspects of early home visiting,* we conducted semistructured face-to-face interviews with new mothers and public health nurses. Using feminist poststructuralism and discourse analysis we inductively analyzed transcripts of the audiotaped interviews to come up with the following themes: 1) understanding institutional tensions

between targeted and universal home visiting programs (Aston et al., 2014); 2) the power of therapeutic relationships between PHNs and mothers (Aston et al., 2015); and 3) shifting the meaning of postpartum health outcomes (Aston et al., 2016). The full report can also be found online at http://tinyurl.com/j7ep8nr.

Mothers told us that becoming a new mother was both exciting and stressful. They also told us that the establishment of a trusting and supportive *relationship* with public health nurses was foundational to helping them feel more confident and thus able to transition into their new role as a mother. Both mothers and public health nurses challenged the meaning and prioritization of *health outcomes*. Similar to dominant practices within the Canadian healthcare system, the Public Health Agency of Canada (2020; 2009) focuses primarily on physical aspects of postpartum, thus perpetuating the hierarchy between physical and psychological/emotional aspects of postpartum. While physical health outcomes such as breastfeeding, back pain, perineal pain, and urinary incontinence are important to address, mothers and public health nurses told us that it was just as important if not more important to include other health outcomes such as self-confidence. Mothers and public health nurses overwhelmingly told us that everyday maternal self-confidence, feeling normal, empowerment, and positive mental health were extremely important indicators of a new mother's ability to adapt to parenting. It also became evident that there were tensions between having targeted and universal programs. Targeted programs for high-risk mothers were prioritized to be more urgent than universal programs for all mothers. This is an issue that continues to be debated globally. Public health nurses and mothers offered insightful examples of how both programs were needed. In particular, PHNs in the universal program had to continually defend their work. Despite strong evidence that PHNs were making a difference in their support of new mothers, PHNs expressed concerns that their work continued to be underappreciated, invisible, and poorly understood.

In our second study, *MUMs: Mapping and understanding mothers' social networks*, we conducted focus groups with mothers across Nova Scotia to examine where and how they sought out information and support. We used feminist poststructuralism and discourse analysis to understand the personal, social, and institutional construction of mothers' experiences and came up with the following themes: 1) Finding normal for baby and mom; 2) Trust your gut; 3) Support and social connections build confidence; 4) How the message is delivered matters; 5) Mothers are savvy when navigating postpartum information (Aston et al., 2018; Price et al., 2018). For more details, you can read our report on our website, www.mumsns.ca (Mapping and understanding mothers' social networks, 2020) as well as watch our video based on research findings (Mommy Dialogues Video, 2019).

Supporting mothers to *find their normal* was a central theme across all interviews. What was normal for the baby and what was normal for mothers was an everyday practice. Normal meant *feeling confident* in their choices to take care of themselves and their babies in the early postpartum period. Sometimes it involved asking other mothers what they did, seeking information from healthcare professionals, talking to friends and family, reading books, or going online. Searching for information was a constant task that at times became overwhelming. To effectively navigate this process it was important to feel supported. Support came in many forms, but ultimately it had to feel right for each mother. Therefore, *trusting your gut* became a central theme and a place to start when building *confidence*, which was clearly an important health outcome. It became clear that it was important to pay attention to how health professionals spoke to new mothers, how public health nurses built trusting relationships, how online chat spaces supported or shamed mothers, and how mothers ultimately came to decisions based on filtering through conflicting information.

I have had the privilege of leading an incredible team of researchers, collaborators, and research assistants. Through my program of research I have been able to collaboratively work with others to publish reports and articles, develop educational videos, share findings at conferences, and ultimately contribute evidence that can be used to make a difference in health delivery by public health nurses and healthcare workers for new mothers, their babies, and families. ∎

REFERENCES

Aston, M., Etowa, J., Price, S., Vukic, A., Hart, C., MacLeod, E., & Randel, P. (2016). Public health nurses and mothers challenge and shift the meaning of health outcomes. *Global Qualitative Nursing Research, 3*, 1–10. https://doi.org/10.1177/2333393616632126.

Aston, M., Price, S., Etowa, J., Vukic, A., Young, L., Hart, C., MacLeod, E., & Randel, P. (2014). Universal and targeted early home visiting: Perspectives of public health nurses and mothers. *Nursing Reports, 4*(1). https://doi.org/10.4081/nursrep.2014.3290.

Aston, M., Price, S., Etowa, J., Vukic, A., Young, L., Hart, C., MacLeod, E., & Randel, P. (2015). The power of relationships: Exploring how public health nurses support mothers and families during postpartum home visits. *Journal of Family Nursing, 21*(1), 11–34. https://doi.org/10.1177/1074840714561524.

Aston, M., Price, S., Monaghan, J., Sim, M., Hunter, A., & Little, V. (2018). Navigating and negotiating information and support: Experiences of first time mothers. *Journal of Clinical Nursing, 27*(3-4), 640–649. https://doi.org/10.1111/jocn.13970.

Aston, M. (2016). Teaching feminist poststructuralism: Founding scholars are still relevant today. *Creative Education, 7*(15), 2251–2267. https://doi.org/10.4236/ce.2016.715220.

Mapping and understanding mothers' social networks. (2020). Report website. www.mumsns.ca.

Mommy Dialogues Video. (2019). https://www.youtube.com/watch?v=G0Z69omZSAY&feature=youtu.be&fbclid=IwAR0YIZuqr6K5ehw-7EKoP72GER-RfMUad4vz-rdFGORMSkPB-Gjv4oemp3A.

Price, S., Aston, M., Monaghan, J., Sim, S., Tomblin Murphy, G., Etowa, J., Pickles, M., Hunter, A., & Little, V. (2018). Maternal knowing and social networks: Understanding first time mothers' search for information and support through online and offline social networks. *Qualitative Health Research, 28*(10), 1552–1563. doi.org/10.1177/1049732317748314.

Public Health Agency of Canada. (2020). Health Pregnancy and Infancy website. https://www.canada.ca/en/public-health/services/health-promotion.html#hp.

Public Health Agency of Canada. (2009). What mothers say: The Canadian Maternity Experiences Survey. https://www.canada.ca/content/dam/phac-aspc/migration/phac-aspc/rhs-ssg/pdf/survey-eng.pdf.

CHAPTER 8

Introduction to Qualitative Research

Sarah Stahlke | Lorraine Thirsk

LEARNING OUTCOMES

After reading this chapter, you will be able to do the following:

- Describe the purposes of qualitative research.
- Describe the general steps of a qualitative research study.
- Identify the links between qualitative research and evidence-informed practice.
- Identify four ways in which qualitative findings can be used in evidence-informed practice.
- Discuss unique features of qualitative research.
- Explain the use of mixed methods to answer research questions.
- Summarize the design and purpose of systematic reviews of qualitative research.

KEY TERMS

bracketing	"grand tour" question	qualitative research
context dependent	inclusion criteria	reflexivity
data saturation	inductive	snowball sampling
deductive	metasynthesis	text
exclusion criteria	naturalistic setting	triangulation
focus group	purposive sample	

STUDY RESOURCES

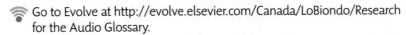 Go to Evolve at http://evolve.elsevier.com/Canada/LoBiondo/Research for the Audio Glossary.

FUNDAMENTAL TO NURSING IS an understanding of human experience. In order to provide excellent patient care and to offer leadership in health care, nurses must be able to recognize and understand the meanings that people give to their health experiences as well as the meanings and perceptions nurses attach to their work. Imagine you wanted to know about homeless people's issues and needs in accessing health care (as did Ramsay et al., 2019), how family caregivers grieve in anticipation of loss (Coelho et al., 2020), how nurses use and manage their emotions when caring for critical ill infants (Cricco-Lizza, 2014), why people do not adhere to medication regimes (Yeh et al., 2019), or what educational needs parents of children with leukemia have (Aburn & Gott, 2014). Qualitative research explores these kinds of questions. Qualitative research is mainly used to delve deeply into human experience (patient, family, nurse) as a means of contributing to practice knowledge, but is also used to develop conceptual frameworks and theories or provide deeper explanations behind the findings of quantitative studies.

In this chapter, the basic tenets of qualitative research are reviewed, the steps of a qualitative study are outlined, the contributions of qualitative research to evidence-informed practice are explored, and the unique features of qualitative research are examined. In addition, we review two trends in research: mixed methods and qualitative synthesis.

WHAT IS QUALITATIVE RESEARCH?

Qualitative research is a systematic, interactive, and experience-based research method used to describe and give meaning to human phenomena. This broad term encompasses several methodologies that share many similarities in the conduct of such research. According to Denzin and Lincoln (2011), "qualitative researchers study things in their natural settings, attempting to make sense of, or interpret, phenomena in terms of the meanings people bring to them" (p. 3). A **naturalistic setting** is one that people live in every day. In many cases, the qualitative researcher goes wherever the participants are: their homes, schools, workplaces, communities, and, sometimes, the hospital or an outpatient setting. There are occasions when qualitative researchers interact with participants in arranged settings such as meeting rooms or public places, but the key point is that they do not attempt to create artificial control groups or other non-natural structures in their research.

Qualitative research has a long history in the social sciences, but until the 1990s, nursing solidly embraced the scientific method and attempted to quantify almost all topics of interest to nursing. For many years, doctoral nursing students were dissuaded from conducting qualitative studies; the push was for a traditional quantitative approach, which was viewed by many as being more credible (Hutchinson, 2001). Thus, as nursing gained its foothold in academics, doctoral students were urged to conduct research by using quantitative methods to help nursing gain legitimacy in academia. It took the efforts of pioneering nursing researchers to promote qualitative research as a highly relevant approach to knowledge generation for nursing. Although quantitative studies do yield valuable information that contributes to practice, their predominance sometimes can obscure the valuable contribution qualitative research can make. As the value of qualitative research has become recognized, contemporary nurse scholars are trained in qualitative methods. Students are encouraged to use the method that best answers their research questions, instead of using methods that might add a veneer of scientific legitimacy to conducting the research but do not answer the research question at hand. The best method is the most suitable method for the topic, which is not necessarily the quantitative method.

Qualitative research is discovery oriented; it is explanatory, descriptive, and interpretive in nature. Words, as opposed to numbers, are used to explain a phenomenon. The data gathered in qualitative research are text-based. The term **text** used in this context means that data are in narrative form, words written from interviews that were recorded and then transcribed or notes written from the researcher's observations. It can also be interpreted very broadly if text is understood as the way people speak of or express themselves, which allows for poetry, photography, art, and artifacts to be regarded as textual qualitative data. Qualitative research gives voice to human experience and lets us see the world through the eyes of another: the parent of a child with leukemia, the emotionally exhausted nurse, the homeless person in need of care. Through qualitative research, nurses can understand these experiences if they interact with people who are having an experience and consider the context in which the experiences take place.

Qualitative research is often based on the premise that in understanding human experience there are multiple realities. For example, although there may be some common aspects of the experience of being a parent of a child with leukemia, it is never entirely the same for any two people. Another foundational perspective in qualitative research is that reality is socially constructed and **context dependent**—that is, the meaning of an observation is defined by its circumstance or the environment. For example, in managing the emotional aspects of their work, neonatal intensive care unit (NICU) nurses with different social supports or different levels of experience may have different needs or coping capacity (Cricco-Lizza, 2014). Qualitative researchers work with text-based data in natural contexts to discover aspects of the human condition and describe and interpret them in rich detail. Ideally, the reader, if even slightly acquainted with the phenomenon, would have an "Aha!" moment in reading a well-written qualitative report.

Many nurses feel a connection to qualitative research and feel comfortable with this approach because they are trained in how to talk to people about the health issues concerning them and are used to listening well (Roper & Shapira, 2000). It has been argued that qualitative research is the best fit for nursing's humanist orientation and the most appropriate for the topics of interests to nurses (Hutchinson, 2001). However, while we generally accept that qualitative research is equal to quantitative research in the search for knowledge for nursing practice, the most important consideration for any research study is whether the methodology fits the question. It must fit, or else the study will contribute little to the scientific knowledge base for practice. This is also the first question you should ask yourself when you read studies and are considering them as evidence on which to base your practice: Does the methodology fit with the research question under study?

 Research Hint _____

All research is based on a paradigm, but the paradigm is seldom specifically identified in a research report.

GENERAL STEPS IN CONDUCTING QUALITATIVE RESEARCH

The general steps of qualitative research can be found in Box 8.1. Further information about each of these steps can be found in the related chapters throughout the text. Here we present an overview to specifically address the unique processes that occur in qualitative research.

Review of the Literature

After a researcher has determined that a qualitative approach is the best way to answer the research question, a review of the relevant literature is required. The literature review builds a picture of what is known about a particular topic and provides a foundation of knowledge for the study the researcher is planning. It also reveals the gaps in knowledge in terms of the kinds of questions that have been asked about a topic, the populations that have been studied (or not), the methods that have been used to inquire about the phenomenon, and changing contexts and ideologies in society and health care. When little is known about a topic, the literature search

---

BOX 8.1

STEPS IN THE QUALITATIVE RESEARCH PROCESS

- Review of the literature
- Study design
- Sample
- Setting: recruitment and data collection
- Data collection
- Data analysis
- Findings
- Conclusions

may require creativity on the author's part because published research on the phenomenon in question may not exist. The researcher can frame their study by looking for studies with similar participants, with the same patient population, or on a closely related concept.

Research by Coelho et al. (2020) helps to illustrate the purpose of a literature review. These researchers were interested in how family caregivers anticipated loss and grief when caring for a loved one with cancer. They found that the concept of anticipatory grief was unclear and had been inappropriately researched, leading to misunderstandings about bereavement. By grounding their study in the literature, they were able to clarify the concept and contribute new knowledge about the experience. In another example, Ramsey et al. (2019) used their literature review to summarize statistics that demonstrated the extent of homelessness in their region and some of the key findings of previous studies about barriers to health care access for homeless people. They explained in their review that a shift in the system toward patient-focused care might have an impact on homeless people's experiences with accessing and navigating the health care system. The change in the context of care raised new qualitative research questions for them to study. Finally, Cricco-Lizza (2014), in her study of emotional labour in NICU, explained that the concept had emerged from sociology and discussed how it had been studied in nursing to a limited extent, but never in NICU, making it necessary to seek understanding about this experience for these nurses. These examples show the different ways that a literature review can be used to provide the background for and/or justify a new qualitative study. While it is most common that qualitative researchers conduct a literature review, it should be noted that there are a few instances (for example, in grounded theory) when qualitative researchers conduct a very limited review because they want to be amenable to discovering and learning about the phenomenon under study and

not be swayed or otherwise influenced by previous findings in the field.

Study Design

The study design is the approach that will be taken to go about answering the research question. In qualitative research, there may simply be a descriptive or naturalistic design, in which the researchers adhere to the general tenets of qualitative research but do not commit to a particular method. However, there are also specific types of qualitative methods, which are discussed in Chapter 9. The researcher should be clear in their mind about what approach they are taking so that the study design is congruent with the philosophical foundations and common characteristics of qualitative research, and the specific steps associated with particular methods. Generally, a qualitative study should be designed to tap into the perspectives and insights of people who are immersed in an experience, with the goal of describing that experience, developing a concept or framework, or describing the nature of a phenomenon, such as pain, change, or caregiving.

Sample

Qualitative research employs particular sampling strategies to ensure that rich data are collected from the appropriate participants. In qualitative studies, the researchers are usually looking for a **purposive sample**: a group consisting of particular people who can elucidate the phenomenon they want to study. Because a common goal of qualitative research is rich description and understanding of human experience, it is critical to ensure that study participants are able to discuss the experience or phenomenon in depth. Random sampling, which is vital in quantitative research, is not appropriate for qualitative research because a random sample would not necessarily contain people who know about the research topic. Qualitative researchers also rely on a sampling procedure called **snowball sampling**. In this sampling processes, people who have already participated in the research refer other people who could speak knowledgeably about the topic and might want to participate in the study. This is helpful and practical for researchers. The referral helps to establish trust and makes it easier for researchers to find people who have had the experience they are studying.

When recruiting the sample, qualitative researchers establish clear criteria for participation in the study in order to find people who are best able to shed light on the phenomenon in question. These parameters are known as inclusion criteria (criteria that people must satisfy to participate in a study) and exclusion criteria (criteria used to exclude people from participating in a study). To illustrate this, Ramsey and colleagues (2019) specifically sought "participants who self-identified as experiencing homelessness, were aged 18 years or older, and ha[d] had an interaction with a health care provider within the health care system during the time they were experiencing homelessness" (p. 1841). Aburn and Gott (2014), who studied the educational needs of parents with children with leukemia, specifically excluded parents of children who were still in the hospital since the study aimed to explore perceptions about discharge teaching. At times, researchers seek samples that include **maximum variation** so they can obtain a range of perspectives on a phenomenon. For example, Cricco-Lizza (2014), in her study of nurses' emotional labour, sampled NICU nurses that varied in age, gender, race, education, and length of experience to provide a "wide-angle picture of their everyday practices, emotions, and coping strategies" (p. 616). Ramsey et al. (2019) also sought variation in their sample by recruiting homeless people with both positive and negative experiences with the health care system. Researchers' decisions about recruitment criteria should be based on sound rationale and should be aimed at gathering the best data to answer the research question.

In qualitative research, there is no set sample size and samples tend to be fairly small. Qualitative researchers seek rich descriptions of a phenomenon or experience rather than specific numbers of participants and they recruit participants until **data saturation** occurs. While each participant can offer new insights, there is a point in each study at which the information being shared with the researcher from participants becomes largely repetitive; in other words, the ideas shared by the participants have been shared by previous participants and few new ideas emerge. This is when data saturation is said to have occurred. Determining the point of saturation can be difficult. It can be difficult to judge the point at which there is conceptual completeness and to convey how that was ascertained. It might be, therefore, more useful for a researcher to consider whether the data offer a sufficient depth of understanding that allows them to interpret and theorise (Nelson, 2017).

Setting: Recruitment and Data Collection

The setting may incorporate both the setting from which participants are recruited and the setting in which data are collected, although often these may be the same. Data are usually collected in a naturalistic setting, which generally means that participants take part in the research within the environment of interest to the researcher. As noted earlier, though, actual interviews may take place outside of the setting of interest for the sake of privacy or convenience. The interview location should be selected carefully to ensure privacy, lack of interruption, and quiet and should be a neutral location that will ensure participant comfort. When the setting for data collection is the environment that the researcher aims to focus on, it can include the participant's home, workplace, community, care unit, school, and so on. Being allowed into a setting that is important to a participant can offer an incredible window into aspects of the participant's life and experience, which can expand on what the researcher is able to see and understand.

It is possible that interview settings may be remote and utilize telephone or video conferencing technology. This allows researchers to include participants who are located in settings of interest that are practically inaccessible to the researcher, such as for study topics that involve remote participants or those in international locations. This has become more common in response to the COVID-19 pandemic. For example, Aburn and Gott (2014) interviewed parents of children with leukemia while they were at the outpatient clinic for their child's appointment, but they also interviewed some parents by telephone when they lived out of town and were not able to extend their time at the clinic to participate in the research.

Data Collection

In a qualitative study, typical data collection strategies include interviews, observation, and document analysis, although there are others. Interviews are a feature of almost every qualitative study. They allow engagement with participants and the gathering of rich experiential data. The researcher may interview an individual or interview a group of people in what is called a **focus group**. The researcher asks the participant(s) questions about the phenomenon of interest and then listens to them as they share aspects of their experience in response. Interview questions should be clear and straightforward and elicit what the researcher wants to know. In qualitative studies, there may be a broad opening or **grand tour question**. For example, when studying the emotional work of NICU nurses, Cricco-Lizza (2014) began with broad interview questions "about the nature of their work and their feelings about their role as a NICU nurse" (p. 617). Similarly, Coelho et al. (2020) asked their participants, "How has your experience been as a caregiver for your relative?" (p. 694). These kinds of questions allow participants to begin their responses from a point that they determine. More specific probing questions can follow so the interviewer can obtain details about the experience that relate to the overall research questions.

Most qualitative researchers use audio recorders to ensure that they have captured the participant's exact words. This also takes some of the pressure off researchers to remember huge volumes of detail or write down every single word, and it frees them up to listen fully. The recordings are usually transcribed verbatim, and then the researcher who conducted the interviews listens to the recordings for accuracy.

Data may also be collected through observation. This takes place when the researcher spends time in the study setting to observe individuals and/or groups of people as they go about their daily activities, such as giving medications, visiting a health professional in a clinic, participating in an educational session, or caring for a sick child. Observational data helps to put the interview data into context and can generate insights about how things work in a particular study environment. Usually, the researcher will take extensive field notes, jotting down observations about the physical setting, relationships, verbal and nonverbal interactions, the flow of activities, and so on. Documents and artifacts may also be reviewed, such as charting systems, policies, posters, memos, and artwork, as these also help the researcher to understand the context of the experience they are studying.

Data collection cannot begin until informed consent is obtained.

Data Analysis

Data analysis involves the interpretation of the raw data, which are usually verbatim transcripts of the recorded interviews in a qualitative study and may also include field notes. Qualitative research can involve high volumes of textual data. Many qualitative researchers use computer-assisted data analysis programs to help with the task of data management (e.g., NVivo, MAXQDA, Atlas.ti, Dedoose). Some researchers prefer to print their transcripts and physically cut apart and group sections of the transcripts that relate to each other. No matter how the researcher handles the data, they are actively involved in reading the data, looking for keywords and phrases. The goal is to find commonalities and differences in the interviews and then to group these into broader, more abstract, overarching categories of meaning, called themes, that capture much of the data (Mayan, 2009).

To illustrate, Yeh et al. (2019), in their study about adherence to medication regimes among youth with multiple sclerosis, had participants who talked about visual cues to take their medication, such as seeing the pill bottle, disruptions to routine that made them forget to take their medication, and the use of alarms or calendar reminders. The researchers captured these pieces of data within the theme "remembering versus forgetting." Thus, it is possible to find a term that encompasses a group of specific participant descriptions. Analyzing the data into themes assists the research user in understanding the most significant aspects of an experience. Nursing researchers usually make it clear when reporting their findings whether they are describing a process, or a list of circumstances that are functioning in some way, a set of conditions that must be present for something to occur, or a description of what it is like to go through some health-related transition or experience. This is by no means an all-inclusive list but rather examples to help you understand what analyzed qualitative findings can look like. After the data are analyzed, the findings of a qualitative study are then compared to the existing literature. The researchers will describe how their findings are similar to or different from what is already known and how their study contributes to knowledge on the topic. They will usually also make suggestions regarding how to use the findings in practice and will discuss whether the findings and subsequent recommendations are transferable to other patients and settings. Because of its exploratory nature, qualitative research can produce results that were not anticipated, and this can provide the foundation for new research questions and studies.

Chapter 16 includes a more in-depth exploration on qualitative data analysis methods.

Research Hint

Values are involved in all research. It is important, however, that they be acknowledged and identified so their influence on the results can be managed and understood.

EVIDENCE-INFORMED PRACTICE

Because nursing is a practice discipline, the most important purpose of nursing research is to use research findings to improve the care of patients. The findings of qualitative nursing research can also be used to improve nurses' working environments and the functioning of the health care system. The best way to start to answer questions that have not been addressed or when a new perspective is needed in practice is through the use of qualitative methods. The answers to questions provided by qualitative data reflect important evidence that may offer the first systematic insights about a phenomenon and the setting in which it occurs. Therefore, broadening evidence models beyond a narrow hierarchical perspective is imperative.

Qualitative research is particularly well suited to studying the human experience of health, a central concern of nursing science. Because qualitative methods focus on the whole of human experience and the meaning ascribed by individuals living the experience, these methods extend understanding of health beyond traditionally measured units to include the complexity of the human health experience as it occurs in everyday life. This closeness to what is "real" and "everyday" holds the promise of guidance for nursing practice.

UNIQUE FEATURES OF QUALITATIVE RESEARCH

Emergent Nature of the Design

The emergent nature of the research design means that the researcher must always be considering the approach to the research and adapting it as circumstances change. For example, there may be a significant change in the research setting that makes the research project more challenging, such as a restructuring of care delivery or the introduction of new equipment and procedures. At times, the change may be so overwhelming that the research must be put on hold, such as when increased demand is placed on caregivers and the health care system during a pandemic. During the course of a study, conditions change, and what was agreeable at the beginning may become intrusive. In some situations, the researcher might find that recruitment is difficult and that different strategies are needed, or different participants must be sought. Other times, as data collection proceeds and new information emerges, the study shifts in a new direction; preliminary data can indicate to the researcher that there is a related but slightly better approach to the research or the need for a revised research question. This may mean that different participants are required or that the research has become something other than what original participants agreed to take part in. Changes to the study design may necessitate updated ethics committee approval.

Researcher–Participant Interaction

In qualitative research, the researcher forms a relationship with the participant. Basic differences exist between the intention of the nurse when conducting research and when engaging in practice (Smith & Liehr, 2003), which has implications for the research relationship. In practice, the nurse has caring–healing intentions. In research, the nurse intends to understand the perspective of the participant about an experience or phenomenon. It may indeed be a therapeutic experience for the participant to describe and share their experience. Sometimes talking to a caring listener about things that matter energizes healing, even if this result is incidental. From an ethical perspective, the qualitative researcher is promising only to listen and to encourage the participant's story. If this experience is therapeutic for the participant, it becomes an unplanned benefit of the research.

Another point to consider regarding the researcher–participant relationship is the balance of power within it. Glesne (2011) has described several roles that the qualitative researcher may assume, such as exploiter, intervener or reformer, advocate, and friend. All researchers "use" participants to some extent to tap into people's experiences and thus answer their research questions, with no recognition of the participants. Although the researcher is usually in a position of power, researchers do not tend to abuse their power. Nevertheless, the power differentials in the research relationship must be carefully considered and managed. Some researchers conduct collaborative research projects that build in power-sharing (e.g., participatory action research; Indigenous methods). Often, the involvement of participants in a study is rationalized by the good that may come of sharing the knowledge obtained from the research. There are some risks for the researcher in the relationship as well. The researcher may be distressed by hearing what the participant says or may have expectations placed upon them that they advocate for a cause or promote a specific agenda in the research (Stahlke, 2018).

Finally, as trust and respect are established, researchers may find themselves in the role of confidant, which may, in some cases, lead to friendship. Although some qualitative researchers find the role of friend acceptable if it is based on trust, caring, and collaboration, an inherent danger exists that the data are given in the context of friendship and not for the purposes of research (Glesne, 2011). Investigators may also find it difficult to end the relationship and say goodbye to participants. Fournier and colleagues (2006) indicated that more attention needs to be given to psychological preparation, focused on exiting the relationship. In participatory action research, the researcher also needs to consider whether there are any long-term obligations to sustain the project (Fournier et al., 2006).

Research Hint

Researchers are privileged to enter the lives of other people and must treat the ensuing relationship with the utmost respect.

Researcher as Instrument

Researchers, whether they are doing qualitative or quantitative studies, bring their own personal history, experiences, and knowledge to their research. Qualitative researchers consider the impact this has on research processes and outcomes because of their unique involvement in the research setting. The responsibility to remain true to the data requires that the researchers acknowledge their **positionality** and interpret findings in a way that accurately reflects the participant's reality. Qualitative researchers frequently write in personal journals during their research activity to monitor and become aware of their personal perspectives and feelings (Glesne, 2011). Through this process of **reflexivity** in qualitative research, researchers constantly challenge themselves to understand how their perspective may be shaping the method, interviews, analysis, and interpretations. Patton (2015) reminds us that, as a researcher, one needs "to be attentive to and conscious of the cultural, political, social, linguistic, and economic origins of one's own perspective and voice as well as the perspective and voices of those one interviews and those to whom one reports" (p. 70).

Research questions can often arise from a nurse researcher's professional background, which means that, at times, the researcher might be conducting research in an area with which they are familiar and in which they may know people (e.g.,

their care unit, clinic, town, school of nursing). Their familiarity makes them an **insider** but their researcher status distances them from the field and makes them an **outsider**. Being an insider helps the researcher to avoid culture shock when studying a new area, eases communication, and improves acceptance of the researcher's presence (Roper & Shapira, 2000). It can also assist the researcher to understand what is going on in the setting. The distance that comes with being an outsider can ensure that the researcher does not take for granted the events taking place in the setting and is able to analyze the research data with fresh eyes.

Streubert and Carpenter (2011) recommend that researchers identify their own thoughts, feelings, and perceptions by compartmentalizing them in the process, referred to as bracketing, in which personal biases about the phenomenon of interest are identified in order to clarify how personal experience and beliefs may influence what is heard and reported. Bracketing is based on the assumption that people can separate their research about a specific phenomenon from their personal experiences and background. While some researchers see the researcher's self as a potential danger to the research, Chesney (2001) argues that, rather than hold oneself at a distance, it is more helpful for the researcher to be honest about their background, answer questions truthfully, and use their knowledge to "spark insight and understanding" (p. 131).

Triangulation

Triangulation can be defined as the act of bringing more than one source of data to bear on a single point (Marshall & Rossman, 2011). Data from different sources can be used to corroborate, elaborate, or illuminate the phenomenon in question. The use of multiple data sources is common in qualitative research. You will recall that earlier it was noted that data collection in qualitative research often involves interviews, observation, and document analysis. These varied sources of data support each other and allow the researcher to develop a broad perspective on the context of the experience or phenomenon they are studying. Triangulation can also be accomplished by having multiple researchers analyze the same data and arrive at a consensus about its meaning or by referring to theory that provides another perspective on what is in the data. Mixed method research, which combines qualitative and quantitative approaches (see next section), can also be considered a form of triangulation.

Evidence-Informed Practice Tip

- Triangulation offers an opportunity for researchers to increase the strength and consistency of evidence provided by the use of multiple sources of data.
- The combination of stories with numbers (qualitative and quantitative research approaches) through use of mixed method research enhances the completeness of the picture of the phenomenon being studied and, therefore, can provide sound evidence for guiding practice.

Four types of triangulation have been described (Carter, Bryant-Lukosius, DiCenso, Blythe, & Neville, 2014):

1. Data triangulation: the use of a variety of data sources in a study. For example, the researcher collects data at different times, in different settings, and from different groups of people.
2. Investigator triangulation: the collaboration of several different researchers or evaluators from divergent backgrounds
3. Theory triangulation: the use of multiple perspectives to interpret a single set of data
4. Methodological triangulation: the use of multiple methods to study a single problem (mixed methods)

MIXED METHODS

Use of mixed methods, as defined by Creswell (2014), "involves combining or integration of qualitative and quantitative research and data in a research study" (p. 14). Mixed methods approaches allow researchers to study the complex and multifaceted problems encountered in healthcare and answer research questions that cannot be addressed using a singular method (Doyle, Brady, & Byrne, 2009). It requires a "purposeful mixing of methods in data collection, data analysis, and interpretation" (Shorten & Smith, 2017, p. 74).

The design of the research is based on the research question. For example, if the purpose of the study is to describe, discover, or explore, then the theoretical drive is **inductive** (generalizing from specific data), with principal methods that are qualitative. Observations lead to the development of generalizations and, in some cases, theory to explain the phenomenon. However, if the purpose of the research is to confirm a theory or hypothesis, the underpinning of the research is **deductive** (concluded from data) and, subsequently, a quantitative drive will be used. Theory is tested by the development of a hypothesis and the gathering of data to accept or reject it. Mixed-methods research provides researchers with a wider range of tools and options to study phenomena.

There are three general types of "mixing" in mixed-methods research, and this may occur within a single study, or across a program of research (Sandelowski, 2014):

- *Used together:* One or more qualitative element and one or more quantitative element are used
- *Linking:* One or more qualitative element and one or more quantitative element are collected and compared
- *Integration:* Qualitative and quantitative elements are converted and integrated

In spite of the complexity of mixing methodologies and methods, serious readers of nursing research do not take long to determine that approaches and methods are being combined to contribute to theory building, to guide practice, and to facilitate instrument development. Several mixed-methodology research designs have been developed, many from the seminal work of nurse researchers such as Morgan (1998) and Morse (1991).

Morgan (1998) identified several models: for example, (1) small, preliminary, qualitative data providing information useful in the development

TABLE 8.1

TYPES OF MULTIMETHOD DESIGNS

DESIGN	ORDER	COMMENTS
INDUCTIVE PARADIGM		
Qualitative + qualitative	Simultaneous	One method is dominant and forms the basis for the study; paradigm is used when more than one perspective is required
Qualitative → qualitative	Sequential	One method is dominant and forms the basis for the study; the second supplements the first
Qualitative + quantitative	Simultaneous	Inductive drive; paradigm is used when some portion of the phenomenon can be measured
Qualitative → quantitative	Sequential	Inductive drive; paradigm can confirm earlier qualitative findings
DEDUCTIVE PARADIGM		
Quantitative + quantitative	Simultaneous	One method is dominant and forms the basis for the study; paradigm validates the finding of each instrument used
Quantitative → quantitative	Sequential	One method is dominant and forms the basis for the study; paradigm is used to elicit further details
Quantitative + qualitative	Simultaneous	Deductive theoretical drive; paradigm is used when some aspect of the phenomenon is not measurable
Quantitative → qualitative	Sequential	Deductive theoretical drive; paradigm is often used when the findings are unexpected, and the qualitative method is used to find explanations

of a larger quantitative study; (2) limited use of quantitative methods to guide the researcher in decisions pertaining to the larger qualitative project; (3) qualitative methods used to interpret results from a quantitative study; and (4) quantitative methods used to confirm results from the qualitative study. Morse (2003) identified eight different types of multimethod designs with simultaneous or sequential use of qualitative and quantitative methods (Table 8.1).

A mixture of methods is also encouraged when studying complex interventions—which are argued to be common in nursing practice (Richards & Borglin, 2011). Quantitative methods are used to test hypotheses and measure key variables and outcomes; qualitative methods are used to capture changes in implementation, experiences of the intervention, understand unanticipated outcomes, and generate further hypotheses or theory (Moore et al., 2015). A combination of methods

and elements will enable researchers to develop and implement better interventions. These various components are often reported across several studies from a research project, or in a program of research. Several examples of mixed methods research are presented in Table 8.2.

Premji et al. (2017, 2018), Dosani et al. (2017), and Currie et al. (2018) provide a good example of how mixed methods can be used in a program of research. This group of researchers published four articles related to late preterm infants (LPIs), exploring several aspects of both parents' and nurses' experiences of caring for LPIs in the community. The research project involved a sample of 122 mothers of LPIs and 10 public health nurses. Dosani et al. (2017) used an exploratory mixed methods design to examine both mother's and public health nurse's experiences of caring for LPIs in relation to breastfeeding. A unique feature of this study was the researchers' ability to triangulate

TABLE 8.2

RESEARCH USING MIXED METHODS APPROACHES

AUTHOR, YEAR	CONCEPTUAL FOCUS	RESEARCH DESIGN	STUDY PURPOSE	CONTRIBUTION TO THEORY	PRACTICE IMPLICATIONS	INSTRUMENT DEVELOPMENT IMPLICATIONS
Dosani et al. (2017)	Breastfeeding	Exploratory mixed methods; quantitative data on demographics, characteristics of mothers and infants, breastfeeding practices; interpretive thematic analysis of interviews	What is the mother's experience of caring for LPIs with respect to breastfeeding? What is the PHNs experience of caring for LPIs with respect to breastfeeding	—	Yes	—
Premji et al. (2018)	Mothers' experiences, stress, and confidence	Sequential explanatory method; questionnaire on maternal confidence, parenting stress, social support, postpartum depression; phenomenological analysis of semi-structured interviews	Understanding what it means to be a mother of a LPI including a mother's level of confidence and stress	—	Yes	—
Premji et al. (2017)	Mothers experiences of community-based care	Descriptive phenomenology	What does it mean to be a mother of a LPI?	—	Yes	—
Currie et al. (2018)	Public health nurses experiences	Descriptive phenomenology	Understand the lived experience of PHNs in caring for LPIs and supporting families in the postpartum period	—	Yes	—
Kaasalainen et al. (2019)	Pain management in long-term care	Mixed methods: controlled before-after study and focus group interviews with thematic content analysis	Evaluation of an NP-led, interprofessional pain management team in long-term care	—	Yes	—

Continued

TABLE 8.2

RESEARCH USING MIXED METHODS APPROACHES—cont'd

AUTHOR, YEAR	CONCEPTUAL FOCUS	RESEARCH DESIGN	STUDY PURPOSE	THEORY-BUILDING IMPLICATIONS	PRACTICE IMPLICATIONS	INSTRUMENT DEVELOPMENT IMPLICATIONS
					Yes	—
					Yes	—
					—	Yes
					—	Yes
					—	Yes
					Yes	Yes
St-Amant et al. (2014)	Professionalizing familial care	Phase 1 correlational survey design Phase 2 emergent grounded theory approach	Examine the processed by which registered nurses enact professional care work within the familial care domain	Yes	Yes	—
Stewart et al. (2015)	To design and evaluate a social support intervention for refugee new parents	Conducted group and in-depth individual interviews to explore impacts of the social support intervention. Secondly, several quantitative instruments were used to measure the impact of the intervention on support needs, loneliness and isolation, coping, and parenting stress index	To design and evaluate a social support intervention for refugee new parents	Yes	Yes	Yes

information generated from the mothers and the public health nurses to understand the phenomenon further. Premji et al. (2018) used a sequential explanatory mixed methods design to understand what it means to be a mother of an LPI, as well as the mothers' levels of confidence and stress. The semi-structured interviews, which followed questionnaire data, allowed for exploration and explanation of the changes in confidence scores amongst the mothers. Premji et al. (2017) used a descriptive phenomenological design to understand the experiences and meaning of being a mother of a LPI. Lastly, Currie et al. (2018) reported on the experiences of public health nurses in caring for LPIs using descriptive phenomenology. Details of these studies can be found in Table 8.2.

Kaasalainen et al. (2016) reported a mixed methods study on the effectiveness of pain management in long-term care. The goals of this study were to evaluate the effectiveness of a nurse practitioner (NP)–led pain management team in terms of resident outcomes and health care providers outcomes. In addition, the research team wanted to explore staff perceptions of implementation of this intervention. To address the first goal of establishing effectiveness, Kassalainenen et al. used a controlled before-and-after design across two intervention groups and a control group. The data collection for the quantitative component included four assessment tools for pain, as well as validated and reliable instruments to measure functional status, depression, and agitation for residents. Data regarding health care provider data were collected from chart reviews. In total, 345 long-term care residents participated in the study. There were significant improvements in pain and functional status across both intervention groups (Kaasalainen et al., 2016).

The qualitative component, described as a thematic content analysis, was used to evaluate the intervention at the end of the study (Kaasalainen et al., 2016). Focus groups were conducted with pain management team members, other health care team members, and administrators. In total,

29 health care providers participated in the qualitative interviews. Three themes were identified including: benefits of having access to a NP, benefits of the pain team, and barriers to pain management. The qualitative analysis was useful in further understanding *why* the intervention was effective—it improved teamwork, collaboration, and access to primary care; another finding that was thought to contribute to success of the program was the approachability and dependability of the NP (Kaasalainen et al., 2016). This knowledge may be useful for further interventions as well as implementation of the intervention in other facilities.

St-Amant et al. (2014; see Table 8.2) used a sequential-methods design to study how professional caregivers (RNs) provided care to an elderly relative. They initially used a quantitative survey design to examine the domain of professional and familial caregiving. In the second phase, the researchers used a qualitative grounded theory approach to examine the negotiating strategies utilized by the caregivers.

Stewart et al. (2015) used a mixed-method study design to develop and evaluate a social support intervention for Zimbabwean and Sudanese refugee new parents. The social support intervention focused on the use of face-to-face support groups co-led by a peer mentor. Qualitative methods such as group and in-depth individual interviews were conducted to explore the impact of the social support intervention. Several quantitative instruments were used to measure the impact of the intervention on support needs, loneliness and isolation, coping, and parenting stress index.

The mixed methods field continues to evolve as nurse researchers strive to determine which research combinations can deliver an enhanced understanding of human complexity and a substantial contribution to nursing science. As a research user, being well versed in a variety of methods will enable you to understand the usefulness and contribution of a variety of methods and tools and evaluate their use in answering specific research questions.

SYSTEMATIC REVIEWS OF QUALITATIVE EVIDENCE: METASYNTHESIS

The volume of qualitative research has grown exponentially over the last 30 years, leading researchers to become interested in bringing together the knowledge and insights generated from multiple studies (Thorne, 2019). Qualitative **metasynthesis** is a type of systematic review applied to qualitative research. Unlike quantitative research, in which statistical approaches are used to aggregate or average data by means of meta-analysis, metasynthesis involves integrating qualitative research findings on a topic and is based on comparative analysis and interpretative synthesis of qualitative research findings, whereby the researcher seeks to retain the essence and unique contribution of each study (Sandelowski & Barroso, 2007). There are several approaches to synthesizing numerous qualitative studies, in a systematic way, including meta-ethnography (Noblit & Hare 1988), meta-study (Paterson et al., 2001), and metasynthesis (Sandelowski & Barroso, 2007).

The data provided in quantitative research can be more easily aggregated and analyzed. In qualitative research, which draws on many different methods, the aggregation of data is sometimes more difficult. These systematic reviews of qualitative research often include an analysis of the types of methods used to study a topic, in addition to the "raw data" that has been published, and a synthesis of the interpretations and analysis that has been previously conducted. A key feature of these qualitative metasyntheses is that they should involve work of interpretation, interrogation, and inductive reasoning, with meaningful outputs and conclusions (Thorne, 2019).

As an example, Carr et al. (2019) reported the results of a qualitative metasynthesis that integrated the findings of qualitative studies of women's experiences of mastectomies after a breast cancer diagnosis. Using the methods of qualitative metasynthesis (see Sandelowski & Barroso, 2007), they reviewed and analyzed 16 qualitative studies retrieved from multiple databases.

On the basis of the synthesis process detailed in the article, the authors developed a taxonomy of concepts related to delayed surgery or immediate surgery. Findings emphasized the important role that health care providers have in providing information to patients.

Keeping-Burke et al. (2020) wished to explore the experiences of nursing students in residential aged care facilities, using the methodology ascribed by the Joanna Briggs Institute for systematic reviews of qualitative evidence. They reviewed 14 qualitative studies that had been published between 2003–2018. After synthesizing the articles, the authors concluded that students need to have knowledge of how to care for older people, as well as how to deal with difficult resident behaviour, prior to the clinical. In addition, across the studies it was concluded that students needed knowledge of the different roles in aged care facilities, including regulated and unregulated care providers (Keeping-Burke et al., 2020).

Essentially, metasynthesis provides a way for researchers to build up a critical amount of qualitative research evidence that is relevant to clinical practice. Sandelowski (2004) cautioned that the use of qualitative metasynthesis is laudable and necessary but that researchers who use metasynthesis methods must clearly understand qualitative methodologies and the nuances of the various qualitative methods. Given the contributions that qualitative research makes to nursing practice, it is important to consider the new knowledge that is contributed through these syntheses. It will be interesting for research consumers to follow the progress of researchers who seek to develop criteria for appraising a set of qualitative studies and to use those criteria to guide the incorporation of these studies into systematic literature reviews.

Evidence-Informed Practice Tip

Qualitative research findings can be used in many ways, including improving ways clinicians communicate with patients and with each other.

CRITICAL THINKING CHALLENGES

- Discuss how a researcher's values could influence the results of a study. Include an example in your answer.
- What is the value of qualitative research in evidence-informed practice? Give an example.
- Discuss how you could apply the findings of a qualitative research study about coping with a mastectomy.

CRITICAL JUDGEMENT QUESTIONS

1. What is a unique consideration for qualitative research?
   a. The process is not consistent across methods
   b. Values influence the research process
   c. The literature review is done before the research
   d. There are different types of relationships developed with participants

2. Why would a mixed methods approach be selected?
   a. When it fits the research question
   b. When triangulation of data from a variety of sources is important
   c. When the researcher needs more data
   d. When developing and testing a theory

3. Why are systematic reviews of qualitative research needed?
   a. To synthesize a growing body of research
   b. To compete with quantitative systematic reviews
   c. To ensure the best possible evidence for practice
   d. To document a variety of methods

KEY POINTS

- All research is based on philosophical beliefs, a worldview, or a paradigm.
- Qualitative research encompasses different methodologies.

- Qualitative researchers are interested in human experiences that are socially constructed and context dependent.
- Researchers' values should be kept as separate as possible from the conduct of research.
- Qualitative research, like quantitative research, follows a process, but the components of the process vary.
- Qualitative research contributes to evidence-informed practice.
- Ethical issues in qualitative research involve issues related to the naturalistic setting, the emergent nature of the design, researcher–participant interaction, and the researcher as instrument.

🛜 FOR FURTHER STUDY

Go to Evolve at http://evolve.elsevier.com/Canada/LoBiondo/Research for the Audio Glossary.

REFERENCES

Aburn, G., & Gott, M. (2014). Education given to parents of children newly diagnosed with acute lymphoblastic leukemia: The parent's perspective. *Pediatric Nursing, 40*(5), 243–256.

Carr, T., Groot, G., Cochran, D., & Holtslander, L. (2019). Patient information needs and breast reconstruction after mastectomy: A qualitative meta-synthesis. *Cancer Nursing, 42*, 229–241. https://doi.org/10.1097/NCC.0000000000000599.

Carter, N., Bryant-Lukosius, D., DiCenso, A., Blythe, J., & Neville, A. (2014). The use of triangulation in qualitative research. *Oncology Nursing Forum, 41*(5), 545–547.

Chesney, M. (2001). Dilemmas of self in the method. *Qualitative Health Research, 11*(1), 127–135.

Coelho, A., de Brito, M., Teixeira, P., Frade, P., Barros, L., & Barbosa, A. (2020). Family caregivers' anticipatory grief: A conceptual framework for understanding its multiple challenges. *Qualitative Health Research, 30*(5), 693–703.

Creswell, J. W. (2014). *Research design: Qualitative, quantitative and mixed methods approaches* (4th ed.). Thousand Oaks, CA: Sage.

Cricco-Lizza, R. (2014). The need to nurse the nurse: Emotional labor in neonatal intensive care. *Qualitative Health Research, 24*(5), 615–628.

Currie, G., Dosani, A., Premji, S. S., Reilly, S. M., Lodha, A. K., & Young, M. (2018). Caring for late preterm infants: public health nurses' experiences. *BMC Nursing, 17*(1), 16. https://doi.org/10.1186/s12912-018-0286-y.

Dosani, A., Hemraj, J., Premji, S. S., Currie, G., Reilly, S. M., Lodha, A. K., Young, M., & Hall, M. (2017). Breastfeeding the late preterm infant: experiences of mothers and perceptions of public health nurses. *International Breastfeeding Journal, 12*(1), 23. http://doi.org/10.1186/s13006-017-0114-0.

Denzin, N. K., & Lincoln, Y. (2011). *The Sage handbook of qualitative research* (4th ed.). Thousand Oaks, CA: Sage.

Doyle, L., Brady, A., & Byrne, G. (2009). An overview of mixed methods research. *Journal of Research in Nursing, 14*(2), 175–185. doi:10.1177/1744987108093962.

Fournier, B., Mill, J., Kipp, W., et al. (2006). Discovering voice: A participatory action research study with nurses in Uganda. *International Journal of Qualitative Methods, 6*(2). Retrieved from http://www.ualberta.ca/,http://iiqm/backissues/6_2/fournier.pdf.

Glesne, C. (2011). *Becoming qualitative researchers: An introduction* (4th ed.). Toronto: Pearson.

Hutchinson, S. A. (2001). The development of qualitative health research: Taking stock. *Qualitative Health Research, 11*(4), 505–521.

Kaasalainen, S., Wickson-Griffiths, A., Akhtar-Danesh, N., Brazil, K., Donald, F., Martin-Misener, R., DiCenso, A., Hadjistavropoulos, T., & Dolovich, L. (2016). The effectiveness of a nurse practitioner-led pain management team in long-term care: A mixed methods study. *International journal of nursing studies, 62*, 156–167. http://dx.doi.org/10.1016/j.ijnurstu.2016.07.022.

Keeping-Burke, L., McCloskey, R., Donovan, C., Yetman, L., & Goudreau, A. (2020). Nursing students' experiences with clinical placement in residential aged care facilities: a systematic review of qualitative evidence. *JBI Evidence Synthesis, 18*(5), 986–1018. https://doi.org/10.11124/JBISRIR-D-19-00122.

Lombardo, A. P., Angus, J. E., Lowndes, R., et al. (2014). Women's strategies to achieve access to healthcare in Ontario, Canada: A meta-synthesis. *Health and Social Care in the Community, 22*(6), 575–587.

Marshall, C., & Rossman, G. B. (2011). *Designing qualitative research* (5th ed.). Los Angeles, CA: Sage.

Mayan, M. (2009). *Essentials of qualitative inquiry.* Walnut Creek, CA: Left Coast Press.

Morgan, D. (1998). Practical strategies for combining qualitative and quantitative methods: Applications to health research. *Qualitative Health Research, 8*, 362–377.

Morse, J. M. (1991). Approaches to qualitative-quantitative research methodological triangulation. *Nursing Research, 40*, 120–123.

Morse, J. M. (2003). Principles of mixed methods and multimethod research design. In A. Tashakkori, & C. Teddlie (Eds.), *Handbook of mixed methods in social & behavioural research* (pp. 189–208). Thousand Oaks, CA: Sage.

Nelson, J. (2017). Using conceptual depth criteria: Addressing the challenge of reaching saturation in qualitative research. *Qualitative Research, 17*(5), 554–570.

Noblit, G. W., & Hare, R. D. (1988). *Meta-ethnography.* Thousand Oaks, CA: Sage.

Paterson, B. L., Thorne, S. E., Canam, C., & Jillings, C. (2001). *Meta-study of qualitative health research: A practical guide to meta-analysis and meta-synthesis.* Thousand Oaks, CA: Sage.

Patton, M. (2015). *Qualitative research & evaluation methods* (4th ed.). Thousand Oaks, CA: Sage.

Premji, S. S., Currie, G., Reilly, S., Dosani, A., Oliver, L. M., Lodha, A. K., & Young, M. (2017). A qualitative study: Mothers of late preterm infants relate their experiences of community-based care. *PLoS ONE, 12*(3), Article e0174419. https://doi.org/10.1371/journal.pone.0174419.

Premji, S. S., Pana, G., Currie, G., Dosani, A., Reilly, S., Young, M., Hall, M., Williamson, T., & Lodha, A. K. (2018). Mother's level of confidence in caring for her late preterm infant: A mixed methods study. *Journal of Clinical Nursing, 5–6*, 1120. https://0-doi-org.aupac.lib.athabascau.ca/10.1111/jocn.14190.

Roper, J., & Shapira, J. (2000). *Ethnography in nursing research.* Thousand Oaks, CA: Sage.

Ramsay, H., Hossain, R., Moore, M., Milo, M., & Brown, A. (2019). Health care while homeless: Barriers, facilitators, and the lived experiences of homeless individuals accessing health care in a Canadian regional municipality. *Qualitative Health Research, 29*(13), 1839–1849.

Sandelowski, M. (2004). Using qualitative research. *Qualitative Health Research, 14*(10), 1366–1386.

Sandelowski, M. (2014). Unmixing mixed-methods research. *Research in Nursing & Health, 37*, 3–8.

Sandelowski, M., & Barroso, J. (2007). *Handbook for synthesizing qualitative research.* Philadelphia: Springer.

Shorten, A., & Smith, J. (2017). Mixed methods research: Expanding the evidence base. *Evidence Based Nursing, 20*(3), 74–75.

Smith, M. J., & Liehr, P. (2003). The theory of attentively embracing story. In M. J. Smith, & P. Liehr (Eds.), *Middle range theory for nursing* (pp. 167–187). New York: Springer.

St-Amant, O., Ward-Griffin, C., Brown, J. B., et al. (2014). Professionalizing familiar care: Examining nurses' unpaid family care work. *Advances in Nursing Science, 37*(2), 117–131.

Stahlke, S. (2018). Expanding on notions of ethical risks to qualitative researchers. *International Journal of Qualitative Methods, 17.* doi:10.1177/1609406918787309.

Stewart, M., Makwarimba, E., Letourneau, N. L., et al. (2015). Impacts of support intervention for Zimbabwean and Sudanese refuges parents: "I am not alone". *Canadian Journal of Nursing Research, 47*(4), 113–140.

Streubert, H. J., & Carpenter, D. (2011). *Qualitative research in nursing: Advancing the humanistic imperative* (5th ed.). New York: Wolters Kluwer.

Thorne, S. (2019). On the evolving world of what constitutes qualitative synthesis. *Qualitative Health Research, 29*(1), 3–6. https://0-doi-org.aupac.lib.athabascau.ca/10.1177/1049732318813903.

Yeh, E. A., Chiang, N., Darshan, B., Nejati, N., Grover, S. A., Schwartz, C. E., Slater, R., & Finlayson, M. (2019). Adherence in youth with multiple sclerosis: A qualitative assessment of habit formation, barriers, and facilitators. *Qualitative Health Research, 29*(5), 645–657.

CHAPTER 9

Qualitative Approaches to Research

Lorraine Thirsk | Sarah Stahlke

LEARNING OUTCOMES

After reading this chapter, you will be able to do the following:

- Identify the processes of qualitative research methods such as phenomenology, grounded theory, ethnography, and participatory action research.
- Outline the appropriate use of community-based participatory research methods.
- Define variety of qualitative methods including qualitative description, interpretive description, and narrative inquiry.
- Summarize the similarities and differences among the various qualitative methods.
- Compare the purposes and processes of selected methods on a similar topic.
- Apply critiquing criteria to evaluate a report of qualitative research.

KEY TERMS

community-based
    participatory research
    (CBPR)
constant comparative
    method
context
culture
data saturation
domains
emic perspective

ethnographic method
ethnography
etic perspective
external criticism
grounded theory method
hermeneutics
interpretive description
intersubjectivity
key informants
lived experience

narrative inquiry
participatory action
    research (PAR)
phenomenological
    method
phenomenology
propositions
qualitative descriptive
snowball sampling
theoretical sampling

STUDY RESOURCES

Go to Evolve at http://evolve.elsevier.com/Canada/LoBiondo/Research
for the Audio Glossary.

QUALITATIVE RESEARCH is becoming increasingly prevalent in health sciences and is increasingly recognized as making a valuable contribution (Brookfield et al., 2019). "Qualitative research offers rich and compelling insights into the real worlds, experiences, and perspectives of patients and health care professionals in ways that are completely different to, but also sometimes complimentary to, the knowledge we can obtain through quantitative methods" (Braun & Clark, 2014, p. 1). Thorne (2020, p. 1) identified the following objectives for qualitative research:

- fill in gaps that quantitative studies have left exposed
- insert patient perspectives into objective clinical understanding
- consider meaningful similarities and differences among people's experiences with common situations, and
- understand something in clinical practice that is incomplete or puzzling

In examining health care interventions, qualitative research is used to capture experiences of the interventions, explain and explore unanticipated or complex causal pathways, and generate new theory or hypotheses (Moore et al., 2015).

This chapter describes a variety of qualitative research methods that are commonly used by nurse researchers. These include phenomenology, grounded theory, ethnography, participatory action research, qualitative description, interpretive description, and narrative inquiry. This is not an exhaustive list of all the qualitative methods that nurse researchers use, but it will give you an overview of how different methods frame the phenomenon of interest and approach the research. You are encouraged to use the researcher's standpoint as each method is introduced—to imagine how it would be to study an issue of interest from the perspective of each of these methods. For example, recall from Chapter 2 that framing research under a critical paradigm means that the focus of the question will likely be on uncovering and understanding how power structures operate and impact people,

and challenging the taken-for-granted or status quo. No matter which method a researcher uses, there is a demand to embrace the wholeness of humans, focusing on the human experience in natural settings.

In general, qualitative researchers value the differing perspectives that individuals have regarding their experiences with a certain phenomenon or topic of interest. They recognize that these experiences are shaped by social and historical **contexts**, and that exploring these experiences can make a meaningful contribution to nursing knowledge. Qualitative methods tend to look at breadth and depth of a few people's experiences, whereas quantitative research captures a few components across many participants. For example, for the adolescent with rheumatoid arthritis, the researcher interested in studying the adolescent's lived experience of pain spends time in the adolescent's natural settings, such as the home and school. Efforts are directed at uncovering the experience of pain as it extends beyond the number of medications taken or a rating on a pain scale. The meaning of the adolescent's pain emerges within the context of personal history, current relationships, and future plans as the adolescent lives daily life in dynamic interaction with the environment.

The researcher using qualitative methods begins by collecting bits of information and piecing them together, building a mosaic or a picture of the human experience being studied. As with a mosaic, when one steps away from the work, the whole picture emerges. This whole picture transcends the bits and pieces and cannot be known from any one piece. In presenting study findings, the researcher strives to capture the human experience and present it so that other people can understand it.

Research Hint

The International Institute of Qualitative Methodology is located at the University of Alberta in the Faculty of Nursing. It serves qualitative researchers from around the world and across disciplines. It also supports the publication of the *International Journal of Qualitative Methods,* which is an open access journal focused on development and innovation in qualitative methods.

QUALITATIVE RESEARCH METHODS

Thus far, the overview of the qualitative research approach (see Chapter 8) has focused on the importance of evidence offered by qualitative research for nursing science. This overview highlighted how the choice of a qualitative approach is reflective of the research question, which aligns with a research paradigm. The topics addressed in the overview provide a foundation for examining the qualitative methods discussed in this chapter. The Critical Thinking Decision Path introduces you to a process for recognizing various qualitative methods by distinguishing areas of interest for each method and noting how the research question might be introduced for each distinct method. The philosophical foundation and assumptions of these methods are discussed in Chapter 2. In addition to the methods listed in the Critical Thinking Decision Path, several other qualitative research methods are used in nursing research. In each of the following sections, we introduce a research article that provides an example of the use of each method.

Phenomenology as Research

Phenomenology is grounded in philosophy and psychology and is concerned with describing the **lived experiences** of humans (Polit & Beck, 2017). Phenomenological research has typically examined things such as "perception, imagination, body-awareness, attention, intentionality, social cognition, and self-consciousness" (Zahavi & Martiny, 2019, p. 158). This method is most useful when the task is to understand an experience in the way that people having the experience understand it and is well suited to the study of phenomena important to nursing. Phenomenology can be useful in nursing research for several reasons (Zahavi & Martiny, 2019, p. 161):

- Recognition of the importance of the lifeworld
- Insistence on developing an open-minded and non-biased attitude
- Interest in human existence
- Recognition of people as embodied and socially and culturally embedded beings-in-the-world

Phenomenological research is based on phenomenological philosophy, which has changed

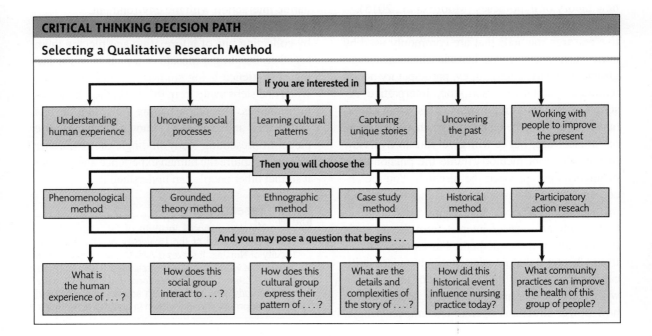

CRITICAL THINKING DECISION PATH

Selecting a Qualitative Research Method

If you are interested in

| Understanding human experience | Uncovering social processes | Learning cultural patterns | Capturing unique stories | Uncovering the past | Working with people to improve the present |

Then you will choose the

| Phenomenological method | Grounded theory method | Ethnographic method | Case study method | Historical method | Participatory action reseach |

And you may pose a question that begins . . .

| What is the human experience of . . . ? | How does this social group interact to . . . ? | How does this cultural group express their pattern of . . . ? | What are the details and complexities of the story of . . . ? | How did this historical event influence nursing practice today? | What community practices can improve the health of this group of people? |

over time and with different philosophers. Descriptive phenomenology, which focuses on rich detailed descriptions of the lived world, is based on Edmund Husserl's philosophy. Heideggerian phenomenology expands description to understanding achieved through searching for the relationships and meanings of phenomena.

Closely related to phenomenology, **hermeneutics** focuses on interpretation of phenomena. Researchers using hermeneutics use the lived experience "as a tool for better understanding the social, cultural, political, or historical context in which those experiences occur" (Polit & Beck, 2017, p. 465). Hermeneutic researchers believe that interpretation cannot be absolutely correct or true but must be viewed from the perspective of the historical or cultural context and the original purpose of the text.

Patton (2015) described many of the different phenomenological approaches in his text *Qualitative Research & Evaluation Methods*. Although he acknowledged the complexity and differing traditions of these approaches, he also states their similarities:

> What these various phenomenological approaches share in common is a focus on exploring how human beings make sense of experience and transform experience into consciousness, both individually and as shared meaning. This requires methodically, carefully, and thoroughly capturing and describing how people experience some phenomenon—how they perceive it, describe it, feel about it, judge it, remember it, make sense of it, and talk about it with others. To gather such data, one must take undertake in-depth interviews with people who have directly experienced the phenomenon of interest; that is, they have "lived experience" as opposed to second-hand experience. (p. 115)

The five important concepts or values in phenomenological research (Cohen, 1987) are as follows:

1. The phenomenological method is a process of learning and constructing the meaning of human experience through intensive dialogue with persons who are living the experience. This method was developed to understand meanings.

2. Phenomenology was based on a critique of positivism, or the positivist view, which was seen as inappropriate in the study of some human concerns.

3. The object of study is the "life world" (*Lebenswelt*), or lived experience, not contrived situations. In other words, as the philosopher Husserl said, researchers are concerned with the appearance of things (*phenomena*) rather than the things themselves (*noumena*).

4. Intersubjectivity—a person's belief that other people share a common world with him or her—is an important tenet in phenomenology. Although phenomena differ, they also share similarities that are based on the similarities in people. The most fundamental of those similarities is that every person has a body in space and time. In other words, the physical body and historical sense lead to similarities in how people experience phenomena. The basic elements, or an essence, of the shared experience are common among people or members of a specific society.

5. The phenomenological reduction, also called *bracketing*, is controversial and more important in some phenomenological approaches than in others. Phenomenological reduction means that researchers must be aware of and examine their prejudices or values.

Whatever the form of phenomenological research, you will find the researcher asking a question about the lived experience.

Identifying the Phenomenon

Because the focus of the phenomenological method is the lived experience—the undergoing of events and circumstances, as opposed to thinking about these events and circumstances—the researcher is likely to choose this method when studying some dimension of day-to-day existence for a particular group of people. An example of hermeneutic phenomenology is a study by Currie and Szabo (2019) about parents' experiences of caring for children with neurodevelopmental disease.

Structuring the Study

For the purpose of describing structuring in a phenomenological study, the following topics are addressed: the research question, the researcher's perspective, and sample selection. The issue of human participants' protection in research was discussed generally with ethics in Chapter 8.

RESEARCH QUESTION. The question that guides phenomenological research always concerns some human experience. It guides the researcher to ask the participant about some past or present experience. The research question is not exactly the same as the question used to initiate dialogue with the participant, often called a grand tour question, but often these questions are very similar. Currie and Szabo's (2019) research question was "What are parents' perceptions and experiences of support from health and social service communities when living with a child with a rare neurodevelopmental disease (NDD)?" (p. 1253).

RESEARCHER'S PERSPECTIVE. In some phenomenological research traditions, bracketing is encouraged as a way for the researcher to identify personal biases about the phenomenon of interest in order to clarify how personal experience and beliefs may influence what is heard and reported. The researcher is expected to set aside personal biases—to bracket them—when engaging with the participants. By becoming aware of personal biases, the researcher is more likely to be able to pursue issues of importance introduced by the participant, rather than leading the participant to issues the researcher deems important. As mentioned previously, this is a contentious issue in phenomenology research. While reflexivity in the research is important, researchers using other phenomenological or hermeneutic methods argue that bracketing is not only impossible, but unnecessary. Bracketing is impossible because it is the beliefs and biases that we are unaware of that affect us the most; it

is unnecessary because our existing knowledge and experience is what allows us to access and understand the world (Moules, 2002). Furthermore, the way that bracketing was described in philosophical phenomenology has been used erroneously in its application to phenomenology as research (Zahavi, 2019).

> ### Research Hint
> Managing personal bias is an expectation of researchers who use all the methods discussed in this chapter. All researchers bring their biases; qualitative researchers explicitly acknowledge and discuss this.

> ### Research Hint
> Although the research question may not always be explicitly reported, you may identify it by evaluating the study's purpose or the question/statement posed to the participants.

SAMPLE SELECTION. As you read a report of a phenomenological study, you will find that the selected participant is either living the experience the researcher is querying about or has lived the experience in the past. Because phenomenologists believe that each individual's history is a dimension of the present, a past experience exists in the present moment. Even when a participant is describing an experience occurring in the present, remembered information is being gathered. The 15 participants in the study by Currie and Szabo (2019) were 11 mothers and 4 fathers, aged 30–45 years. Participants were recruited through several pediatric outpatient clinics and parent support groups in Western Canada. All of the participants had a child aged 11 years old or younger who had been diagnosed with a rare NDD (defined by the Rare Disease Foundation of Canada as occurring in <1 in 2,000 live births).

> ### Research Hint
> Qualitative studies often involve the use of purposive sampling (see Chapter 8).

Data Gathering

Written or oral data may be collected when the phenomenological method is used. The researcher may pose the query in writing and ask for a written response or may schedule a time to interview the participant and record the interaction. In either case, the researcher may return to ask for clarification of written or recorded transcripts. To some extent, the particular data-collection procedure is guided by the choice of a specific analysis technique. Various analysis techniques require different numbers of interviews. In general, open-ended questions—such as "What comes to mind when you think of . . . ?"—guide the participants to describe their lived experience. During the interview, the researcher attempts to gather more information by asking clarifying questions.

Several criteria may be used to determine that enough data have been collected. **Data saturation** typically means that no new ideas are being generated through further interviews. Other phenomenology projects may stop data collection when several new ideas have been generated or a complex idea or theory has been flushed out. Many times, resources for conducting interviews will restrict the amount of data that can be collected. For example, Currie and Szabo (2019) stopped recruiting when their analysis "expanded understanding" (p. 1253).

Data Analysis

As data are collected, data analysis begins. Several techniques are available for data analysis when the phenomenological method is used. Detailed information about specific techniques can be found in the original sources (Colaizzi, 1978; Giorgi et al., 1975; Spiegelberg, 1976; van Kaam, 1969). Although the techniques are slightly different from each other, there is a general pattern of moving from the participant's description to the researcher's synthesis of all participants' descriptions. The steps generally include the following:

1. Thorough and sensitive reading of presence with the entire transcription of the participant's description

2. Identification of shifts in participant thought, resulting in division of the transcription into thought segments
3. Specification of significant phrases in each thought segment, in the participant's own words
4. Distillation of each significant phrase to express the central meaning of the segment in the researcher's words
5. Grouping together of segments that contain similar central meanings for each participant
6. Preliminary synthesis of grouped segments for each participant with a focus on the essence of the phenomenon being studied
7. Final synthesis of the essences that have surfaced in all participants' descriptions, resulting in an exhaustive description of the lived experience

Whereas some phenomenological approaches will report common ideas or meanings found across participants, others will focus on interesting or significant reports from participants and expand on understanding that case. In hermeneutic research, this is known as the "fecundity of the individual case" (Gadamaer, 2004; Jardine, 1992).

Currie and Szabo (2019) described their process of data management: all interviews were transcribed and the transcripts were checked for accuracy. Then the researchers read the interviews multiple times, reflected on them, and re-read them, making interpretive notes. They noted impressions, divergent patterns, insights, and interpretations, and constructed insights into the parents' experience (Currie & Szabo, 2019).

Describing the Findings

When using the phenomenological method, the nurse researcher constructs a path of information leading from the research question through samples of participants' words and the researcher's interpretation to the final synthesis that elaborates the lived experience. When reading the report of a phenomenological study, you should find that detailed descriptive language is used to convey the complex meaning of the lived experience. Currie and Szabo (2019) provided numerous quotations from participants to support their findings. They identified three themes, or insights, into parenting a child with rare NDD: *Disconnect; In the Ring;* and *Self-Sacrifice.* For example, a quotation exemplifying the theme of "In the Ring" is as follows:

> It feels like a fight every day. We fight for her. We fight the system, and we fight for any support we can actually get. It's very isolating and very lonely and very frustrating.... It's terribly soul crushing. (p. 1255) https://doi.org/10.11124/JBISRIR-D-19-00122

Direct quotations from participants enable the reader to evaluate the connection between what the participant said and the researcher's interpretation or analysis.

Evidence-Informed Practice Tip

Phenomenological research is an important approach for accumulating evidence when researchers study a new topic about which little is known and when trying to uncover and challenge common assumptions.

Grounded Theory Method

In the grounded theory method, a systematic set of procedures is used to explore the social processes that guide human interaction and to inductively develop a theory on the basis of those observations. The grounded theory method is based on the sociological tradition of the Chicago School of Symbolic Interactionism, a tradition that reflects on issues related to human behaviour. Glaser and Strauss (1967) developed the method of grounded theory and published the classic first text describing the methodology: *The Discovery of Grounded Theory*. According to Strauss and Corbin (1990), grounded theory

> is one that is inductively derived from the study of the phenomenon it represents. That is, it is discovered, developed, and provisionally verified through systematic data collection and analysis of data pertaining to that phenomenon. Therefore, data collection, analysis, and theory stand in reciprocal relationship with each other.

> One does not begin with a theory, then prove it. Rather one begins with an area of study and what is relevant to that area is allowed to emerge. (p. 23)

In many qualitative research traditions, explanatory models and theories are described and developed in relation to a human phenomenon under study; grounded theory is distinctive from the other traditional qualitative research methods because its primary focus is on generating theory about dominant social processes. The three major premises that continue to underlie grounded theory research are outlined in Box 9.1.

The purpose of grounded theory, as the name implies, is to generate a theory from data. Grounded theory has contributed substantively to the body of knowledge in the field of nursing. Often, the theories generated from grounded research are then tested empirically. Qualitative data are gathered through interviews and observation. Through analysis of the data, substantive codes are generated and then are clustered into categories. Propositions link the concepts to create a foundation that guides further data collection. Additional data that are thought likely to answer generated hypotheses are collected until all categories are "saturated"—that is, no new information is generated. The goal of generating a theory implies that laws drive at least some portion of reality. The truth is sought from relevant groups, for example, patients who are dying.

BOX 9.1

MAJOR PREMISES OF GROUNDED THEORY

1. Humans act toward objects on the basis of the meaning that those objects have for them. Meaning is embedded in context and, therefore, cannot be separated from the context or from the consequences of the meanings in a particular setting.
2. Social meanings arise from social interactions with other people over time and are embedded socially, historically, culturally, and contextually. Therefore, the focus of grounded theory is on social interactions.
3. People use interpretive processes to handle and change meanings in dealing with their situations.

The context is very important, as was shown in a classic work by Glaser and Strauss (1965). They noted that, at the time of their work, patients were unwilling to talk openly about the process of their own dying, physicians were unwilling to disclose the imminence of death to patients, and nurses were expected not to make these disclosures. This lack of communication led Glaser and Strauss (1965) to their study of the problem of awareness of dying. They described various types of awareness contexts, problems of awareness, and practical uses of awareness theory. Their early fieldwork led to hypotheses and the gathering of additional data, and the framework was refined with further analysis until they formed a systematic substantive theory.

As stated earlier, constructive grounded theory emerged from the seminal work by Glaser and Strauss (1967). While Glaser and Strauss focused on discovering theory as emerging from data that were separate from the researcher, Charmaz (2014) argued,

> neither data nor theories are discovered. Rather, we are part of the world we study and the data we collect. And the analyses we produce. We construct our grounded theories through our past and present involvements and interactions with people, perspectives, and research practices. (p. 30)

Identifying the Phenomenon

Researchers typically use the grounded theory method when they are interested in either social processes from the perspective of human interactions or patterns of action and interaction between and among various types of social units (Denzin & Lincoln, 1998). The basic social process is sometimes expressed as a gerund, indicating that change across time as social reality is negotiated. El Hussein et al. (2019) used grounded theory to explore the clinical reasoning processes used by registered nurses (RNs) and licensed practical nurses (LPNs) to recognize delirium. They developed a theory or professional socialization to explain the similarities and differences in reasoning processes.

Structuring the Study

RESEARCH QUESTION. Research questions appropriate for the grounded theory method are those that address basic social processes that shape human behaviour. In a grounded theory study, the research question can be a statement or a broad question that permits in-depth explanation of the phenomenon. The researcher does not always need to identify a problem or research question but chooses an area of interest; the problem is then discovered through the research process (Polit & Beck, 2017).

RESEARCHER'S PERSPECTIVE. In a grounded theory study, the researcher brings some knowledge of the literature to the study, but an exhaustive literature review is not performed (Polit & Beck, 2017). Therefore, theory emerges directly from data and reflects the contextual values that are integral to the social processes being studied. Thus, the theory product that emerges is "grounded in" the data. In the study by El Hussein et al. (2019), the literature review focused on describing delirium and the clinical outcomes associated with underrecognition. In addition, they reviewed evidence about the impact that experience, education, and clinical reasoning might have in noticing clinical problems and improving patient safety.

SAMPLE SELECTION. Sample selection involves (1) choosing participants for a purposive sample who are experiencing the circumstance and "are judged to have good knowledge of the study domain" (Wuest, 2011, p. 235); and (2) selecting events and incidents that are related to the social process under investigation. As problems begin to emerge, the researchers may conduct theoretical sampling, a sampling method used to select experiences that helps the researchers test ideas and gather complete information about developing concepts. In this method, researchers seek participants who can further clarify the emerging concepts. El Hussein et al. (2019) collected data from 28 nurses in total for their study, from two acute care units in large hospitals in western Canada.

After the 10th interview, the researchers engaged in theoretical sampling to seek more data for the emerging theory. Through theoretical sampling, the researchers can target certain groups to test and refine the emerging findings.

Another recruitment strategy, snowball sampling, occurs when a participant recommends other participants from his or her contacts. As more and more participants bring on new recruits, the sample appears to grow like a snowball. Researchers may also include key informants to provide clarification on issues such as regulatory and legal issues. Key informants are individuals who have special knowledge, status, or communication skills and who are willing to teach the researcher about the phenomenon.

Data Gathering

In grounded theory, data are collected through interviews and through skilled observations of individuals interacting in a social setting. Interviews are audio-recorded and then transcribed, and observations are recorded as field notes. Open-ended questions are used initially to identify concepts for further focus. El Hussein et al. (2019) used semi-structured interviews to collect data through interviews in two phases. The first phase uncovered flawed clinical reasoning in RNs that led to under-recognition of delirium. In phase two they included additional RNs and LPNs to validate the subcategories previously developed in the emerging theory.

Data Analysis

A major feature of the grounded theory method is that data collection and analysis occur simultaneously. The process requires systematic, detailed record keeping using field notes and transcribed interview recordings. Hunches about emerging patterns in the data are noted in memos, and the researcher directs activities in the field by pursuing these hunches. This technique of theoretical sampling is used to select participants whose experiences will help the researcher test ideas and gather complete information about developing concepts. The researcher begins by noting indicators or actual events, actions, or words in the data. Concepts, or abstractions, are developed from the indicators (Charmaz, 2000; Strauss, 1987).

The initial analytical process is called *open coding* (Strauss, 1987). Data are examined carefully line by line, categorized into discrete parts, and compared for similarities and differences (Corbin & Strauss, 2008). Data are compared with other data continuously as they are acquired during research. This process is called the **constant comparative method**. Codes in the data are clustered to form categories. The categories are expanded and developed, or they are collapsed into one another. Theory is constructed through this systematic process. As a result, data collection, analysis, and theory generation have a direct reciprocal relationship (Charmaz, 2000; Strauss & Corbin, 1990). El Hussein et al. (2019) analyzed the transcripts line by line, noting, in particular, fallacies and lack of clarity in the participants' reasoning. When they had coded several similar concepts, they collapsed them into subcategories. They continued data collection and analysis until their concepts were verified and saturated. They offered explanations of the relationships between subcategories and tracked their analysis through memos.

Describing the Findings

Grounded theory studies are reported in enough detail to provide the reader with the steps in the process, the logic of the method, and the theory that has emerged. In reports of grounded theory studies, descriptive language and diagrams of the process are used as evidence to ensure that the theory reported in the findings remains connected to the data. Instead of providing a description of people's experiences, the focus is to provide theoretical statements about the relationships between the concepts (Wuest, 2011). El Hussein et al. (2019) described the core category that emerged from their study as "Professional Socialization."

In reporting their findings, they described an existing concept (professional socialization) that had been previously validated and fit their data to explain their findings (see Dinmohammadi et al., 2013). El Hussein et al. further described the RNs' reasoning processes as having the purpose to uncover, whereas LPNs' reasoning processes had the purpose to report. The findings serve to clarify, with examples, the differences the researchers noted between clinical reasoning between RNs and LPNs. They argued that the differences in professional socialization—which includes comprehensive education, competent role models, and adequate field experiences—is what leads to the differences in clinical reasoning (El Hussein et al., 2019).

Evidence-Informed Practice Tip

When you think about the evidence generated by the grounded theory method, consider whether the theory is useful in explaining, interpreting, or predicting the study phenomenon of interest.

Research Hint

In a report of research in which the grounded theory method was used, you can expect to find a diagrammed model of a theory in which the researcher's findings are synthesized in a systematic way.

Ethnography

Ethnographic research has a long history in the qualitative research tradition and is considered by some authorities to be the oldest of the traditions (Patton, 2015). Anthropologists developed the **ethnographic method**, defined as a method of scientifically describing cultural groups. The Greek root *ethnos* means "people" or "a cultural group." **Ethnography** is a "research process of learning *about* people by learning *from* them... to understand and describe why a group of people do what they do" (Roper & Shapira, 2000, p. 1). The aim of ethnographic research is to combine the **emic perspective** (the insider's view of the world) with the **etic perspective** (the view of the

researcher [outsider]) to develop a rich description of the study environment. Although early ethnographic work addressed the cultural patterns of village life in distant locations, the notion of **culture** has expanded far beyond race or ethnicity or "foreignness." Any particular social context or social group can be conceptualized as a culture, such as a university classroom, a clinic, a work team, or a community group. As well, nurses now often conduct focused ethnographic research, such as the study of distinct problems within a specific context among a small group of people, or the study of a group's social construction and understanding of a health or illness experience (Roper & Shapira, 2000).

Ethnography (ethnographic research) is the study of models or patterns of behaviour of people within a culture. Culture is fundamental to ethnographic studies. Culture is observed through a group's patterns of behaviour and customs, its way of life, and what it produces (Roper & Shapira, 2000). More specific cultural elements include ideas, beliefs, values, knowledge, social arrangements, and the workings of power (Fetterman, 1998; Morse & Richards, 2002; Smith, 2001; Wolcott, 1999). Understanding culture requires a holistic perspective that captures the breadth of the beliefs, knowledge, and activities of the group being studied (Roper & Shapira, 2000). To capture cultural experiences, ethnographers generally rely on interviews, participant observation, and document and artifact analysis, although adaptations to the method have changed how these data collection strategies are incorporated.

Other ethnographic approaches used in nursing research include autoethnography, institutional ethnography, visual ethnography, and critical (including feminist) ethnographies. Autoethnography is a method in which the researcher describes and systematically analyzes their personal experience in order to understand that experience in its cultural context (Ellis et al., 2011). Institutional ethnography (IE) is a method of inquiry based on Smith's (2005) sociology, which was influenced by the feminist movement. Using IE, a researcher explores and maps the structural aspects of a cultural setting to determine how people are organized and controlled by those who have power and create practices that serve their power (Campbell & Gregor, 2002).

Critical ethnography does not entail the use of different methods. Based on critical theory, it focuses on "raising consciousness and aiding emancipatory goals in the hope of effecting social change" (Polit & Beck, 2017, p. 480). Critical ethnographic researchers make their values explicit. They explore how dominant social groups oppress those in the minority or those without power and are motivated to promote social justice and social change. For example, Pauly et al. (2015) explored how persons who use illicit drugs encounter stigma and discrimination, resulting in barriers when accessing health care services. Finally, many critical ethnographers consider study participants to be co-investigators and explore problems and possible solutions with them.

Feminist researchers, like critical ethnographers, focus on oppression and power but apply their work to women (although they do examine the ways in which gender ideologies impact other genders as well). They also consider and analyze the effects of race, class, culture, ethnicity, sexual preference, and other identities as forces that cause and sustain oppression (Macquire, 1996).

Identifying the Phenomenon

The phenomenon under investigation in an ethnographic study is a given experience within its cultural context, with the understanding that cultures are everywhere. The local worlds of people such as patients or nurses have cultural, political, economic, institutional, and social–relational dimensions in much the same way that larger, complex societies do. In Campbell and Rankin's (2017) hospital-based study of nurses' use of electronic health records (EHR), an acute care unit that had implemented an EHR was seen as a culture

appropriate for ethnographic study. An ethnographer understands and describes what the experience is like for that given cultural group.

Structuring the Study

RESEARCH QUESTION. When you review a report of ethnographic research, note that questions are asked about particular patterns of behaviour within the social context of a culture or subculture. Ethnographic nursing studies address questions that concern how cultural knowledge, norms, values, and other contextual variables influence a person's health care experience. They may focus on identifying problems, describing facilitators or barriers, or building models or theories about an experience (LeCompte & Schensul, 2010) so research questions may reflect that this is what is sought.

RESEARCHER'S PERSPECTIVE. When a researcher uses the ethnographic method, the researcher's perspective is that of an interpreter entering an unfamiliar world and attempting to make sense of that world from the insider's point of view (Agar, 1986). Like phenomenologists and grounded theory researchers, ethnographers make their own beliefs explicit and may bracket, or set aside, their personal biases as they interpret the findings and seek to understand the worldview of other people. In some cases, such as in ethnographic research that focuses on how power works in a specific culture, researchers will use their perspectives to direct the study toward the goal of emancipation and social change.

SAMPLE SELECTION. The ethnographer selects a cultural group that is experiencing the phenomenon under investigation. Within this culture, the researcher gathers information from general informants and from key informants.

Data Gathering

Ethnographic data gathering involves participant observation or immersion in the setting, interviews of informants, and examination of documents and artifacts within the setting (Morse & Richards, 2002). According to Boyle (1991), ethnographic research in nursing, as in other disciplines, involves interviewing in the natural setting as the major data-collection method. Spradley (1979) identified three categories of questions for ethnographic inquiry: descriptive, or broad, open-ended questions; structural, or in-depth, questions that expand and verify the unit of analysis; and contrast questions, which further clarify and provide criteria for exclusion. Fieldwork is also a major focus of the method. The researchers become immersed in the field by spending extensive time with the group under study. They document their observations, keep a diary of the day's events, and record their impressions and any insights in field notes (Merriam & Tisdell, 2016). In Campbell and Rankin's (2017) study, they used data obtained through participant observation and volunteer informants during a series of studies about nurses' work in acute care hospitals.

Other techniques may include obtaining life histories and collecting documents, artifacts, and other material items reflective of the culture. These may include policies, care plans, equipment and tools, photographs, setting décor, mementos, and books. Reviewing or noticing these items can enrich a researcher's understanding of the culture. For example, Wall (2013), in a focused ethnographic study about nurses in nontraditional roles, described how material items such as art and tapestries created a unique kind of workspace for these nurses, showing how they wanted to shift away from the expected clinic culture with medical posters on the walls.

Data Analysis

As with other qualitative methods, data are collected and analyzed simultaneously. Data analysis proceeds through several levels as the researcher looks for cultural elements and the meaning ascribed to them in the informant's words. Analysis begins with a search for **domains**, or symbolic

categories that include smaller categories. Language is analyzed for semantic relationships, and structural questions are formulated to expand and verify data. Analysis proceeds through increasing levels of complexity until the data, grounded in the informant's reality and synthesized by the researcher, lead to hypothetical propositions about the cultural phenomenon under investigation. Campbell and Rankin (2017) focus on one nurse's interactions with a patient and the EHR, with the goal of exploring the "materials, processes and actions that coordinate those specific activities" (p. 371). Their analysis involves "tracing," which means exploring and understanding the social organization that explains the empirical observations. They examine hospital policy documents, unit processes, EHR workplans, and workload measurement tools to help explain the nurse's interactions with a patient.

Describing the Findings

In ethnographic studies, field notes of observations, interview transcriptions, and sometimes other artifacts such as photographs yield large quantities of data. Rich descriptions are the hallmark of ethnographic research. Wolcott (1994) describes the process of description as sharing "What is going on here?" (p. 12). Charmaz (2000) recommends five techniques in her guidelines for ethnographic writing: pulling the reader in, recreating the experiential mood, adding surprising observations, reconstructing the ethnographic experience, and creating closure for the study. The findings of complete ethnographies may be published as monographs, such as Chambliss' (1996) book about the social organization of ethics in nursing practice. When you read an ethnographic study, you will see that the researcher usually provides examples from data, thorough descriptions of the analytical process, interpretations about the data, and connections of their findings to the literature. They may provide a model or taxonomy that organizes the data.

Campbell and Rankin (2017) describe their findings by presenting an initial case of one nurse and then describe the associated institutional policies and processes that have affected this nurses' work. They include examples of policies, interviews with administrators, and information from the EHR. This is integrated through their article explaining the ruling relations that are present (Campbell & Rankin, 2017).

Evidence-Informed Practice Tip ____

Evidence generated by ethnographic studies answers questions about how cultural knowledge, norms, values, and other contextual variables influence the health experience of a particular patient population in a specific setting.

Action Research

Participatory action research (PAR) and Community-based Participatory Research (CBPR) share characteristics in their conceptual foundations such as critical theory. These methods are labelled action research, because the activity of the research is meant to bring about change, or action. These research projects are typically grounded in an analysis of power structures and involve working with groups or communities that are vulnerable or oppressed (Polit & Beck, 2017). While introduced in this chapter, PAR and CBPR can use a variety of qualitative and quantitative methods to achieve their goals—the methods used will be dependent on the research questions.

Participatory action research (PAR) is a method in which a goal is to change society through a collaborative research process. According to the tenets of PAR, all forms of knowledge, including indigenous knowledge, are of value and can be applied to practical problems. The researcher studies a particular setting to identify areas in which improvements in practice are needed (Glesne, 2011). After possible solutions are identified, action is taken to implement changes in partnership with the "stakeholders." Careful attention is given to evaluating the process to ensure that the changes have the desired effect. PAR requires careful collaboration with the research

participants, in all phases of the research process, and focuses on practical problems that are particular to a practice setting or community (Polit & Beck, 2017). Stringer and Genat (2004) define action research as

> a systematic, participatory approach to inquiry that enables people to extend their understanding of problems or issues and to formulate actions directed towards the resolution of those problems or issues . . . action research seeks local understandings that are specifically relevant to the particular context of a study. (p. 4)

Community-based participatory research (CBPR) is a method by which the voice of a community is systematically accessed in order to plan context-appropriate action. According to Holkup et al. (2004), CBPR

> provides an alternative to traditional research approaches that assume a phenomenon may be separated from its context for purposes of study. . . . CBPR recognizes the importance of involving members of a study population as active and equal participants, in all phases of the research project, if the research process is to be a means of facilitating change. (p. 2)

Change or action is the intended outcome of CBPR, and *action research* is a term related to CBPR. Some scholars would consider CBPR a sort of action research and would group both action research and CBPR within the tradition of critical science (Fontana, 2004).

Evidence-Informed Practice Tip ____

Although qualitative in its approach to research, CBPR leads to an action component in which a nursing intervention is implemented and evaluated for its effectiveness in a specific patient population.

In his book *Action Research*, Stringer (1999) distills the research process into three phases: "look," "think," and "act." Stringer defines the "look" as "building the picture" by getting to know stakeholders so that the problem is defined on their terms and the problem definition is reflective of the community context. The "think" phase addresses interpretation and analysis of what was learned in the "look" phase; the researcher is charged with connecting the ideas of the stakeholders so that they provide evidence that is understandable to the community group (Stringer, 1999). Finally, in the "act" phase, Stringer advocates for planning, implementing, and evaluating, on the basis of information collected and interpreted in the other phases of research.

Identifying the Phenomenon

PAR evolved from the work of Lewin (1948), who viewed action research as a means for solving practical social problems and for enacting change for the improvement of communities. PAR is heavily used as a research methodology in education and, in the health professions, PAR methods are used to improve health care services in communities. PAR has been applied to health and wellness programs, program evaluation, care plans, community nursing, and health care delivery and policy. Studies have ranged from issues and conditions stemming from chronic illness, pregnancy and childbirth, pain management, and incontinence to rehabilitation (Stringer & Genat, 2004). For example, MacDonald et al. (2015) were interested in Mi'kmaq women's experiences with Pap screening. Their study is used in the following section to illustrate PAR.

Structuring the Study

RESEARCH QUESTION. The first step in structuring the PAR study, as in other qualitative methods, is to frame the research question and to identify who is affected by or has an effect on the problem. Because of the emergent nature of PAR, researchers can begin with a tentative problem and questions and then refine or reframe them as they enter the field. Recall the look–think–act cycle of Stringer (1999) described earlier. In the "look" phase, the researcher explores the problem by "asking who is involved, what is happening,

and how, where and when events and activities occur" (p. 36). Reflecting on their observations, researchers, in collaboration with the stakeholders, can fine-tune the final research question, which serves as a guide to the study. As mentioned earlier, MacDonald et al. (2015) explored the experiences of Mi'kmaq women with Pap screening. Utilizing talking circles and individual in-depth interviews with Mi'kmaq women and interviews with health care providers, the researchers explored the historical and social contexts that impacted the women's experiences. The women were considered active participants who provided input into the research process, including the development of the research questions, participant recruitment, data collection, and analysis.

RESEARCHER'S PERSPECTIVE. When using PAR methods, the researcher is no longer the expert but acts more as a consultant. In their case study of Mi'kmaq women's experiences with Pap screening, MacDonald et al. (2015) used participatory methodology, involving pregnant Indigenous women and parenting Indigenous families. MacDonald et al. upheld the principles of PAR and principles of respectful research with Indigenous people by enabling the community to participate, valuing all participants' viewpoints and experiences, and using collaborative decision-making throughout all aspects of the research process, from recruitment to dissemination of findings. In PAR, the participants are co-researchers and are engaged in the research process as it emerges. This involvement requires processes that are democratic, participatory, empowering, and life-enhancing (Stringer & Genat, 2004). PAR investigators, like ethnographers, immerse themselves in the field for deep understanding and to build trust and credibility. For example, MacDonald et al. (2015) frequented the health centre and attended community events.

SAMPLE SELECTION. Because it is not possible to include everyone who may have a "stake" or interest in the research question, researchers purposively select a sample of participants who represent varied perspectives, experiences, and backgrounds. Participants may be people who have the widest range of differences in their experiences, particularly interesting backgrounds or experiences; those who are typical; and those with particular knowledge of the phenomenon under study. For example, MacDonald et al. (2015) worked with community facilitators who assisted in recruitment of the participants, utilizing purposive and snowball sampling. The initial talking-circle participants recruited by the community facilitators were purposefully selected Indigenous women of diverse ages, socioeconomic backgrounds, education, and Pap screening experiences. The purpose of the talking circle was to facilitate collaboration with the community and to co-design the study. This group recruited a few other women to the study. The 16 women who were eventually recruited for the more in-depth interviews had to fit certain criteria, such as identify as Indigenous Mi'kmaq, be between 21 and 75 years of age, and have had at least one Pap screening.

Data Gathering

In the "look" phase, data are gathered from a variety of sources; interviews are the principal means for understanding the experiences of the participants. PAR also includes observation in the field, gathering and reviewing of relevant documents, and the examination of relevant materials and equipment. A literature review may add information to enhance the understanding of the data emerging from the interviews and other sources. MacDonald et al. (2015) interviewed the 16 women to hear their stories about their beliefs, attitudes, and experiences related to Pap screening. All but one woman participated in a second interview in which they reviewed the initial analysis of the first interviews to provide feedback on the data interpretation, preliminary findings, and

emerging themes. This is a hallmark of CBPR: the participants are involved in all steps of the research process.

Research Hint

As mentioned in Chapter 1, there is a growing movement to ensure patients are involved in all aspects of the research process. Qualitative researchers are typically interested in the experience and perspectives of patients; however, patient engagement in research expands this beyond the role of research participants. Patients are now increasingly involved in all steps in the research process—from priority setting and funding decisions to working as co-researchers on projects.

Data Analysis

In the "think" phase, the researchers think about and reflect on all of the data gathered. The purpose of data analysis is to distill and reduce the volume of information into a manageable and organized set of concepts or ideas. The process in PAR must directly capture the experiences of the participants and be distilled in such a way "that it makes sense to them all" (Stringer & Genat, 2004).

Stringer and Genat (2004) have identified two approaches to analysis. The first, based on "epiphanic moments" (Denzin, 1998), focuses on the significant experiences as the primary units of analysis, giving voice to the participants' experiences. A second process involves the categorization and coding of data to reveal patterns and themes. Regardless of the process used, PAR allows the participants to make sense of their experience and then to use the new understanding to make a positive change.

In MacDonald et al.'s (2015) study, the participants read and validated the initial interview and provided input on the analysis. The researchers then changed some of their initial coding and themes based on the participant and community facilitator feedback. Critical to this process was the opportunity for the participants to ensure that the names of the themes and subthemes were appropriately titled from an Indigenous perspective and accurately reflected their experiences.

Describing the Findings

In accordance with Stringer's (1999) look–think–act framework, the next step is to present the outcomes to the participants and other nonparticipant stakeholders so that they understand what is happening. Several dissemination mechanisms may be used because formal academic writing is not accessible for most lay participants. The results may be shared in written reports, oral presentations, or performances. Written narrative accounts and storytelling are often used to describe the findings. The next, and most important, step is to apply the findings to solve the research problem or issue that instigated the study. This action portion of PAR parallels the nursing process of identification of goals and objectives, intervention, and, finally, evaluation. The action plans should include the following (Stringer & Genat, 2004):

Why: A statement of the overall purpose
What: A set of objectives to be obtained
How: A sequence of tasks and steps for each objective
Who: The people responsible for each task and activity
Where: The place where the tasks will be done
When: The time for initiation and completion

The researcher should also arrange for ongoing evaluation of the process. As with the exploratory phase, stakeholders are intimately involved in each step of the action plan, from identifying the plan to implementing it. The participants in MacDonald et al.'s (2015) study identified five themes and subthemes and presented them in a diagram and in excerpts from the data. They found that, despite challenging circumstances, many women still accessed Pap screening. They stated that providers of health care for Indigenous people need to appreciate the impact of historical trauma and interpersonal violence and to individualize Pap screening policies, as the best practice guideline does not always apply to Indigenous people.

Generic Qualitative Research

The previous research designs have various disciplinary, philosophical, or theoretical backgrounds. There are also common qualitative methods that are less specifically tied to a certain worldview. Generic qualitative research, also called basic, descriptive, or interpretive qualitative research, is common and has a place among the different qualitative research methods. Generic qualitative research does not adhere to the strategies of more defined and established methodologies, although they may borrow aspects of them. It is useful for exploratory projects, for novice researchers who are learning basic qualitative research techniques, and for clinicians who have qualitative questions but do not have a methodological background (Caelli et al., 2003).

Critics of generic qualitative research are concerned about whether it is possible to evaluate the quality of generic research without being able to rely on the standards of more established qualitative methods. Some are concerned that rigour can be threatened when researchers borrow bits and pieces from various methods, creating an inconsistent approach. Generic qualitative research is also criticized for being atheoretical (Caelli et al., 2003; Kahlke, 2014). However, generic qualitative approaches may offer the methodological flexibility to allow researchers to "think in new ways or examine new things" (Kahlke, 2014, p. 47).

Evidence-Informed Practice Tip

There is often as much variance within a qualitative method as there is across methods. To further your understanding of the variety in other qualitative methods, try searching for articles that claim to use qualitative description, interpretive description, and narrative inquiry. What similarities or differences do you notice?

Many qualitative researchers use **qualitative description** when they want to provide a comprehensive summary of the experiences of their participants. It is one of the most used qualitative approaches (Polit & Beck, 2017). As Sandelowski (2000) describes, "Researchers conducting qualitative descriptive studies stay close to their data and to the surface of words and events...Qualitative descriptive study is the method of choice when straight descriptions of phenomena are desired" (p. 334). Although all research involves interpretation to some extent as the researcher looks for new insights, Sandelowski (2000) suggested that qualitative description offers a "low-inference" approach that stays closer to the original data. Qualitative description utilizes typical qualitative sampling approaches, especially maximum variation sampling, to develop a broad picture of an experience. Interviews are the most common data collection tool used within this approach (Kahlke, 2014). Qualitative description utilizes "eclectic combinations of sampling, data collection, and data analysis techniques...[and] could never be described as any one method that any one person invented" (Sandelowski, 2000, p. 78).

Another increasingly common approach to generic qualitative research in nursing is **interpretive description**, which was initiated by Thorne and her colleagues (Thorne et al., 1997). They argued that nursing needed a unique method that would fit with its particular clinical and practice needs. Interpretive description focuses on developing research questions from practice and generating evidence that can then be used in the practice setting (Thorne, 2018). Interviews are the primary source of data in this approach. In analyzing the data, researchers using interpretive description aim for broad understanding of the data, rather than a line-by-line understanding of the details. Applicability to the practice setting is emphasized in this method.

Narrative Analysis

When narrative inquiry is used as a form of qualitative research, stories of people are collected and examined as the primary source of data (Duffy, 2011; Patton, 2015). The hermeneutic tradition is extended to include in-depth interview transcripts, memoirs, stories, and creative nonfiction. This discipline also draws from the phenomenological tradition in its interest in the lived experience and perceptions of experience. On the basis of the "stories" of people, at times including those of the researcher, researchers using narrative analysis in an attempt to interpret and understand experiences in terms of cultural and social meanings (Patton, 2002; see Practical Application box). As Patton (2015) notes, storytelling and narrative inquiry are not the same thing: The story is data, whereas the narrative analysis "involves interpreting the story, placing it in context, and comparing it with other stories" (p. 128).

Practical Application

Estefan et al. (2019) used narrative inquiry to examine adolescents and young adults' experiences of sexuality while living with cancer. Data were collected over 14 months from two participants through repeated interviews as well as informal conversations over phone and email. The researchers met with participants and negotiated the narrative accounts, which also evolved into the theoretical and practical perspectives shared in the research report. Estefan et al. described this as a "negotiated process in which researcher and participant work together to determine the stories that need to be told, and how to tell them" (Estefan et al., 2019, p. 195). In discussing the two stories presented, Estefan et al. described how stories can provoke and activate, and encouraged health care providers to explore the narratives of adolescents and give them opportunities to discuss aspects of life like sexuality.

APPRAISING THE EVIDENCE

Qualitative Research

Although general criteria for critiquing qualitative research are proposed in the following Critiquing Criteria box, each qualitative method has unique characteristics that influence what you may expect in the published research report, and journals often have page restrictions that penalize qualitative researchers because it can be difficult to fully explain the research process in a few pages. The criteria for critiquing are formatted to evaluate the selection of the phenomenon, the structure of the study, data gathering, data analysis, and description of the findings. Each question of the criteria focuses on factors discussed throughout the chapter. Appraising qualitative research is a useful activity for learning the nuances of this research approach. You are encouraged to identify a qualitative study of interest and apply the criteria for critiquing. Keep in mind that qualitative methods are the best way to examine questions that previously have not been addressed in research studies or to explain and explore phenomenon in a different way. The answers provided by qualitative data reflect important evidence that may provide the first insights into a patient population or clinical phenomenon.

CRITIQUING CRITERIA

Qualitative Approaches

IDENTIFYING THE PHENOMENON

1. Is the phenomenon clearly described and consistent throughout?

STRUCTURING THE STUDY

Research Question

2. Does the question specify a distinct process, phenomenon, or experience to be studied?
3. Does the question identify the context (participant group/place) that will be studied?
4. Does the choice of a specific qualitative method fit with the research question?

Researcher's Perspective

5. Is the researcher's relationship to participants described?

6. What is the role of the researcher as instrument?

Sample Selection

7. Is it clear that the selected sample is experiencing the phenomenon of interest?
8. Are there other people who would offer differing perspectives on the phenomenon?

DATA GATHERING

9. Are data sources and methods for gathering data specified?
10. Is there evidence that participant consent is an integral part of the data-gathering process?

DATA ANALYSIS

11. Can the dimensions of data analysis be identified and logically followed?

12. Is the participant's reality clearly described?
13. Is participant data (e.g., quotes) shown to substantiate the researcher's interpretation?
14. How did the research team make decisions and proceed through analysis?

DESCRIBING THE FINDINGS

15. Are examples provided to guide the reader from the raw data to the researcher's synthesis?
16. Does the researcher link the findings to existing theory or literature, or is a new theory generated?
17. Are the conclusions and implications for practice appropriate and justified based on the scope of the study?

In summary, the term *qualitative research* is an overriding description of multiple methods with distinct origins and procedures. In spite of distinctions, each method shares a common nature that guides data collection from the perspective of the participants to create a story that synthesizes disparate pieces of data into a comprehensible whole that provides evidence and promises direction for building nursing knowledge. An example of how three of these methods are used to study topics in palliative care is provided in Table 9.1. When reading these abstracts, consider how the research question fits the method that was selected, the different perspectives or worldviews that might be represented by the particular approach, and the different types of knowledge that each research project generated.

TABLE **9.1**

EXAMPLES OF QUALITATIVE METHODS EXPLORING PALLIATIVE CARE

AUTHOR AND TITLE	METHOD	ABSTRACT
Kaasalainen et al. (2019)	Mixed methods with partici-patory action research	The goal of this study was to examine current rates of resident deaths, emergency department (ED) use within the last year of life, and hospital deaths for long-term care (LTC) residents. Using a mixed-methods approach, we compared these rates across four LTC homes in Ontario, Canada and explored potential explanations of variations across homes to stimulate staff reflections and improve performance based on a quality improvement approach. Chart audits revealed that 59% of residents across sites visited EDs during the last month of life and 26% of resident deaths occurred in hospital. Staff expressed surprise at the amount of hospital use during end of life (EOL). Reflections suggested that clinical expertise, comfort with EOL communication, clinical resources (i.e., equipment), and family availability for EOL decision making could all affect nondesirable hospital transfers at EOL. Staff appeared motivated to address these areas of practice following this reflective process.
Schick-Makaroff & Sawatzky (2020)	Interpretive description	The Edmonton Symptom Assessment System (Revised) (ESAS-r) contains nine questions pertaining to symptoms/well-being. It is a standardized patient-reported assessment instrument, but inconsistently used in palliative care. Thus, a problem exists in knowledge translation regarding routine use of the ESAS-r in palliative practice. The objective was to understand clinicians' perspectives on the use of the ESAS-r in palliative care in hospitals and at home. Qualitative focus groups (n = 14 with 46 clinicians) and interviews (n = 24) elicited views regarding use of the ESAS-r in palliative practice. Interpretive description was used as a general approach to this qualitative analysis focused on understanding clinicians' views. Palliative clinicians presented multiple perspectives of the ESAS-r pertaining to their (1) underlying values, (2) disparate purposes, and (3) incommensurate responses toward use in daily practice. Benefits and challenges supported diversity within these themes, highlighting divergence among perspectives and complexity of integrating a standardized tool in patient care. Integration of the ESAS-r in palliative care requires (1) educational support for developing competence; (2) consideration of clinicians' existing, heterogeneous beliefs regarding the use of standardized assessment instruments; and (3) consultation with multidisciplinary practitioners about optimal ways that ESAS-r results can be used in a person-centered approach to palliative care. (p.692)
Sutherland et al. (2017)	Critical ethnography	Evidence of gender differences in the amount and type of care provided by family caregivers in hospice palliative home care suggests potential inequities in health and health care experiences. As part of a larger critical ethnographic study examining gender relations among clients with cancer, their family caregivers and primary nurses, this article describes gendered expectations and exemptions for family caregivers within the sociopolitical context of end-of-life at home. Data were collected from in-depth interviews (n = 25), observations of agency home care visits (n = 9) and analyses of policy and home care agency documents (n = 12). Employing a critical feminist lens, a gender-based analysis revealed that structural discourses emphasizing an artificial divide between public and private spheres constructed end-of-life at home as private and apolitical. Associated with care of home and family, women were most impacted by these public/private discourses underpinning neoliberal values of cost-efficiency. Findings suggest that a critical perspective is needed to assist policy makers and healthcare providers to view how caregiver experiences are shaped by structures that control the availability of resources. Thus, instead of focusing on caregivers' deficits, interventions should be directed at the social, political and economic conditions that shape gendered experiences. (p.1)

CRITICAL THINKING CHALLENGES

- How does the researcher select a specific type of qualitative research method to answer the research question?
- Do findings from qualitative research studies need to be validated in subsequent studies?
- How can a nurse researcher select a qualitative research method when he or she is attempting to accumulate evidence regarding a new topic about which little is known?
- How can a focused ethnography approach to research be applied to evidence-informed practice?

CLINICAL JUDGEMENT QUESTIONS

1. What needs to be considered when engaging patients in research?
   a. All methods can engage patients throughout the entire research process
   b. Patient engagement can only occur with qualitative methods
   c. Patients routinely participate in qualitative research
   d. All methods use patients at a particular step in the research

2. Which method would be most appropriate to study processes?
   a. Participatory action research
   b. Grounded theory
   c. Phenomenology
   d. Institutional ethnography

3. What is a common critique of generic qualitative methods?
   a. They are too complicated for novice researchers
   b. They can lack the rigour found in other methods
   c. The interpretations stay close to the data
   d. There is no data saturation.

KEY POINTS

- Qualitative research is the investigation of human experiences in naturalistic settings, pursuing knowledge that informs theory, practice, instrument development, and further research.
- Qualitative research studies are guided by research questions.
- Data saturation occurs when the information being shared with the researcher becomes repetitive.
- Qualitative research methods include five basic elements: identifying the phenomenon, structuring the study, gathering the data, analyzing the data, and describing the findings.
- The phenomenological method is a process of learning and constructing the meaning of human experience through intensive dialogue with persons who are living the experience.
- The grounded theory method is an inductive approach that implements a systematic set of procedures to arrive at theory about basic social processes.
- The ethnographic method focuses on systematic descriptions of cultural groups.
- CBPR is a method that systematically accesses the voice of a community to plan context-appropriate action.

🛜 FOR FURTHER STUDY

Go to Evolve at http://evolve.elsevier.com/Canada/LoBiondo/Research for the Audio Glossary.

REFERENCES

Agar, M. H. (1986). *Speaking of ethnography*. Beverly Hills, CA: Sage.

Boyle, J. S. (1991). Field research: A collaborative model for practice and research. In J. M. Morse (Ed.), *Qualitative nursing research: A contemporary dialogue*. Newbury Park, CA: Sage.

Braun, V., & Clarke, V. (2014). What can "thematic analysis" offer health and wellbeing researchers? *International Journal of Qualitative Studies on Health and Wellbeing, 9*(1), 26152. doi:10.3402/qhw.v9.26152.

Brookfield, S., Fitzgerald, L., Selvey, L., & Maher, L. (2019). The blind men and the elephant: Meta-ethnography 30 years on. *Qualitative Health Research, 29*(11), 1674–1681. https://doi.org/10.1177/2F1049732319826061.

Caelli, K., Ray, L., & Mill, J. (2003). "Clear as mud": Toward greater clarity in generic qualitative research. *International Journal of Qualitative Methods, 2*(2), 1–24.

Campbell, M., & Gregor, F. (2002). *Mapping social relations: A primer in doing institutional ethnography.* Aurora, ON: Garamond Press.

Campbell, M. L., & Rankin, J. M. (2017). Nurses and electronic health records in a Canadian hospital: Examining the social organisation and programmed use of digitised nursing knowledge. *Sociology of Health & Illness, 39*(3), 365–379. https://doi.org/10.1111/1467-9566.12489.

Chambliss, D. F. (1996). *Beyond caring: Hospitals, nurses, and the social organization of ethics.* Chicago: University of Chicago Press.

Charmaz, K. (2000). Grounded theory: Objectivist and constructivist methods. In N. K. Denzin, & Y. S. Lincoln (Eds.), *Handbook of qualitative research* (2nd ed., pp. 509–535). Thousand Oaks, CA: Sage.

Charmaz, K. (2014). *Constructing grounded theory: A practical guide through qualitative analysis* (2nd ed.). Thousand Oaks, CA: Sage.

Cohen, M. Z. (1987). A historical overview of the phenomenological movement. *Image, 19*(1), 31–34.

Colaizzi, P. (1978). Psychological research as a phenomenologist views it. In R. S. Valle, & M. King (Eds.), *Existential phenomenological alternatives for psychology* (pp. 48–71). New York: Oxford University Press.

Corbin, J., & Strauss, A. (2008). *Basics of qualitative research.* Los Angeles: Sage.

Currie, G., & Szabo, J. (2019). "It would be much easier if we were just quiet and disappeared": Parents silenced in the experience of caring for children with rare diseases. *Health Expectations, 22*(6), 1251–1259. https://doi.org/10.1111/hex.12958.

Denzin, N. K (1998). The practices and politics of interpretation. In N. K. Denzin, & Y. S. Lincoln (Eds.), *Collecting and interpreting qualitative materials* (pp. 458–498). Thousand Oaks, CA: Sage.

Denzin, N. K., & Lincoln, Y. S. (1998). *The landscape of qualitative research.* Thousand Oaks, CA: Sage.

Dinmohammadi, M., Peyrovi, H., & Mehrdad, N. (2013). Concept analysis of professional socialization in nursing. *Nursing Forum, 48,* 26–34. https://doi.org/10.1111/nuf.12006.

Duffy, M. (2011). Narrative inquiry: The method. In P. Munhall (Ed.), *Nursing research: A qualitative perspective* (5th ed., pp. 421–440). Mississauga, ON: Jones & Bartlett Learning.

El Hussein, M., Hirst, S., & Osuji, J. (2019). Professional socialization: A grounded theory of the clinical reasoning processes that RNs and LPNs use to recognize delirium. *Clinical Nursing Research, 28*(3), 321–339. https://doi.org/10.1177/1054773817724961.

Ellis, C., Adams T. E., & Bochner, A. P. (2011). Autoethnography: An overview historical social research. *Historische Sozialforschung, 36*(138), 273–290.

Estefan, A., Moules, N. J., & Laing, C. M. (2019). Composing sexuality in the midst of adolescent cancer. *Journal of Pediatric Oncology Nursing, 36*(3), 191–206. https://doi.org/10.1177/1043454219836961.

Fetterman, D. M. (1998). Ethnography. In L. Bickman, & D. J. Rog (Eds.), *Handbook of applied social research methods* (pp. 473–504). Thousand Oaks, CA: Sage Publications.

Fontana, J. S. (2004). A methodology for critical science in nursing. *Advances in Nursing Science, 27,* 93–101.

Gadamer, H. G. (2004). *Truth and method* (2nd rev. ed.). (Weinsheimer, J., Marshall, D. G., Trans.). New York: Continuum.

Giorgi, A., Fischer, C. L., & Murray, E. L. (1975). *Duquesne studies in phenomenological psychology.* Pittsburgh, PA: Duquesne University Press.

Glaser, B., & Strauss, A. (1965). *Awareness of dying.* Chicago: Aldine de Gruyter.

Glaser, B. G., & Strauss, A. L. (1967). *The discovery of grounded theory: Strategies for qualitative research.* Chicago: Aldine.

Glesne, C. (2011). *Becoming qualitative researchers: An introduction* (4th ed.). Toronto: Pearson.

Holkup, P. A., Tripp-Reimer, T., Salois, E. M., et al. (2004). Community-based participatory research: An approach to intervention research with a Native American community. *Advances in Nursing Science, 27,* 162–175.

Jardine, D. W. (1992). The fecundity of the individual case: Considerations of the pedagogic heart of interpretive work. *Journal of Philosophy of Education, 26,* 51–61. doi:10.1111/j.1467-9752.1992.tb00264.x.

Kahlke, R. M. (2014). Generic qualitative approaches: Pitfalls and benefits of methodological mixology. *International Journal of Qualitative Methods, 13,* 37–52.

Kaasalainen, S., Sussman, T., Durepos, P., McCleary, L., Ploeg, J., & Thompson, G. (2019). What are staff perceptions about their current use of emergency departments for long-term care residents at end of life? *Clinical Nursing Research, 28*(6), 692. https://doi.org/10.1177/1054773817749125.

LeCompte, M. D., & Schensul, J. J. (2010). *Designing and conducting ethnographic research: An introduction*. Lanham, MD: AltaMira Press.

Lewin, K. (1948). *Resolving social conflicts*. New York: Harper.

Lundy, K. S. (2011). Historical research. In P. Munhall (Ed.), *Nursing research: A qualitative perspective* (5th ed., pp. 381–397). Mississauga, ON: Jones & Bartlett Learning.

MacDonald, C., Martin-Misener, R., Steenbeek, A., et al. (2015). Honouring stories: Mi'kmaq women's experiences with Pap screening in Eastern Canada. *Canadian Journal of Nursing Research*, *47*(1), 72–96.

Macquire, P. (1996). Considering more feminine participatory research: What's congruency got to do with it? *Qualitative Inquiry*, *2*, 106–118.

Merriam, S. B., & Tisdell, E. J. (2016). *Qualitative research: A guide to design and implementation*. San Francisco: Jossey-Bass.

Moore, G. F., Audrey, S., Barker, M., Bond, L., Bonell, C., Hardeman, W., ... & Baird, J. (2015). Process evaluation of complex interventions: Medical Research Council guidance. *British Medical Journal*, *350*. https://doi.org/10.1136/bmj.h1258.

Morse, J. M., & Richards, L. (2002). *Readme first for a user's guide to qualitative methods*. Thousand Oaks, CA: Sage.

Moules, N. J. (2002). Hermeneutic inquiry: Paying heed to history and Hermes an ancestral, substantive, and methodological tale. *International Journal of Qualitative Methods*, *1*(3), 1–21. https://journals.sagepub.com/doi/full/10.1177/160940690200100301.

Patton, M. (2002). *Qualitative research & evaluation methods* (3rd ed.). Thousand Oaks, CA: Sage.

Patton, M. (2015). *Qualitative research & evaluation methods* (4th ed.). Thousand Oaks, CA: Sage.

Pauly, B., McCall, J., Browne, A. J., et al. (2015). Toward cultural safety: Nurse and patient perceptions of illicit substance use in a hospitalized setting. *Advances in Nursing Science*, *38*(2), 121–135.

Polit, D., & Beck, C. (2017). *Nursing research: Generating and assessing evidence for nursing practice* (10th ed.). Riverwoods, IL: Wolters Kluwer.

Roper, J., & Shapira, J. (2000). *Ethnography in nursing research*. Thousand Oaks, CA: Sage.

Sandelowski, M. (2000). What ever happened to qualitative description? *Research in Nursing and Health*, *23*, 334–340.

Sandelowski, M. (2010). Whats in a name?: Qualitative description revisited. *Research in Nursing and Health*, *1*, 77. https://0-doi-org.aupac.lib.athabascau.ca/10.1002/nur.20362.

Schick-Makaroff, K., & Sawatzky, R. (2020). Divergent perspectives on the use of the Edmonton Symptom Assessment System (Revised) in palliative care. *Journal of Hospice & Palliative Nursing*, *22*, 75–81. https://doi.org/10.1097/NJH.0000000000000617.

Smith, D. E. (2005). *Institutional ethnography: A sociology for people*. Lanham, MD: AltaMira Press.

Smith, V. (2001). Ethnographies of work and the work of ethnographers. In P. Atkinson, A. Coffey, S. Delamont, J. Lofland, & L. Lofland (Eds.), *Handbook of ethnography* (pp. 220–233). Thousand Oaks, CA: Sage.

Spiegelberg, H. (1976). *The phenomenological movement* (Vols. I–II). The Hague: Martinus Nijhoff.

Spradley, J. P. (1979). *The ethnographic interview*. New York: Holt, Rinehart, & Winston.

Strauss, A. L. (1987). *Qualitative analysis for social scientists*. New York: Cambridge University Press.

Strauss, A., & Corbin, J. (1990). *Basics of qualitative research: Grounded theory procedures and techniques*. Newbury Park, CA: Sage.

Stringer, E. T. (1999). *Action research* (2nd ed.). Thousand Oaks, CA: Sage.

Stringer, E. T., & Genat, W. J. (2004). *Action research in health*. Thousand Oaks, CA: Sage.

Sutherland, N., Ward, G. C., McWilliam, C., & Stajduhar, K. (2017). Structural impact on gendered expectations and exemptions for family caregivers in hospice palliative home care. *Nursing Inquiry*, *24*(1). n/a. https://doi.org/10.1111/nin.12157.

Thorne, S. (2018). What can qualitative studies offer in a world where evidence drives decisions? *Asia-Pacific Journal of Oncology Nursing*, *5*(1), 43–45. https://doi.org/10.4103/apjon.apjon_51_17.

Thorne, S. (2020). Beyond theming: Making qualitative studies matter. *Nursing Inquiry*, *27*, e12343. https://doi.org/10.1111/nin.12343.

Thorne, S., Reimer Kirkham, S., & MacDonald-Emes, J. (1997). Interpretive description: A noncategorical qualitative alternative for developing nursing knowledge. *Research in Nursing & Health*, *2*, 169–177.

van Kaam, A. (1969). *Existential foundations in psychology*. New York: Doubleday.

Wall, S. (2013). Nursing entrepreneurship: Motivators, strategies and possibilities for professional advancement and health system change. *Nursing Leadership*, *26*(2), 29–40. https://doi.org/10.7939/R3VF1G.

Wolcott, H. F. (1994). *Transforming qualitative data: description, analysis and interpretation*. Thousand Oaks, CA: Sage.

Wolcott, H. F. (1999). *Ethnography: A way of seeing.* Lanham, MD: AltaMira Press.

Wuest, J. (2011). Grounded theory: The method. In P. Munhall (Ed.), *Nursing research: A qualitative perspective* (5th ed., pp. 225–256). Mississauga, ON: Jones & Bartlett Learning.

Zahavi, D. (2019). Getting it quite wrong: Van Manen and Smith on phenomenology. *Qualitative Health Research, 29*(6), 900–907.

Zahavi, D., & Martiny, K. M. (2019). Phenomenology in nursing studies: New perspectives. *International Journal of Nursing Studies, 93*, 155–162.

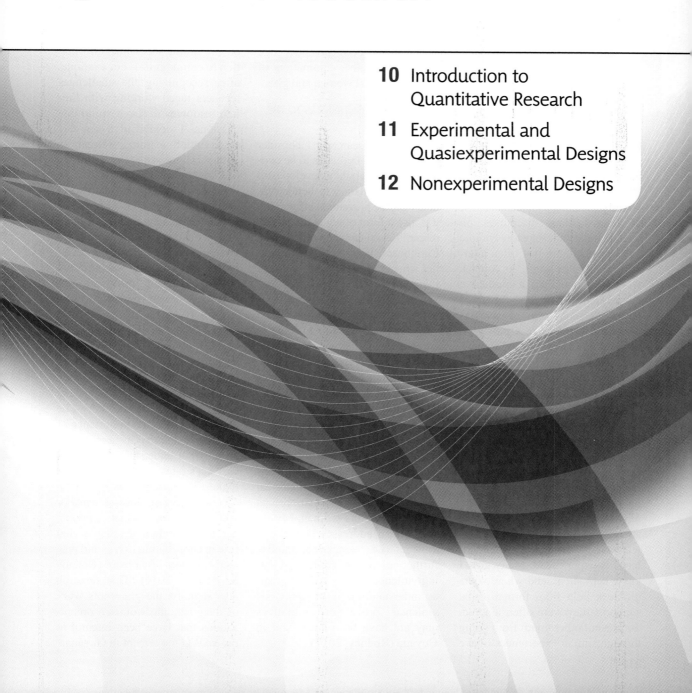

PART FOUR

Quantitative Research

RESEARCH **VIGNETTE**

Why I Focus on Violence Against Women and Girls (VAWG)

Ruth Rodney
Assistant Professor
School of Nursing
York University
Toronto, Ontario

VAWG is a human rights and public health issue that affects one in three women globally (WHO, 2013). Unfortunately, these numbers are even higher in some regions of the world (Contreras-Urbina et al., 2019). Communities can react differently to dating violence because of long-standing discourses on gender, race, age, socioeconomic status, and culture that often intersect in complex ways. As a black woman, a daughter, a mother, a nurse, and a researcher, this topic is very personal to me. I have experienced violence in a past relationship and have assisted friends, acquaintances, and patients (in my role as a frontline nurse) who have experienced violence.

When reflecting on my own youth, I realized that dating violence was common and, to some degree, normalized. For many teenage girls and boys these experiences created an unhealthy starting point for dating and long-term relationships. I also noticed that adolescents faced greater challenges in accessing help when violence is experienced. Many girls I knew kept silent, and when others did seek help from formal social supports, they were often ignored. To prevent other youth from going through similar experiences I have

had or witnessed others go through, I made a conscious decision to contribute to the body of knowledge that supports the elimination of violence against women and girls.

MY RESEARCH CONTRIBUTES TO THE FIELD OF VAWG

As a nurse researcher, I consider the knowledge I produce to be twofold: it informs policy development and implementation to better support violence prevention efforts, and it is also a form of advocacy, as my research is co-created with African Caribbean Black (ACB) communities who are not well represented in literature on dating violence.

Specifically, my doctoral thesis was the first study of its kind completed in Guyana to address adolescent dating violence with adolescents, parents, and teachers. It also contributes to the larger body of knowledge on adolescent dating violence, an area that is lacking within the Caribbean (Rodney, 2017), as it delves into the complexity of how community ideas of gender and respectability are shaped by historical understandings of relationships between men and women. My research also addresses how social systems (i.e., education, family) further complicate adolescent dating violence and provides a greater understanding of why previous violence prevention initiatives may not have been successful in Guyana (Rodney, 2017).

From a social justice perspective, I believe a fundamental component of health research is to ensure that communities who participate in research can access, understand, and utilize the information obtained. This means that my attention is focused not only on academic literature but also on providing accessible information to communities. For example, after recognizing the challenges teachers faced working with limited resources in focus group discussions, I organized a one-day experiential learning retreat in collaboration with the Ministry of Education in Guyana for teachers. The goal of this retreat was to provide teachers with an opportunity to learn new techniques and insights in decreasing negative interactions with students by developing a more positive classroom environment and providing opportunity for self-reflection.

I completed the qualitative component of the first national prevalence study on VAWG in Guyana, supported by UN Women (Contreras-Urbina et al., 2019). This study illustrates the regional difference of VAWG in a Caribbean country. The results highlight the importance of qualitative inquiry as it provides an in-depth understanding of why Guyana's rates of violence may be highest in the region, why women do not always disclose violence or seek help from formal supports, and how communities play a vital role in contributing to risk and protective factors of violence (Rodney & Bobbili, 2019). This research also supports the grassroots work of long-standing women's organizations that have been integral to the VAWG movement in Guyana.

In keeping with my commitment to knowledge translation for diverse communities, my colleague and I conducted three radio interviews about the results of this study with a local radio station, 94.1 BOOM FM. These interviews were recorded on Facebook Live and garnered over 8000 listeners in total. Audience members listened to key findings of the report and were provided with tips on how to continue discussions on VAWG within their own communities. Additionally, we also disseminated findings in a local newspaper to provide greater access to research findings (Bobbili & Rodney, 2019).

Furthermore, given the importance of the topic, the established trust and relationship with the community and the long-term commitment required to effect change for the elimination of VAWG, I continue to maintain a connection with communities in Guyana.

IMPLICATIONS FOR NURSING PRACTICE

Given that most nurses worldwide are women, the implications for nursing practice are significant. First, the global numbers of women's experiences of violence (i.e., one in three women) implies that nurses experience violence in their personal lives, while also supporting patients who experience violence. Acknowledging this reality means ensuring that nurses are provided with access to institutional social supports (Rodney & Bobbili, 2019). Advocating for these resources contributes to the overall safety of the public by supporting the mental and physical health of nurses (Rodney & Bobbili, 2019).

Additionally, identifying gaps in professional policies of VAWG (that may vary based on geographical area and healthcare system) can have greater implications for nursing practice and improve health outcomes for women and their families. Irrespective of country, healthcare plays a critical role in the multidisciplinary effort needed for violence prevention and treatment (UN Women, 2015). The research completed in Guyana illustrates that in the absence of directive policies for care, nurses' interaction with patients offered opportunities to provide violence prevention resources—even if women were not comfortable disclosing violence (Rodney & Bobbili, 2019). This means that nurses are ideally positioned to provide violence prevention resources, offer a safe space for women to disclose if they wish, and continue to contribute to the body of literature that examines VAWG and its elimination.

WHAT ARE MY AREAS OF FUTURE FOCUS?

I am focused on two main areas moving forward. Most of my work to date has been within Guyana. While the understanding of dating violence in Guyana is applicable to a Canadian context given the ACB communities that have migrated from the Caribbean, adolescent dating in a North American context is different. Therefore, I am focusing on how to improve dating relationships within a Canadian context for ACB youth. Secondly, while messages denouncing domestic and dating violence are widespread, communities are not necessarily receiving these messages in the way it was intended (Rodney, 2017; Rodney & Bobbili, 2019). Therefore, I am constantly questioning how to improve knowledge translation with the end goal of changing dominant discourses on violence in Guyana and Canada. ▮

REFERENCES

Bobbili, S., & Rodney, R. (2019, November 25). Violence against women in Guyana: How do we make a change? In the Diaspora. Stabroek Newspaper. https://www.stabroeknews.com/2019/11/25/features/in-the-diaspora/violence-against-women-in-guyana-how-do-we-make-a-change/.

Contreras-Urbina, M., Bourassa, A., Myers, R., Ovince, J., Rodney, R., & Bobbili, S. (2019). Guyana Womens Health and Life Experiences Survey Report: UN Women. https://caribbean.unwomen.org/en/materials/publications/2019/11/guyana-womens-health-and-life-experiences-survey-report.

Rodney, R. (2017). Building healthier relationships within communities: The critical examination of guyanese perspectives on adolescent dating violence and its Prevention. ProQuest Dissertations & Theses Global. (1996230249). Retrieved from: http://ezproxy.library.yorku.ca/login?url=https://search-proquest-.

Rodney, R., & Bobbili, S. (2019). Women's health and life experiences: A qualitative research report on violence against women in Guyana: UN Women. https://caribbean.unwomen.org/en/materials/publications/2019/11/womens-health-and-life-experiences-a-qualitative-research-report-on-violence-against-women-in-guyana.

UN, Women (2015). A framework to underpin action to prevent violence against women: UN Women Library. Retrieved from https://www.un-women.org/en/digital-library/publications/2015/11/prevention-framework.

World Health Organization (WHO). (2013). Global and regional estimates of violence against women: prevalence and health effects of intimate partner violence and nonpartner sexual violence: WHO Library. Retrieved from https://www.who.int/reproductivehealth/publications/violence/9789241564625/en/.

CHAPTER 10

Introduction to Quantitative Research

Ramesh Venkatesa Perumal | Mina D. Singh

LEARNING OUTCOMES

After reading this chapter, you will be able to do the following:

- Define research design.
- Identify the purpose of the research design.
- Define control as it affects the research design.
- Compare and contrast the elements that affect control.
- Begin to evaluate the degree of control that should be exercised in the design.
- Define internal validity.
- Identify the threats to internal validity.
- Define external validity.
- Identify the conditions that affect external validity.
- Identify the links between study design and evidence-informed practice.
- Evaluate the design by using the critiquing questions.

KEY TERMS

accuracy	feasibility	objectivity
attrition	Hawthorne effect	pilot study
bias	history threat	randomization
constancy	homogeneity	reactivity
control	instrumentation threats	selection bias
control group	internal validity	selection effects
experimental group	maturation	testing effect
external validity	measurement effects	
extraneous variable	mortality	

STUDY RESOURCES

 Go to Evolve at http://evolve.elsevier.com/Canada/LoBiondo/Research for the Audio Glossary.

THE WORD "DESIGN" IMPLIES THE ORGANIZATION of elements into a masterful work of art. In the world of art and fashion, the word conjures up images of processes and techniques that are used to express a total concept. When an individual creates something, process and form are employed. The form, process, and degree of adherence to structure depend on the aims of the creator.

The same can be said of the research process. The research process does not need to be a sterile procedure, but it should be one in which the researcher develops a masterful work within the limits of a problem and the related theoretical basis. The organization plan that the researcher creates is the design. When reading a study, the research consumer should be able to recognize that the research problem, purpose, literature review, theoretical framework, and hypothesis all interrelate with, complement, and assist in the operationalization of the design (Figure 10.1). The degree to which a fit exists between these design elements determines the strength of the study and of the consumer's confidence in the evidence provided by the findings and their potential applicability to practice.

Nursing practice is concerned with a variety of activities that require varying degrees of process and form, such as the provision of quality care, cost-effective patient care, responses of patients to disease, and factors that affect caregivers. When nurses administer patient care, they draw on the nursing process. Previous chapters stressed the importance of theory and knowledge of subject matter to research. How a researcher structures, implements, or designs a study affects the results of a research project.

To grasp the implications and the use of research, you need to understand the central issues in the design of a research project. This chapter provides an overview of the meaning, purpose, and issues related to quantitative research design. Chapters 10 and 11 discuss specific types of quantitative designs.

PURPOSE OF THE RESEARCH DESIGN

The purpose of the research design is to provide the plan for answering research questions. These questions can result in research driven by a researcher's curiosity or interest in a theoretical

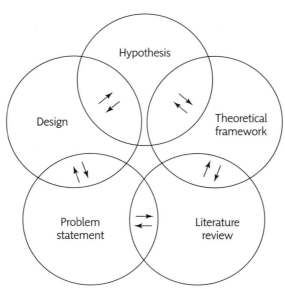

FIG. 10.1 Interrelationships of design, problem statement, literature review, theoretical framework, and hypothesis.

question. This process is called *basic research,* and its motivation is to expand nursing knowledge. In contrast, *applied research* is designed to solve clinical problems rather than to acquire knowledge for knowledge's sake; thus, the goal is to improve the patient's health care condition.

The design in quantitative research then becomes the vehicle for hypothesis testing or answering research questions, whether they are basic or applied. The design involves a *plan,* a *structure,* and a *strategy.* These three design concepts guide a researcher in writing the hypothesis or research questions, conducting the project, and analyzing and evaluating the data. The overall purpose of the research design is twofold: to aid in the solution of research problems and to maintain control (see Practical Application box). All research is an attempt to answer questions. The design, along with the methods and analysis, is the mechanism for finding solutions to research questions. **Control** is defined as the measures that the researcher uses to hold the conditions of the study uniform and avoid possible influence of **bias** (distortion of the results) on the dependent variable or outcome.

Practical Application

A research example that demonstrates how the design can aid in answering a research question and maintain control is the study by Henrique et al. (2018). The main purpose of their study was to test the effect of warm shower therapy and perineal exercises using a ball on pain, anxiety, and stress parameters during childbirth. To maintain control, the researchers had strict sample characteristics. Inclusion criteria were as follows: (1) older than 18 years of age, (2) single live fetus, (3) cephalic presentation, (4) no clinical or obstetric pathology, (5) cervical dilation between 3 and 8 cm, (6) gestational term, and (7) pain score ≥ 5. The exclusion criteria were as follows: (1) caesarean indication on admission, (2) analgesia, (3) smoker, (4) mental disorder, (5) caffeine intake equal to or less than 10 hours, (6) drug user, (7) less than 6 prenatal visits, and (8) without corticosteroids and analgesics in the previous 6 hours. By establishing the specific sample criteria and the participant's eligibility, the researchers were able to maintain control over the study's condition and answer the research question appropriately.

Various considerations, including the type of design, affect the accomplishment of the study. These considerations include **objectivity**—the use of facts without distortion by personal feelings or bias—in the conceptualization of the problem; accuracy; feasibility; control of the experiment; internal validity; and external validity. Statistical principles underlie the many forms of control, but it is more important that the research consumer have a clear conceptual understanding of statistics and how they inform the research questions.

The type of design used in a study also affects its application to practice. Chapters 11 and 12 present a number of experimental, quasiexperimental, and nonexperimental designs. The type of design used in a study is linked to the level of evidence, and, in turn, the contribution of a study's findings is linked to evidence-informed practice. As discussed in Chapter 1, the term *evidence-informed practice* is currently being used instead of *evidence-based practice* because it is more inclusive in that it encompasses many forms of evidence, such as clinical experience and judgement with research utilization. As you critically appraise the design, take into account other aspects of a study's design, which are reviewed in this chapter.

OBJECTIVITY IN THE CONCEPTUALIZATION OF THE PROBLEM

In the conceptualization of the problem, objectivity is derived from a review of the literature and development of a theoretical framework (see Figure 10.1). Using the literature, the researcher assesses the depth and breadth of available knowledge about the problem. The literature review and theoretical framework should show that the researcher reviewed the literature critically and objectively (see Chapters 2 and 5), because this conceptualization of the problem affects the type of design chosen. For example, for a question about the relationship of the length of a breastfeeding education program, either an experimental or a correlational design may be recommended (see

Chapters 10 and 11), whereas for a question regarding the physical changes in a woman's body during pregnancy and the maternal perception of the unborn child, a survey or correlation study may be advised (see Chapter 11). The literature review should reflect the following:

- When the problem was studied
- The aspects of the problem that were studied
- Where the problem was investigated
- By whom the problem was investigated
- The gaps or inconsistencies in the literature

Research Hint

A review that incorporates the aspects presented here allows the research consumer to judge the objectivity of the problem area and therefore whether the design chosen is suitable for investigating the problem.

ACCURACY

Accuracy in determining the appropriate design is also accomplished through the theoretical framework and review of the literature (see Chapters 2 and 5). **Accuracy** means that all aspects of a study systematically and logically follow from the research problem. The beginning researcher is wise to answer a question involving few variables that does not require the use of sophisticated designs. The simplicity of a research project does not render it useless or of a lesser value for practice. Although the project is simple, the researcher should not forgo accuracy. The research consumer should believe that the researcher chose a design that was consistent with the research problem and offered the maximum amount of control.

Many clinical problems have not yet been researched, so a preliminary, or pilot, study is a wise approach to testing the accuracy of a study design before a larger study is undertaken. A **pilot study** is a small, simple study conducted as a prelude to a larger study. The key is the accuracy, validity, and objectivity used by the researcher in attempting to answer the question. Accordingly, you should read various types of research reports and assess whether and how the criteria for each

step of the research process were followed. Many nursing journals publish not only sophisticated clinical research projects but also smaller clinical studies whose results can be applied to practice.

FEASIBILITY

When you, as a consumer of research, critique the study design, you must also be aware of the pragmatic consideration of feasibility. Feasibility is the capability of the study to be successfully carried out. Sometimes, the reality of feasibility does not truly sink in until the researcher begins the study. When you review a study, you should consider feasibility, including availability of the participants, timing of the research, time required for the participants to take part in the study, costs, and analysis of the data (Table 10.1). Studies in which researchers are testing feasibility are also called *pilot studies* (see Practical Application box).

An example of a feasibility study is one conducted by Tryphonopoulos and Letourneau (2020). This feasibility study examined the effectiveness of the original protocol for a video feedback interaction guidance intervention designed to improve maternal–infant interaction quality, maternal depressive symptoms, and cortisol patterns of depressed mothers and their infants. The results of this study are used to support the implementation of a large-scale randomized controlled trial.

Practical Application

Santiago et al. (2019) conducted a pilot study to explore the feasibility of using a tablet equipped with a communication app in assisting with communication of patients in the intensive care unit. The results indicated that it was feasible for patients to use the tablet equipped with a communication app as an adjunct to communication.

Before a large experimental study (such as a randomized clinical trial) is conducted, it is helpful to first conduct a pilot study with a small number of participants to determine the feasibility of participant recruitment, the intervention, the

TABLE 10.1

PRAGMATIC CONSIDERATIONS IN DETERMINING THE FEASIBILITY OF A RESEARCH PROBLEM

FACTOR	PRAGMATIC CONSIDERATION
Time	The research problem must be able to be studied within a realistic period of time. All researchers have deadlines for completion of a project. The scope of the problem must be circumscribed enough to provide ample time for the completion of the entire project. Research studies generally take longer than anticipated to complete.
Participant availability	The researcher must determine whether a sufficient number of eligible participants will be available and willing to take part in the study. If a researcher has a "captive" audience (e.g., students in a classroom), it may be relatively easy to enlist their cooperation. When a study involves the participants' independent time and effort, they may be unwilling to participate when they will receive no apparent reward for doing so. Other potential participants may have fears about harm or confidentiality and be suspicious of the research process in general. Participants with unusual characteristics, such as rare diseases, are often difficult to locate. People are generally cooperative about taking part in a study, but a researcher must consider needing a larger participant pool than will actually participate. At times, when reading a research report, the researcher may note how the procedures were liberalized or the number of participants was altered—probably as a result of some unforeseen pragmatic consideration.
Facility and equipment availability	All research projects require some kind of equipment, such as questionnaires, telephones, stationery, stamps, technical equipment, or another apparatus. Most research projects also require the availability of a facility for the work, such as a hospital site for data collection, a laboratory space, or a computer centre for data analysis.
Money	Many research projects require some expenditure of money. Before embarking on a study, the researcher probably itemized the expenses and estimated the total cost of the project. This estimation of cost provides a clear picture of the budgetary needs for items such as books, stationery, postage, printing, technical equipment, telephone and computer charges, and salaries. These expenses can range from about $200 for a small-scale student project to hundreds of thousands of dollars for a large-scale federally funded project.
Researcher experience	The selection of the research problem should be based on the nurse's experience and interest. It is much easier to develop a research study related to a topic that is either theoretically or experientially familiar. Selecting a problem that is of interest to the researcher is essential for maintaining enthusiasm when the inevitable successes and failures occur.
Ethics	Research problems that place unethical demands on participants are not feasible for study. Researchers must take ethical considerations seriously. The consideration of ethics may affect the choice of the design and the methodology.

data-collection protocol, the likelihood that participants will complete the study, the reliability and validity of new measurement tools, and the costs of the study. These pragmatic considerations are not presented as a step in the research process, as are the theoretical framework and methods, but they do affect every step of the process and

therefore should be considered when you assess a study. For example, the student researcher may or may not have funding or accessible services. When you critique a study, note the credentials of the author or authors and whether the investigation was part of either a student project or a fully funded grant project. If the project was a student project, the standards of critiquing are applied more liberally than for projects conducted by an experienced researcher or clinician with a doctoral degree. Finally, the pragmatic issues raised affect the scope and breadth of an investigation and, therefore, its generalizability.

CONTROL

When developing a study, a researcher attempts to use a design to maximize the degree of control over the tested variables. Control involves holding the conditions of the study constant and establishing specific sampling criteria to reduce variability in the sample characteristics that may influence the outcome under investigation, as described by Hall et al. (2019) in a study of the feasibility of implementing a yoga intervention for participants with chronic pain. The intervention consisted of weekly 1-hour session for 10 weeks. The authors ensured homogeneity of the sample by using the inclusion and exclusion criteria. Adult patients (above the age of 18) suffering with chronic pain (with a recommendation from their therapist) and who could speak English were included in the study. Patients who have had some surgery in the past or scheduled in the future, who are pregnant, and who are enrolled in some other yoga course were excluded from the study.

An efficient design can maximize results, decrease errors, and control pre-existing conditions that may affect outcome. To accomplish these tasks, the research design and methods should demonstrate the researcher's efforts at control. For example, in a study to assess the effectiveness of Hernia Repair Education Intervention (HREI) for patients following inguinal hernia repair, the researchers had a specific inclusion and exclusion criteria to ensure homogeneity of the samples (Sawhney et al., 2017).

When research designs are critiqued, the issue of control is always raised, but with varying levels of flexibility. The issues discussed here will become clearer as you review the various types of designs.

Control is accomplished by ruling out extraneous variables that compete with the independent variables as an explanation for a study's outcome. An **extraneous variable** (also called a *mediating variable*) interferes with the operations of the phenomena being studied (e.g., age and gender). Means of controlling extraneous variables include the following:

- Use of a homogeneous sample
- Use of consistent data-collection procedures
- Manipulation of the independent variable
- Randomization

An investigator might be interested in how a new smoking cessation program (independent variable) affects smoking behaviour (dependent variable). The independent variable is assumed to affect the outcome, or dependent variable. An investigator needs to be relatively sure that the decrease in smoking is truly related to the smoking cessation program rather than to another variable, such as motivation.

The following example illustrates and defines these concepts further. In a study to assess the effectiveness of an electronic nursing intervention in improving mood and decreasing stress during first six months postpartum, the authors used a three-arm randomized controlled trial. To rule out the effects of extraneous variables on mood and stress, demographic information was collected, including if mothers had experienced depression or anxiety during or before pregnancy and if they were receiving treatment. This demographic information was then included in the statistical hypothesis testing to check if there were any differences between the groups (McCarter et al., 2019).

Although the design of the research study alone does not inherently provide control, an appropriately designed study with the necessary controls can increase an investigator's ability to answer a research question.

Evidence-Informed Practice Tip

As you read a report, assess whether the study includes a tested intervention and whether the report contains a clear description of the intervention and how it was controlled. If the details are not clear, the intervention may have been administered differently among the participants, which would affect the interpretation of the results.

Homogeneous Sampling

In the example of smoking cessation, extraneous variables may affect the dependent variable. The characteristics of a study's participants are common extraneous variables. Age, gender, length of time smoked, amount smoked, and even smoking rules may affect the outcome in the smoking cessation example, even though they are extraneous or outside the study's design. As a control for these and other similar problems, the researcher's participants should demonstrate **homogeneity**, or similarity with regard to the extraneous variables relevant to the particular study (see Chapter 12). Extraneous variables are not fixed but must be reviewed, and their inclusion in the analyses is based on the study's purpose and theoretical base. By using a sample of homogeneous participants, the researcher has used a straightforward step of control.

In a randomized controlled trial, Lee et al. (2020) pilot tested an educational intervention to reduce fatigue among HIV clients. In order to have a homogenous sample and to reduce heterogeneity, the authors used a specific sampling criterion. The specific inclusion and exclusion criteria were: (a) diagnosed with HIV/AIDS, (b) at least 45 years of age, (c) unemployed, retired, or on disability, (d) with a phone or email for communicating with research staff, and (e) who stated they had experienced fatigue during the past week. Individuals with cognitive impairment, obesity, and sleep disorders were excluded from the study. In addition to the inclusion and exclusion criteria, the researchers included samples who had the potential confounding factors, such as adults 45 years and older who were unemployed or retired, as varying employment schedules. By this control step, authors limited the generalizability of the outcomes to other populations

(see Chapter 17). The results can then be generalized only to a similar population of individuals. Homogeneity could be considered limiting, but not necessarily, because no treatment or program is applicable to all populations and educated consumers of research must take into consideration the differences in populations.

Research Hint

When reviewing studies, remember that it is better to have a "clean" study, whose results can be used to make generalizations about a specific population, than a "messy" study, whose results may be poorly or not at all generalizable.

If the researcher believes that one of the extraneous variables is important, it may be included in the design. In the smoking cessation example, if individuals are working in an area where smoking is not allowed and this condition is considered to be important to the study, the researcher could account for it in the design and set up a control condition for it. This condition can be established by comparing two different work areas: one where smoking is allowed and one where it is not. Of importance is that before the data are collected, the researcher should have identified, planned for, and controlled the important extraneous variables.

Constancy in Data Collection

Another basic but critical component of control is constancy in data-collection procedures. **Constancy** refers to the ability of the data-collection design to hold the conditions of the study to a cookbook-like recipe. In other words, for the purpose of collecting data for the study, each participant is exposed to the same environmental conditions, timing of data collection, data-collection instruments, and data-collection procedures (see Chapter 13).

An example of constancy in data collection is illustrated in the study by Boitor et al. (2019). The objective of this randomized controlled trial was to assess the effect of hand massage on the pain intensity and pain-related interference with functioning of cardiac surgery patients. The interventions were standardized across patients and provided by one registered nurse trained in massage therapy at the same time of the day to patients. This type of control aided the investigators' ability to draw conclusions, discuss the findings, and cite the need for further research in this area. For the consumer, constancy demonstrates a clear, consistent, and specific means of data collection.

In a study to assess the effectiveness of video feedback intervention on improving the quality of interaction between mothers with postpartum depression and their infants, researchers used an intervention checklist to ensure accurate implementation of the intervention or implementation fidelity (Tryphonopoulos & Letourneau, 2020). All study designs should demonstrate constancy (fidelity) of data collection, but studies that test an intervention require the highest level of intervention fidelity.

Manipulation of the Independent Variable

A third means of control is manipulation of the independent variable. *Manipulation* refers to the administration of a program, treatment, or intervention to only one group within the study but not to the other participants in the study. The first group is known as the **experimental group**, and the other group is known as the **control group**, or comparison group. In a control group, the variables under study are held at a constant or comparison level. For example, in a randomized control trial, authors examined the effect of lanolin on nipple pain among breastfeeding women with damaged nipples. The experimental group received 40 gm tube of Lansinoh® along with a pamphlet. Participants were asked to apply lanolin over the damaged nipples following every feeding for 7 days. The mothers in the control group were not provided with the intervention (Jackson & Dennis, 2017).

Experimental and quasiexperimental designs involve manipulation, whereas in nonexperimental designs, the independent variable is not manipulated. This lack of manipulation does not decrease the usefulness of a nonexperimental design. The use of a control group in an experimental or quasiexperimental design is related to the research question and, again, its theoretical framework.

Blinding is a technique used in experimental and quasiexperimental research in which the participants are not aware of whether they are receiving the intervention. *Double blinding* is a technique in which both the researchers and the participants are not aware of who is receiving the intervention and who is in the control group. For example, Evans et al. (2018) conducted a double blind randomized controlled trial assessing the effectiveness of ginger aromatherapy in relieving chemotherapy-induced nausea in children with cancer, compared with a placebo. The participants were randomly assigned to one of the three groups, namely control group (no intervention), placebo intervention group, and the experimental group with ginger aromatherapy. In this study both the children and the nurse who collected the data were blinded to group assignment.

Research Hint
Be aware that the lack of manipulation of the independent variable does not mean that the study is weaker. The level of the problem, the amount of theoretical work, and the research that has preceded the project affect the researcher's choice of the design. If the problem is amenable to a design in which the independent variable can be manipulated, the power of a researcher to draw conclusions will increase, provided that all of the considerations of control are equally addressed.

Randomization

Researchers may also choose other forms of control, such as randomization. **Randomization** is a participant selection procedure in which each participant in a population has an equal chance of being assigned to either the experimental group or the control group. Randomization eliminates bias, aids in the attainment of a representative sample, and can be used in various designs. In a randomized controlled trial to assess the effectiveness of Hernia Repair Education Intervention (HREI), the researchers assigned the eligibility participants to either the experimental group or the control group. Randomization occurred in a private office to minimize contamination (Sawhney et al., 2017). Randomization may be especially important in longitudinal studies, in which bias from giving the same instrument to the same participants on a number of occasions can be a problem (see Chapter 12).

QUANTITATIVE CONTROL AND FLEXIBILITY

The same level of control cannot be exercised in all types of designs. At times, when a researcher wants to explore an area in which little or no literature on the concept exists, the researcher will probably use an exploratory design. In this type of study, the researcher is interested in describing or categorizing a phenomenon in a group of individuals. Freeman et al. (2020) used an exploratory cross-sectional design to investigate palliative care nurse attitudes towards medical assistance in dying, as the scholarly literature on this topic was limited. The researchers concluded that the palliative care nurses have moderate attitude overall (based on the aggregated scores) towards MAID. In critiquing this type of study, the issue of control should be applied in a highly flexible manner because of the novelty of the nature of study.

If from a review of a study you determine that the researcher intended to conduct a correlational study (an examination of the relationship between or among the variables), then the issue of control takes on more importance. Control must be exercised as strictly as possible. At this intermediate level of design, it should be clear to the reviewer that the researcher considered the extraneous variables that may affect the outcomes.

All aspects of control are strictly applied to studies that use an experimental design. The reader should be able to locate in the research report how the researcher met these criteria: whether the conditions of the research were constant throughout the study, the assignment of participants was random, and experimental and control groups were used. Because of the control exercised in the study, the reader can determine that all issues related to control were considered and the extraneous variables were addressed.

Evidence-Informed Practice Tip ___

Remember that establishing evidence for practice is determined by assessing the validity of each step of the study, assessing whether the evidence assists in planning patient care, and assessing whether patients respond to the evidence-informed care.

INTERNAL AND EXTERNAL VALIDITY

Consumers of research must believe that the results of a study are valid, based on precision, and faithful to what the researcher wanted to measure. To form the basis of further research, practice, and theory development, a study must be credible and dependable. The two important criteria for evaluating the credibility and dependability of the results are internal validity and external validity. Threats to validity are listed in Box 10.1, and a discussion of each threat follows.

BOX **10.1**

THREATS TO VALIDITY

INTERNAL VALIDITY
History threats
Maturation effects
Testing effects
Instrumentation threats
Mortality (attrition)
Selection bias

EXTERNAL VALIDITY
Selection effects
Reactive effects
Measurement effects

Internal Validity

Internal validity is the degree to which the experimental treatment, not an uncontrolled condition, resulted in the observed effects. To establish internal validity, the researcher rules out other factors or threats as rival explanations of the relationship between the variables. Threats to internal validity may be numerous and are considered by researchers in planning a study and by consumers before implementing the results in practice (Campbell & Stanley, 1996). Research consumers should note that the threats to internal validity are most clearly applicable to experimental designs, but attention to factors that can compromise outcomes should be considered to some degree in all quantitative designs. If these threats are not considered, they could negate the results of the research by affecting the design. Threats to internal validity include history threats, maturation effects, testing effects, instrumentation threats, mortality (attrition), and selection bias. Table 10.2 provides examples of these threats.

History Threats

Not only the independent variable but also another specific concurrent event may affect the dependent variable, either inside or outside the experimental setting. This threat to internal validity is referred to as the **history threat**. For example, in a study on the effects of a breastfeeding education program on the length of time of breastfeeding, government-sponsored breastfeeding promotions on television and in newspapers could affect the length of time of breastfeeding and would be considered a threat of history (see Table 10.2).

Maturation Effects

Maturation refers to the developmental, biological, or psychological processes that operate within an individual as a function of time; these processes are external to the events of the investigation. For example, suppose that a researcher wished to evaluate the effect of a specific teaching method on the achievements of baccalaureate students on a skills test. The investigator would record the students' abilities before and after the teaching method. Between the pretest and the posttest, the students would have grown older and wiser. The growth or change is unrelated to the investigation, and the differences between the two testing periods may be explained by such maturation rather than by the experimental treatment.

Maturation effects could also occur in a study of the relationship between two methods of teaching about children's knowledge of self-care measures. Posttests of student learning must be conducted relatively soon after the teaching sessions are completed. Such a short interval allows the investigator to conclude that the results were the outcome of the design of the study and not maturation in a population of children who are learning new skills rapidly. Maturation is more than change that results from an age-related developmental process; maturation can also be related to physical changes (see Table 10.2).

Testing Effects

Taking the same test repeatedly could influence participants' responses the next time the test is completed. For example, the effect on the participant's posttest score as the result of having taken a pretest is known as a **testing effect**. The effect of taking a pretest may sensitize an individual and improve the score on the posttest. Individuals generally score higher when they take a test a second time regardless of the treatment. The differences between posttest and pretest scores may be a result not of the independent variable but rather of the experience gained through the testing. For example, in one study the researchers used identical pretests and posttests based on a case scenario to assess the effect of simulation on Undergraduate Nursing Students' Knowledge of Nursing Ethics Principles (Donnelly et al., 2017). Whether the increase in scores of posttests regarding the knowledge of nursing ethics principles resulted from the teaching and learning strategies or was the effect

TABLE **10.2**

EXAMPLES OF INTERNAL VALIDITY THREATS

THREAT	EXAMPLE
History threat	A study tested a teaching intervention in one hospital and compared outcomes to those of another hospital in which usual care was given. During the final months of data collection, the control hospital implemented a heart failure critical pathway; as a result, data from the control hospital (cohort) was not included in the analysis.
Maturation effect	If the change or difference in the outcome variable is due to the natural development process and not solely due to the effect of an independent variable that is considered as maturation effect.
Testing effect	A researcher wishes to measure acute pain with a repeated-measures design during a lengthy procedure. The researcher must consider the results in view of the possible bias of repeating the pain measurements over a short period of time. The measurements may prime the patients' responses, and the practice of reporting pain repeatedly on the same instrument during a procedure may influence the results. In a randomized controlled trial pilot study to assess the adolescent mothers perceptions of a phone-based peer support intervention designed to prevent postpartum depression, the researchers used a self-reported questionnaire to collect data. The researchers noted that though self-reported questionnaire has good psychometric properties, use of self-report is a possible limitation (Chyzzy et al., 2020).
Instrumentation threat	Boitor et al. (2019) discussed issues that possibly affected instrumentation such as reliance on patients recall of interference in the preceding 24 hours and the ability of patients in the critical units who are at risk of having disturbances in their circadian rhythm to recall the events correctly.
Mortality (attrition)	In a randomized controlled trial to test the effectiveness of psychotherapeutic intervention to relieve anxiety, the researchers noted that they had loss of samples (31% attrition) in the intervention group owing to lack of motivation or poor acceptability of the intervention. The authors also noted that similar attrition rates are found in studies where the length of therapy is specified at the outset (Sampaio et al., 2018).
Selection bias	In a study to assess the self-perceived palliative care competence of nurses and care aides working in settings that do not specialize in palliative care, the researchers reported that the sample may not be a representative sample. They also reported that there could be a self-selection bias among the samples favouring those who were interested or amenable to the integration of palliative care (Sawatzky et al., 2019).

of taking the test more than once was difficult to determine. Table 10.2 provides another example of a testing effect.

Instrumentation Threats

Instrumentation threats are changes in the variables or observational techniques that may account for changes in the obtained measurement. For example, a researcher may wish to study various types of thermometers (e.g., tympanic, digital, electronic, chemical indicator, plastic strip, and mercury) to compare the accuracy of the mercury thermometer with the other temperature-taking methods. To prevent instrumentation threats, the researcher must check the calibration of the thermometers according to the manufacturer's specifications before and after data collection.

Another example concerns techniques of observation or data collection. If a researcher has several raters collecting observational data, they all must be trained in a similar manner. If they are not similarly trained, or even if they are similarly trained but unable to conduct the study as planned, a lack of consistency may occur in their ratings; therefore, a threat to internal validity will occur.

To avoid instrumentation threats and to maintain consistency in data collection, researchers in a study to validate the functional pain scale for hospitalized adults provided the initial training to the research assistants. After the initial training, the researcher and the research assistant assessed patients concurrently to ensure 90% interrater reliability before the research assistant was ready to collect data independently. The researchers also met with the research assistants once a month to assess if the research assistants needed additional training to maintain consistency in data collection (Arnstein et al., 2019). (For another example, see Table 10.2.) Although the researcher can take steps to prevent problems of instrumentation, the threat of instrumentation may still occur. When a research critiquer finds such a threat, it must be evaluated within the total context of the study.

Mortality/Attrition

Mortality or attrition is the loss of study participants from the first data-collection point (pretest) to the second data-collection point (posttest). If the participants who remain in the study are not similar to those who dropped out, the results could be affected. The loss of participants may be from the sample as a whole or, in a study that has both an experimental group and a control group, more of the participants may drop out from one group than from the other group; this effect is known as *differential loss of participants*. For example, in a study of the ways in which a media campaign affects the incidence of breastfeeding, if most dropouts were non–breastfeeding women, the perception given could be that exposure to the media campaign increased the number of breastfeeding women, whereas the effect of experimental attrition led to the observed results. See Table 10.2 for an example of a study in which mortality (attrition) may have influenced the results.

Selection Bias

If precautions are not used to gain a representative sample, selection bias—the threat to internal validity that arises when pretreatment differences exist between the experimental group and the control group—could result from the way the participants were chosen. Selection effects are a problem in studies in which the individuals themselves decide whether to participate in a study. Suppose an investigator wishes to assess whether a new smoking cessation program contributes to smoking cessation. If the new program is offered to all smokers, chances are that only individuals who are more motivated to stop smoking will take part in the program. Assessment of the effectiveness of the program is problematic because the investigator cannot know for certain whether the new program encouraged smoking cessation behaviours or whether only highly motivated individuals joined the program. To avoid selection bias, the researcher could randomly assign participants to either the new teaching method group or a control group that receives a different type of instruction. Table 10.2 provides another example of selection bias.

Research Hint
The list of threats to internal validity is not exhaustive. More than one threat can be found in a study, depending on the type of study design. Finding a threat to internal validity in a study does not invalidate the results and is usually acknowledged by the investigator in the "Results" or "Discussion" section of the study.

Evidence-Informed Practice Tip
Avoiding threats to internal validity in clinical research can be difficult. However, this reality does not render studies that have threats useless. It is important to take the threats into consideration and weigh the total evidence of a study for not only its statistical meaningfulness but also its clinical meaningfulness.

External Validity

External validity concerns the generalizability of an investigation's findings to additional populations and to other environmental conditions and hence internal validity must be established prior to establishing external validity. To achieve external validity, variation in the conditions and the types of participants should lead to the same results. The goal of the researcher is to select a design that maximizes both internal and external validity, although attaining this goal is not always possible. If it is not possible, the researcher must attain the minimum criterion of external validity.

The factors that may affect external validity are related to the selection of participants, study conditions, and type of observations. These factors are termed *selection effects, reactive effects,* and *testing effects.* You may notice the similarity in the names of the factors of selection and testing and those of the threats to internal validity. When considering factors as internal threats, the reader assesses them as they relate to the *independent* and *dependent* variables within the study; when assessing them as external threats, the reader considers them in terms of the generalizability, or use outside the study with other populations and settings.

The Critical Thinking Decision Path displays the ways in which threats to internal and external validity can interact. This path is not, however, exhaustive with regard to the type of threats and their interaction. In comparison with problems of internal validity, generalizability issues are typically more difficult to deal with because they mean that the researcher is assuming that other populations are similar to the one being tested.

Selection Effects

Selection concerns the generalizability of the results to other populations. An example of **selection effects** is when the researcher cannot attain the ideal sample population. At times, the number of available participants may be low, or they may not be accessible to the researcher. The researcher may then need to choose a nonprobability method of sampling, not a probability method. Therefore, the type of sampling method used and how participants are assigned to research conditions will affect the generalizability

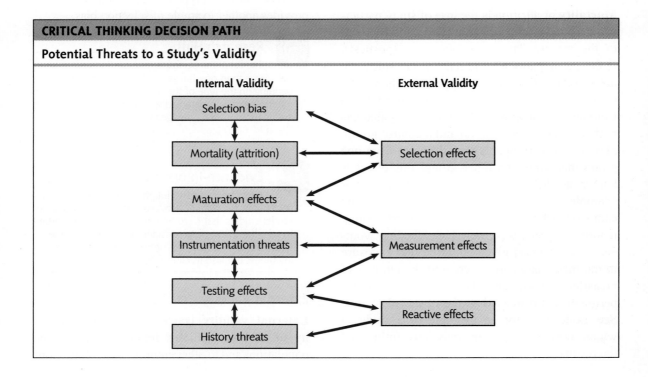

of findings to other groups, or the external validity. In the following quotations, the authors have noted selection effects:

- "The study was limited from a sample size perspective (n = 12), due to limited resources and difficulties faced in getting the samples" (Tryphonopoulos & Letourneau, 2020)
- "The mothers who participated in this study are highly educated compared to the provincial average of education. This reduces the generalizability" (Letourneau et al., 2019)
- "The modest group size of each staff position limits overall generalizability, calls for replication and extension, and positions the present findings as preliminary" (Ezeobele et al., 2019).
- "The online survey design limited the participation to only those with Internet access, thus not representing potential participants without Internet connectivity. Also, the online survey relied on self-report and is therefore subject to self-report bias. While this study examined previous breastfeeding experience as a potential variable influencing breastfeeding self-efficacy, the survey strictly identified the length of previous breastfeeding experience. More meaningful results could have been obtained had the survey included questions examining the quality of previous breastfeeding experience." (Corby et al., 2019)

These remarks are cautionary, but they also point out the usefulness of the findings for practice and for future research aimed at building the data in these areas.

Reactive Effects

Reactivity is defined as the participants' responses to being studied. Participants may behave in a certain way with the investigator not because of the study procedures but merely as an independent response to being studied. This response is also known as the **Hawthorne effect**, named after Western Electric Corporation's Hawthorne plant, where a study of working conditions was conducted in the 1930s. The researchers developed several different working conditions, such as turning up the lights, piping in music loudly or softly, and changing work hours. They found that no matter what was done, the workers' productivity increased. They concluded that production increased as a result of the workers' knowing that they were being studied rather than because of the experimental conditions.

For example, in a randomized controlled study, Yang et al. (2019) tested the feasibility and acceptability of an online mindfulness intervention for pregnant women as an approach to reduce depressive and anxious symptoms. They also reported that the differences in the scores of the experimental group could also be due to the effect of increased attention and interaction of the experimental group members compared to the control group members with the researchers. The researchers recommend that the further research should use a properly matched control group.

Measurement Effects

Administration of a pretest in a study affects the generalizability of the findings to other populations; the resulting changes are known as **measurement effects**. Just as pretesting affects the posttest results within a study, pretesting affects the posttest results and generalizability outside the study. For example, suppose a researcher wants to conduct a study with the aim of changing attitudes toward acquired immune deficiency syndrome (AIDS). To accomplish this task, an education program on the risk factors for AIDS is incorporated. To test whether the education program changes attitudes toward AIDS, tests are given before and after the teaching intervention. The pretest on attitudes allows the participants to examine their attitudes regarding AIDS. The participants' responses on follow-up testing may differ from those of individuals who were given the education program and did not see the pretest. Therefore, when a study is conducted and a pretest is given, it may prime the participants and affect their subsequent answers, which in turn can affect the generalizability of the findings.

Research Hint

When you review a study, be aware of the internal and external threats to validity. These threats do not render a study useless; instead, they make it more useful to you. Recognition of the threats allows researchers to build on data and allows consumers to think through what part of the study can be applied to practice. Specific threats to validity depend on the type of design and generalizations that the researcher hopes to make.

Other threats to external validity depend on the type of design and methods of sampling used by the researcher but are beyond the scope of this text. Campbell and Stanley (1996) offered detailed coverage of the issues related to internal and external validity.

APPRAISING THE EVIDENCE

Quantitative Research

Critiquing the design of a study requires knowledge of the overall implications of a particular design for the study as a whole (see Critiquing Criteria box). Researchers want to consider the level of evidence provided by the design and how the study can be used to improve or change practice. Minimizing threats to internal and external validity enhances the strength of evidence for any quantitative design. The concept of the research design is all-inclusive and parallels the concept of the theoretical framework. The research design is similar to the theoretical framework in that it deals with a piece of the research study that affects the whole. This chapter has introduced the meaning, purpose, and important factors of design choice, as well as the vocabulary that accompanies these factors. Several criteria for evaluating the design can be drawn from this chapter. Remember that the criteria are applied differently with various designs. Differences in application do not mean that the research consumer will find a haphazard approach to design but rather that each design has particular criteria that allow the consumer to classify the design by type (e.g., experimental or nonexperimental). These criteria must be met and addressed in conducting an experiment. The particulars of specific designs are addressed in Chapters 10 and 11. The following discussion primarily pertains to the overall evaluation of a quantitative research design.

The research outcome should demonstrate that an objective review of the literature and the establishment of a theoretical framework guided the choice of the design. No explicit statement regarding these areas is made in a research article. A consumer can evaluate the design by critiquing the theoretical framework (see Chapter 2) and

literature review (see Chapter 5). Is the question new and not extensively researched? Has a great deal of research been conducted on the question, or is the question a new or different way of looking at an old question? Depending on the level of the question, the investigators make certain choices. These choices enable researchers to look for differences in a controlled, comparative manner.

The research consumer should be alert for the methods that investigators use to maintain control (e.g., homogeneity in the sample, consistent data-collection procedures, manipulation of the independent variable, and randomization). As discussed in Chapter 10, all of these criteria must be met for an experimental design. As you begin to understand the types of designs (i.e., experimental, quasiexperimental, and nonexperimental designs, such as survey and relationship designs), you will find that control is applied in varying degrees or—as in the case of a survey study—the independent variable is not manipulated (see Chapter 11). The level of control and its applications presented in Chapters 10 and 11 provide the remaining knowledge for fully critiquing the aspects of a study's design.

Once you have established whether the necessary control or uniformity of conditions has been maintained, you must determine whether the study is believable or valid. You should ask whether the findings are the result of the variables tested—and thus internally valid—or whether another explanation is possible. To assess this aspect, you should review the threats to internal validity. If the investigator's study was systematic, was well grounded in theory, and followed the criteria for each of the processes, you will probably conclude that the study is internally valid.

APPRAISING THE EVIDENCE—*cont'd*

Quantitative Research

In addition, you must know whether a study has external validity or generalizability to other populations or environmental conditions. External validity can be claimed only after internal validity has been established. If the credibility of a study (internal validity) has not been established, a study has no generalizability to other populations (external validity). Determination of external validity is related directly to the sampling method (see Chapter 12). If the study is not representative of any one group or phenomenon of interest, external validity may be limited or not present. The establishment of internal and external validity requires not only knowledge of the threats to internal and external validity but also knowledge of the phenomena being studied, which allows critical judgements to be made about the linkage of theories and variables for testing. You should find that the design follows from the theoretical framework, literature review, research question, and hypotheses. You should believe, on the basis of clinical knowledge and knowledge of the research process, that the investigators are not, as the expression goes, comparing apples with oranges.

CRITIQUING CRITERIA

1. Is the type of study design employed appropriate?
2. Does the researcher use the various concepts of control that are consistent with the type of design chosen?
3. Does the design seem to reflect feasibility?
4. Does the design flow from the proposed research question, theoretical framework, literature review, and hypothesis?
5. What are the threats to internal validity?
6. What are the controls for the threats to internal validity?
7. What are the threats to external validity?
8. What are the controls for the threats to external validity?
9. Is the design appropriately linked to the levels of evidence hierarchy?

CRITICAL THINKING CHALLENGES

- Consider the following statement: "All research attempts to solve problems." How would you support or refute this statement?
- As a consumer of research, you recognize that control is an important concept in the issue of research design. You are critiquing an assigned experimental study as part of your "open-book" midterm examination. From what is written, you cannot determine how the researchers kept the conditions of the study constant. How does this characteristic affect the study's use in an evidence-informed practice model?
- Box 10.1 lists six major threats to the internal validity of an experimental study. Prioritize them and defend the one that you deem the essential, or number one, threat to address in a study.

- You are critiquing the research design of an assigned study as a consumer of research. How does the research design influence the findings of evidence in the study?
- How do threats to external validity contribute to the strength and quality of evidence provided by the findings of a research study?

CRITICAL JUDGEMENT QUESTIONS

1. How would an investigator ensure that the sample is homogenous?
   a. Restrict eligibility criteria to limit extraneous variables relevant to the study
   b. Randomly assign subjects to either the experimental or the control group
   c. Assign one research assistant to collect all data
   d. Collect all data at the same time of day

2. Which situation represents a threat to internal validity in an experimental study measuring the effect of an online post-op education for patients being discharged after coronary artery bypass graft surgery?
   a. Both men and women were included as subjects in the study
   b. Two new surgeons began performing the coronary artery bypass graft surgeries
   c. Patients in the experimental group gave the link to patients in the usual care control group
   d. Data collection took 1 year
3. COVID-19 outbreak in 2020 would represent what type of threat to internal validity in a longitudinal study that started on January 1, 2018 examining mortality rates due to respiratory infection?
   a. Maturation
   b. Instrumentation
   c. Selection bias
   d. History

should also reflect how the investigator attempted to control threats to both internal and external validity.
- Internal validity must be established before external validity can be established. Both are considered within the sampling structure.
- No matter which design the researcher chooses, it should be evident to the reader that the choice was based on a thorough examination of the research question within a theoretical framework.
- The design, research question, literature review, theoretical framework, and hypothesis should all be interrelated.
- The choice of the design is affected by pragmatic issues. At times, two different designs may be equally valid for the same question.
- The choice of design affects the study's level of evidence.

FOR FURTHER STUDY

Go to Evolve at http://evolve.elsevier.com/Canada/LoBiondo/Research for the Audio Glossary.

KEY POINTS

- The purpose of the design is to provide the format of masterful and accurate research.
- Many types of designs exist. No matter which type of design the researcher uses, the purpose remains the same.
- The research consumer should be able to locate within the study a sense of the question that the researcher wished to answer. The question should be proposed with a plan or scheme for the accomplishment of the investigation. Depending on the question, the consumer should be able to recognize the steps taken by the investigator to ensure control.
- The choice of the specific design depends on the nature of the question. To specify the nature of the research question, the design must reflect the investigator's attempts to maintain objectivity, accuracy, pragmatic considerations, and, most important, control.
- Control affects not only the outcome of a study but also its future use. The design

REFERENCES

Arnstein, P., Gentile, D., & Wilson, M. (2019). Validating the functional pain scale for hospitalized adults. *Pain Management Nursing, 20*(5), 418–424. https://doi.org/10.1016/j.pmn.2019.03.006.

Boitor, M., Martorella, G., Maheu, C., Laizner, A. M., & Gélinas, C. (2019). Does hand massage have sustained effects on pain intensity and pain-related interference in the cardiac surgery critically ill? A randomized controlled trial. *Pain Management Nursing, 20*(6), 572–579. https://doi.org/10.1016/j.pmn.2019.02.011.

Campbell, D., & Stanley, J. (1996). *Experimental and quasi-experimental designs for research*. Chicago: Rand-McNally.

Chyzzy, B., Nelson, L. E., Stinson, J., Vigod, S., & Dennis, C.-L. (2020). Adolescent mothers' perceptions of a mobile phone-based peer support intervention. *Canadian Journal of Nursing Research, 52*(2), 129–138. https://doi.org/10.1177/0844562120904591.

Corby, K., Kane, D., & Dayus, D. (2019). Investigating predictors of prenatal breastfeeding self-efficacy.

Canadian Journal of Nursing Research, 53(1), 56–63. https://doi.org/10.1177/0844562119888363.

Donnelly, M. B., Horsley, T. L., Adams, W. H., Gallagher, P., & Zibricky, C. D. (2017). Effect of simulation on undergraduate nursing students' knowledge of nursing ethics principles. *Canadian Journal of Nursing Research, 49*(4), 153–159. https://doi.org/10.1177/0844562117731975.

Evans, A., Malvar, J., Garretson, C., Pedroja Kolovos, E., & Baron Nelson, M. (2018). The use of aromatherapy to reduce chemotherapy-induced nausea in children with cancer: A randomized, double-blind, placebo-controlled trial. *Journal of Pediatric Oncology Nursing, 35*(6), 392–398. https://doi.org/10.1177/1043454218782133.

Ezeobele, I. E., McBride, R., Engstrom, A., & Lane, S. D. (2019). Aggression in acute inpatient psychiatric care: A survey of staff attitudes. *Canadian Journal of Nursing Research, 51*(3), 145–153. https://doi.org/10.1177/0844562118823591.

Freeman, L. A., Pfaff, K. A., Kopchek, L., & Liebman, J. (2020). Investigating palliative care nurse attitudes towards medical assistance in dying: An exploratory cross-sectional study. *Journal of Advanced Nursing, 76*(2), 535–545. https://doi.org/10.1111/jan.14252.

Hall, S. F., Wiering, B. A., Erickson, L. O., & Hanson, L. R. (2019). Feasibility trial of a 10-week adaptive yoga intervention developed for patients with chronic pain. *Pain Management Nursing, 20*(4), 316–322. https://doi.org/10.1016/j.pmn.2019.01.001.

Henrique, A. J., Gabrielloni, M. C., Rodney, P., & Barbieri, M. (2018). Non-pharmacological interventions during childbirth for pain relief, anxiety, and neuroendocrine stress parameters: A randomized controlled trial. *International Journal of Nursing Practice, 24*(3), 1–8. https://doi.org/10.1111/ijn.12642.

Jackson, K. T., & Dennis, C. L. (2017). Lanolin for the treatment of nipple pain in breastfeeding women: a randomized controlled trial. *Maternal and Child Nutrition, 13*(3), 1–10. https://doi.org/10.1111/mcn.12357.

Lee, K. A., Jong, S. S., & Gay, C. L. (2020). Fatigue management for adults living with HIV: A randomized controlled pilot study. *Research in Nursing and Health, 43*(1), 56–67. https://doi.org/10.1002/nur.21987.

Letourneau, N. L., de Koning, A. P. J., Sekhon, B., Ntanda, H. N., Kobor, M., Deane, A. J., Morin, A. M., Dewey, D., Campbell, T. S., & Giesbrecht, G. F. (2019). Parenting interacts with plasticity genes in predicting behavioral outcomes in preschoolers. *Canadian Journal of Nursing Research.* 084456211986361. https://doi.org/10.1177/0844562119863612.

McCarter, D. E., Demidenko, E., Sisco, T. S., & Hegel, M. T. (2019). Technology-assisted nursing for postpartum support: A randomized controlled trial. *Journal of Advanced Nursing, 75*(10), 2223–2235. https://doi.org/10.1111/jan.14114.

Sampaio, F. M. C., Araújo, O., Sequeira, C., Lluch Canut, M. T., & Martins, T. (2018). A randomized controlled trial of a nursing psychotherapeutic intervention for anxiety in adult psychiatric outpatients. *Journal of Advanced Nursing, 74*(5), 1114–1126. https://doi.org/10.1111/jan.13520.

Santiago, C., Roza, D., Porretta, K., & Smith, O. (2019). The use of tablet and communication app for patients with endotracheal or tracheostomy tubes in the medical surgical intensive care unit: A pilot, feasibility study. *Canadian Journal of Critical Care Nursing, 30*(1), 17–23.

Sawatzky, R., Roberts, D., Russell, L., Bitschy, A., Ho, S., Desbiens, J.-F., Chan, E. K. H., Tayler, C., & Stajduhar, K. (2019). Self-perceived competence of nurses and care aides providing a palliative approach in home, hospital, and residential care settings: A cross-sectional survey. *Canadian Journal of Nursing Research, 53*(1), 64–77. https://doi.org/10.1177/0844562119881043.

Sawhney, M., Watt-Watson, J., & McGillion, M. (2017). A pain education intervention for patients undergoing ambulatory inguinal hernia repair: A randomized controlled trial. *Canadian Journal of Nursing, 49*(3), 108–117. https://doi.org/10.1177/0844562117714704.

Tryphonopoulos, P. D., & Letourneau, N. (2020). Promising results From a video-feedback interaction guidance intervention for improving maternal–infant interaction quality of depressed mothers: A feasibility pilot study. *Canadian Journal of Nursing Research, 52*(2), 74–87. https://doi.org/10.1177/0844562119892769.

Yang, M., Jia, G., Sun, S., Ye, C., Zhang, R., & Yu, X. (2019). Effects of an online mindfulness intervention focusing on attention monitoring and acceptance in pregnant women: A randomized controlled trial. *Journal of Midwifery and Women's Health, 64*(1), 68–77. https://doi.org/10.1111/jmwh.12944.

CHAPTER 11

Experimental and Quasiexperimental Designs

Ramesh Venkatesa Perumal | Mina D. Singh

LEARNING OUTCOMES

After reading this chapter, you will be able to do the following:

- List the criteria necessary for inferring cause-and-effect relationships.
- Distinguish the differences between experimental and quasiexperimental designs.
- Define problems with internal validity that are associated with experimental and quasiexperimental designs.
- Describe the use of experimental and quasiexperimental designs for evaluation research.
- Critically evaluate the findings of selected studies in which cause-and-effect relationships were tested.
- Apply levels of evidence to experimental and quasiexperimental designs.
- Differentiate causation from association.

KEY TERMS

a priori
after-only design
after-only nonequivalent
    control group design
antecedent variable
attrition
control
dependent variable
evaluation research
experiment
experimental design
experimental group

formative evaluation
independent variable
intervening variable
manipulation
mortality
nonequivalent control
    group design
one-group pretest–
    posttest design
posttest–only control
    group design
pre-experimental design

quasiexperiment
quasiexperimental
    design
randomization
Solomon four-group
    design
summative evaluation
testing effects
time series design
true experiment

STUDY RESOURCES

 Go to Evolve at http://evolve.elsevier.com/Canada/LoBiondo/Research for the Audio Glossary.

CHAPTER 10 PROVIDED AN OVERVIEW OF the meaning, purpose, and issues related to quantitative research design. This chapter provides a discussion of specific types of quantitative designs, inasmuch as choosing the correct design is crucial for hypothesis testing or answering research questions. The design involves a *plan*, a *structure*, and a *strategy*, which guide a researcher in writing the hypothesis or research questions, conducting the project, and analyzing and evaluating the data. Each design has specific characteristics to maintain control: for example, homogeneity in the sample, consistent data-collection procedures, manipulation of the independent variable, and randomization.

One of the fundamental purposes of scientific research in any profession is to determine cause-and-effect relationships. Nurses, for example, are concerned with developing effective approaches to maintaining and restoring wellness. Testing such nursing interventions to determine how well they actually work—that is, evaluating the outcomes in terms of efficacy and cost-effectiveness—is accomplished with the use of experimental and quasiexperimental designs. These designs differ from nonexperimental designs in one important way: The researcher actively seeks to bring about the desired effect and does not passively observe behaviours or actions. In other words, the researcher is interested not merely in observing customary patient care but in making something beneficial happen. Experimental and quasiexperimental studies are also important to consider in relation to evidence-informed practice because they provide level II and level III evidence. The findings of such studies provide the validation of clinical practice and the rationale for changing specific aspects of practice (see Chapter 20).

Experimental designs are particularly suitable for testing cause-and-effect relationships because they help eliminate potential alternative explanations (threats to validity) for the findings. Inferring causality requires that the following three criteria be met:

1. The causal variable and effect variable must be associated with each other.

2. The cause must precede the effect.
3. The relationship must not be explainable by another variable.

When you critique studies in which experimental and quasiexperimental designs were used, the primary focus is on the validity of the conclusion that the experimental treatment, or the **independent variable**, caused the desired effect on the outcome, or **dependent variable**. The validity of the conclusion depends on how well the researcher controlled the other variables that may explain the relationship studied. Thus, the focus of this chapter is to explain how various types of experimental and quasiexperimental designs control extraneous variables.

The purpose of this chapter is to acquaint you with the issues involved in interpreting studies that have an **experimental design** (characterized by three properties: randomization, control, and manipulation) or a **quasiexperimental design** (in which random assignment is not used, but the independent variable is manipulated, and certain mechanisms of control are used). Examples of these designs are listed in Box 11.1. The Critical Thinking Decision Path shows an algorithm that influences a researcher's choice of experimental or quasiexperimental design.

BOX 11.1

SUMMARY OF EXPERIMENTAL AND QUASI-EXPERIMENTAL RESEARCH DESIGNS

EXPERIMENTAL DESIGNS

1. True experimental (pretest–posttest control group) design
2. Solomon four-group design
3. After-only design

QUASIEXPERIMENTAL DESIGNS

1. Nonequivalent control group design
2. After-only nonequivalent control group design
3. One-group pretest–posttest design
4. Time series design

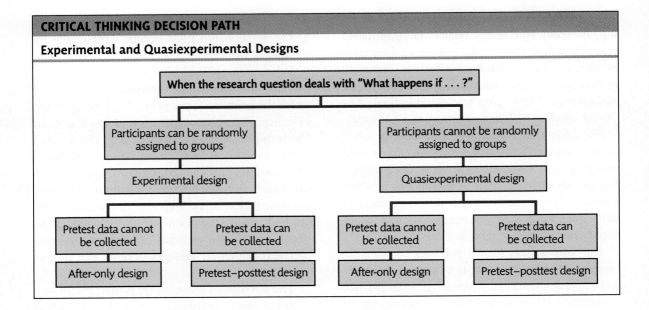

CRITICAL THINKING DECISION PATH

Experimental and Quasiexperimental Designs

When the research question deals with "What happens if . . . ?"

Participants can be randomly assigned to groups

Experimental design

Pretest data cannot be collected

After-only design

Pretest data can be collected

Pretest–posttest design

Participants cannot be randomly assigned to groups

Quasiexperimental design

Pretest data cannot be collected

After-only design

Pretest data can be collected

Pretest–posttest design

TRUE EXPERIMENTAL DESIGN

An **experiment** is a scientific investigation that makes observations and collects data according to explicit criteria. A **true experiment**—also known as a *pretest–posttest control group design* or *classic experiment*—has three identifying properties: randomization, control, and manipulation. These properties allow for other explanations of the phenomenon to be ruled out and thereby provide the strength of the design for testing cause-and-effect relationships.

A research study in which an experimental design is used is commonly called a *randomized control trial* (RCT). An RCT or experimental design is considered to be the best research design, "the gold standard," for providing information about cause-and-effect relationships. An individual RCT generates level II evidence because only minimal bias is introduced by this design. The higher level of evidence that a design produces, the more likely the results are to offer an unbiased estimate of the effect of an intervention and the more confident you can be that the intervention will be effective and produce the same results over and over again.

An example of an RCT is a study conducted by Sawhney et al. (2017) to assess the effectiveness of an individualized hernia repair education intervention (HREI) for patients following hernia repair. Patients undergoing ambulatory inguinal hernia repair were randomly assigned preoperatively either to the intervention group (those who received HREI) or to the control group (those received usual care). Authors concluded with positive findings on the effectiveness of HREI in reducing postoperative pain.

Randomization

Randomization, or random assignment to a group, is required for a study to be considered a true experimental design. It involves the assignment of participants to either the experimental or the control group on a purely random basis. In other words, each participant has an equal and known probability of being assigned to any group. Random assignment may be performed individually or by groups (for examples, see Tryphonopoulos & Letourneau, 2020; Anis et al., 2020; Page-cutrara & Turk, 2017). Random assignments to experimental or control groups allows for the elimination of any systematic bias that may affect the dependent variable being studied. In randomization, it is assumed that any important intervening variable (a condition that occurs during the study that affects the dependent variable) will occur in an equal distribution between the groups. Randomization ensures an equal opportunity for participants to be included in the experimental group and decreases selection bias. Participants are randomly assigned to groups through several procedures, such as a table of random numbers or computer-generated number sequences. Whatever method is used, it is important that the process be truly random, that it be tamper-proof, and that the group assignment is concealed. Note that random assignment to groups is different from the random sampling discussed in Chapter 13.

Control

Control refers to the introduction of one or more constants into the experimental situation. Control is acquired by manipulating the causal or independent variable, randomly assigning participants to a group, carefully preparing experimental protocols, and using comparison groups. In experimental research, the comparison group is the control group, or the group that receives the usual treatment rather than the innovative, experimental treatment.

Manipulation

As discussed previously, experimental designs are characterized by the researcher "doing something" to at least some of the participants. The experimental treatment is administered to some participants in the study but not to others, or different amounts of it are administered to different groups. This difference in how the treatment is provided is the **manipulation** of the independent variable. The independent variable might be a treatment, a teaching plan, or a medication. The effect of this manipulation is measured to determine the result of the experimental treatment.

The concepts of control, randomization, and manipulation and their application to experimental design are sometimes confusing for students. These concepts allow researchers to have confidence in the causal inferences they make by allowing them to rule out other potential explanations.

Consider the use of control, randomization, and manipulation in the following example. In a randomized control trial, the researchers tested the effect of child health parent training programs on parent–child interaction quality and child development. In this pilot study, the researchers randomly assigned 20 families to an experimental or to a control group. The randomization was performed by a random assignment schedule created by an independent research staff (Anis et al., 2020).

The use of random assignment meant that all patients who met the study criteria had an equal and known chance of being assigned to the **control group** or the **experimental group**. The use of random assignment to groups helps ensure that the two study groups are comparable with regard to pre-existing factors that might affect the outcome of interest, such as violence among families, depression prevalence, and the nature of parent–child interaction. Also, the researchers in the above study (Anis et al., 2020) checked statistically whether the procedure of random assignment did, in fact, produce groups that were similar at baseline.

Evidence-Informed Practice Tip

In health care research, the term *randomized control trial (RCT)* often refers to a true experimental design. These designs are being used more frequently in nursing research, which is critical to evidence-informed practice initiatives.

The degree of control exerted over the experimental conditions in Tryphonopoulos and Letourneau's (2020) study is illustrated by its detailed description of the implementation of video feedback intervention. This control helped ensure that all members of the experimental group received similar treatment and helps readers understand the process of experiment. The control group provided a comparison against which the experimental group could be judged.

In Tryphonopoulos and Letourneau's (2020) study, receiving the video feedback intervention was the manipulated treatment. The study aimed to assess the effectiveness of a video feedback intervention on improving the quality of interaction between depressed mothers and their infants. The results of the pilot feasibility study is positive and hence the authors could claim that video feedback intervention improved the quality of interaction between mothers with postpartum depression and their infants.

The use of the experimental design allows researchers to rule out many of the potential threats to internal validity of the findings, such as selection bias, history, and maturation effects (see Chapter 10). The strength of the true experimental design lies in its ability to help the researcher control the effects of any extraneous variables—alternative events that could explain the findings—that might constitute threats to internal validity. Such extraneous variables can be either *antecedent* or *intervening*.

The **antecedent variable** occurs before the study but may affect the dependent variable and confound the results. Factors such as age, gender, socioeconomic status, and health status might be important antecedent variables in nursing research because they may affect dependent variables, such as recovery time and ability to integrate health care behaviours. Antecedent variables that might have affected the dependent variables in the study by Tryphonopoulos and Letourneau (2020) include being on antidepressant or antipsychotic medication or having other therapies such as counselling. Random assignment to groups ensures that the groups are similar with regard to these variables so that differences in the dependent variable may be attributed to experimental treatment. The researchers also have compared both groups with regard to the above variables and reported in the study.

An **intervening variable** is a condition that occurs during the course of the study and is not part of the study; however, the intervening variable affects the dependent variable and can affect the study outcomes. An example of an intervening variable that might have affected the outcomes of Tryphonopoulos and Letourneau's (2020) study is the effect of antipsychotic medication. This can lead to changes in the primary outcome measured in the study.

Types of Experimental Designs

Several different experimental designs exist (Campbell & Stanley, 1966). Each is based on the classic design called the *true experiment*, diagrammed in Figure 11.1. Above the description diagram, symbolic notations are routinely used:

- R represents random assignment (for both the experimental group and the control group).
- O signifies observation through data collection on the dependent variable.
- O_1 signifies pretest data collection.
- O_2 represents posttest data collection.
- X represents exposure to the intervention.

Therefore, in Figure 11.1, note that the participants were assigned randomly (R) to the experimental or the control group. The experimental treatment (X) was given only to participants in the experimental group, and the pretests (O_1) and posttests (O_2) are the measurements of the dependent variables that were made before and after the experimental treatment was performed. In all true experimental designs, participants are randomly assigned to groups, an experimental treatment is introduced to some of the participants, and the effects of the treatment are observed. The variation in designs primarily concerns the number of observations that are made.

As shown in Figure 11.1, participants are randomly assigned to the two groups, experimental and control, so that antecedent variables are controlled. Next, pretest measurements or observations are made so that the researcher has a baseline for determining the effect of the

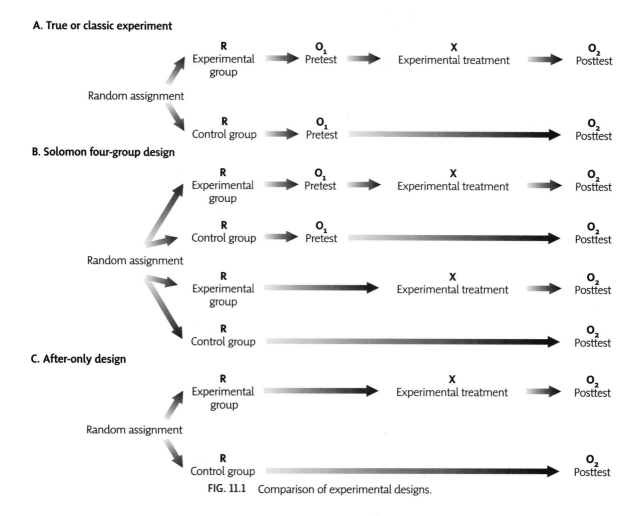

FIG. 11.1 Comparison of experimental designs.

independent variable. The researcher then introduces the experimental variable to one of the groups and measures the dependent variable again to see whether it has changed. The control group receives no experimental treatment, but the dependent variable in that group is also measured later for comparison with the experimental group. The degree of difference between the two groups at the end of the study indicates the confidence the researcher has that a causal link exists between the independent and dependent variables. Because random assignment and the control inherent in this design minimize the effects of many threats to internal validity, the

true experimental design is a strong design for testing cause-and-effect relationships.

However, the design is not perfect. Some threats cannot be controlled in true experimental studies (see Chapter 10). People tend to drop out of studies that require their participation over an extended period. The influence over the outcome of an experiment of people dropping out or dying is commonly known as **attrition** or **mortality**. If the number or type of people who drop out of the experimental group differs from that of the control group, a mortality/attrition effect might explain the findings. When you read such a work, examine the sample and the results carefully to see whether dropouts or deaths occurred.

Testing effects—the effects on the scores of a posttest as the result of having taken a pretest—also can be a problem in these studies because the researcher is usually administering the same test twice, and participants tend to score better the second time just by learning the test. Researchers can circumvent this problem in one of two ways: They might use different forms of the same test for the two measurements, or they might use a more complex experimental design called the Solomon four-group design.

The **Solomon four-group design**, shown in Figure 11.1, consists of two groups that are identical to those used in the classic experimental design plus two additional groups: an experimental after-group and a control after-group. As the diagram shows, all four groups have randomly assigned (*R*) participants, as in all experimental studies. However, the addition of these latter two groups helps rule out testing threats to internal validity that the before- and after-groups may experience. For example, suppose a researcher is interested in the effects of counselling on the self-esteem of patients with chronic illness. Just taking a test of self-esteem (O_1) may influence how the participants report themselves. The items might make the participants think more about how they view themselves so that the next time they fill out the questionnaire (O_2), their self-esteem might appear to have improved. In reality, however, their self-esteem may be the same as it was before; the scores are different only because the participants had previously taken the test. The use of this design with the two groups that do not receive the pretest allows for evaluating the effect of the pretest on the posttest in the first two groups. (See Practical Application box for another example of use of the Solomon four-group design.)

Although this design helps evaluate the effects of testing, the threat of mortality/attrition remains a problem, as in the classic experimental design.

Practical Application

Williams (2019) used the Solomon four-group design to test the effectiveness of high-fidelity simulation (HFS) as a teaching pedagogy for baccalaureate nursing students in a historically black college and university (HBCU). The author hypothesized that the students who received the focused respiratory assessment scenario through HFS would have higher scores in their posttest (measured through HESI). The study participants were randomly assigned to one of four groups.
1. Pretest, HFS intervention and posttest
2. No pretest, HFS intervention and posttest
3. Pretest, no intervention and posttest
4. No pretest, no intervention, only posttest

The study found that although there was an increase in the posttest scores of the group with the pretest, it was not statistically significant.

A less frequently used experimental design is the **after-only design**, shown in Figure 11.1. This design, which is sometimes called the **posttest–only control group design**, is composed of two randomly assigned groups (*R*), but in contrast to the true experimental design, neither group is given a pretest or other measures. Again, the independent variable is introduced to the experimental group (*X*) and not to the control group. The process of randomly assigning the participants to groups is assumed to be sufficient to ensure a lack of bias so that the researcher can still determine whether the treatment (*X*) created significant differences between the two groups (O_1 and O_2). This design is particularly useful when testing effects are expected to be a major problem and the number of available participants is too limited for a Solomon four-group design.

An example of this design would be a study of an intervention on postoperative pain management, inasmuch as pain cannot be measured before surgery and only an after-only design is required.

Research Hint

Remember that mortality/attrition is a problem in most experimental studies because data are usually collected more than once. The researcher should demonstrate that the groups are equivalent both when they enter the study and at the final analysis.

Field and Laboratory Experiments

Experiments also can be classified by setting. Field experiments and laboratory experiments share the properties of control, randomization, and manipulation and involve the same design characteristics but are conducted in different environments. Laboratory experiments take place in an artificial setting created specifically for the purpose of research. In the laboratory, the researcher has almost total control over the features of the environment, such as temperature, humidity, noise level, and participant conditions. Conversely, field experiments are exactly what the name implies: experiments that take place in a real, pre-existing social setting, such as a hospital or clinic, where the phenomenon of interest usually occurs.

Because most experiments in the nursing literature are field experiments and control is such an important element in the conduct of experiments, studies conducted in the field are subject to treatment contamination by factors specific to the setting that the researcher cannot control. However, studies conducted in the laboratory are by nature "artificial" because the setting is created for the purpose of research. Thus, laboratory experiments, although stronger with regard to internal validity questions than field studies are, have more problems with external validity. For example, a participant's behaviour in the laboratory may be quite different from the person's behaviour in the real world; this dichotomy presents problems in generalizing findings from the laboratory to the real world. Therefore, when you read research reports, you need to consider the possible effect of the experiment's setting on the findings of the study.

Consider a hypothetical study on different types of wound treatment gels and creams for the management of pressure ulcers. This study could be performed in a laboratory with animals, which would have allowed complete control over the external environment of the study—a variable that might be important in studying wound healing.

However, researchers cannot guarantee that the results found in a study in a laboratory would be applicable to human patients in hospital settings; thus, some external validity would be lost.

Advantages and Disadvantages of the Experimental Design

As previously discussed, experimental designs are the most appropriate design for testing cause-and-effect relationships because the design enables the researcher to control the experimental situation. Therefore, experimental designs offer better corroboration than if the independent variable is manipulated in such a way that certain consequences can be expected. Such studies are important because one of nursing's major research priorities is documenting outcomes to provide a basis for changing or supporting current nursing practice.

Experimental designs are not commonly used in nursing research, for several reasons. First, experimentation is conducted under the assumption that all the relevant variables involved in a phenomenon have been identified. For many areas of nursing research, this is simply not the case, and descriptive studies need to be completed before experimental interventions can be applied. Second, these designs have some significant disadvantages. One problem with an experimental design is that many variables important in predicting outcomes of nursing care are not amenable to experimental manipulation. It is well known that health status varies with age and socioeconomic status. No matter how careful a researcher is, no one can assign participants randomly by age or a certain level of income. In addition, it may be technically possible to manipulate some variables, but their nature may preclude their actually manipulation.

For example, if a researcher tried to randomly assign groups to study the effects of cigarette smoking and asked the experimental group to smoke two packs of cigarettes a day, that researcher's ethics would be seriously questioned. It is also potentially true that such a study would not work because nonsmokers randomly assigned to the smoking group would be unlikely to comply with the research task. Thus, sometimes even when a researcher plans to conduct a true experiment, participants dropping out of the study or other factors may, in effect, make the study a quasiexperiment.

Quasiexperimental designs are considered when it is not possible to randomly assign participants or when a control group is lacking. For example, Verkuyl et al. (2019) assessed the effects of three different debriefing methods (self-debrief only, self-debrief followed by a small group debriefing session, and self-debrief followed by a large group debrief) on improving the knowledge and debriefing experience after playing a gaming simulation. Randomly assigning students to control and experimental groups was not feasible; therefore, researchers randomly assigned the groups of students (based on lab sections) to the control group or to the intervention groups.

Another problem with experimental designs is that they may be difficult or impractical to perform in field settings. It may be quite difficult to randomly assign patients on a hospital floor to different groups when they might talk to each other about the different treatments. Experimental procedures also may be disruptive to the usual routine of the setting. If several nurses are involved in administering the experimental program, it may be impossible to ensure that the program is administered in the same way to each participant.

Because of these problems in carrying out true experiments, researchers frequently turn to another type of research design to evaluate cause-and-effect relationships. Such designs, because they seem experimental but lack some of the control of the true experimental design, are called *quasiexperiments*.

QUASIEXPERIMENTAL DESIGNS

Quasiexperimental designs are intended to test cause-and-effect relationships; however, in a quasi-experimental design, full experimental control is not possible. A **quasiexperiment** is a research design in which the researcher initiates an experimental treatment, but some characteristic of a true experiment is lacking. Control may not be possible because of the nature of the independent variable or the nature of the available participants. Quasi-experimental designs usually lack the element of true randomization, as described earlier with the Verkuyl et al. (2019) study. In other cases, the control group may be missing. However, like experiments, quasiexperiments involve the introduction of an experimental treatment.

In comparison with the true experimental design, quasiexperimental designs are used similarly. Both types of designs are used when the researcher is interested in testing cause-and-effect relationships. However, the basic problem with the quasiexperimental approach is a weakened confidence in making causal assertions. Because of the lack of some controls in the research situation, quasiexperimental designs are subject to contamination by many, if not all, of the threats to internal validity discussed in Chapter 10.

Types of Quasiexperimental Designs

Many different quasiexperimental designs exist. Only the ones most commonly used in nursing research are discussed in this book. To illustrate, the symbols and notations introduced earlier in the chapter are used. Refer to the true experimental design shown in Figure 11.1 and compare it with the **nonequivalent control group design** shown in Figure 11.2. Note that the latter design looks exactly like that of the true experiment except that participants are not randomly assigned to groups.

For example, suppose a researcher is interested in the effects of a new diabetes education program on the physical and psychosocial outcomes of patients with newly diagnosed diabetes. If the conditions were right, the researcher might be able to randomly assign participants to either the group receiving the new program or the group receiving the usual program, but for any number of reasons,

A. Nonequivalent control group design

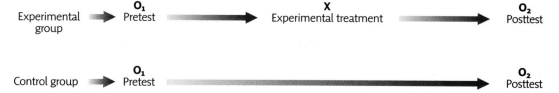

B. After-only nonequivalent control group design

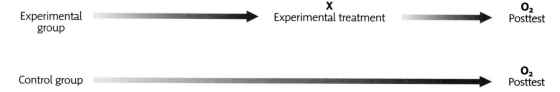

C. One-group pretest–posttest design

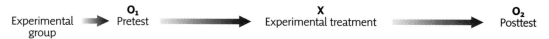

D. Time series design

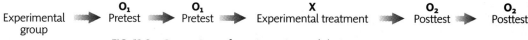

FIG. 11.2 Comparison of quasiexperimental designs.

that design might not be possible (e.g., nurses on the unit where patients are admitted might be so excited about the new program that they cannot help but include the new information for all patients). Thus, the researcher has two choices: to abandon the experiment or to conduct a quasi-experiment. To conduct a quasiexperiment, the researcher might find a similar unit where the new program has not been introduced and study the patients with newly diagnosed diabetes who are admitted to that unit as a comparison group. The study would then involve the quasiexperimental type of design because it lacks randomization.

Studies in which both quantitative and qualitative methods are used are called *mixed-methods studies*.

 Research Hint

Remember that researchers often make trade-offs and sometimes use a quasiexperimental design instead of an experimental design because it may be pragmatically impossible to randomly assign participants to groups. The fact that the design is not "pure" does not decrease the value of the study, although the utility of the findings may be decreased.

The nonequivalent control group design is commonly used in nursing research studies conducted in field settings. The basic problem with the design is the weakening of the researcher's confidence in assuming that the experimental and comparison groups are similar at the beginning of the study. Threats to internal validity, such as selection bias, maturation effects, testing effects, and mortality (attrition), are possible with this design. However, the design is relatively strong because the gathering of the data at the time of the pretest allows the researcher to compare the equivalence of the two groups on important antecedent variables before the independent variable is introduced.

An example of the nonequivalent control group design is that of Sezgin and Esin (2018). The purpose of this project was to evaluate the effects of PRECEDE-PROCEED model of ergonomic risk management program in reducing musculoskeletal symptoms of ICU nurses. The Ergonomic Risk Management Program (ERMP) intervention was the health promotion program based on PRECEDE-PROCEED model that included video training, personal interviews, provision of exercise mats, and regular text messages for six months. A total of 30 ICU nurses in the intervention group and 31 ICU nurses in control group were recruited for the study. The nurses were chosen randomly and not through randomization. As a nonequivalent control group design, the pretest done in the study was a baseline measurement of musculoskeletal symptoms and risks assessments (environment, predisposing factors, and upper rapid upper risk assessment) through surveys. These measurements were then compared with posttest measurements in order to determine the effectiveness of the intervention.

An example of the nonequivalent control group design is that of Kim and Kim (2020). The purpose of this study was to evaluate the effectiveness of electrocardiography training program using team-based learning for early-stage nurses in intensive care units. Thirty-six participants in the intervention group and 29 participants in the control group were recruited for the study. The participants were chosen considering their convenience to participate in the study. The intervention (Team Based Learning) was implemented in three stages over a 5-week period on selected topics whereas the control group received only a lecture on the same topics. As a nonequivalent

control group design, the pretest done in the study was assessment of the knowledge of EKG and reading ability of bedside EKG monitoring and 12-lead EKG. These assessments were then compared with the posttest measurements in order to determine the effectiveness of the intervention.

Suppose that the researcher did not measure the participants' responses before the introduction of the new treatment (or the researcher was hired after the new program began) but later decided that data demonstrating the effect of the program would be useful. Perhaps, for example, a third party asks for such data to determine whether it should pay the extra cost of the new teaching program. Sometimes the outcomes simply cannot be measured before the intervention, as with prenatal interventions that are expected to affect birth outcomes. The study that could be conducted would have an **after-only nonequivalent control group design**, illustrated in Figure 11.2. This design is similar to the after-only experimental design, but randomization is not used to assign participants to groups. In this design, the two groups are assumed to be equivalent and comparable before the introduction of the independent variable (X). Thus, the soundness of the design and the confidence that the researchers can have in the findings depend on the soundness of this assumption of preintervention comparability. Often, the assumption that the two nonrandomly assigned groups are comparable at the outset of the study is difficult to assert because the validity of the statement cannot be assessed.

In the example of the teaching program for patients with newly diagnosed diabetes, measuring the participants' motivation after the teaching program would not reveal whether their motivations differed before they received the program, and it is possible that the teaching program would motivate individuals to learn more about their health problem. Therefore, the researcher's conclusion that the teaching program improved physical status and psychosocial outcome would be subject to the alternative conclusion that the results were an effect of pre-existing motivations (selection effect) in combination with greater learning by participants so motivated (selection–maturation interaction). Nonetheless, this design is frequently used in nursing research because opportunities for data collection are often limited and because this design is particularly useful when testing effects may be problematic.

An approach used by researchers when only one group is available is to study that group over a longer period—that is, to test participants before an intervention and again afterwards. This quasiexperimental design is called a **time series design** and is illustrated in Figure 11.2. Time series designs are useful for determining trends as in a study on the effectiveness of a concussion workshop among the youth of First Nations community, their parents, and coaches in improving their knowledge and attitude (Hunt et al., 2018). The participants completed the same survey at three points (before intervention, immediately post workshop, and six months after the workshop). The survey had questions that measured the knowledge and attitude related to concussion. Sometimes data are collected many times before the introduction of the treatment to establish a baseline point of reference on outcomes. The experimental treatment is then introduced, and data are collected multiple times afterwards to determine a change from baseline. The broad range and number of data-collection points help rule out alternative explanations, such as history effects. However, a testing threat to internal validity is ever present because of multiple data-collection points, and without a control group, the threats of selection bias and maturation effects cannot be ruled out (see Chapter 10).

To rule out some alternative explanations for the findings of a one-group pretest–posttest design, researchers typically measure the phenomenon of interest over a longer period and introduce the experimental treatment sometime during the course of the data-collection period (see Figure 11.2). Even with the absence of a control group, the broader range of data-collection points helps rule out threats to validity such as history threats. Obviously, the earlier example of teaching patients with diabetes does not lend itself to this design because researchers do not have access to the patients before the diagnosis.

Research Hint

One of the reasons replication is so important in nursing research is that many problems cannot be subjected to experimental methods. Therefore, the consistency of findings across many patient populations helps support a cause-and-effect relationship even when an experiment cannot be conducted.

Advantages and Disadvantages of Quasiexperimental Designs

Because of the problems inherent in interpreting the results of studies with quasiexperimental designs, you may wonder why anyone would use them. Quasiexperimental designs are used frequently because they are practical and feasible, and the results are generalizable. These designs are more adaptable to the real-world practice setting than controlled experimental designs. In addition, for some hypotheses, these designs may be the only way to evaluate the effect of the independent variable of interest.

The weaknesses of the quasiexperimental approach involve mainly the inability to establish clear cause-and-effect relationships. However, if the researcher can rule out any plausible alternative explanations for the findings, such studies can lead to increased knowledge about causal relationships. Researchers have several options for ruling out these alternative explanations. They may control extraneous variables **a priori** (before initiating the intervention) by design.

Researchers can also use methods to control extraneous variables statistically. In some cases, common-sense knowledge of the problem and the population can suggest that a particular explanation is not plausible. Nonetheless, replicating such studies is important to support the causal assertions developed through the use of quasiexperimental designs.

The literature on cigarette smoking is an excellent example of how findings from many studies, experimental and quasiexperimental, can be linked to establish a causal relationship. A large number of well-controlled experiments with laboratory animals randomly assigned to smoking and nonsmoking conditions have documented that lung disease does develop in "smoking" animals. Although such evidence is suggestive of a link between smoking and lung disease in humans, it is not directly transferable because animals and humans are different. Because humans cannot be randomly assigned to smoking and nonsmoking groups, for ethical and other reasons, researchers interested in this problem must use quasiexperimental data to test their hypotheses about smoking and lung disease.

Several different quasiexperimental designs have been used to study this problem, and all have yielded similar results: A causal relationship does exist between cigarette smoking and lung disease. Note that the combination of results from both experimental and quasiexperimental studies led to the conclusion that smoking causes lung disease, because the studies together meet the causal criteria of relationship, timing, and lack of an alternative explanation.

The tobacco industry has argued that because the studies on humans are not true experiments, another explanation is possible for the relationships that have been found. For example, these relationships suggest that the tendency to smoke is linked to the tendency for lung disease to develop, and smoking is merely an unimportant intervening variable. The reader needs to review the evidence from studies to determine whether the cause-and-effect relationship postulated is believable.

Evidence-Informed Practice Tip

Findings from studies with experimental designs are considered level II evidence, and those from studies with quasiexperimental designs are considered level III evidence. Quasiexperimental designs are lower on the hierarchy of evidence because of a lack of a research control, which limits the ability to establish confident cause-and-effect statements that influence clinical decision-making.

PRE-EXPERIMENTAL DESIGNS

Pre-experimental designs follow similar experimental steps but do not include a control or comparison group. There is only a single group, with no comparison with an equivalent or nonequivalent nontreatment group. Examples are the one-group pretest–posttest $(O_1 \rightarrow X \rightarrow O_2)$ and the one-group posttest-only $(X \rightarrow O_1)$ designs, where X is the treatment or intervention and O is the data-collection points.

In the one-group pretest–posttest design, data are collected before and after an experimental treatment on this one group of participants. In this type of design, the participants act as their own controls, and no randomization occurs. Because controls and randomization are important characteristics that enhance the internal validity of the study, the evidence generated by the findings of this type of pre-experimental design needs to be interpreted with careful consideration of the design limitations.

The advantage of these designs is that they can be used to evaluate treatments, ruling out ineffective treatments before large-scale experimental or quasiexperimental studies are initiated. The disadvantage of this design is that without a control or comparison group, it is difficult to make any conclusions as to whether the treatment, (X), really caused the outcomes or changes.

Practical Application

Hickin et al. (2017) conducted a one-group pretest–posttest design study to check if the focused educational intervention for critical care nurses is effective in increasing long-term delirium knowledge and improving perception and rates of routine delirium screening in the ICU. The ICU nurses were provided with PowerPoint presentations on various aspects of delirium and assessments tools during their annual ICU refresher. Each participant acted as his own control by being tested thrice: before the educational intervention and then 3 and 18 months after the interventions. Findings revealed that the educational intervention led to an increase in the knowledge and the frequency of delirium assessment of patients in ICU.

EVALUATION RESEARCH AND EXPERIMENTATION

As the science of nursing expands and the cost of health care rises, nurses and other health care providers have become increasingly concerned with the ability to document the costs and the benefits of nursing care (see Chapter 1). This task is a complex process, but at its heart is the ability to evaluate or measure the outcomes of nursing care to inform health care decision-making. Such studies usually are associated with quality assurance, quality improvement, and evaluation. Studies of evaluation or quality assurance do exactly what the name implies: They are concerned with the determination of the quality of nursing and health care and with the assurance that the public is receiving high-quality care.

Quality assurance and quality improvement in nursing are current and important topics for nursing care. Many early studies of quality assurance documented whether nursing care met predetermined standards. The goal of quality improvement studies is to evaluate the effectiveness of nursing interventions and to provide direction for further improvement in the achievement of quality clinical outcomes and cost-effectiveness.

Evaluation research is the use of scientific research methods and procedures to evaluate a program, treatment, practice, or policy. In evaluation research, analytical means are used to document the worth of an activity such as an intervention, but such research is not a different design. Both experimental and quasiexperimental designs (as well as nonexperimental designs) are used to determine the effect or outcomes of a program. When these designs are used in evaluating a program, the term *evaluation research* is used. Bigman (1961) listed the following purposes and uses of evaluation research:

1. To discover whether and how well the objectives are being fulfilled
2. To determine the reasons for specific successes and failures
3. To direct the course of the experiment with techniques for its effectiveness

4. To reveal principles that underlie a successful program
5. To base further research on the reasons for the relative success of alternative techniques
6. To redefine the means to be used for attaining objectives and to redefine subgoals in view of research findings

According to Clarke (2001), the following four levels of evaluation research are being highlighted in health care, especially nursing research: evaluation of the effectiveness of clinical interventions; evaluation of the effect of new ways of delivering health care; evaluation of structured programs aimed at specific patient groups; and evaluation of the quality of service. In many evaluation research studies, investigators use mixed methods, with both quantitative and qualitative information.

Evaluation studies may be either formative or summative. In **formative evaluation**, a program is assessed as it is being implemented; usually, the focus is on evaluation of the process of a program rather than the outcomes. In **summative evaluation**, the outcomes of a program are assessed after completion of the initial program.

Fraser et al. (2017) used a summative evaluation to assess the effects of an adult and feedback delivered to care providers on home care client outcomes. In contrast Vanstone et al. (2020) used a formative evaluation to evaluate the implementation of a 3 Wishes Project (3WP) in the ICUs. Knowledge related to summative (outcomes) and formative (process) evaluation of programs is important in translating research into clinical practice.

The use of experimental and quasiexperimental designs in studies of quality improvement and evaluation enables researchers to determine not only whether care is adequate but also which method of care is best under certain conditions. Furthermore, such studies can be used to determine whether a particular type of nursing care or intervention is cost-effective—that is, that the care or intervention does what it is intended to do but at lower or equivalent cost. Cost studies are usually incorporated into the evaluation of an intervention. For example, Conway et al. (2019) reported that implementation of a thermal care bundle for treating inadvertent perioperative hypothermia reduced cost and improved quality of life of patients undergoing surgery.

In an era of health care reform and cost containment for health expenditures, evaluating the relative costs and benefits of new programs of care has become increasingly important. Relatively few studies in nursing and medicine have been dedicated to such evaluation, but in terms of outcomes, nursing costs and cost savings will be important in future studies.

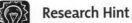 **Research Hint**

According to Gaudine and Lamb (2015), the term *quality assurance* in health care has been replaced with the term *quality improvement (QI)*, as quality can be improved, not assured. The purpose of QI is thus to bring about immediate improvement to processes and outcomes by using a systematic, evidence-informed approach and compare organizations' quality to standards or benchmarks. QI projects in health care focus on improving patient, staff, and institutional outcomes. The steps are to identify which outcomes need to be improved, discern how they will be improved, and develop a strategy to implement and evaluate QI outcomes. Thus, QI projects include an evaluation. These projects are site specific, and the results may not be generalizable knowledge to other groups or sites.

APPRAISING THE EVIDENCE

Experimental and Quasiexperimental Designs

As discussed earlier in the chapter, various designs for research studies differ in the amount of control the researcher has over the antecedent and intervening variables that may affect the results of the study. True experimental designs, which yield level II evidence, offer the most possibility for control, whereas nonexperimental designs, which yield level IV, V, or VI evidence, offer the least. Quasiexperimental designs, which yield level III evidence, offer evidence that lies somewhere in between. Research designs must balance the needs for internal validity and external validity in order to produce useful results. In addition, judicious use of design requires that the chosen design be appropriate to the problem, free of bias, and capable of answering the research question.

Questions that you should pose when reading studies that test cause-and-effect relationships are listed in the Critiquing Criteria box. All of these questions should help you judge, with confidence, whether a causal relationship exists.

For studies in which either experimental or quasiexperimental designs are used, first try to determine the type of design that was used. Often, a statement describing the design of the study appears in the abstract and in the "Methods" section of the article. If such a statement is not present, you should examine the study for evidence of the following three characteristics: control, randomization, and manipulation. If all are discussed, the

design is probably experimental. Conversely, if the study involves the administration of an experimental treatment but does not involve the random assignment of participants to groups, the design is quasiexperimental. Next, try to identify which of the variations within these two types of designs was used. Determining the answer to these questions gives you a head start because inherent in each design are particular threats to validity, and this step makes it easier to critically evaluate the study. The next question to ask is whether the researcher required a solution to a cause-and-effect problem. If so, the study is suited to these designs. Finally, think about the conducting of the study in the setting. Is it realistic to think that the study could be conducted in a clinical setting without some contamination?

The most important question to ask as you read experimental studies is "What else could have happened to explain the findings?" Thus, the author must provide adequate accounts of how the procedures for randomization, control, and manipulation were carried out. The study should include a description of the procedures for random assignment to such a degree that the reader can determine the likelihood for any one participant to be assigned to a particular group. The description of the independent variable also should be detailed. The inclusion of this information helps the reader decide whether the treatment given to some participants in the experi-

APPRAISING THE EVIDENCE—*cont'd*

Experimental and Quasiexperimental Designs

mental group might differ from what was given to others in the same group. In addition, threats to validity, such as testing effects and mortality (attrition), should be addressed. Otherwise, the conclusions of the study could potentially be erroneous and less believable to the reader.

This question of potential alternative explanations or threats to internal validity for the findings is even more important when you critically evaluate a quasiexperimental study because these study designs cannot possibly control for many plausible alternative explanations. A well-written report of a quasiexperimental study systematically reviews potential threats to the validity of the findings. Then your work as the reader is to decide whether the author's explanations make sense. When critiquing

evaluation research, you should look for a careful description of the program, policy, procedure, or treatment being evaluated. In addition, you may need to determine the design used to evaluate the program and assess the appropriateness of the design for the evaluation. Once you have discerned the design, you can assess threats to validity for the appropriate design in determining the appropriateness of the author's conclusions in relation to the outcomes. As with all research, the results of studies with these designs need to be generalizable to a larger population of people than was actually studied. Thus, researchers need to decide whether the experimental protocol eliminated some potential participants and whether this weakness affected not only internal validity but also external validity.

CRITIQUING CRITERIA

1. What design is used in the study?
2. Is the design experimental or quasiexperimental?
3. Is the problem one of a cause-and-effect relationship?
4. Is the method used appropriate to the problem?
5. Is the design suited to the setting of the study?

EXPERIMENTAL DESIGNS

1. What experimental design is used in the study, and is it appropriate?
2. How are randomization, control, and manipulation applied?
3. Are there reasons to believe that alternative explanations exist for the findings?
4. Are all threats to validity, including mortality (attrition), addressed in the report?

5. Whether the experiment was conducted in the laboratory or a clinical setting, are the findings generalizable to the larger population of interest?

QUASIEXPERIMENTAL DESIGNS

1. What quasiexperimental design is used in the study, and is it appropriate?
2. What are the most common threats to the validity of the findings of this design?
3. What are the plausible alternative explanations, and have they been addressed?
4. Are the author's explanations of threats to validity acceptable?
5. What does the author say about the limitations of the study?

6. Do other limitations related to the design exist that are not mentioned?

EVALUATION RESEARCH

1. Do the authors identify a specific problem, practice, policy, or treatment that they will evaluate?
2. Do the authors identify the outcomes to be evaluated?
3. Is the problem analyzed and described?
4. Is the program to be analyzed described and standardized?
5. Do the authors identify the measurement of the degree of change (outcome) that occurs?
6. Do the authors determine whether the observed outcome is related to the activity or to one or more other causes?

CRITICAL THINKING CHALLENGES

- Discuss the barriers to nurse researchers in meeting the three criteria of a true experimental design.

- How is it possible to have a research design that includes an experimental treatment intervention and a control group and yet is not considered a true experimental study? How does this affect the usefulness of the findings in an evidence-informed practice?

- Argue your case for supporting or not supporting the following claim: "The fact that true experimental design is not used does not decrease the value of the study, even though it may decrease the utility of the findings in practice." Include examples with your rationale.

- Respond to the following question: Why are experimental studies considered the best evidence for an evidence-informed practice model? Justify your answer.

CRITICAL JUDGEMENT QUESTIONS

1. What aspect should be the primary consideration in critiquing the research report of an experimental study and determining the validity of the conclusions presented?
   a. How well the researcher controlled for extraneous variables
   b. The direction of the relationship between the dependent and independent variables
   c. The credentials and previous experience of the researcher
   d. The number of persons involved in the data collection process

2. In a study to help people avoid overdosing on opioids, one group of participants received a single supportive phone call 10 days after attending a program on harm reduction approaches. A second group received a weekly supportive phone call for 6 weeks after attending the same program, and a third group received no supportive phone calls after attending the program. What property of experimental research did the researcher employ in this study?
   a. Quasiexperimental research—no control group
   b. Random assignment to research groups
   c. Manipulation of the intervention
   d. Controlling for extraneous variables

3. In a study to assess the effect of a videotape format teaching method on the learning of adolescent males about the warning signs of testicular cancer, why would a nurse researcher select to

implement a quasiexperimental study design instead of an experimental study design?
   a. The study is planned to be conducted in a laboratory setting
   b. An experimental treatment is not part of the study
   c. The researcher has not conducted research before
   d. Full experimentational control is not possible

KEY POINTS

- Experimental designs or randomized clinical trials provide the strongest evidence (level II) in terms of whether an intervention or treatment affects patient outcomes.
- Two types of design commonly used in nursing research to test hypotheses about cause-and-effect relationships are experimental and quasiexperimental designs. Both are useful for the development of nursing knowledge because they test the effects of nursing actions and lead to the development of prescriptive theory.
- True experiments are characterized by the ability of the researcher to control extraneous variation, manipulate the independent variable, and randomly assign participants to research groups.
- Experiments conducted in clinical settings or in the laboratory provide the best evidence in support of a causal relationship because the following three criteria can be met: (1) the independent and dependent variables are related to each other; (2) the independent variable chronologically precedes the dependent variable; and (3) the relationship cannot be explained by the presence of a third variable.
- Researchers frequently use quasiexperimental designs to test cause-and-effect relationships because experimental designs are often impractical or unethical.
- Quasiexperiments may lack either randomization or the comparison group, or both, which are characteristics of true experiments. Their

usefulness in studying causal relationships depends on the ability of the researcher to rule out plausible threats to the validity of the findings, such as history threats, selection bias, and maturation and testing effects.
- The level of evidence (level III) provided by quasiexperimental designs weakens confidence that the findings were the result of the intervention rather than extraneous variables.
- The overall purpose of critiquing such studies is to assess the validity of the findings and to determine whether these findings are worth incorporating into the nurse's personal practice.

 ## FOR FURTHER STUDY

Go to Evolve at http://evolve.elsevier.com/Canada/ LoBiondo/Research for the Audio Glossary.

REFERENCES

Anis, L., Letourneau, N. L., Benzies, K., Ewashen, C., & Hart, M. J. (2020). Effect of the attachment and child health parent training program on parent–child interaction quality and child development. *Canadian Journal of Nursing Research, 52*(2), 157–168. https://doi.org/10.1177/0844562119899004.

Bigman, S. K. (1961). Evaluating the effectiveness of religious programs. *Review of Religious Research, 2,* 99–110.

Campbell, D., & Stanley, J. (1996). *Experimental and quasiexperimental designs for research.* Chicago: Rand-McNally.

Clarke, A. (2001). Evaluation research in nursing and health care. *Nurse Researcher, 8*(3), 4–14.

Conway, A., Gow, J., Ralph, N., Duff, J., Edward, K., Alexander, K., Munday, J., & Bräuer, A. (2019). Implementing a thermal care bundle for inadvertent perioperative hypothermia: A cost-effectiveness analysis. *International Journal of Nursing Studies, 97,* 21–27. https://doi.org/10.1016/j.ijnurstu.2019.04.017.

Fraser, K. D., Sales, A. E., Baylon, M. A. B., Schalm, C., & Miklavcic, J. J. (2017). Data for Improvement and Clinical Excellence: A report of an interrupted time series trial of feedback in home care. *Implementation Science, 12*(66), 1–10. https://doi.org/10.1186/s13012-017-0600-1.

Gaudine, A., & Lamb, M. (2015). *Nursing leadership and management: Working in Canadian healthcare organizations.* North York, ON: Pearson.

Hickin, S. L., White, S., & Knopp-sihota, J. (2017). Nurses' knowledge and perception of delirium screening and assessment in the intensive care unit: Long-term effectiveness of an education-based knowledge translation intervention. *Intensive & Critical Care Nursing, 41,* 43–49. https://doi.org/10.1016/j.iccn.2017.03.010.

Hunt, C., Michalak, A., Lefkimmiatis, C., Johnston, E., Macumber, L., Jocko, T., & Ouchterlony, D. (2018). Exploring concussion awareness in hockey with a First Nations community in Canada. *Public Health Nursing, 35*(3), 202–210. https://doi.org/10.1111/phn.12407.

Kim, S., & Kim, C. (2020). Effects of an electrocardiography training program: Team-based learning for early-stage intensive care unit nurses. *The Journal of Continuing Education in Nursing, 51*(4), 174–180. https://doi.org/10.3928/00220124-20200317-07.

Page-cutrara, K., & Turk, M. (2017). Impact of prebriefing on competency performance, clinical judgment and experience in simulation: An experimental study. *Nurse Education Today, 48,* 78–83. https://doi.org/10.1016/j.nedt.2016.09.012.

Sawhney, M., Watt-Watson, J., & McGillion, M. (2017). A pain education intervention for patients undergoing ambulatory inguinal hernia repair: A randomized controlled trial. *Canadian Journal of Nursing Research, 49*(3), 108–117. https://doi.org/10.1177/0844562117714704.

Sezgin, D., & Esin, M. N. (2018). Effects of a PRECEDE-PROCEED model based ergonomic risk management programme to reduce musculoskeletal symptoms of ICU nurses. *Intensive & Critical Care Nursing, 47,* 89–97. https://doi.org/10.1016/j.iccn.2018.02.007.

Tryphonopoulos, P. D., & Letourneau, N. (2020). Promising results from a video-feedback interaction guidance intervention for improving maternal–infant interaction quality of depressed mothers: A feasibility pilot study. *Canadian Journal of Nursing Research, 52*(2), 74–87. https://doi.org/10.1177/0844562119892769.

Vanstone, M., Neville, T. H., Clarke, F. J., Swinton, M., Sadik, M., Takaoka, A., Smith, O., Baker, A. J., Leblanc, A., & Foster, D. (2020). Compassionate end-of-life care: Mixed-methods multisite evaluation of the 3 Wishes Project. *Annals of Internal Medicine, 172,* 1–12. https://doi.org/10.7326/M19-2438.

Verkuyl, M., Hughes, M., Atack, L., McCulloch, T., Lapum, J. L., Romaniuk, D., & St-Amant, O. (2019). Comparison of self-debriefing alone or in combination with group debrief. *Clinical Simulation in Nursing, 37,* 32–39. https://doi.org/10.1016/j.ecns.2019.08.005.

Williams, T. (2019). Using high fidelity simulation to prepare baccalaureate nursing students enrolled in a historically Black college and university. *ABNF Journal, 30*(2), 37–43. http://search.ebscohost.com/login.aspx?direct=true&db=rzh&AN=136798779&site=ehost-live.

CHAPTER 12

Nonexperimental Designs

Mina D. Singh | Ramesh Venkatesa Perumal

LEARNING OUTCOMES

After reading this chapter, you will be able to do the following:

- Describe the overall purpose of nonexperimental designs.
- Describe the characteristics of survey and relationship/difference designs.
- Define the differences between survey and relationship/difference designs.
- List the advantages and disadvantages of surveys and each type of relationship/difference design.
- Identify methodological, secondary analysis, and meta-analysis research.
- Identify the purposes of methodological, secondary analysis, and meta-analysis research.
- Discuss relational inferences versus causal inferences as they relate to nonexperimental designs.
- Identify the criteria used to critique nonexperimental research designs.
- Apply the critiquing criteria to the evaluation of nonexperimental research designs as they appear in research reports.
- Apply levels of evidence to nonexperimental designs.

KEY TERMS

cohort
correlational study
cross-sectional study
descriptive/exploratory
survey
developmental study
epidemiological study
ex post facto study

hierarchical linear modelling
(HLM)
incidence
longitudinal study
meta-analysis
methodological research
nonexperimental research design
prediction study

prevalence
prospective study
psychometrics
relationship/difference study
retrospective data
retrospective study
secondary analysis
survey study

STUDY RESOURCES

Go to Evolve at http://evolve.elsevier.com/Canada/LoBiondo/Research
for the Audio Glossary.

MANY PHENOMENA OF INTEREST AND RELEVANCE to nursing do not lend themselves to an experimental design. For example, nurses studying pain may be interested in knowing the amount of pain, variations in the amount of pain, and patients' responses to postoperative pain. The investigator would not design an experimental study that would potentially intensify a patient's pain just to study the pain experience; that would be unethical. Instead, the researcher would use a nonexperimental design to examine the factors that contribute to the variability in a patient's postoperative pain experience. Nonexperimental research designs are used in studies when the researcher wishes to construct a picture of a phenomenon; examine events, people, or situations as they naturally occur; or test relationships and differences among variables. Nonexperimental designs may enable the researcher to understand how a phenomenon occurs at one point or over a period of time.

In experimental research, the independent variable is manipulated; in a nonexperimental research design, the independent variable is not manipulated. In nonexperimental research, the independent variables have occurred naturally, and the investigator cannot directly control them by manipulation. In contrast, in an experimental design, the researcher actively manipulates one or more variables. The researcher in a nonexperimental design explores relationships or differences among the variables. Nonexperimental research requires a clear, concise research problem or hypothesis that is based on a theoretical framework. Even though the researcher does not actively manipulate the variables, the concepts of control (see Chapter10) should be considered as much as possible.

Researchers do not agree on how to classify nonexperimental studies. A continuum of quantitative research designs is shown in Figure 12.1. This chapter divides nonexperimental designs into *survey studies* and *relationship/difference studies*, as illustrated in Box 12.1. These categories are flexible; nonexperimental studies may be classified in a different way in other sources. Some studies belong exclusively to one of these categories, whereas other studies have the characteristics of more than one category or more than one design label. As you read the research literature, you will often find that researchers who are conducting a nonexperimental study use several design classifications. This chapter introduces the various types of nonexperimental designs, their advantages and disadvantages, the use of nonexperimental research, the issues of causality, and the critiquing process as it relates to nonexperimental research. The Critical Thinking Decision Path outlines the path to the choice of a nonexperimental design.

Evidence-Informed Practice Tip
When you critically appraise nonexperimental studies, be aware of possible sources of bias that can be introduced at any point in the study.

BOX 12.1

SUMMARY OF NONEXPERIMENTAL RESEARCH DESIGNS

SURVEY STUDIES
- Descriptive
- Exploratory
- Comparative

RELATIONSHIP/DIFFERENCE STUDIES
- Correlational
- Developmental
- Cross-sectional
- Longitudinal or prospective
- Retrospective or ex post facto

Nonexperimental ⟹ Quasiexperimental ⟹ Experimental

FIG. 12.1 Continuum of quantitative research designs.

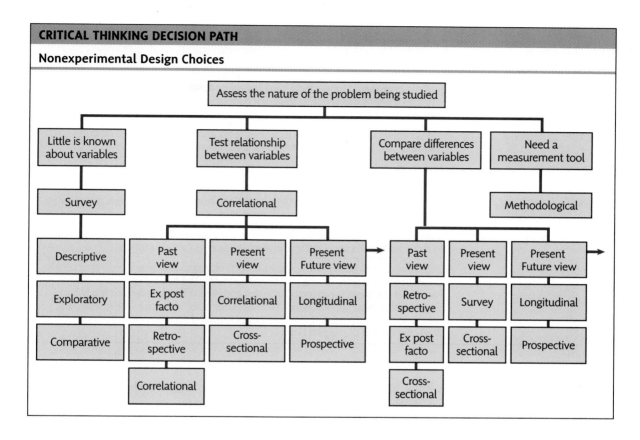

SURVEY STUDIES

The broadest category of nonexperimental designs is the survey study. In a survey study—further classified as *descriptive, exploratory*, or *comparative*—detailed descriptions of existing variables are collected, and the data are used to justify and assess current conditions and practices or to make more plans for improving health care practices. When you read research, you will find that the terms *exploratory, descriptive, comparative*, and *survey* may be used either alone, interchangeably, or together to describe the design of a study (Table 12.1). For example, investigators may use a descriptive/exploratory survey to search for accurate information about the characteristics of particular participants, groups, institutions, or situations or about the frequency of a phenomenon's occurrence, particularly when little is known about the phenomenon. The data are

used to justify or assess current conditions or to make plans for improvement of conditions. Qualitative researchers also use the term *descriptive* in their reports, as in the study by Arnaert et al. (2019), who used a qualitative descriptive design to explore the experiences of midwives and community health workers using mHealth to improve services to pregnant women in rural Burkina Faso. You will be able to determine the difference in study type by checking in the analysis and findings sections, inasmuch as the qualitative descriptive study entails the use of the analyses outlined in Chapter 16, whereas the descriptive correlational or survey studies entail the use of descriptive and inferential statistical analyses.

In survey studies, the types of variables of interest can be classified as opinions, attitudes, or facts. For example, Covell and colleagues (2017) conducted a Pan-Canadian survey to describe

TABLE **12.1**

EXAMPLES OF STUDIES WITH MORE THAN ONE DESIGN LABEL

DESIGN TYPE	STUDY'S PURPOSE
Observational, cross-sectional	Della Pelle et al. (2018) conducted a study to assess Italian nurses' knowledge and attitudes towards gay and lesbian sexual orientation and lesbian, gay, bisexual, and transgender (LGBT) patients.
Descriptive, correlational	This descriptive correlational study examines relationship among change fatigue, resilience, and job satisfaction of hospital staff nurses (Brown et al., 2018).
Cross-sectional, descriptive	This study describes the knowledge and attitudes about pain management among nursing students (Hroch et al., 2019).
Explanatory, correlational	This study's aim was to determine the associations between staffing hours and quality of care indicators in long-term care (Boscart et al., 2018).
Retrospective, cross-sectional	The purpose of this investigation was to explore the barriers and facilitators to exercise in individuals with cancer in Ontario (Fernandez et al., 2015).
Prospective, cohort	Adhikari Dahal et al. (2017) followed two cohorts of pregnant women, beginning about 0–24 weeks gestation, until 4 months postpartum. The two cohorts were All OUR Families and Alberta Pregnancy Outcomes and Nutrition datasets. Each study had similar recruitment periods, which were between 2008 and 2012. The researchers were interested in predicting whether neighbourhood socioeconomic status predicted the risk of preterm birth.

a demographic and human capital profile of Internationally Educated Nurses (IENs) and to identify the key human capital characteristics and types of assistance that predict IENs' professional recertification and employment as regulated nurses. The human capital characteristics (fact variables) were nursing education, professional experience, and language proficiency. In another example, Freeman et al. (2020) investigated palliative care nurses' attitudes towards medical assistance in dying using a secure online survey platform.

Often, the terms survey and questionnaire are used interchangeably, but they are not the same. A survey is a data collection tool that includes both a questionnaire and/or an interview, whereas a questionnaire is a written set of questions (see Chapter 14). Surveys are also thought of as an approach to collecting data, being inclusive of both the tool (questionnaire) and the process of collecting, followed by the analysis of those questions. For example, Dahlke et al. (2019) used a survey, a questionnaire only, to obtain student nurses' perceptions of older people. Another example is

the study by Schofield, Forchuk, Montgomery, and associates (2016), who used a face-to-face structured interview to compare personal health practices between individuals with mental illness and the general Canadian population.

Survey researchers study either small or large samples of participants recruited from defined populations. The sample can be either broad or narrow and can be made up of people or institutions. For example, if a primary care rehabilitation unit based on a case-management model is to be established in a hospital, researchers might survey prospective applicants' attitudes with regard to case management before the unit staff members are selected. In a broader example, if a hospital is contemplating converting all patient care units to a case-management model, a survey might be conducted to determine the attitudes of a representative sample of nurses in the hospital toward case management. The data might provide the basis for projecting the in-service needs of nursing with regard to case management. The scope and depth of a survey are a function of the nature of the problem.

In surveys, investigators attempt only to relate one variable to another or to assess differences between variables; they do not attempt to determine causation. The two major advantages of surveys are the great deal of information that can be obtained from a large population in a more economical manner than face-to-face interviews and the surprising accuracy of survey research information. If a sample is representative of the population (see Chapter 13), a relatively small number of participants can accurately represent the views of the population.

However, survey studies have several disadvantages. First, the information obtained in a survey tends to be superficial. The breadth rather than the depth of the information is emphasized. Second, conducting a survey requires a great deal of expertise in various research areas. The survey investigator must have skills in sampling techniques, questionnaire construction, interviewing, and data analysis to elicit reliable and valid data. Third, large-scale surveys can be time consuming and costly, although the use of on-site personnel can reduce costs.

Research Hint

Research consumers should recognize that a well-constructed survey can provide a wealth of data about a particular phenomenon of interest, even though causation is not being examined.

Evidence-Informed Practice Tip

Evidence obtained from a survey population may be coupled with clinical expertise and applied to a similar population to develop an educational program to enhance knowledge and skills in a particular clinical area. For example, a survey designed to measure nursing staff's knowledge and attitudes about evidence-informed practice may yield data that are used to develop a staff development course in evidence-informed practice.

RELATIONSHIP/DIFFERENCE STUDIES

Investigators endeavour to trace the relationships or differences between variables that can provide a deeper insight into a phenomenon. This type of study can be classified as a relationship/difference study. The following types of relationship/difference studies are discussed here: *correlational studies* and *developmental studies*.

Correlational Studies

In a correlational study, an investigator examines the relationship between two or more variables. The researcher is not testing whether one variable causes another variable or how different one variable is from another variable. Instead, the researcher is testing whether the variables covary; in other words, as one variable changes, does a related change occur in the other variable? The researcher using this design is interested in quantifying the strength of the relationship between the variables or in testing a hypothesis about a specific relationship. The positive or negative direction of the relationship is also a central concern (see Chapter 17 for an explanation of the correlation between variables).

In their correlational study, Levya et al. (2019) described nursing faculty attitudes and beliefs about caring for people living with HIV/AIDS. They explored the relationships between prejudice, stereotype, and discrimination. These researchers were not testing a cause-and-effect relationship.

Another example of correlational research is the study by Rayan (2019), who explored the relationship between mindfulness, self-efficacy, and stress among final-year nursing students. They found that stress was significantly and negatively associated with mindfulness and self-efficacy.

Correlational studies offer researchers and research consumers the following advantages:
- An increased flexibility when investigating complex relationships among variables
- An efficient and effective method of collecting a large amount of data about a problem
- A potential for practical application in clinical settings
- A potential foundation for future experimental research studies
- A framework for exploring the relationship between variables that cannot be inherently manipulated

The correlational design has a quality of realism and is particularly appealing because it suggests the potential for practical solutions to clinical problems. However, there are disadvantages of correlational studies:

- Inability to manipulate the variables of interest
- No randomization in the sampling procedures because the study deals with pre-existing groups; therefore, generalizability is decreased
- Inability to determine a causal relationship between the variables because of the lack of manipulation, control, and randomization

One of the most common misuses of a correlational design is the researcher's conclusion that a causal relationship exists between the variables. In their correlational study, Winsett et al. (2016) explored the nurse work environment by evaluating the self-report of missed nursing care and the reasons for the missed care. They correctly determined that staffing adequacy was found to have an inverse relationship with communication, material resource, and labor resource. They recommended that "additional staffing may not always be feasible; but rethinking approaches to the nursing care delivery system, using the current staff in more efficient ways is certainly within reach" (p. 132).

Correlational studies may be further labelled *descriptive correlational* or *predictive correlational*. An example of a descriptive correlational study is by Jin et al. (2017) where they described relationships among perceptions of functional deficits, mood states, and empathic responses in family caregivers for patients with strokes.

The inability to draw causal statements should not lead you to conclude that a nonexperimental correlational study has a weak design. In terms of evidence for practice, researchers—on the basis of the literature review and their findings—frame the utility of the results in view of previous research and therefore help establish supportive evidence of the applicability of the results to a specific patient population. A correlational design is very useful for clinical research studies because many of the phenomena of clinical interest are beyond the researcher's ability to manipulate, control, and randomize.

Developmental Studies

Nonexperimental designs in which a time perspective is used can be further subclassified. A developmental study is concerned not only with the existing status and the relationship and differences among phenomena at one point in time but also with changes that occur as a function of time. The following three types of developmental study designs are discussed here: *cross-sectional, longitudinal* or *prospective*, and *retrospective* or *ex post facto*. Remember that in the literature, studies may be designated by more than one design name. This practice is accepted because many studies have elements of several nonexperimental designs. Table 12.1 provides examples of studies classified with more than one design label.

Cross-Sectional Studies

In a cross-sectional study, researchers examine data at one time; in other words, the data are collected on only one occasion with the same participants rather than with the same participants at several times.

An example of a cross-sectional study is provided by Freeman et al. (2020) who investigated palliative care nurse attitudes towards medical assistance in dying. In another example, Rochefort et al. (2016) explored the rationing of nursing care interventions and its associations with nurse-reported outcomes in the neonatal intensive care unit. Wall et al. (2018) conducted a cross-sectional study to explore the relationship between psychosocial health (anxiety, stress, depression) and preterm birth in Tanzanian women.

Evidence-Informed Practice Tip

Replication of significant findings in nonexperimental studies, with similar or different populations, or both, increases your confidence in the conclusions offered by the researcher and the strength of evidence generated by consistent findings from more than one study.

Longitudinal or Prospective Studies

In contrast to the cross-sectional design, the longitudinal study or prospective study (also referred to as *repeated-measures* studies) involves collecting data from the same group at different times. Researchers also use longitudinal studies to explore differences and relationships. For example, the investigator conducting a study with children with diabetes could use a longitudinal design. In that case, the investigator could collect yearly data or monitor the same children over a number of years to compare changes in the variables at different ages. By collecting data from each participant at yearly intervals, the investigator obtains a longitudinal perspective of the diabetic process.

An example of a prospective cohort study is where the researchers examined and compared risk factors for postpartum depression among: (1) recent (less and equal to 5 years) migrant and Canadian-born women, and (2) refugee, asylum-seeking, and non-refugee immigrant women. Women completed questionnaires at 1–2 weeks and at 16 weeks postpartum (Dennis et al., 2017). Castonguay et al. (2017) conducted a prospective study over 6 months to test body-related shame and guilt as predictors of breast cancer survivors' moderate to vigorous intensity physical activity.

Cross-sectional and longitudinal designs have many advantages and disadvantages. When assessing the appropriateness of a cross-sectional study versus a longitudinal study, the research consumer should first assess the researcher's goal in view of the theoretical framework. For example, in a hypothetical study of infant colic, the researchers are investigating a developmental process; therefore, a longitudinal design seems more appropriate. However, the disadvantages inherent in a longitudinal design also must be considered. The period of data collection may be long because of the time the participants take to progress to each data-collection point. In the infant colic study, it might take the researchers between 12 and 18 months to collect the data from the total

sample. Threats to internal validity, such as testing and attrition, also are ever-present and unavoidable in a longitudinal study (see Chapter 17). As a result, longitudinal designs are costly in terms of time, effort, and money. Moreover, confounding variables could affect interpretation of the results. Participants in these studies may respond in a socially desirable way that they believe is congruent with the investigators' expectations (see discussion of the Hawthorne effect, in Chapter 10).

Despite the pragmatic constraints imposed by a longitudinal study, the researcher should proceed with this design if the theoretical framework supports a longitudinal developmental perspective. The advantages of a longitudinal study are that participants are monitored separately and thereby serve as their own controls; an increased depth of responses can be obtained; and early trends in the data can be analyzed. The researcher can assess changes in the variables of interest over time and explore both relationships and differences between variables.

Cross-sectional studies, in comparison with longitudinal studies, are less time consuming and less expensive and are thus more manageable for the researcher. Because large amounts of data can be collected at one time, the results are more readily available. In addition, the confounding variable of maturation, which results from the passage of time, is not present. However, the investigator's ability to establish an in-depth developmental assessment of the interrelationships of the phenomena being studied is reduced. Thus, the researcher is unable to determine whether the change that occurred is related to the change that was predicted because the same participants were not monitored over a period of time. In other words, the participants are unable to serve as their own controls (see Chapter 11).

In summary, longitudinal studies begin in the present and end in the future, and cross-sectional studies encompass a broader perspective of a cross-section of the population at one specific time.

Retrospective or Ex Post Facto Studies

A retrospective study is essentially the same as an ex post facto study. Epidemiologists primarily use the term *retrospective*, whereas social scientists prefer the term *ex post facto*. In either case, the dependent variable has already been affected by the independent variable, and the investigator attempts to link current events to past events.

When scientists wish to explain causality or the factors that determine the occurrence of events or conditions, they prefer to use an experimental design. However, they cannot always manipulate the independent variable or use random assignments. In cases in which experimental designs cannot be employed, ex post facto studies may be used. *Ex post facto* literally means "from after the fact." These studies also are known as *causal-comparative* studies or *comparative* studies. As this design is discussed further, you will see that ex post facto research is similar to quasiexperimental research because in both, differences between variables are examined.

In retrospective studies, a researcher hypothesizes, for example, that variable X (cigarette smoking) is related to and a determinant of variable Y (lung cancer), but X, the presumed cause, is not manipulated, and participants are not randomly assigned to groups. Instead, the researcher chooses a group of participants who have experienced X (cigarette smoking) in a normal situation and a control group of participants who have not experienced X. The behaviours, performances, or conditions (lung tissue) of the two groups are compared in order to determine whether the exposure to X had the effect predicted by the hypothesis. Table 12.2 illustrates this example and reveals that although cigarette smoking appears to be a determinant of lung cancer, the researcher is still not able to conclude that a causal relationship exists between the variables because the independent variable has not been manipulated and the participants were not randomly assigned to groups.

Another example of a retrospective study is that of Dall'Ora et al. (2019) who investigated whether working 12-hr shifts is associated with increased sickness absence among registered nurses and health care assistants (HCAs). They conducted a retrospective longitudinal study analyzing data on all shifts scheduled for RNs and HCAs over a 3-year period. They found that 1,689 staff (86%) experienced at least one sickness episode during the 3-year study. The sickness episodes ranged from 1 day to 496 days in length; the most common length of sickness episodes was 2 days (n = 1,221, 15.1%). 2,532 (31.3%) sickness episodes lasted 7 or more days and were classified as long-term sickness episodes, while 5,555 sickness episodes lasting less than 7 days were classified as short-term sickness episodes. Another example is the study by Strazzieri-Pulido et al. (2019) who estimated the incidence of pressure injury and its predictors including nursing workload in critical patients. They studied a retrospective cohort of 766 patients in nine intensive care

TABLE 12.2		
PARADIGM FOR THE EX POST FACTO DESIGN		
GROUPS (NOT RANDOMLY ASSIGNED)	**INDEPENDENT VARIABLE (NOT MANIPULATED BY INVESTIGATOR)**	**DEPENDENT VARIABLE**
Exposed group: cigarette smokers	X: cigarette smoking	Y_e: lung cancer
Control group: nonsmokers		Y_c: no lung cancer

units of two university hospitals over a 3-month period. Pressure injury was present in 143 patients totalling an incidence of 18.7% within 766 patients. On average, pressure injuries developed in 6.9 days (SD = 5.9), with a median of 4 days and a variation of 2–30 days (p.303). The significant predictors of the pressure injury incidence were length of hospitalization, mechanical ventilation, palliative care, age, and nursing activities (p. 307).

The advantages of the retrospective design are similar to those of the correlational design. The additional benefit of the retrospective design is that it offers a higher level of control than a correlational study. For example, in a cigarette smoking study, the lung tissue samples from nonsmokers and smokers could be compared. This comparison would enable the researcher to establish the existence of a differential effect of cigarette smoking on lung tissue. However, the researcher would remain unable to draw a causal link between the two variables. This inability is the major disadvantage of the retrospective design.

Another disadvantage of retrospective research is that an alternative hypothesis may be the reason for the documented relationship. If the researcher obtains data from two existing groups of participants, such as one that has been exposed to X and one that has not, and the data support the hypothesis that X is related to Y, the researcher cannot be sure whether X or an extraneous variable is the cause of the occurrence of Y. Finding naturally occurring groups of participants who are similar in all ways except for their exposure to the variable of interest is very difficult. The possibility always exists that the groups differ in another way (e.g., in exposure to another lung irritant, such as asbestos), which can affect the findings of the study and produce spurious results. Consequently, when you read about such a study, you need to cautiously evaluate the conclusions drawn by the investigator.

Research Hint _____

When you read research reports, you will find that, at times, researchers classify a study's design with more than one design label. This classification is correct because research studies often reflect aspects of more than one design.

Longitudinal or prospective (cohort) studies are less common than retrospective studies because it can take a long time for the phenomenon of interest to become evident in a prospective study. For example, if researchers were studying pregnant women who regularly consume alcohol, it would take 9 months for the effect of low birth weight in the participants' infants to become evident. The problems inherent in a prospective study are therefore similar to those of a longitudinal study. However, longitudinal or prospective studies are considered stronger than retrospective studies because of the degree of control that can be imposed on extraneous variables that might confound the data.

Research Hint _____

Remember that nonexperimental designs can test relationships, differences, comparisons, or predictions, depending on the purpose of the study.

PREDICTION AND CAUSALITY IN NONEXPERIMENTAL RESEARCH

Researchers and research consumers are concerned with the issues of prediction and causality in explaining cause-and-effect relationships. Historically, researchers have said that only experimental research can support the concept of causality. For example, nurses are interested in discovering what causes anxiety in many settings. If nurses can uncover the causes, they can perhaps develop interventions that would prevent or decrease the anxiety. Causality makes it necessary to order events chronologically; therefore, if nurses find in a randomized experiment that event 1 (stress) occurs before event 2 (anxiety) and that participants who experienced stress were anxious, whereas those in the unstressed group were not, then the hypothesis that stress causes anxiety is supported. If these results occurred in a nonexperimental study in which some participants underwent the stress of surgery and were anxious, whereas others did not have surgery and were not anxious, an association or relationship would be said to exist between stress (surgery) and anxiety. The results of a nonexperimental study, however, do not imply that the stress of surgery caused the anxiety.

Many variables (e.g., anxiety) that nurse researchers wish to study to explore causation cannot be manipulated, nor would it be wise to try to manipulate the variables. However, studies that can assert a predictive or causal sequence are needed. In view of this need, many nurse researchers use several analytical techniques that can explain the relationships among variables to establish predictive or causal links. These techniques are called *causal modelling, model testing*, path analysis, and *associated causal analysis*.

> ### ▶ Practical Application
> Fox et al. (2018) used structural equation modelling to test the direct and indirect relationships between geriatric practice environment, geriatric nursing practice, and overall quality of care for older adults and their families, while controlling for nurse and hospital characteristics. One of their findings is that the geriatric practice environment is directly associated with quality of care.

You will also find the terms path analysis, LISREL, analysis of covariance structures, structural equation modelling (SEM) (see Practical Application box), and hierarchical linear modelling (HLM) (Raudenbush & Bryk, 2002) used to describe the statistical techniques (see Chapter 17) used in these studies. An HLM is a type of regression analysis that allows for analysis of hierarchically structured data simultaneously at all levels (see the following Practical Application box for an example of the use of HLM).

> ### ▶ Practical Application
> An example of HLM appeared in a study by Pien et al. (2019) who validated the Chinese version Psychosocial Safety Climate Scale (PSC-12) and examined the associations between PSC, workplace violence, and self-rated health (SRH). In the hierarchical linear model, they found that participants from hospitals with the lowest PSC score had twofold risks of having poor SRH (p. 584).

In a prediction study, a model may be tested to assess which independent variables can best explain one or more dependent variables in order to make a forecast or prediction derived from particular phenomena. For example, Stephenson, DeLongis, Steele, and colleagues (2017) examined the role of maternal posttraumatic growth in changes in behavioural problems among siblings of children with complex chronic health conditions. Results from a time-lagged multilevel regression revealed that higher levels of maternal posttraumatic growth predicted subsequent declines in parent-reported internalizing, externalizing, and total behavioural problems among healthy siblings.

> ### ◆ Research Hint
> Nonexperimental clinical research studies have progressed to the point at which prediction models are used to explore or test relationships between independent variables and dependent variables.

As nurse researchers develop their programs of research in a specific area, more tests of models will be available. The statistics used in model-testing studies are advanced, but the beginning research consumer should be able to read the article, understand the purpose of the study, and determine whether the model generated was logical and developed with a solid basis from the literature and past research.

A full description of the techniques and principles of causal modelling is beyond the scope of this text.

Evidence-Informed Practice Tip ____

Research studies that entail the use of nonexperimental designs and provide level IV evidence can build the foundation for a program of research that leads to experimental designs in which the effectiveness of nursing interventions can be tested.

ADDITIONAL TYPES OF QUANTITATIVE STUDIES

Other types of quantitative studies complement the science of research. These additional designs provide a means of viewing and interpreting phenomena to provide further breadth and knowledge to nursing science and practice. These types of quantitative studies are methodological research, systematic review, meta-analysis, integrative review, secondary analysis, and epidemiological studies.

Methodological Research

Methodological research is the development and evaluation of data-collection instruments, scales, and techniques. As noted in Chapters 14 and 15, methodology has a strong influence on research. The most significant and important aspect of methodological research addressed in measurement development is psychometrics—the theory and development of measurement instruments (such as questionnaires) and measurement techniques (such as observational techniques) through the research process. Thus, psychometrics is concerned with the measurement of a concept, such as anxiety or interpersonal conflict, with reliable and valid tools. (See Chapter 15 for a discussion of reliability and validity.)

Nurse researchers have used the principles of psychometrics to develop and test measurement instruments that focus on nursing phenomena. Nurse researchers also use instruments developed in other disciplines, such as psychology and sociology, in which tools have been psychometrically tested. Sound measurement tools are critical for the reliability and validity of a study.

A study's purpose, problems, and procedures may be clear, and the data analysis may be correct and consistent, but if the measurement tool has inherent psychometric problems, the findings will be rendered questionable or of limited utility.

The main problem for nurse researchers is locating appropriate measurement tools. Many of the phenomena of interest in nursing practice and research are intangible, such as interpersonal conflict, caring, coping, and maternal–fetal attachment. The intangible nature of various phenomena, and yet the need to measure them, places methodological research in an important position in research. Methodological research differs from other designs of research. First, it does not include all of the research process steps discussed in Chapter 3. Second, to implement methodical research techniques, the researcher must have a sound knowledge of psychometrics or must consult with a researcher knowledgeable in psychometric techniques. The methodological researcher is not interested in the relationship of the independent variable to a dependent variable or in the effect of an independent variable on a dependent variable. Instead, the methodological researcher is interested in identifying an intangible construct (concept) and making it tangible with a paper-and-pencil instrument or observation protocol.

A methodological study includes the following steps:

- Defining the construct, or concept, or behaviour to be measured
- Formulating the tool's items
- Developing instructions for users and respondents
- Testing the tool's reliability and validity

A sound, specific, and exhaustive literature review is necessary to identify the theories underlying the steps in this construct. The literature review provides the basis of item formulation. Once the items have been developed, the researcher assesses the tool's reliability and validity (see Chapter 15). Various aspects of these procedures may differ according to the tool's use, purpose, and stage of development.

In an example of methodological research, Boscart et al. (2018) documented the evaluation of the psychometric properties of the Team Member Perspectives of Person-Centered Care (TM-PCC) Survey. Another example is the study by Vincelette et al. (2018), where the researchers developed and validated the Nurse Cardiopulmonary Resuscitation Survey (NCRS) among intensive care unit nurses.

Common considerations that researchers incorporate into methodological research are outlined in Table 12.3. Psychometric or methodological studies are found primarily in journals that report research. The *Journal of Nursing Measurement* is devoted to the publication of information on instruments, tools, and approaches for measurement of variables.

TABLE **12.3**

COMMON CONSIDERATIONS IN THE DEVELOPMENT OF MEASUREMENT TOOLS

CONSIDERATION	COMMENT
The well-constructed scale, test, interview schedule, or other form of index should consist of an objective, standardized measure of samples of a behaviour that has been clearly defined. Observations should be made on a small but carefully chosen sampling of the behaviour of interest, thus creating confidence that the samples are representative.	A new tool should be based on a thorough review of previous theoretical and research literature to ensure validity.
The tool should be standardized; that is, a set of uniform items and response possibilities are uniformly administered and scored.	Without specific criteria and rating procedures, the evaluations of the items would be based on the subjective impressions, which may have varied significantly between observers and conditions.
The items of a measurement tool should be unambiguous; they should be clear-cut, concise, exact statements with only one idea per item. Negative stems or items with negatively phrased response possibilities result in ambiguity in meaning and scoring.	For example, in constructing a tool to measure job satisfaction, a nurse scientist writes the following item: "I never feel that I don't have time to provide good nursing care." The response format consists of "Agree," "Undecided," and "Disagree." A response of "Disagree" will likely not reflect the respondent's true intention because of the confusion that is created by the double-negative phrasing "never . . . don't."
The type of items used in any one test or scale should be restricted to a limited number of variations. Participants who are expected to shift from one kind of item to another may fail to provide a true response as a result of the distraction of making such a change.	Mixing true-or-false items with questions that require a yes-or-no response and items that provide a response format of five possible answers can lead to a high level of measurement error.
Items should not provide irrelevant clues. Unless carefully constructed, an item may furnish an indication of the expected response or answer. Furthermore, the correct answer or expected response to one item should not be given by another item.	An item that provides a clue to the expected answer may contain value words that convey cultural expectations, such as "A good wife enjoys caring for her home and family."
The items of a measurement tool should not be made difficult by requiring unnecessarily complex or exact operations. Furthermore, the difficulty of an item should be appropriate to the level of the participants being assessed. Limiting each item to one concept or idea helps accomplish this objective.	A test constructed to evaluate learning in an introductory course in research methods may contain an item that is inappropriate for the designated group, such as "A nonlinear transformation of data to linear data is a useful procedure before a hypothesis of curvilinearity is tested."

TABLE **12.3**

COMMON CONSIDERATIONS IN THE DEVELOPMENT OF MEASUREMENT TOOLS—cont'd

CONSIDERATION	COMMENT
The diagnostic, predictive, or measurement value of a tool depends on the degree to which it serves as an indicator of a relatively broad and significant area of behaviour, known as the *universe of content* for the behaviour. As already emphasized, a behaviour must be clearly defined before it can be measured. The definition is developed from the universe of content: that is, the information and research findings that are available for the behaviour of interest. The items should reflect that definition. The extent to which the test items appear to accomplish this objective is an indication of the validity of the instrument.	Two nurse researchers are studying the construct of quality of life. Each nurse has defined this construct in a different way. Consequently, the measurement tool that each nurse devises will include different questions. The questions on each tool will reflect the universe of content for quality of life as defined by each researcher.
The instrument also should adequately cover the defined behaviour. The primary consideration is whether the number and nature of items in the sample are adequate. If the sample has too few items, the accuracy or reliability of the measure must be questioned. In general, the sample should have a minimum of 10 items for each independent aspect of the behaviour of interest.	For example, few people would be satisfied with an assessment of intelligence if the scale were limited to three items.
The measure must prove its worth empirically through tests of reliability and validity.	The researcher should demonstrate to the reader that the scale is accurate and measures what it purports to measure (see Chapter 15).

The specific procedures of methodological research are beyond the scope of this book, but you are urged to look closely at the tools used in studies.

Systematic Review

A *systematic review* is a summation and assessment of research studies found in the literature based on a clearly focused question that uses systematic and explicit methods to identify, select, critically appraise, and analyze relevant data from the selected studies to summarize the findings in a focused area (see Chapter 3). The strength of evidence provided by systematic reviews is a key component for developing a practice based on evidence. The qualitative counterpart to a systematic review is meta-synthesis, which uses qualitative principles to assess qualitative research and is described in Chapter 5. In a systematic review,

statistical methods such as a meta-analysis may or may not be used to analyze the studies reviewed. A systematic review provides the most powerful and useful evidence available to guide practice: level I evidence (see Chapter 3). Systematic reviews that use multiple randomized clinical trials (RCTs) to combine study results offer stronger evidence (level I) in estimating the magnitude of an effect for an intervention.

You will also find reviews of an area of research or theory synthesis termed *integrative reviews*, discussed later in the chapter. Systematic and integrative reviews are not designs per se, but methods for searching and integrating the literature related to a specific clinical issue. These methods take the results of many studies in a specific area, assesses the studies critically for reliability and validity (quality, quantity, and consistency), and synthesize findings to inform practice.

Meta-analysis provides level I evidence—the highest level of evidence, as it involves statistically analyzing and integrating the results of many studies. Systematic reviews and meta-analyses also grade the level of design or evidence of the studies reviewed. Of all the review types, a meta-analysis provides the strongest summary support because it summarizes studies using data analysis. Box 12.2 outlines the path for completing a systematic review.

The components of a systematic review are the same as in a meta-analysis (Box 12.3) except for the analysis of the studies. An example of a systematic review is that by Richards et al. (2018)

BOX 12.2

COMPLETING A SYSTEMATIC REVIEW

A systematic review is a summary of the quantitative research literature that used similar designs based on a focused clinical question. The goal is to bring together all of the studies concerning a focused clinical question and, using rigorous inclusion and exclusion criteria, assess the strength and quality of the evidence provided by the chosen studies in relation to:
- Sampling issues
- Internal validity (bias) threats
- External validity
- Data analysis

The purpose is to report, in a consolidated fashion, the most current and valid research on intervention effectiveness and clinical knowledge, which will ultimately be the basis for evidence-informed decision-making about the applicability of findings to clinical practice.

Once the studies in a systematic review are gathered from a comprehensive literature search (see Chapter 5), they are assessed for quality and synthesized according to quality or focus; then practice recommendations are made and presented in an article. More than one person independently evaluates the studies to be included or excluded in the review. Generally, the articles critically appraised are discussed in the article and presented in a table format within the article, which helps you to easily identify the specific studies gathered for the review and their quality. The most important principle to assess when reading a systematic review is how the author(s) of the review identified the studies to evaluate and how they systematically reviewed and appraised the literature that leads to the reviewers' conclusions.

BOX 12.3

SYSTEMATIC REVIEW COMPONENTS WITH OR WITHOUT META-ANALYSIS

- Introduction
- Review rationale and a clear clinical question (PICOT)
- Methods
- Information sources, databases used, and search strategy identified: how studies were selected and data extracted as well as the variables extracted and defined
- Description of methods used to assess risk of bias, summary measures identified (e.g., risk, ratio); identification of how data are combined, if studies are graded what quality appraisal system was used (see Chapters 1, 18, and 19)
- Results
- Number of studies screened and characteristics, risk of bias within studies, if a meta-analysis, there will be a synthesis of results including confidence intervals, risk of bias for each study, and all outcomes considered
- Discussion
- Summary of findings including the strength, quality, quantity, and consistency of the evidence for each outcome
- Any limitations of the studies, conclusions, and recommendations of findings for practice
- Funding
- Sources of funding for the systematic review

---

on the effect of nursing care interventions for nutrition, elimination, mobility, and hygiene, where the authors:

- Synthesized the literature from studies on the effect of each of nutrition, elimination, mobility, and hygiene
- Included a clear clinical question; all of the sections of a systematic review were presented; in addition, there was a statistical meta-analysis (combination of studies data) of the studies as a whole.

Each study in this review was considered individually, not collectively, for its sample size, effect size, and its contribution to knowledge in the area, based on a set of criteria.

Another systematic review was conducted by Jones et al. (2019) to determine the predictors of infant care competence among women with postpartum depression.

Although systematic reviews are highly useful, they also have to be reviewed for potential bias. Thus the studies in a review need to be carefully critiqued for scientific rigour in each step of the research process.

Meta-Analysis

A meta-analysis is a systematic summary using statistical techniques to assess and combine studies of the same design to obtain a precise estimate of effect (impact of an intervention on the dependent variable/outcomes or association between variables). The terms *meta-analysis* and *systematic review* are often used interchangeably, and this is incorrect. The main difference is that, as noted earlier, a meta-analysis includes a statistical assessment of the studies reviewed. Meta-analysis involves statistically analyzing the data from each of the studies, treating all the studies reviewed as one large data set in order to obtain a precise estimate of the effect (impact) of the results (outcomes) of the studies in the review.

Meta-analysis involves a rigorous process of summary and determining the impact of a number of studies rather than the impact derived from a single study alone (see Chapter 11). After the clinical question is identified and the search of the review of published and unpublished literature is completed, a meta-analysis is conducted in two phases:

Phase I: The data are extracted (i.e., outcome data, sample sizes, and measures of variability from the identified studies).

Phase II: The decision is made as to whether it is appropriate to calculate what is known as a pooled average result (effect) of the studies reviewed.

Effect sizes are calculated using the difference in the average scores between the intervention and control groups from each study. Each study is considered a unit of analysis. A meta-analysis takes the effect size (see Chapter 13) from each of the studies reviewed to obtain an estimate of the population (or the whole) to create a single effect size of all the studies. Thus the effect size is an estimate of how large a difference there is between intervention and control groups in the summarized studies.

In addition to calculating effect sizes, authors of meta-analyses use multiple statistical methods to present and depict the data from studies reviewed (see Chapters 20 and 21). One of these methods is a forest plot, sometimes called a blobbogram. A forest plot graphically depicts the results of analyzing a number of studies. Figure 12.2 is an example of a forest plot from the study by Rose et al. (2016) where they reviewed prenatal maternal anxiety as a risk factor for preterm birth.

Evidence-Informed Practice Tip

Evidence-informed practice methods such as meta-analysis increase your ability to manage the ever-increasing volume of information produced to develop the best evidence-informed practices.

Figure 12.2 displays the studies that compared the type of anxiety (anxiety disorder, pregnancy-specific disorder, state anxiety, general anxiety) and its relationship to having a spontaneous preterm birth. Each study analyzed is listed on the left under Study ID. To the right of the listed study is a horizontal line that identifies the risk ratio of anxiety, which is set at 1. The box on the vertical line represents the weight of each study, while the line is the confidence interval, and the diamond is the significance of the combined studies. The boxes to the left of the 1 line mean that anxiety did not produce a significant risk in preterm birth. The box to the right of the line indicates studies anxiety was significant in preterm birth. The diamond is a more precise estimate of the interventions, as it combines the data from the studies. The exemplar provided is basic, as meta-analysis is a sophisticated methodology.

A well-done meta-analysis assesses for bias in studies and provides clinicians a means of deciding the merit of a body of clinical research. Besides the repository of meta-analyses found in The Cochrane Library, published by The Cochrane Collaboration, meta-analyses can be found published in journals.

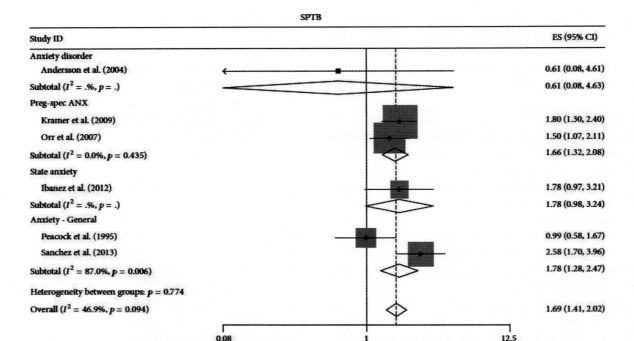

FIG. 12.2   An example of a forest plot. *CI*, confidence interval; *df*, degrees of freedom; *IV*, independent variable; *SD*, standard deviation.

The Cochrane Collaboration

The largest repository of meta-analyses is the Cochrane Collaboration/Review. The Cochrane Collaboration is an international organization that prepares and maintains a body of systematic reviews that focus on health care interventions (Box 12.4). The reviews are found in the Cochrane Database of Systematic Reviews. The Cochrane Collaboration collaborates with a wide range of health care individuals with different skills and backgrounds for developing reviews. These partnerships assist with developing reviews that minimize bias while keeping current with assessment of health care interventions, promoting access to the database, and ensuring the quality of the reviews (Higgins & Green, 2011). The steps of a Cochrane Report mirror those of a standard meta-analysis except for the plain language summary. This useful feature is a straightforward summary of the meta-analysis. The Cochrane Library also publishes several other useful databases (Box 12.5).

BOX 12.4

COCHRANE REVIEW SECTIONS

- Review information: Authors and contact person
- Abstract
- Plain language summary
- The review
- Background of the question
- Objectives of the search
- Methods for selecting studies for review
- Type of studies reviewed
- Types of participants, types of intervention, types of outcomes in the studies
- Search methods for finding studies
- Data collection
- Analysis of the located studies, including effect sizes
- Results including description of studies, risk of bias, intervention effects
- Discussion
- Implications for research and practice
- References and tables to display the data
- Supplementary information (e.g., appendices, data analysis)

Integrative Review

Critical reviews of an area of research without a statistical analysis or a theory synthesis are termed *integrative reviews*. An integrative review is the broadest category of review. It can include theoretical literature, research literature, or both. An integrative review may include methodology studies, a theory review, or the results of differing research studies with wide-ranging clinical implications. An integrative review can include quantitative or qualitative research, or both. Statistics are not used to summarize and generate conclusions about the studies (see Chapter 3).

Secondary Analysis

Secondary analysis also is not a design but a form of research in which the previously collected and analyzed data from one study are reanalyzed for a secondary purpose. The original study may be either an experimental, a nonexperimental design, or Canadian national surveys; for example, Scott et al. (2016) conducted a study using the 2012 Canadian Community Health Survey – Mental Health data to describe the relationship between sexual orientation and depression in the Canadian population. Another method of obtaining secondary data is from a previous study that the researchers conducted; for example, Sidani et al. (2018) examined the extent to which participant characteristics (age,

gender, education, race, employment), treatment type and method, and self-reported outcome factors contributed to satisfaction with the process and outcome attributes of therapies for insomnia. This study consists of a secondary analysis of data obtained from a partially randomized preference trial.

Epidemiological Studies

In an epidemiological study, factors affecting the health and illness of populations are examined in relation to the environment. The purview of public health for many years, epidemiological studies are investigations of the distribution, determinants, and dynamics of health and disease. In these studies, investigators attempt to link effects with cause; however, a clear understanding of the causes is often not possible, especially when the illness or problem has already occurred and the method is to look retrospectively at the evidence.

Some of the questions that epidemiological researchers attempt to answer are "Did exposure to a certain environment affect health?" and "Does staff shortage or do organizational issues affect burnout?" Research cannot answer such questions directly but can establish a statistically significant association between exposure to causative factors and disease or the effects of ill health.

Two frequently conducted types of epidemiological studies are studies of prevalence (the number of people affected by a disease or health problem) and studies of incidence (the number of cases occurring in a particular period).

TOOLS FOR EVALUATING INDIVIDUAL STUDIES

As the importance of practising from a base of evidence has grown, so has the need to have tools or instruments available that can assist practitioners in evaluating studies of various types. When evaluating studies for clinical evidence, it is first important to assess whether the study is valid. At the end of each chapter of this text are critiquing questions that will aid you in assessing whether studies are valid and whether the results are applicable to your practice. In addition to these questions, there are standardized appraisal tools that can assist with appraising the evidence. The international collaboration Critical Appraisal Skills Programme (CASP), whose focus is on teaching critical appraisal, developed tools known as Critical Appraisal Skills Programme Checklists that provide an evidence-informed approach for assessing the quality, quantity, and consistency of specific study designs (CASP, 2018). These instruments are part of an international network that provides consumers with specific questions to help assess study quality. Each checklist has a number of general questions as well as design-specific questions. The tools centre on assessing a study's methodology, validity, and reliability. The questions focus on the following:

1. Are the study's results valid? Understanding the steps of research methodology, especially threats to internal validity as described in the previous and subsequent chapters, will assist in this process (see Chapters 10 through 17).
2. What are the results? This means, can you rely on the results (analysis) or the study's findings (see Chapters 17 and 18)?
3. Are the findings applicable to your practice? Chapters 20 and 21 are aimed at helping you with this decision.

Each CASP guideline is divided into one of the above three areas in a study. There are eight critical appraisal checklists. The checklist with instructions can be found the at CASP website at https://casp-uk.net/casp-tools-checklists/. The design-specific CASP tools with checklists are available online and include the following:

- Systematic reviews
- Randomized controlled studies
- Cohort studies
- Diagnostic studies
- Case-control studies
- Economic evaluations
- Qualitative studies
- Clinical prediction rule

CLINICAL PRACTICE GUIDELINES

Clinical practice guidelines are systematically developed statements or recommendations that link research and practice and serve as a guide for practitioners. Guidelines have been created to assist in bridging practice and research and are developed by professional organizations, government agencies, institutions, or convened expert panels. Guidelines provide clinicians with an algorithm for clinical management, to assist in decision-making for specific diseases (e.g., colon cancer), or for treatments (e.g., pain management). Not all guidelines are well developed and, like research, must be assessed before implementation (see Chapter 10). Guidelines should present scope and purpose of the practice, detail who the development group included, demonstrate scientific rigour, be clear in their presentation, demonstrate clinical applicability, and demonstrate editorial independence. An example is the National Comprehensive Cancer Network, which is an interdisciplinary consortium of 30 cancer centres across the world. Interdisciplinary groups develop practice guidelines for practitioners and education guidelines for patients. These guidelines are accessible at https://www.nccn.org.

The research findings in a clinical practice guideline need to be evaluated for quality, quantity, and consistency. Practice guidelines can be either expert-based or evidence-informed. Evidence-informed practice guidelines are those developed using a scientific process. This process includes first assembling a multidisciplinary group of experts in a specific field. This group is charged with completing a rigorous search of the literature and completing an evidence table that summarizes the quality and strength of the evidence on which the practice guideline is derived (see Chapters 20 and 21). For various reasons, not all areas of clinical practice have a sufficient research base; therefore, expert-based practice guidelines are developed. Expert-based guidelines depend on having a group of nationally known experts in the field who meet and solely use opinions of experts along with whatever research evidence is developed to date. If limited research is available for such a guideline, a rationale should be presented for the practice recommendations.

Many national organizations develop clinical practice guidelines. It is important to know which one to apply to your patient population. For example, there are numerous evidence-informed practice guidelines developed for the management of pain. These guidelines are available from organizations such as the Oncology Nurses Society, American Academy of Pediatrics, National Comprehensive Cancer Network, National Cancer Institute, American College of Physicians, and American Academy of Pain Medicine.

The Agency for Healthcare Research and Quality (AHRQ) supports the National Guideline Clearinghouse (NGC). The NGC's mission is to provide health care providers from all disciplines with objective, detailed information on clinical practice guidelines and measures that are disseminated, implemented, and issued. Specific guidelines can be found on the AHRQ Effective Health Care Program website at https://www.ahrq .gov/programs/index.html?search_api_views_ fulltext=&field_program_topics=14174.

Evaluating Clinical Practice Guidelines

As the number of evidence-informed practice guidelines increases, it becomes more important that you critique these guidelines with regard to the methods used for guideline formulation and consider how they might be used in practice. Critical areas that should be assessed when critiquing evidence-informed practice guidelines include the following:

- Date of publication or release and authors
- Endorsement of the guideline
- Clear purpose of what the guideline covers and patient groups for which it was designed
- Types of evidence (research, nonresearch) used in guideline formulation

- Types of research included in formulating the guideline (e.g., "We considered only randomized and other prospective controlled trials in determining efficacy of therapeutic interventions")
- Description of the methods used in grading the evidence
- Search terms and retrieval methods used to acquire evidence used in the guideline
- Well-referenced statements regarding practice
- Comprehensive reference list
- Review of the guideline by experts
- Whether the guideline has been used or tested in practice and, if so, with what types of patients and what types of settings

Evidence-informed practice guidelines that are formulated using rigorous methods provide a useful starting point for nurses to understand the evidence base of practice. However, more research may be available since the publication of the guideline, and refinements may be needed. Although information in well-developed, national, evidence-informed practice guidelines are a helpful reference, it is usually necessary to localize the guideline using institution-specific evidence-informed policies, procedures, or standards before application within a specific setting.

There are several tools for appraising the quality of clinical practice guidelines. The Appraisal of Guidelines for Research and Evaluation II (AGREE II) instrument (2013) is one of the most widely used tools to evaluate the applicability of a guideline to practice (Brouwers et al., 2010). The AGREE II was developed to assist in evaluating variability in guideline quality, provide a methodological strategy for guideline development, and inform practitioners about what information should be reported in guidelines and how it should be reported. The AGREE II is available online and replaces the original AGREE tool. The instrument focuses on six domains with a total of 23 questions rated on a 7-point scale and two final assessment items that require the appraiser to make overall judgments of the guideline based on how the 23 items were rated. Along with the instrument itself, the AGREE Enterprise website offers guidance on tool usage and development. The AGREE II has been tested for reliability and validity. The guideline assesses the following components of a practice guideline:

1. Scope and purpose of the guideline

2. Stakeholder involvement
3. Rigour of guideline development
4. Clarity of presentation of the guideline
5. Applicability of the guideline to practice
6. Demonstrated editorial independence of the developers

APPRAISING THE EVIDENCE

Systematic Reviews and Clinical Practice Guidelines

For each of the review methods described—systematic review, meta-analysis, integrative review, and clinical practice guidelines—think about each method as one that progressively sifts and sorts research studies and the data until the highest quality of evidence is used to arrive at the conclusions. First the researcher combines the results of all the studies that focus on a specific question. The studies considered of lowest quality are then excluded and the data are reanalyzed. This process is repeated sequentially, excluding studies until only the studies of highest quality available are included in the analysis. An alteration in the overall results as an outcome of this sorting and separating process suggests how sensitive the conclusions are to the quality of studies included. No matter which type of review is completed, it is important to understand that the research studies reviewed still must be examined through your evidence-informed practice lens. This means that evidence that you have derived through your critical appraisal and synthesis or through other researchers' review must be integrated with an individual clinician's expertise and patients' wishes. The criteria for critiquing systematic reviews and clinical practice guidelines are presented in the Critiquing Criteria boxes.

CRITIQUING CRITERIA

SYSTEMATIC REVIEWS

1. Does the PICOT (Population, Intervention, Comparison, Outcome, Time) question used as the basis of the review match the studies included in the review?
2. Are the review methods clearly stated and comprehensive?
3. Are the dates of the review's inclusion clear and relevant to the area reviewed?
4. Are the inclusion and exclusion criteria for studies in the review clear and comprehensive?
5. What criteria were used to assess each of the studies in the review for quality and scientific merit?
6. If studies were analyzed individually, were the data clear?
7. Were the methods of study combination clear and appropriate?
8. If the studies were reviewed collectively, how large was the effect?
9. Are the clinical conclusions drawn from the studies relevant and supported by the review?

Clinical practice guidelines, though they are systematically developed and make explicit recommendations for practice, may be formatted differently. Practice guidelines should reflect the components listed. Guidelines can be located on an organization's website, on the Registered Nurses' Association of Ontario website (http://rnao.ca/bpg), on the AHRQ website (https://www.AHRQ.gov), or on MEDLINE (see Chapters 3 and 21). Well-developed guidelines are constructed using the principles of a systematic review.

CRITIQUING CRITERIA

CLINICAL PRACTICE GUIDELINES

1. Is the date of publication or release current?
2. Are the authors of the guideline clear and appropriate to the guideline?
3. Is the clinical problem and purpose clear in terms of what the guideline covers and

patient groups for which it was designed?

4. What types of evidence (research, nonresearch) were used in formulating the guideline, and are they appropriate to the topic?

5. Is there a description of the methods used to grade the evidence?

6. Were the search terms and retrieval methods used to acquire research and nonresearch evidence used in the guideline clear and relevant?

7. Is the guideline well referenced and comprehensive?

8. Are the recommendations in the guideline sourced according to the level of evidence for its basis?

9. Has the guideline been reviewed by experts in the appropriate field of discipline?

10. Who funded the guideline development?

Evidence-informed practice requires that you determine—based on the strength and quality of the evidence provided by the systematic review, coupled with your clinical expertise and patient values—whether or not you would consider a change in practice.

Evidence-Informed Practice Tip ____

Evidence-informed practice methods, such as systematic reviews, increase a nurse's ability to manage the ever-increasing volume of information produced to develop the best practices that are evidence informed.

Research Hint _____

As you read the literature, you will find studies with labels such as *outcomes research, needs assessments, evaluation research,* and *quality assurance.* These studies are not designs per se; instead, these studies are conducted with either experimental or nonexperimental designs. Studies with these labels are designed to test the effectiveness of health care techniques, programs, or interventions. When reading such a research study, you should assess which design was used and whether the principles of the design, sampling strategy, and analysis are consistent with the study's purpose.

APPRAISING THE EVIDENCE

Nonexperimental Designs

The criteria for critiquing nonexperimental designs are presented in the Critiquing Criteria box. When you critique nonexperimental research designs, keep in mind that such designs offer the researcher the least amount of control. The first step in critiquing nonexperimental research is to determine which type of design was used in the study. Often, a statement describing the design of the study appears in the abstract and in the "Methods" section of the report. If such a statement is not present, you should closely examine the report for evidence of which type of design was employed. You should be able to discern that either a survey or a relationship design was used, as well as the specific subtype. For example, you would expect an investigation of self-concept development in children from birth to 5 years of age to be a relationship study with a longitudinal design.

Next, you should evaluate the theoretical framework and underpinnings of the study to determine whether a nonexperimental design was the most appropriate approach to the problem. For example, in many of the studies on pain discussed throughout this text, the relationship between pain and any of the independent variables under consideration cannot be manipulated. For such studies, a nonexperimental correlational, longitudinal, or cross-sectional design is appropriate. Investigators use one of these designs to examine the relationship between the variables in naturally occurring groups. Sometimes, you may think that it would have been more appropriate for the investigators to use an experimental or a quasiexperimental design. However, you must recognize that pragmatic or ethical considerations also may have guided the researchers in their choice of design (see Chapters 6 and 11).

You should assess whether the problem is at a level of experimental manipulation. Often, researchers merely wish to examine whether relationships exist between

Continued

APPRAISING THE EVIDENCE—cont'd

Nonexperimental Designs

variables. Therefore, when you critique such studies, you should be able to determine the purpose of the study. If the purpose of the study does not include the expectation of a cause-and-effect relationship, you need not look for one. However, be wary when the researcher in a nonexperimental study suggests a cause-and-effect relationship in the findings.

Finally, the factor or factors that influence changes in the dependent variable are often ambiguous in nonexperimental designs. As with all complex phenomena, multiple factors can contribute to variability in the participants' responses. When an experimental design is not used for controlling some of these extraneous variables that can influence results, the researcher must strive to provide as much control of these variables as possible within the context of a nonexperimental design.

When it has not been possible to randomly assign participants to treatment groups as an approach to controlling an independent variable, the researcher may use a strategy of matching participants for identified variables. For example, in a study of birth weight, pregnant women could be matched with regard to variables such as weight, height, smoking habits, drug use, and other factors that might influence the birth weights of their infants. The independent variable of interest, such as the type of

prenatal care, would then be the major difference in the groups. You would then feel more confident that the only difference between the two groups was the differential effect of the independent variable because the other factors in the two groups were theoretically the same. However, you should also remember that other influential variables—such as income, education, and diet—might have been present but were not considered in matching. Threats to internal and external validity represent a major influence on the interpretation of a nonexperimental study because they impose limitations on the generalizability of the results.

If you are critiquing one of the additional types of research discussed, you must first identify the type of research used; then you must understand its specific purpose and format. The format and methods of secondary analysis, methodological research, and meta-analysis vary; knowing how they vary allows you to assess whether the process was applied appropriately. Some of the basic principles of these methods were presented in this chapter. The specific criteria for evaluating these designs are beyond the scope of this text; the references provided can assist you in this process. Even though the format and methods vary, all research has a central goal: to answer questions scientifically.

CRITIQUING CRITERIA

1. Which nonexperimental design is used in the study?
2. In accordance with the theoretical framework, is the rationale for the type of design evident?
3. How is the design congruent with the purpose of the study?
4. Is the design appropriate for the research problem?
5. Is the design suited to the data-collection methods?
6. Does the researcher present the findings in a manner congruent with the design used?
7. Does the researcher theorize beyond the relational parameters of the findings and erroneously infer cause-and-effect relationships between the variables?
8. Are alternative explanations for the findings possible?
9. How does the researcher discuss the threats to internal and external validity?
10. How does the researcher deal with the limitations of the study?

CRITICAL THINKING CHALLENGES

- Discuss which type of nonexperimental design might help validate the defining characteristics of a particular nursing diagnosis you use in practice.

Do you think it is possible for nurses and patients to serve as the participants in this type of study?

- The midterm group (five-student) assignment for your research class is to critique an assigned quantitative study. To proceed, you must first decide the study's overall type. You think it is an ex post facto nonexperimental design, whereas the other students think it is an experimental design because the study has several explicit hypotheses. How would you convince the other students that you are correct?

- You are completing your senior practicum on a surgical step-down unit. The nurses completed an evidence-informed practice protocol for patient-controlled analgesics. Some of the nurses want to implement it immediately, whereas others want to implement it with only some patients. You think that it should be implemented as a research study. Could either of the ways the nurses want to implement the protocol be considered in a research study?

- You are part of a journal club at your hospital. Your group has been examining a phenomenon specific to your patient population and noticed that 20 correlational studies on the topic have been published. Your group decides to perform a meta-analysis of the data. What steps need to be considered in performing the meta-analysis? What level of evidence would you expect to obtain with this method? Explain your answer.

- In reviewing a clinical practice guideline, think about what types of evidence (research, nonresearch) were used in formulating the guideline and whether they are appropriate to the topic. Is there a description of the methods used to grade the evidence? Were the search terms and retrieval methods that were used to acquire research and nonresearch evidence in the guideline clear and relevant? Is the guideline well referenced and comprehensive? Are the recommendations in the guideline sourced according to the level of evidence for its basis?

CRITICAL JUDGEMENT QUESTIONS

1. Which study title suggests a cross-sectional design?
   a. Effect of prenatal parenting classes on infant care knowledge in the early post-partum period
   b. Change in self-esteem over time among women participating in a weight loss support group
   c. Relationship between self-esteem and successful breastfeeding at 1 month and 6 months after birth
   d. Women's appraisal of the diagnosis of breast cancer within the first 48 hours after cancer diagnosis

2. Which title is most suggestive of a longitudinal study?
   a. Effect of prenatal parenting classes on maternal–infant bonding in the early postpartum period
   b. Change in self-esteem over time among women participating in a weight loss support group
   c. Relationship between self-esteem and successful breastfeeding at 1 month, 3 months, and 6 months after birth
   d. Women's appraisal of the diagnosis of breast cancer within the first 48 hours after initial cancer diagnosis

3. In a study of psychosocial adjustment to breast cancer, data collection instruments were sent to the same sample of women at six different times during the first year of living with breast cancer. What type of study design does this exemplify?
   a. Cross-sectional
   b. Retrospective
   c. Longitudinal
   d. Correlational

KEY POINTS

- Nonexperimental research designs are used in studies that make an account of events as they naturally occur. The major difference between nonexperimental and experimental research is that in nonexperimental designs, the independent variable is not actively manipulated by the investigator.
- Nonexperimental designs can be classified either as survey studies or as relationship/difference studies.
- Survey studies and relationship/difference studies are both descriptive and exploratory in nature.

- In survey research, the investigator collects detailed descriptions of existing phenomena and uses the data either to justify current conditions and practices or to make more intelligent plans for improving them.
- In relationship/difference studies, researchers endeavour to explore the relationships or differences between variables in order to provide deeper insight into the phenomena of interest.
- In correlational studies, researchers examine relationships.
- Developmental studies are further divided into categories of cross-sectional, longitudinal (prospective), and retrospective (ex post facto) studies.
- Methodological research, secondary analysis, meta-analysis, epidemiological studies, and clinical practice guidelines are examples of other means of adding to the body of nursing research. Both the researcher and the reader must consider the advantages and disadvantages of each design.
- Nonexperimental research designs do not enable the investigator to establish cause-and-effect relationships between the variables. You must be wary of nonexperimental studies in which researchers make causal claims about the findings, unless a causal modelling technique is used.
- Nonexperimental designs offer the researcher the least amount of control. Threats to validity represent a major influence on the interpretation of a nonexperimental study because they impose limitations on the generalizability of the results and, as such, should be fully assessed by the critical reader.
- The critiquing process is directed toward evaluating the appropriateness of the selected nonexperimental design in relation to factors such as the research problem, the theoretical framework, the hypothesis, the methodology, and the data analysis and interpretation.
- Although nonexperimental designs do not provide the highest level of evidence (level I), they do provide a wealth of data that become useful for formulating both level I and level II studies that are aimed at developing and testing nursing interventions.

🛜 FOR FURTHER STUDY

Go to Evolve at http://evolve.elsevier.com/Canada/LoBiondo/Research for the Audio Glossary.

REFERENCES

Arnaert, A., Ponzoni, N., Debe, Z., Meda, M. M., Nana, N. G., & Arnaert, S. (2019). Experiences of women receiving health-supported antenatal care in the village from community health workers in rural Burkina Faso, Africa. *Digital Health, 10*(3), 57–64. https://doi.org/10.1177/2055207619892756.

Boscart, V. M., Davey, M., Ploeg, J., Heckman, G., Dupuis, S., Sheiban, L., Luh Kim, J., Brown, P., & Sidani, S. (2018). Psychometric evaluation of the Team Member Perspectives of Person-Centered Care (TM-PCC) survey for long-term care homes. *Healthcare, 6*(2), 59. https://doi.org/10.3390/healthcare6020059.

Brouwers, M., Kho, M. E., Browman, G. P., Burgers, J. S., Cluzeau, F., Feder, G., Fervers, B., Graham, I. D., Grimshaw, J., Hanna, S., Littlejohns, P., Makarski, J., & Zitzelsberger, L. (2010). AGREE Next Steps Consortium. AGREE II: Advancing guideline development, reporting and evaluation in healthcare. *Canadian Medical Association Journal, 182*(18), E839–E842. https://doi.org/10.1503/cmaj.090449.

Castonguay, A., Wrosch, C., Pila, E., & Sabiston, C. (2017). Body-related shame and guilt predict physical activity in breast cancer survivors over time. *Oncology Nursing Forum, 44*(4), 465–475. https://doi.org/10.1188/17.ONF.465-475.

Covell, C. L., Primeau, M-D., Kilpatrick, K., & St-Pierre, I. (2017). Internationally educated nurses in Canada: Predictors of workforce integration. *Human Resources for Health, 15*(1), 1–16. https://doi.org/10.1186/s12960-017-0201-8.

Critical Appraisal Skills Programme (CASP). (2018). Critical appraisal skills programme: Making sense of evidence. https://casp-uk.net/casp-tools-checklists/.

Dahlke, S., Davidson, S., Duarte Wisnesky, U., Kalogirou, M. R., Salyers, V., Pollard, C., Fox, M. T., Hunter, K. F., & Baumbusch, J. (2019). Student nurses' perceptions about older people. *International Journal of Nursing Education Scholarship*(1), 16. https://doi.org/10.1515/ijnes-2019-0051.

Dall'Ora, C, Ball, J, Redfern, O, et al. (2019). Are long nursing shifts on hospital wards associated with sickness absence? A longitudinal retrospective observational study. *Journal of Nursing Management, 27*, 19–26. https://doi-org.ezproxy.library.yorku.ca/10.1111/jonm.12643.

Della Pelle, C., Cerratti, F., Di Giovanni, P., Cipollone, F., &. Cicolini, G. (2018). Attitudes Towards and Knowledge About Lesbian, Gay, Bisexual, and Transgender Patients Among Italian Nurses: An Observational Study. *Journal of Nursing Scholarship, 50*(4), 367–374. https://doi.org/10.1111/jnu.12388.

Dennis, C., Merry, L., & Gagnon, A. (2017). Postpartum depression risk factors among recent refugee, asylum-seeking, non-refugee immigrant, and Canadian-born women: Results from a prospective cohort study. *Social Psychiatry and Psychiatric Epidemiology, 52*(4), 411–422. https://doi.org/10.1007/s00127-017-1353-5.

Fernandez, S., Franklin, J., Amlani, N., DeMilleVille, C., Lawson, D., & Smith, J. (2015). Physical activity and cancer: A cross-sectional study on the barriers and facilitators to exercise during cancer treatment. *Canadian Oncology Nursing Journal = Revue Canadienne de Nursing Oncologique, 25*(1), 37–48. https://doi.org/10.5737/236880762513742.

Fox, M., McCague, H., Sidani, S., & Butler, J. (2018). The relationships between the geriatric practice environment, nursing practice, and the quality of hospitalized older adults' care. *Journal of Nursing Scholarship, 50*(5), 513–521. https://doi.org/10.1111/jnu.12414.

Freeman, L. A., Pfaff, K. A., Kopchek., L, & Liebman, J (2020). Investigating palliative care nurse attitudes towards medical assistance in dying: An exploratory cross-sectional study. *Journal of Advanced Nursing, 76*, 535–545. https://doi.org/10.1111/jan.14252.

Higgins, J. P. T., & Green, S. (2011). *Cochrane handbook for systematic reviews of interventions version 5.1.0.* Retrieved from http://handbook.cochrane.org.

Jin, C., Lobchuk, M., Chernomas, W., & Pooyania, S. (2017). Examining associations of functional deficits and mood states with empathic responses of stroke family caregivers. *Journal of Neuroscience Nursing, 49*(1), 12–14. https://doi.org/10.1097/JNN.0000000000000250.

Jones, D., Letourneau, N., & Duffett-Leger, L. (2019). Systematic review of predictors of infant care competence among women with postpartum depression. *Journal of Nursing Education and Practice, 9*(5), 118–128. https://doi.org/10.5430/jnep.v9n5p118.

Leyva-Moral, J. M., Dominguez-Cancino, K. A., Guevara-Vasquez, G. M., Edwards, J. E., & Palmieri, P. A. (2019). Faculty attitudes about caring for people living with HIV/AIDS: a comparative study. *Journal of Nursing Education, 58*(12), 712–717.

Pien, L.-C., Cheng, Y., & Cheng, W.-J. (2019). Psychosocial safety climate, workplace violence and self-rated health: A multi-level study among hospital nurses. *Journal of Nursing Management, 27*, 584–591. https://doi-org.ezproxy.library.yorku.ca/10.1111/jonm.12715.

Raudenbush, S. W., & Bryk, A. S. (2002). Hierarchical linear models: Applications and data analysis methods. (Vol. 1). Sage.

Rayan, A. (2019). Mindfulness, self-efficacy, and stress among final-year nursing students. *Journal of Psychosocial Nursing, 57*(4), 49–55. https://doi.org/10.3928/02793695-20181031-01.

Richards, D. A., Hilli, A., Pentecost, C., Goodwin, V. A., & Frost, J. (2018). Fundamental nursing care: A systematic review of the evidence on the effect of nursing care interventions for nutrition, elimination, mobility and hygiene. *Journal of Clinical Nursing, 27*(11-12), 2179–2188. https://doi.org/10.1111/jocn.14150.

Rochefort, C. M., Rathwell, B. A., & Clarke, S. P. (2016). Rationing of nursing care interventions and its association with nurse-reported outcomes in the neonatal intensive care unit: A cross-sectional survey. *BMC Nursing, 15*, 46. https://doi.org/10.1186/s12912-016-0169-z.

Rose, M. S., Pana, G., & Premji, S. (2016). Prenatal maternal anxiety as a risk factor for preterm birth and the effects of heterogeneity on this relationship: A systematic review and meta-analysis. *BioMed Research International, 2016*, Article 8312158. https://doi.org/10.1155/2016/8312158.

Schofield, R., Forchuk, C., Montgomery, P., Rudnick, A., Edwards, B., Meier, A., & Speechley, M. (2016). Comparing personal health practices: Individuals with mental illness and the general Canadian population. *Canadian Nurse, 112*(5), 23–27.

Scott, R., Lasiuk, G., & Norris, C. (2016). Sexual orientation and depression in Canada. *Canadian Journal of Public Health, 107*(6), e545–e549. https://doi.org/10.17269/CJPH.107.5506.

Sidani, S., Epstein, D. R., Fox, M., & Collins, L. (2018). The contribution of participant, treatment, and outcomes factors to treatment satisfaction. *Research in Nursing and Health, 41*(6), 572–582. https://doi.org/10.1002/nur.21909.

Stephenson, E., DeLongis, A., Steele, R., et al. (2017). Siblings of children with a complex chronic health condition: Maternal posttraumatic growth as a predictor of changes in child behavior problems. *Journal of Pediatric Psychology, 42*(1), 104–113.

Strazzieri-Pulido, K. C., Carol, C. V., Nogueira, P. C., Padilha, K. G., & Vera, V. L. C. (2019). Pressure injuries in critical patients: Incidence, patient-associated factors, and nursing workload. *Journal of Nursing Management, 27*(2), 301–310. https://doi.org/10.1111/jonm.12671.

Vincelette, C., Lavoie, S., Fortin, O., & Quiroz-Martinez, H. (2018). Intensive care unit nurses' knowledge, skills and attitudes regarding three resuscitation procedures: A cross-sectional survey. *Canadian Journal of Critical Care Nursing, 29*(4), 29–35.

Wall, V., Premji, S. S., Letourneau, N., McCaffrey, G., & Nyanza, E. C. (2018). Factors associated with pregnancy-related anxiety in Tanzanian women: A cross sectional study. *BMJ Open, 8*(6), 1–8. https://doi.org/10.1136/bmjopen-2017-020056.

Winsett, R. P., Rottet, K., Schmitt, A., Wathen, E., & Wilson, D. (2016). Medical surgical nurses describe missed nursing care tasks—Evaluating our work environment. *Applied Nursing Research, 32*, 128–13388. https://doi.org/10.1016/j.apnr.2016.06.006.

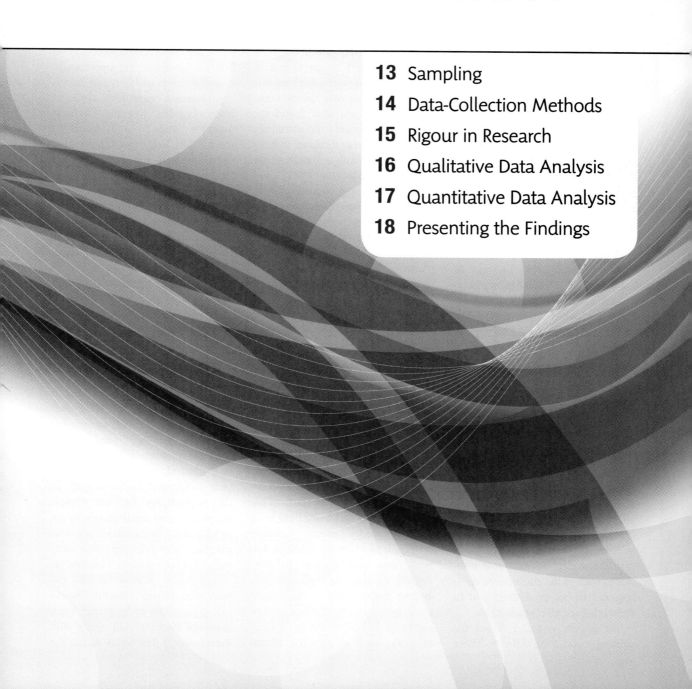

PART **FIVE**

Processes Related to Research

RESEARCH **VIGNETTE**
Nursing Workforce

Mélanie Lavoie-Tremblay, BScN, MScN, PhD
Associate Professor
Ingram School of Nursing
McGill University
Montréal, Quebec

Though university nursing programs do their best to provide adequate instruction in theory and practice to their students, it is well documented that newly graduated nurses (NGNs) still feel unprepared for their transition into the work environment, which contributes to an alarming number of new nurses quitting the profession (Duchscher, 2009; Lavoie-Tremblay, O'Brien-Pallas, Gélinas, Desforges, & Marchionni, 2008; Marleau & Lapointe, 2014). Healthcare organizations have been facing this challenge for many years, which has spurred the development of several interventions, such as mentorship programs, to help NGNs acclimate to the clinical environment. However, even with these interventions in place, when NGNs begin to work independently, they continue to experience multifactorial challenges when providing nursing care, be they professional, organizational, or personal in nature (Kelly & Ahern, 2009; Murray, Sundin, & Cope, 2019). As such, it is important to study the experience of new nurses in order to find what can be done to ease the student-to-nurse role transition, both in the educational environment before graduation and in the workplace after graduation.

As a new nurse, I found the working conditions difficult. There was a significant gap between what I learned at school and the reality of the workplace, and I was asking myself if I should stay or quit the nursing profession. I began to realize that I was not alone in thinking this way, as the other new nurses working alongside me also found the start of their careers to be extremely challenging. I was fortunate to have discussed this with a clinical nurse specialist at the hospital where I was working, who suggested that I help them review their orientation program to help new nurses have a better transition at work. This is why I started my Master's in nursing, as part of an effort to modernize their orientation program for new nurses. With the leader of the nursing team, we completed a participatory action research study and were able to improve the orientation program based on new nurses' needs. This work eventually led to the publication of my first manuscript in 2002, entitled "How to facilitate the orientation of new nurses into the workplace."

After finishing my Master's program, I realized that we can increase retention of new nurses in their first years of work by having a healthier workplace. This led me to undertake my PhD with a participatory action research program, in order to optimize the workplace and reduce psychological distress and absenteeism among nurses. This research gave me a better understanding of key concepts linked to being healthy at work, such as rewards, social support, autonomy, and empowerment. In order to foster a healthy work environment, it is also imperative to understand the nature of the constraints in the workplace, and to involve nurses and other healthcare professionals in proposing solutions.

Since I began my career as a professor at McGill University in 2005, I have had the opportunity to collaborate with several health organizations on projects aimed at improving the working environment for nurses. In 2017, as chair of the McGill Nursing Collaborative for Education and Innovation in Patient- and Family-Centred Care, I helped to establish the *Nightingale Fellows Project*, a group mentorship experience aimed at helping graduating students have an easier transition into clinical practice. This program, which is offered to all McGill nursing students in their final year of study, has two main goals: to provide educational and experiential support to students as they prepare to pass from student to nurse, and to provide a safe environment where students can discuss this process with experienced clinicians, thereby increasing their understanding of the knowledge and skills they will need to succeed as graduate nurses working in a clinical unit. Each academic year, students who participate in the Nightingale Fellows Project are placed into small groups of six to eight students, each of which is assigned to one of nine nurse mentors. These mentors, known as "Nightingale Fellows," are all experienced nurses currently working in hospitals in Montreal. Each group of students then meets with their mentors four times during the spring semester and once more the following fall, and at each meeting they discuss topics related to entering the workforce, such as preparing for their licensure exam, finding a job after graduation, managing workload and stress, and adjusting to organizational culture. Now in its fourth year of existence, this program has helped over 200 students with their transition from student to nurse (Lavoie-Tremblay, Sanzone, Primeau & Lavigne, 2019).

IN SUMMARY

Several initiatives can be implemented to promote attraction and retention of new nurses, to ensure a smooth transition from student to nurse, and to create healthy workplaces for nurses and patients. It is crucial to involve students, nurses, and patients in creating healthy workplaces, so that we can co-construct solutions that are suitable and sustainable in the long-term. ■

REFERENCES

Duchscher, J. E. B. (2009). Transition shock: The initial stage of role adaptation for newly graduated registered nurses. *Journal of Advanced Nursing, 65*(5), 1103–1113. https://doi.org/10.1111/j.1365-2648.2008.04898.x.

Kelly, J., & Ahern, K. (2009). Preparing nurses for practice: A phenomenological study of the new graduate in Australia. *Journal of Clinical Nursing, 18*(6), 910–918.

Lavoie-Tremblay, M., O'Brien-Pallas, L., Gélinas, C., Desforges, N., & Marchionni, C. (2008). Addressing the turnover issue among new nurses from a generational viewpoint. *Journal of Nursing Management, 16*(6), 724–733. https://doi.org/10.1111/j.1365-2934.2007.00828.x.

Lavoie-Tremblay, M., Sanzone, L., Primeau, G., & Lavigne, G. L. (2019). Group mentorship programme for graduating nursing students to facilitate their transition: A pilot study. *Journal of Nursing Management, 27*(1), 66–74. https://doi.org/10.1111/jonm.12649.

Marleau, D., & Lapointe, J. (2014). *Portrait de la relève infirmière: 2013–2014.* (Report No. 293S (13-14)). Quebec: Ordre des infirmières et infirmiers du Quebec.

Murray, M., Sundin, D., & Cope, V. (2019). Benner's model and duchscher's theory: Providing the framework for understanding new graduate nurses' transition to practice. *Nurse Education in Practice, 34*, 199–203. https://doi.org/10.1016/j.nepr.2018.12.003.

CHAPTER 13

Sampling

Mina D. Singh | Ramesh Venkatesa Perumal

LEARNING OUTCOMES

After reading this chapter, you will be able to do the following:

- Identify the purpose of sampling.
- Define population, sample, and sampling.
- Compare a population and a sample.
- Discuss the eligibility criteria for sample selection.
- Define nonprobability sampling and probability sampling.
- Identify the types of strategies for both nonprobability and probability sampling.
- Identify the types of qualitative sampling.
- Compare the advantages and disadvantages of specific nonprobability and probability sampling strategies.
- Discuss the contribution of nonprobability and probability sampling strategies to the strength of evidence provided by study findings.
- Discuss the factors that influence determination of sample size.
- Discuss the procedure for drawing a sample.
- Identify the criteria for critiquing a sampling plan.
- Use the critiquing criteria to evaluate the "Sample" section of a research report.

KEY TERMS

accessible population
cluster sampling
convenience sampling
data saturation
delimitations
effect size
element
eligibility criteria
heterogeneity
homogeneous
matching

multistage sampling
network sampling
nonprobability sampling
pilot study
population
probability sampling
purposive sampling
quota sampling
random selection
representative sample
sample

sampling frame
sampling interval
sampling unit
simple random
    sampling
snowball effect sampling
stratified random
    sampling
systematic sampling
target population
theoretical sampling

STUDY RESOURCES

 Go to Evolve at http://evolve.elsevier.com/Canada/LoBiondo/Research for the Audio Glossary.

SAMPLING IS THE PROCESS OF SELECTING representative units of a population for study in a research investigation. Although sampling is a complex process, it is a familiar one. In their daily lives, people gather knowledge, make decisions, and formulate predictions on the basis of sampling procedures. For example, nursing students may make generalizations about the overall quality of nursing professors as a result of their exposure to a sample of nursing professors during their undergraduate programs. Patients may make generalizations about a hospital's food or quality of nursing care during a 1-week hospital stay. Limited exposure to a limited portion of these phenomena forms the basis of people's conclusions, so much of their knowledge and many of their decisions are based on their experience with samples.

Researchers also derive knowledge from samples. Many questions in scientific and naturalistic research cannot be answered without the use of sampling procedures. For example, when the effectiveness of a new education intervention for diabetic patients is tested, the intervention is administered to a sample of the population. The researcher must come to some conclusions without giving the intervention to the entire population of diabetic patients. To obtain the experiences or outcomes of engaging in this education, the researcher needs to select the appropriate sampling strategy in accordance with the research design and question. This is done to avoid erroneous conclusions or making generalizations from a nonrepresentative sample. Thus, research methodologists have expended considerable effort to develop sampling theories and procedures that produce accurate and meaningful information. Essentially, researchers sample representative segments of the population because sampling the entire population of interest to obtain relevant information is rarely feasible or necessary.

This chapter will familiarize you with the basic concepts of sampling as they pertain to the principles of quantitative and qualitative research designs, nonprobability and probability sampling, sample size, and the related critiquing process.

SAMPLING CONCEPTS

Population

A **population** is a well-defined set that has certain specified properties or characteristics from which data can be gathered and analyzed. A population can be composed of people, animals, objects, or events. For example, if a researcher is studying undergraduate nursing students, the type of educational preparation of the population must be specified. In this example, the population consists of undergraduate students enrolled in a generic baccalaureate nursing program. Examples of other possible populations might be all female patients admitted to a certain hospital for lumpectomies for treatment of breast cancer during 2016, all children with asthma in the province of Alberta, or all men and women with a diagnosis of schizophrenia in North America. These examples illustrate that a population may be broadly defined and potentially involve millions of people, or it may be narrowly specified to include only a few people. The target population is the entire population of interest, while the accessible population is the portion of the target population that is available to the researcher.

When you read a research report, you should consider whether the researcher has identified the population descriptors that form the basis for the inclusion (eligibility) or exclusion criteria (delimitations) that are used to select the sample from the array of all possible units, whether people, objects, or events. Consider the population previously defined as undergraduate nursing students enrolled in a generic baccalaureate program. Would this population include both part-time and full-time students? Would it include students who had previously attended another nursing program? What about international students? At which level (first year through senior year) would students qualify? As much as possible, the researcher must specifically delineate the exact criteria used to decide whether an individual would be classified as a member of a given population. The population descriptors that provide the basis for inclusion (eligibility) criteria should be evident in the sample; in other words, the characteristics of the population and the sample should be congruent. The degree of congruence is evaluated to assess the representativeness of the sample. For example, if a population is defined as full-time, Canadian-born, senior-level nursing students enrolled in a generic baccalaureate nursing program, the sample would be expected to reflect these characteristics.

Think about the concept of inclusion criteria, or **eligibility criteria** (characteristics of a population that meet requirements for inclusion in a study), applied to a research study in which the participants are patients. For example, in an investigation of the effects of music on dyspnea during exercise in individuals with chronic obstructive pulmonary disease (COPD), the participants had to meet all of the following inclusion (eligibility) criteria:

1. A confirmed medical diagnosis of COPD (i.e., chronic bronchitis, emphysema, or both)
2. Ability to speak and read English
3. Ability to ambulate independently
4. Experiencing dyspnea at least once a week
5. An increase in the level of dyspnea of at least two points on the Borg scale after a 6-minute walk

In their study to better understand the unique narratives of social exclusion for mothers experiencing homelessness, Benbow et al. (2019) had the following inclusion criteria: the participants had to (a) self-identify as mothers (with or without physical custody of their child(ren)), (b) self-identify as experiencing homelessness currently or within the last year, and (c) be aged 18 years and older.

Examples of exclusion criteria, or **delimitations** (characteristics that restrict the population to a homogeneous group of participants), include gender, age, marital status, socioeconomic status, religion, ethnicity, level of education, age of children, health status, and diagnosis. In a study examining and comparing risk factors for postpartum depression among recent refugee, asylum-seeking, non-refugee immigrant, and Canadian-born women, the exclusion criteria were if women (1) had a major mental illness (schizophrenia, other psychoses, or profound, previously existing depression) or cognitive impairment that precluded informed consent; (2) were visitors to Canada; (3) had given the infant up for adoption; or (4) had a stillbirth delivery or infant death (p. 413).

As another example, in a randomized control trial, Jackson and Dennis (2017) in Appendix B had strict inclusion and exclusion criteria to study the effects of applying lanolin for the treatment of nipple pain in breastfeeding. Inclusion criteria were breastfeeding women who: (1) had nipple pain and visible nipple damage; (2) delivered a full-term (greater than 37 weeks), singleton infant within the previous 72 hours; and (3) were able to speak English. The exclusion criteria included: (1) infants not expected to be discharged home with their mother; (2) infants with a congenital abnormality that would impair breastfeeding, or ankyloglossia (tongue-tie); (3) maternal allergy to lanolin; (4) maternal health condition(s) that might interfere with breastfeeding; and (5) maternal aversion to, or, strong desire to use lanolin (p. 2).

The **heterogeneity**, or dissimilarities, of a sample group inhibits the researchers' ability to interpret the findings meaningfully and to make generalizations. It is much wiser to study only one **homogeneous** group—that is, a group with limited variation in attributes or characteristics, or to include specific groups as distinct subsets of the sample and study the groups comparatively, as was the case in Dennis et al. (2017) study on examining risk factors for postpartum depression among recent refugee, asylum-seeking, non-refugee immigrant, and Canadian-born women. They found that recent migrant women had significantly higher rates of depression at 16 weeks postpartum than Canadian-born women (p. 411).

Remember that exclusion criteria or delimitations are not established in a casual or meaningless way but are established to control for extraneous variability or bias. Each exclusion criterion should have a rationale, presumably related to a potential contaminating effect on the dependent variable. Carefully established sample exclusion criteria increase the precision of the study and contribute to accuracy while constraining the generalizability or transferability of the findings (see Chapter 10).

The population criteria establish the **target population**—that is, the entire set of cases about which the researcher would like to make generalizations. A target population might include all undergraduate nursing students enrolled in generic baccalaureate programs in Canada. Because of time, money, and personnel, however, using a target population is often not feasible. An **accessible population**—one that meets the population criteria and is available—is used instead. For example, an accessible population might include all full-time generic baccalaureate students attending school in Manitoba. Pragmatic factors must also be considered in identifying a potential population of interest.

Research Hint

Often, researchers do not clearly identify the population under study, or the population is not clarified until the "Discussion" section, when an effort is made to discuss the group (population) to which the study findings can be generalized.

A population is not restricted to human participants. The population may consist of hospital records; blood, urine, or other specimens taken from patients at a clinic; historical documents; or laboratory animals. For example, a population might consist of all urine specimens collected from patients in the Mount Sinai Hospital antepartum clinic or all patient charts on file at a day surgery centre. A population can be defined in a variety of ways. Of importance is that the basic unit of the population be clearly defined, because the generalizability of the findings is a function of the population criteria.

Evidence-Informed Practice Tip

Consider whether the sample selection was biased, thereby influencing the validity of the evidence provided by the outcomes of the study.

Samples and Sampling

Sampling is a process of selecting a portion or subset of the designated population to represent the entire population. A **sample** is a set of elements that make up the population; an **element** is the most basic unit about which information is collected. A sampling frame is another name for the list of elements from which the sample will be chosen from. The most common element in nursing research is individuals, but other elements (e.g., places or objects) can form the basis of a sample or population. For example, a researcher plans a study to compare the effectiveness of different nursing interventions on reducing falls in older adults in long-term care facilities. Four facilities, each of which having a different treatment protocol, are identified as the sampling units—not the nurses themselves or the treatment alone. A sampling unit can be an organization, a group, or an individual person.

The purpose of sampling is to increase the efficiency of a research study. Examining every element or unit in the population would not be feasible. When sampling is done properly, the researcher can draw inferences and make generalizations about the population without examining each unit in the population.

In qualitative research, the results can also have good generalizability to the population under study. Sampling procedures that entail the formulation of specific criteria for selection ensure that the characteristics of the phenomena of interest will be, or are likely to be, present in all of the elements being studied. The researcher's efforts to ensure that the sample is representative of the target population provide a stronger position from which to draw conclusions from the sample findings that are generalizable to the population (see Chapter 10).

After reviewing a number of research studies, you will recognize that samples and sampling procedures vary in terms of merit. The foremost criterion in evaluating a sample is its representativeness. A **representative sample** has key characteristics that closely approximate those of the population. For instance, if 70% of the population in a study of child-rearing practices consisted of women and 40% were full-time employees, a representative sample should reflect these characteristics in the same proportions.

The representativeness of a sample cannot be guaranteed without access to a database about the entire population. Because it is difficult and inefficient to assess an entire population, the researcher must employ sampling strategies that minimize or control for sample bias. If an appropriate sampling strategy is used, the sample data will almost always enable a reasonably accurate understanding of the phenomena under investigation.

Evidence-Informed Practice Tip

Determining whether the sample is representative of the population being studied in journal articles will influence both your interpretation of the evidence provided by the findings and your decision-making about the findings' relevance to the your patient population and practice setting.

SAMPLING STRATEGIES USED IN QUANTITATIVE RESEARCH

Sampling strategies are generally grouped into two categories: *nonprobability sampling* and *probability sampling*. In **nonprobability sampling**, elements are chosen through nonrandom methods. The drawback of this strategy is that each element's probability of being included in the samples cannot be estimated. In other words, ensuring that every element has a chance for inclusion in the nonprobability sample is not possible. In **probability sampling**, some form of random selection is used when the sample units are chosen. This type of sample enables the researcher to estimate the probability that each element of the population will be included in the sample. Probability sampling is the more rigorous sampling strategy used in quantitative research and is more likely to result in a representative sample.

The remainder of this section is devoted to a discussion of different types of nonprobability and probability sampling strategies. A summary of sampling strategies appears in Table 13.1. You may refer to this table as the various nonprobability and probability strategies are discussed in the following sections. Note that if there is bias in sampling, it will distort the analysis and the findings of the study.

Research Hint

Research articles are not always explicit about the type of sampling strategy that was used. If the sampling strategy is not specified, assume that in a quantitative study, a convenience sample was used and that in a qualitative study, a purposive sample was used.

Nonprobability Sampling

Because of a lack of random selection, the nonprobability sampling strategy is less generalizable than probability sampling because it tends to produce less representative samples. Such samples are more feasible for the researcher to obtain, however, and most samples—in nursing

TABLE **13.1**

SUMMARY OF SAMPLING STRATEGIES

SAMPLING STRATEGY	EASE OF DRAWING A REPRESENTATIVE SAMPLE	RISK OF BIAS	REPRESENTATIVENESS OF THE SAMPLE
NONPROBABILITY			
Convenience	Very easy	Greater than in any other sampling strategy	Because samples tend to be self-selecting, representativeness is questionable
Quota	Relatively easy	Contains an unknown source of bias that affects external validity	Builds in some representativeness by using knowledge about the population of interest
Purposive	Relatively easy	Bias increases with greater heterogeneity of the population; conscious bias is also a danger but is offset with maximal variation	Very limited ability to generalize because the sample is handpicked from a quantitative view, but this approach is necessary for the qualitative researcher to choose participants on the basis of the phenomenon under study
Network	Can be easy if the network is accessible	Minimal if a thorough sampling plan is developed	Represents the event, incident, or experience being studied
Theoretical	Requires a two-stage process; can be prolonged	Minimal if a thorough sampling plan is developed	Typically begins with another type of sampling, such as convenience or criterion sampling aimed at variation in the phenomenon, and thus represents aspects of the theory being constructed
PROBABILITY			
Simple random	Laborious	Low	Maximized; the probability of nonrepresentativeness decreases with increased sample size
Stratified random	Time-consuming	Low	Enhanced
Cluster	Less time-consuming than simple or stratified sampling	Subject to more sampling errors than is simple or stratified sampling	Less representative than simple or stratified sampling
Systematic	More convenient and efficient than is simple, stratified, or cluster sampling	Bias in the form of nonrandomness can be inadvertently introduced	Less representative if bias occurs as a result of coincidental nonrandomness

research and the research of other disciplines—are nonprobability samples. When a nonprobability sample reflects the target population through the careful use of inclusion and exclusion criteria, you can have more confidence in the representativeness of the sample and the external validity of the findings. The major types of nonprobability sampling used in quantitative research are *convenience sampling* and *quota sampling*.

Convenience Sampling

Convenience sampling is the use of the most readily accessible persons or objects as participants in a study. The participants may include volunteers, the first 25 patients admitted to a certain hospital with a particular diagnosis, all of the people who enrolled in a certain program during the month of September, or all of the students enrolled in a certain course at a particular university during 2021. The participants are convenient and accessible to the researcher; hence the term *convenience sample*.

As an example, Dosani et al. (2017) recruited a convenience sample of 122 mothers to study the experiences of mothers breastfeeding the late preterm infant and perceptions of public health nurses. In another study, Chan et al. (2019) used a convenience sample of 69 nursing students to investigate the influence nursing students' self-efficacy (confidence) related to medication administration and medication errors using an electronic administration record in clinical simulation.

The advantage of a convenience sample is that it can be an easy way for the researcher to obtain participants. The researcher may need to be concerned only with obtaining a sufficient number of participants who meet the same criteria. The major disadvantage of a convenience sample is that the risk of bias is greater than in any other type of sample (see Table 13.1). Because convenience samples entail voluntary participation, the probability that researchers will recruit people who feel strongly about the issue being studied is increased, which may favour certain outcomes of the study. The problem of bias is related to the tendency of convenience samples to be self-selecting; in other words, the researcher obtains information only from the people who volunteer to participate. In this case, the following questions must be raised:

- What motivated some of the people to participate and others not to participate?
- What kind of data would have been obtained if nonparticipants had also responded?
- How representative of the population are the people who did participate?

For example, a researcher may stop people on a street corner to ask their opinion on an issue; place advertisements in the newspaper; put signs in local churches, community centres, or supermarkets; or search specific agencies websites to recruit volunteers for a particular study. To study the influence of visible physical signs on caregiver's patient-centred and empathetic behaviours in chronic pain, Paul-Savoie et al. (2018) used a convenience sample of 21 nurses and 21 physicians recruited through advertisements and referrals. To assess the degree to which a convenience sample approximates a random sample, a researcher can compare the convenience sample data with the known demographic information and examine variability around the mean. In this manner, the researcher checks for the representativeness of the convenience sample and the extent to which bias is or is not evident.

Because recruiting research participants is crucial for nurse researchers, innovative recruitment strategies are sometimes used. For example, a researcher may offer to pay the participants for their time. A relatively new method of accessing and recruiting participants is through online computer networks (e.g., disease-specific chat rooms and bulletin boards).

In evaluating a research report, you should recognize that the convenience sample strategy, although the most common, is the weakest form of sampling strategy in quantitative research in terms of generalizability. When a convenience sample is used, researchers should analyze and interpret the data cautiously. When you critique a research study in which this sampling strategy was used, you should be skeptical about the external validity of the findings (see Chapter 10).

Quota Sampling

Quota sampling refers to a form of nonprobability sampling in which knowledge about the population of interest is used to ensure some representativeness about the sample (see Table 13.1). Through quota sampling, the researcher identifies a particular strata of the population, and the quota sample proportionally represents the strata. For example, the data in Table 13.2 reveal that of the 5,000 nurses in a particular city, 20% are diploma graduates, 40% are post–RN degree graduates, and 40% are baccalaureate graduates. Each of these strata should be proportionately represented in the sample. In this case, the researcher used a proportional quota sampling strategy and decided to include 10% of a population of 5,000 (i.e., 500 nurses). On the basis of the proportion of each stratum in the population, 100 diploma graduates, 200 post-RN graduates, and 200 baccalaureate graduates were the quotas established for the three strata. The researcher recruited participants who met the eligibility criteria of the study until the quota for each stratum was filled. In other words, once the researcher obtained the necessary 100 diploma graduates, 200 post-RN graduates, and 200 baccalaureate graduates, the sample was complete with regard to both the research design and other pragmatic matters, such as economy.

The researcher systematically ensures that proportional segments of the population are included in the sample. For example, in Im et al. (2012) study exploring midlife women's attitudes toward physical activity, the researchers stratified a quota sample of 542 subjects by ethnicity and socioeconomic status. An example of nonproportional quota sampling is in the study by Fox et al. (2010), who examined differences in sleep complaints among adults with varying amounts of bed rest who were residing in extended-care facilities for chronic disease management. The three cohorts (comparative, moderate, and high) reflected different amounts of bed rest that were naturally occurring. To ensure equal representation of the different amounts of bed rest, nonproportional quota sampling was used.

The characteristics chosen to form the strata are selected according to a researcher's judgement on the basis of knowledge of the population and the literature review. The criterion for selection should be a variable that reflects important differences in the independent variables under investigation. Age, gender, religion, ethnicity, medical diagnosis, socioeconomic status, level of completed education, and occupation are among the variables that are likely to be important in stratifying samples in nursing research investigations.

In critiquing a research strategy, you need to determine whether the sample strata appropriately reflect the population under consideration and whether the variables used are homogeneous enough to ensure a meaningful comparison. Even when the researcher has addressed these factors, you must remember that a quota strategy is a nonprobability sample and thus includes an unknown source of bias that affects the external validity. The people who choose to participate may not be typical of the population in terms of the variables being measured, and assessing the possible biases that may be operating is not possible. When the phenomena being investigated are relatively similar within the population, the risk of bias may be minimal; however, in heterogeneous populations, the risk of bias is greater.

TABLE **13.2**			
NUMBERS AND PERCENTAGES OF STUDENTS IN STRATA OF A QUOTA SAMPLE OF 5,000 GRADUATES OF NURSING PROGRAMS IN A PARTICULAR CITY			
CATEGORIES	**DIPLOMA GRADUATES**	**PRACTICAL NURSES**	**BACCALAUREATE GRADUATES**
Strata	1000 (20%)	2000 (40%)	2000 (40%)
Quota sample	100	200	200

Evidence-Informed Practice Tip ____

When you think about applying study findings to your clinical practice, consider whether the participants in the sample are similar to your own patients.

Probability Sampling

The primary characteristic of probability sampling is the random selection of elements from the population. In **random selection**, each element of the population has an equal and independent chance of being included in the sample. In the hierarchy of evidence, probability sampling represents the strongest type of sampling strategy. That means there is greater confidence that the sample is representative rather than biased and that it more closely reflects the characteristics of the population of interest. Nevertheless, there will always be differences between the sample and the population; this difference is called sampling error. Four commonly used probability sampling strategies are *simple random sampling, stratified random sampling, cluster sampling*, and *systematic sampling.*

Random selection of sample participants should not be confused with random assignment of participants. As discussed in Chapter 11, *randomization* refers to the assignment of participants to either an experimental or a control group on a purely random basis.

Simple Random Sampling

Simple random sampling is a laborious and carefully controlled process. Because the principles of simple random sampling are incorporated in the more complex probability designs, the principles of this strategy are presented.

In **simple random sampling**, the researcher defines the population (a set), lists all units of the population (a **sampling frame**), and selects a sample of units (a subset) from which the sample will be chosen. For example, if Canadian hospitals specializing in the treatment of cancer were the sampling unit, a list of all such hospitals

would be the sampling frame. If certified adult nurse practitioners constituted the accessible population, a list of those nurses would be the sampling frame.

Once a list of the population elements has been developed, the best method of selecting a sample is to employ a table of random numbers containing columns of digits, as shown in Figure 13.1. Such tables can be generated by computer programs. For example, Tryphonopoulos and Letourneau (2020) tested a video-feedback interaction guidance intervention designed to improve maternal–infant interaction, depressive symptoms, and cortisol patterns of depressed mothers and their infants. Participants were allocated into either the intervention or control group using an online randomization program (http://www.random.org/sequences/) with the number 1 denoting intervention group placement and the number 2 denoting control group placement. Once pre-test data were collected, the program was used to generate one of these two integers randomly, and subsequent group placement was assigned accordingly (pp. 3–4). The system generated a random blocking table, which ensured even distribution of the control and experimental group in all four sites of the study. After assigning consecutive numbers to units of the population, the researcher starts at any point on the table of random numbers and reads consecutive numbers in any direction (i.e., horizontally, vertically, or diagonally). When a number is read that corresponds with the written unit on a card, that unit is chosen for the sample. The investigator continues to read until a sample of the desired size is drawn. As an example, Henrique et al. (2018) randomly allocated 128 patients into one of the following interventions groups: warm shower hydrotherapy, perineal exercises with a ball, and the combination of interventions of warm shower hydrotherapy with perineal exercises with a ball (p. 2).

The advantages of simple random sampling are as follows:

- The sample selection is not subject to the conscious biases of the researcher.

1000 random integers between 0 and 99

40	23	0	29	10	94	17	58	12	85	13	25	80	84	72	74	54	63	55	31
32	98	59	23	74	97	51	42	21	87	48	64	54	38	84	68	14	17	35	48
84	34	84	14	53	65	67	37	2	45	84	21	71	34	10	80	72	27	11	13
86	37	24	89	23	4	44	40	72	81	44	69	25	44	34	34	34	75	50	50
50	58	85	8	22	24	73	20	63	35	60	87	91	92	96	80	19	22	87	24
1	87	43	82	9	31	40	88	33	28	82	73	18	6	48	64	59	45	34	3
21	19	42	76	84	67	29	68	8	66	93	89	96	28	12	14	38	47	52	65
32	66	33	21	81	97	39	76	67	27	97	22	76	89	41	11	91	29	6	66
16	82	42	75	35	42	92	90	77	24	21	8	36	16	5	54	89	51	57	85
74	32	63	65	93	96	18	36	82	72	39	69	37	97	51	17	36	71	38	30
50	94	4	66	17	37	10	53	8	29	67	74	88	38	11	59	60	91	56	17
71	47	81	18	53	98	7	87	29	37	22	93	13	6	95	7	95	71	14	6
71	93	48	16	33	19	46	21	60	44	52	91	52	58	10	9	41	31	35	18
20	94	13	99	45	6	53	54	1	25	79	28	1	48	36	26	68	37	59	7
75	22	69	56	62	40	64	45	40	99	94	14	98	84	22	38	24	87	43	71
16	87	41	0	88	83	11	37	71	78	22	39	43	37	75	84	84	11	55	58
92	90	80	2	30	37	84	55	56	50	3	71	24	13	62	74	82	44	90	32
96	89	31	32	37	45	70	67	80	55	58	9	55	60	61	55	86	44	27	77
38	29	36	94	65	39	56	29	29	65	88	13	71	38	71	8	81	66	31	44
20	6	61	66	90	13	70	60	92	53	87	49	34	42	14	47	75	33	26	9
63	44	94	21	14	13	41	80	39	72	29	3	25	89	44	88	13	49	18	58
13	32	93	90	31	75	86	95	18	51	61	59	84	95	67	54	40	30	29	63
26	35	48	81	19	24	36	36	76	16	46	5	93	41	97	46	79	54	95	49
89	74	96	95	94	69	31	60	16	69	76	42	28	71	69	34	46	55	20	42
50	39	28	64	20	68	60	33	92	82	61	70	5	68	95	88	12	85	18	94
55	86	5	96	87	69	75	93	54	79	0	57	45	8	86	59	25	21	9	29
75	35	1	2	86	62	70	83	85	13	97	37	13	73	16	38	36	23	54	11
74	50	1	77	87	92	68	87	57	36	17	47	0	97	78	72	72	45	54	51
34	24	35	13	26	42	22	75	47	2	34	87	15	50	65	27	5	72	28	68
73	33	42	65	91	24	44	84	71	55	70	1	27	30	8	61	65	61	18	92
7	55	12	6	61	17	23	95	91	58	60	30	35	61	34	27	75	44	35	64
10	94	18	4	3	19	21	37	28	55	76	25	10	29	80	64	8	81	20	32
20	48	92	87	95	58	57	73	42	1	12	81	94	85	63	97	24	19	93	51
81	10	92	49	70	15	76	4	36	92	62	99	78	32	86	74	43	22	98	46
66	67	82	94	67	75	16	88	84	98	0	52	37	0	43	9	0	51	2	62
84	92	36	11	3	52	44	65	45	67	97	86	92	2	50	5	93	66	73	40
36	29	98	46	88	23	28	44	8	71	69	43	53	16	87	21	56	23	37	24
15	11	82	30	59	94	23	30	40	25	87	26	24	30	44	53	33	65	72	55
89	57	49	79	83	88	42	45	41	93	38	24	15	80	97	18	61	12	13	42
23	36	65	9	64	26	93	37	26	44	42	17	45	68	27	77	74	56	49	34
9	93	90	61	45	40	75	85	64	66	36	89	72	43	99	90	92	10	10	85
53	94	30	31	62	92	82	30	94	56	40	4	50	53	9	74	87	2	36	36
18	69	77	38	89	78	30	68	71	92	22	93	91	74	52	1	97	69	71	42
50	20	76	36	6	20	75	56	36	5	14	70	9	78	23	33	91	33	25	72
30	46	1	10	16	72	69	26	94	39	80	36	36	68	92	74	22	74	41	42
59	47	7	92	77	55	2	12	5	24	0	30	25	62	83	36	92	96	36	75
93	22	3	20	82	44	16	69	98	72	30	57	77	15	90	29	32	38	3	48
9	55	27	41	40	94	77	14	54	10	25	75	1	74	72	15	69	80	33	58
70	8	3	5	46	89	28	86	40	6	25	40	81	26	63	97	87	48	26	41
19	6	89	31	80	60	13	89	17	69	38	93	58	55	54	69	74	33	8	55

FIG. 13.1 A table of random numbers.

- The representativeness of the sample is maximized in relation to the population characteristics.
- The differences in the characteristics of the sample and the population are purely a function of chance.
- The probability of choosing a nonrepresentative sample decreases as the size of the sample increases.

You must remember, however, that although a researcher may use a carefully controlled sampling procedure that minimizes error, no guarantee exists that the sample will be representative. Factors such as sample heterogeneity and participant dropout may jeopardize the representativeness of the sample despite the most stringent random sampling procedure. In examining the relationship between critical care nurses' information-seeking behaviour, perception of personal control, training, and the nonroutineness of tasks, Newman, Doran, and Nagle (2014) drew the sample from a population of critical care nurses working in hospitals in Ontario, Canada, to reduce heterogeneity. A random sample was drawn from the College of Nurses of Ontario database.

The major disadvantage of simple random sampling is that it is a time-consuming and inefficient method of obtaining a random sample. (Consider the task of listing all baccalaureate nursing students in Canada.) With random sampling, it may also be impossible to obtain an accurate or complete listing of every element in the population. Imagine, for example, trying to obtain a list of all completed suicides in Toronto for 2021. Although suicide may have been the cause of death, another cause (e.g., cardiac failure) often appears on the death certificate. It would be difficult to estimate how many elements of the target population would be eliminated from consideration. Bias would definitely be an issue, despite the researcher's best efforts. Thus, the evaluator of a research article must exercise caution in generalizing from reported findings, even when random sampling is the stated strategy, if the target population has been difficult or impossible to list completely.

Stratified Random Sampling

Stratified random sampling requires that the population be divided into strata or subgroups. The subgroups or subsets that the population is divided into are homogeneous. An appropriate number of elements from each subset is randomly selected on the basis of the proportion in the population. The goal of this strategy is to achieve a greater degree of representativeness. Stratified random sampling is similar to the proportional stratified quota sampling strategy discussed earlier in this chapter. The major difference is that stratified random sampling involves a random selection procedure for obtaining sample participants. Figure 13.2 illustrates the use of stratified random sampling.

The population is stratified according to any number of attributes, such as age, gender, ethnicity, religion, socioeconomic status, or level of education completed. The variables selected to make up the strata lead to subgroups that share one or more of the attributes being studied (see Practical Application box). The following questions can be asked in the selection of a stratified sample:

- Does a critical variable or attribute exist that provides a logical basis for stratifying the sample?
- Does the population list contain sufficient information about the attributes that will be used to divide the sample into subsets?
- Is it appropriate for each subset to be equal in size, or is it more appropriate for each subset to be proportionally stratified on the basis of the proportion of each subset in the population?
- If proportional sampling is being used, is the number of participants in each subset sufficient as a base for meaningful comparisons?
- Once the subset comparison has been determined, are random procedures used for selection of the sample?

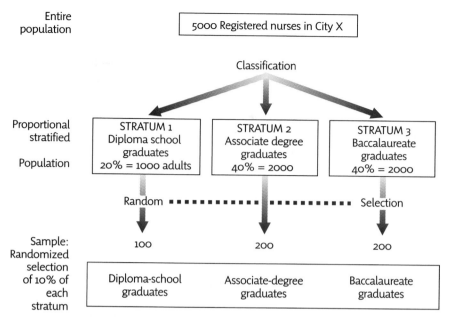

FIG. 13.2 Participant selection through the use of a proportional stratified random sampling strategy.

Practical Application

Koopman et al. (2016) explored the relationship between hope, coping, and quality of life in adults with myasthenia gravis. The researchers stratified a sample of 100 patients to match the proportion of these patients according to the type of myasthenia gravis in the population: 25% ocular myasthenia gravis and 75% generalized myasthenia gravis.

As illustrated in Table 13.1, a stratified random sampling strategy has the following advantages: (1) the representativeness of the sample is enhanced, and (2) the risk of bias is low (i.e., the researcher has a valid basis for making comparisons among subsets if information about the critical variables has been available). A third advantage is that the researcher is able to oversample a disproportionately small stratum to adjust for the researchers' underrepresentation, statistically weigh the data accordingly, and continue to make legitimate comparisons.

The obstacles encountered by a researcher in using this strategy include (1) the difficulty of obtaining a population list containing complete critical variable information; (2) the time-consuming effort of obtaining multiple enumerated lists; (3) the challenge of enrolling proportional strata; and (4) the time and money involved in carrying out a large-scale study with a stratified sampling strategy. In critiquing the study, you must question the appropriateness of this sampling strategy for the problem under investigation.

Havaei et al. (2016) used a proportionate stratified random sample, based on health authorities and employment status, to describe and compare registered nurse (RN) and licensed practical nurse (LPN) emotional exhaustion, intention to leave, and reasons for leaving. It is appropriate for the researcher to strive to represent all strata proportionately in the study sample.

Multistage Sampling (Cluster Sampling)

Multistage sampling, or **cluster sampling**, involves a successive random sampling of units (clusters) that meet sample eligibility criteria; this sampling progresses from large to small. A **sampling unit** is an element or set of elements used for selecting the sample. The first-stage sampling unit consists of large units or clusters. The second-stage sampling unit consists of smaller units or clusters. Third-stage sampling units are even smaller.

Consider an example in which a sample of nurse practitioners is desired. The first sampling unit is a random sample of hospitals, obtained from a provincial nurses' association list, that meet the eligibility criteria (e.g., size, type). The second-stage sampling unit consists of a list of acute care nurse practitioners (ACNPs) practising at each hospital selected in the first stage (i.e., the list obtained from the vice president for nursing at each hospital). The criteria for inclusion in the list of ACNPs are as follows: (1) participants must be certified ACNPs with at least 2 years' experience as an ACNP; (2) at least 75% of the ACNPs' time must be spent in providing care directly to patients in acute or critical care practices; and (3) the participants must be in full-time employment at the hospital. The second-stage sampling strategy calls for random selection of two ACNPs from each hospital who meet the eligibility criteria.

When multistage sampling is used in relation to large national surveys, provinces are used as the first-stage sampling unit, followed by successively smaller units (such as counties, cities, districts, and blocks) as the second-stage sampling unit and then households as the third-stage sampling unit.

Sampling units or clusters can be selected by simple random or stratified random sampling methods (see Practical Application box). Suppose that the hospitals described in the preceding example are grouped into four strata according to size (i.e., number of beds) as follows: (1) 200 to 299; (2) 300 to 399; (3) 400 to 499; and (4) 500 or more. Stratum 1 comprises 25% of the population; stratum 2 comprises 30% of the population; stratum 3 comprises 20% of the population; and stratum 4 comprises 25% of the population. Thus, either a simple random or a proportional stratified sampling strategy can be used to randomly select hospitals that would proportionately represent the population of hospitals in the provincial nurses' association list. An example of cluster sampling being used is the study by Rostad et al. (2018), where the researchers assessed whether regular pain assessment using a pain assessment tool is associated with changes in (1) pain scores and (2) analgesic use in nursing home residents with severe dementia. A cluster was defined as a single nursing home, and it was used to decrease the risk of contamination effects (see Chapter 17).

The main advantage of cluster sampling, as stated in Table 13.1, is that it is considerably more economical in terms of time and money than other types of probability sampling, particularly when the population is large and geographically dispersed or when a sampling frame of the elements is not available. However, cluster sampling has two major disadvantages: (1) more sampling errors tend to occur than with simple random or stratified random sampling, and (2) the appropriate handling of the statistical data from cluster samples is very complex.

In critiquing a research report, you need to consider whether the use of cluster sampling is justified in light of the research design, as well as other pragmatic matters, such as economy.

Practical Application

Sawatzky et al. (2019) used a two-stage clustered and stratified sampling strategy. Stage 1 involved a random selection of 114 sites from five health authorities in BC, which included both urban and rural jurisdictions. The sampling of sites was clustered by health authority and stratified by type of site (39 acute medical units, 37 home care settings, and 38 residential care facilities), size of site (based on a median split of the sizes of sites within each health authority), and, for acute medical care units, whether the site was specialized or general medical unit.

Laschinger, Read, Wilk, et al. (2014) used a cluster sample of 525 nurses in 49 nursing units in 25 acute care hospitals, across all regions in Ontario, to study the influence of nursing unit empowerment and social capital on unit effectiveness and nurse perceptions of patient care quality.

Systematic Sampling

Systematic sampling is a sampling strategy that involves the selection of every "*k*th" case drawn from a population list at fixed intervals, such as every 10th member listed in the directory of the College and Association of Registered Nurses of Alberta (CARNA). Systematic sampling might be used to recruit every "*k*th" person who enters a hospital lobby or who is hospitalized with a diagnosis with the COVID-19 infection in 2020. When systematic sampling is used, the population must be narrowly defined (e.g., as consisting of all people entering or leaving the hospital lobby) for the sample to be considered a probability sample. If older adults were sampled systematically on entering a hospital lobby, the resulting sample would not be a probability sample because not every older adult would have a chance of being selected. As such, systematic sampling can sometimes represent a nonprobability sampling strategy.

Systematic sampling strategies can be designed, however, to fulfill the requirements of a probability sample. First, the listing of the population (sampling frame) must be random in relation to the variable of interest. For example, suppose that participants were being selected from every 10th hospital room for a study on patient satisfaction with nursing care. In the hospital where the study was being conducted, every 10th room happened to be a private room. Patients in private rooms might respond differently regarding their satisfaction than patients in semiprivate rooms. Because of the nonrandom arrangement of the rooms, bias may be introduced.

Second, the first element or member of the sample must be selected randomly. In this case, the researcher—who has a population list, or sampling frame—first divides the population *(N)* by the size of the desired sample *(n)* to obtain the sampling interval width *(k)*. The **sampling interval** is the standard distance between the elements chosen for the sample. For example, to select a sample of 50 family nurse practitioners from a population of 500 family nurse practitioners, the sampling interval would be as follows:

$$k = \frac{500}{50} = 10$$

Essentially, every 10th case on the family nurse practitioner list would be sampled. Thus, if the starting point was participant 5, the next person chosen would be 15th, then 25th, etc.

Once the sampling interval has been determined, the researcher uses a table of random numbers (see Figure 13.1) to obtain a starting point for the selection of the 50 participants. If the population size is 500 and a sample size of 50 is desired, a number between 1 and 500 is randomly selected as the starting point. In this instance, if the first number is 51, the family nurse practitioners corresponding to numbers 51, 61, 71, and so forth would be included in the sample of 50.

Another procedure recommended in many texts is to randomly select the first element from within the first sampling interval. If the sampling interval is 5, a number between 1 and 5 is selected as the random starting point. For example, the number 3 is randomly chosen. Keeping in mind the sampling interval of 5, the next elements selected would correspond to the numbers 8, 13, 18, and so on, until the sample was obtained. Although this procedure is technically correct, choosing a random starting point from across the total population of elements is more attractive because every element has a chance to be chosen for the sample during the first selection step.

Systematic sampling and simple random sampling are essentially the same type of procedure. The advantage of systematic sampling is that the results are obtained in a more convenient and efficient manner (see Table 13.1). The disadvantage of systematic sampling is that bias in the form of nonrandomness can be inadvertently introduced into the procedure. This problem may occur if the population list is arranged so that a certain type of element is listed at intervals that coincide with the sampling interval. For example, if every 10th nursing student on a population list of all types of nursing students in Ontario was a baccalaureate student and the sampling interval was 10, baccalaureate students would be overrepresented in the sample.

Cyclical fluctuations are also a factor in systematic sampling. For example, if a list is kept of nursing students using the college library each day to do computer literature searches, a biased sample would probably be obtained if every seventh day, such as Sunday, is chosen as the sampling interval because probably fewer and perhaps different nursing students use the library on Sundays than on weekdays. Therefore, caution must be exercised about departures from randomness because they affect the representativeness of the sample and, as a result, the external validity of the study.

You should note whether a satisfactory random selection procedure was performed. If randomization was not used, the systematic sampling may have become a nonprobability quota sample. You need to be cognizant of this issue because the implications related to interpretation and generalizability are drastically altered when a nonprobability sample is involved.

For example, in their study, Ridout, Aucoin, Browning, and associates (2014) explored the incidence of failure to communicate vital information as patients progressed through the six phases of the perioperative process. One thousand eight hundred fifty-eight eligible surgical cases were identified, and 293 charts needed to be reviewed to achieve a power of 0.8 and determine a difference at the 0.05 level. Every sixth record that met the criteria was used for the study. Because randomization was not used at any phase of this multilevel sampling procedure, you would consider this study to be a nonprobability stratified sample with the external validity limitations of that sampling strategy (see Chapter 10).

Evidence-Informed Practice Tip

The sampling strategy, whether probability or nonprobability, must be appropriate for the study design and evaluated in relation to the level of evidence provided by the design.

Special Sampling Strategies

Several special sampling strategies are used in nonprobability sampling. **Matching** is a special strategy used to construct an equivalent comparison sample group by filling it with participants who are similar to each participant in another sample group in terms of pre-established variables, such as age, gender, level of education, medical diagnosis, or socioeconomic status. Theoretically, any variable other than the independent variable that could affect the dependent variable should be matched. In reality, the more variables matched, the more difficult it is to obtain an adequate sample size.

For example, Graziotti, Hammond, Messinger, and colleagues (2012) examined strategies to maximize retention in longitudinal studies involving high-risk families. The researchers conducted a follow-up study of 1388 children, half of whom were initially identified as cocaine or opiate exposed ($n = 658$), who were then matched to a non-cocaine- or non-opiate-exposed control ($n = 730$), based on gestational age, race, and gender.

SAMPLING STRATEGIES USED IN QUALITATIVE RESEARCH

Because nonprobability sampling is the best method of obtaining individuals who are key informants of a phenomenon, these sampling methods are widely used in qualitative research. As described in Chapter 7, qualitative research methods are conducted to gain both insights into and in-depth meaning about experiences, incidents, or events. In qualitative research, the sampling procedure is governed by the methodology used.

Many sampling strategies are used in qualitative sampling, but the most common approaches are *convenience sampling, network sampling, purposive sampling*, and *theoretical sampling*.

Convenience Sampling

Convenience sampling is also used in qualitative research to access participants of a particular phenomenon. Buck-McFadyen and MacDonnell (2017) used a purposeful convenience sampling strategy to recruit nurses and nursing students who had an interest in political activism and who represented a diversity of practice settings, educational backgrounds, and generational cohorts to obtain their sample of 13 educators and 14 nursing students.

Network Sampling

Network sampling, sometimes referred to as **snowball effect sampling** or *snowballing*, is a strategy used for locating samples that are difficult or impossible to locate in other ways. This sampling strategy takes advantage of social networks and the tendency of friends to share characteristics. When a few participants with the necessary eligibility criteria are found, the researcher asks for their assistance in getting in touch with other people with similar characteristics that meet these criteria.

Network sampling was described by O'Byrne et al. (2014), who studied how gay and bisexual men perceived the criminal prosecution of persons living with HIV and who do not disclose their HIV status. They recruited participants by raising awareness of the project within AIDS service agencies, distributed posters in venues frequented by gay men, and used snowball sampling by giving participants a supply of the research assistant's business cards to pass on to others who might be willing to participate.

In a qualitative study, Pesut et al. (2019) explored the implications of a legislated approach to assisted death for nurses' experiences and nursing

practice (see Appendix A). Fifty-nine registered nurses and nurse practitioners were recruited using convenience, purposive, and snowball sampling. The researchers advertised through the Canadian Nurses' Association, through health regions, and through the Canadian Association of MAiD Assessors and Providers (p. 3).

Today, online computer networks, as described in the following section on purposive sampling, can be used to assist researchers in recruiting participants who are otherwise difficult to locate, thereby taking advantage of the networking or snowball effect. The Critical Thinking Decision Path illustrates the relationship between the type of sampling strategy and the appropriate generalizability.

Purposive Sampling

Purposive sampling is an increasingly common strategy in which the researcher's knowledge of the population and its elements is used to handpick the cases to be included in the sample. The researcher usually selects participants who are considered typical of the population.

For example, Currie and Szabo (2020) used purposive sampling to recruit 15 parents (11 mothers and 4 fathers) from medical genetic, endocrine, and neuropsychiatry clinics to study social isolation and exclusion in parents who are caring for children with rare neurodevelopmental disorders.

A purposive sample is also used when a highly unusual group is being studied, such as a population with a rare genetic disease (e.g., Tay-Sachs disease). In this case, the researcher would describe the sample characteristics precisely to ensure that the reader will have an accurate picture of the participants in the sample. This type of sample can also be used to study the differential effect of risk factors in a specific population longitudinally. In another situation, the researcher may wish to interview individuals who reflect a particular characteristic. For example, Guruge et al. (2019) used purposive sampling to clarify older immigrants' social needs, networks, and support and how they shape their capacity, resilience, and independence in aging well in Ontario.

Ganann et al. (2019) used two types of qualitative sampling strategies in their study to explore provider perspectives on facilitators and barriers to accessible service provision for immigrant women with postpartum depression. A stratified purposeful sampling (i.e., by profession, years in practice, practice settings) was employed to select

the initial knowledge users, who were the service providers and administrators, and provided further contacts. Then snowball sampling was used to recruit more knowledge users (p. 192).

Today, computer networks (e.g., online services) can be of great value in helping researchers access and recruit participants for purposive samples. For instance, Balneaves and Alraja (2019) used letters of invitation via e-mails to eligible participants to explore the perspectives of Nurse Practitioner nursing regulatory bodies regarding

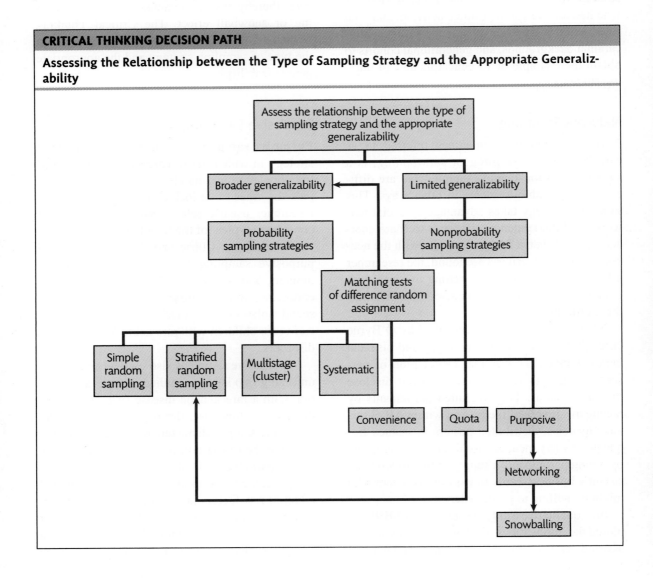

CRITICAL THINKING DECISION PATH

Assessing the Relationship between the Type of Sampling Strategy and the Appropriate Generalizability

practice and policy issues related to medical cannabis.

The researcher who uses a purposive sample assumes that errors of judgement in overrepresenting or underrepresenting elements of the population in the sample will tend to balance each other. The validity of this assumption, however, cannot be determined objectively. You must be aware that the more heterogeneous the population, the greater the chance that bias is introduced in the selection of a purposive sample. As indicated in Table 13.1, conscious bias in the selection of participants remains a constant concern. Therefore, the findings from a study involving a purposive sample should be regarded with caution. As with any nonprobability sample, the ability to generalize is very limited. The following are several instances when a purposive sample may be appropriate:

- The effective pretesting of newly developed instruments with a purposive sample of diverse types of people
- The validation of a scale or test with a known-groups technique
- The collection of exploratory data in relation to an unusual or highly specific population, particularly when the total target population remains unknown to the researcher
- The collection of descriptive data (e.g., as in qualitative studies) with which researchers seek to describe the lived experience of a particular phenomenon (e.g., postpartum depression, caring, hope, or surviving childhood sexual abuse)
- The focus of the study population when it is related to a specific diagnosis (e.g., type 1 diabetes, multiple sclerosis), a specific condition (e.g., legal blindness, terminal illness), or a specific demographic characteristic (e.g., same-sex twin pairs)

Many types of purposive sampling exist (Palys, 2008), but the following three types of cases are the most often used:

1. Typical cases: cases that are "normal" or "average" among those being studied

2. Deviant or extreme cases: cases that represent unusual manifestations of the phenomenon of interest
3. Confirming or disconfirming cases: cases that are exceptions, that represent variation, or for which an initial elaborate analysis is necessary

In any type of purposive sampling, sampling is stopped when **data saturation** occurs—that is, when the information being shared with the researcher becomes repetitive.

Criterion sampling is also a form of purposive sampling. The researcher needs to have a set of criteria for a sample, and all cases that meet these criteria are selected. It is important that the criteria are established so that cases that are chosen will yield rich data relevant to the research problem being explored—for example, all patients who were in a smoking cessation program and have resumed smoking. This criterion would enable an understanding of what is needed to support individuals who wish to quit smoking.

Theoretical Sampling

Theoretical sampling is associated with grounded theory research. As you learned in Chapter 8, the goal of grounded research is theory generation; thus, a theoretical sampling strategy is used to fully elaborate and validate variations in the data by finding examples of a theoretical construct (Sandelowski, 1995). In theoretical sampling, the researcher selects experiences that will help test ideas and gather complete information about developing concepts. Sampling is stopped when theory saturation or redundancy occurs.

Convenience and theoretical sampling were used by King-Shier et al. (2019) who examined the process that South Asians undergo when managing their hypertension. The initial sample was from those who volunteered, then theoretical sampling was used where participants were screened based on: 1) additional criteria to ensure adequate reflection of the group being studied (e.g., sex, age, language, and time since immigration); and 2) emergence of the theory and category. Sampling continued until theoretical saturation occurred, that is, no new data were revealed (p. 322).

Research Hint

Look for a brief discussion of a study's sampling strategy in the "Methods" section of a research article. Some articles have a separate subsection with the heading "Sample," "Participants," or "Study Participants." A statistical description of the characteristics of the actual sample often does not appear until the "Results" section of a research article.

SAMPLE SIZE: QUANTITATIVE

No single rule can be applied to the determination of a sample's size. When researchers estimate sample size, they must consider many factors, such as the following:

- The type of design used
- The type of sampling procedure used
- The type of formula used for estimating the optimal sample size
- The degree of precision required
- The heterogeneity of the attributes under investigation
- The relative frequency at which the phenomenon of interest occurs in the population (i.e., a common versus a rare health problem)
- The projected cost of using a particular sampling strategy
- The homogeneity of the population
- The anticipated response rate of participants
- The attrition rate, especially in longitudinal studies with multiple data collection points

The sample size should be determined before the study is conducted. A general rule is always to use the largest sample possible. The larger the sample, the more likely it is to be representative of the population; smaller samples produce less accurate results.

An exception to the rule about sample size is the **pilot study**, which is a small sample study conducted as a prelude to a larger-scale (parent) study. The pilot study typically is conducted with similar methods and procedures that both yield preliminary data for determining the feasibility of conducting a larger-scale study and establish that sufficient scientific evidence exists to justify subsequent, more extensive research.

Hertzog (2008) summarized methods for justifying sample sizes on the basis of the aim of the pilot study. This author suggests that a sample size as small as 10 to 15 participants per group may be sufficient for the decisions being made but cautions that this is not a simple or straightforward issue as these types of studies are influenced by many factors as noted above. For pilot studies involving group comparisons, 10 to 20 participants per group may be enough. On the other hand, if a researcher is developing or testing an instrument, it is suggested that each group comprise 35 to 40 participants. For example, Santiago et al. (2019) conducted a pilot study to (1) measure the feasibility of implementing a tablet equipped with a communication app (TalkRocketGoTM) for patients with an endotracheal or tracheostomy tube who are unable to communicate using verbal speech, and (2) determine if bedside clinicians find a tablet equipped with a communication app a useful device in clinician-patient communication interactions (p. 18); the sample size was 20 patients. Billingham et al. (2013) concluded in their review of sample sizes for pilot and other feasibility studies that these type of studies do not necessarily require a sample size calculation, but researchers should be able to justify their chosen sample size. There are also other methods of ascertaining sample sizes in a pilot study based on a simple formula with a chosen level of confidence, problems that may arise with a given probability (Viechtbauer et al., 2015).

The principle of "larger is better" holds true for both probability and nonprobability samples. Results based on small samples (fewer than 10 participants) tend to be unstable; the values fluctuate from one sample to the next. Small samples tend to increase the probability of obtaining a markedly nonrepresentative sample. As the sample size increases, the mean more closely approximates the population values; thus, fewer sampling errors are introduced.

An example of this concept is illustrated by a study in which the average monthly consumption of sleeping pills was investigated for patients on a rehabilitation unit after a cerebrovascular accident. The data in Table 13.3 indicate that the population consisted of 20 patients whose average consumption of sleeping pills was 15.2 per month. The population of 20 patients was divided into sets of two simple random samples with sizes of 2, 4, 6, and 10. Each sample average in the right column represents an estimate of the population average, which is known to be 15.15. In most cases, the population value was unknown to the researchers, but because the population is so small, it could be calculated. In Table 13.3, note that with a sample size of two, the estimate might have been wrong by as much as eight sleeping pills in sample 1B. As the sample size increases, the averages get closer to the population value, and the differences in the estimates between samples A and B also get smaller. Large samples permit the principles of randomization to work effectively (i.e., to counterbalance atypical values in the long run).

The sample size can be estimated with the use of a statistical procedure known as *power analysis* (see Chapter 17). A simple example illustrates this concept. Suppose that a researcher wants to determine the effect of nurse preoperative teaching on patient postoperative anxiety. Patients are randomly assigned to an experimental group or a control group. How many patients should be used in the study? When using power analysis, the researcher must estimate how large a difference will be observed between the groups (i.e., the difference in the mean amount of postoperative anxiety after the experimental preoperative teaching program). This difference is called the **effect size**. If a small difference is expected, the sample must be large (in this case, 196 patients in each group) to ensure that the differences will be revealed in a statistical analysis. If a medium-size difference is expected, the total sample size would be 128 (64 in each group). When expected differences are large, a small sample size can ensure that differences will be revealed through statistical analysis.

An example is illustrated by the study of Penz et al. (2018) who tested a conceptual model of confidence and competence in rural and remote nursing practice. Before data collection, they

TABLE **13.3**

COMPARISON OF POPULATION AND SAMPLE VALUES AND AVERAGES IN A STUDY OF SLEEPING PILL CONSUMPTION

NUMBER IN GROUP	GROUP	NUMBER OF SLEEPING PILLS CONSUMED (VALUES EXPRESSED MONTHLY)	AVERAGE
20	Population	1, 3, 4, 5, 6, 7, 9, 11, 13, 15, 16, 17, 19, 21, 22, 23, 25, 27, 29, 30	15.2
2	Sample 1A	6, 9	7.5
2	Sample 1B	21, 25	23.0
4	Sample 2A	1, 7, 15, 25	12.0
4	Sample 2B	5, 13, 23, 29	17.5
6	Sample 3A	3, 4, 11, 15, 21, 25	13.3
6	Sample 3B	5, 7, 11, 19, 27, 30	16.5
10	Sample 4A	3, 4, 7, 9, 11, 13, 17, 21, 23, 30	13.8
10	Sample 4B	1, 4, 6, 11, 15, 17, 19, 23, 25, 27	13.8

conducted a power analysis, with an alpha value set at .05 and the power set at .80; the power analysis indicated that a minimum sample size of 1889 would be required to detect a significant effect (with a small effect size of 0.1). Alpha is the probability of making a type I error (rejecting the null hypothesis when the null hypothesis is true). Another example is provided by Tryphonopoulos and Letourneau (2020), who conducted a feasibility pilot study to test a video-feedback interaction guidance intervention designed to improve maternal–infant interaction, depressive symptoms, and cortisol patterns of depressed mothers and their infants. At the outset of the study, original power calculations (20 per group, alpha .05, power .080) would have been sufficient to detect a moderate effect in the primary outcome of maternal–infant interaction. Instead their recruitment was slow, and they obtained only 12 participants, 6 in each group. Therefore, all analyses were underpowered, leading to possible Type II error, which means that no group differences were found when there could possibly be differences (see Chapter 17).

Power analysis is an advanced statistical technique that is commonly used by researchers and is a requirement for external funding. When power analysis is not used, research studies may be based on samples that are too small, which may lead to a lack of support for the researcher's hypotheses and to a type I error (rejecting a null hypothesis when it should have been accepted); in other words, the researcher finds significant results when none exist (see Chapter 17). A researcher may also commit a type II error (accepting a null hypothesis when it should have been rejected) if the sample is too small; in other words, the sample is too small to detect treatment effects (see Chapter 17).

Despite the principles related to determining sample size that have been identified in this chapter, you should be aware that large samples do not ensure representativeness or accuracy. A large sample cannot compensate for faulty research design. The proportion of the population that is sampled does not provide a guarantee of accurate results. Accurate results can be obtained from only a small fraction of a large population. For example, a 10% probability sample of a population containing 1500 elements will yield more precise results than will a nonprobability .01% sample of a population with 100,000 elements.

You should evaluate the sample size in terms of (1) how representative the sample is of the target population and (2) to which population the researcher wishes to generalize the results of the study. The goal of sampling is to gather a sample as representative as possible with as few sampling errors as possible.

SAMPLE SIZE: QUALITATIVE

In qualitative research, no power analyses are conducted a priori to determine sample size requirements, but there is discussion around thinking of a priori sample size (Sim et al., 2018; Turner-Bowker et al. 2018). According to Sandelowski (1995), sample size is determined by the purpose and type of the sampling and the research method to be used. Morse (1994) recommended about six participants for phenomenological studies and about 30 to 50 cases for ethnographies and grounded theory studies. Creswell (1998) suggests 5 to 25 cases for phenomenology and 20–30 cases for a grounded theory. As you can see, these are suggestions and do not constitute a hard-and-fast rule because a one-person case study may be sufficient for a phenomenological study. When you critique a study, you need to note how the researcher has explained the sampling plan, how data saturation was met, and what limitations have been stated. Participants are added to the sample until data saturation is reached (i.e., new data no longer emerge during the data-collection process). The fittingness of the data is a more important concern than the representativeness of participants (see Chapter 15).

Research Hint

Remember to look for some rationale about the sample size and the strategies that the researcher has used (e.g., matching, test of differences on demographic variables) to ascertain or build in sample representativeness.

Evidence-Informed Practice Tip

Research designs and types of samples are often linked. You would expect to see experimental designs in which probability sampling strategies were used; if a nonprobability purposive sampling strategy is used to recruit participants to such a study, you would expect the participants to then be randomly assigned to intervention and control groups.

SAMPLING PROCEDURES

The criteria for selecting a sample vary according to the sampling strategy. Regardless of which strategy is used, the procedure must be systematically organized. Such organization will eliminate the bias that occurs when sample selection is carried out inconsistently. Bias in sample representativeness and generalizability of findings are important sampling issues that have generated national concern.

For example, many of the landmark adult health studies (e.g., the Framingham Heart Study and the Baltimore Longitudinal Study of Aging) historically excluded women as participants. The findings of these studies were generalized from men to all adults despite the lack of female representation in the samples. Findings based on Euro-American or Euro-Canadian data cannot be generalized to Punjabis, Chinese, West Indians, or any other cultural group. Consequently, careful identification of the target population is a crucial step in the process. For example, Donnelley et al. (2017) conducted a study to determine if participation in an ethics consultation simulation increased nursing students' knowledge of nursing ethics principles compared to students who were taught ethics principles in the traditional didactic format. The researchers noted that the sample consisted of students from three United States Midwest colleges/universities and that these students may not be representative of all United States students (p. 158).

In order to establish conclusions about, for example, psychosocial stressors related to all patients with a first-time myocardial infarction, both men and women must be included in the target population. As another example, to establish conclusions about the incidence of extrapyramidal adverse effects of haloperidol (Haldol) in a psychiatric ward among Chinese patients in comparison with Euro-Canadians, the target population must be diverse. Sometimes, however, the target population must be gender specific, as when breast or prostate cancer or aspects of pregnancy or menopause are studied.

Several general steps (Figure 13.3) ensure the identification of a consistent approach by the researcher. Initially, the target population (i.e., the entire group of people or objects about whom the researcher wants to establish conclusions or make generalizations) must be identified. The target population may consist, for example, of all female patients with a first-time diagnosis of breast cancer, all children with asthma, all pregnant teenagers, or all doctoral nursing students in Canada.

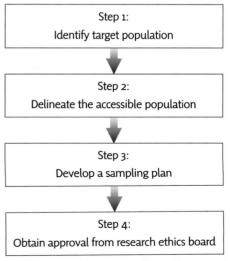

FIG. 13.3 Summary of the general sampling procedures.

Next, the accessible portion of the target population must be delineated. An accessible population might consist of all nurse practitioners in the province of New Brunswick, all older patients with COVID-19 admitted to a certain hospital during 2020, all pregnant teenagers in a specific prenatal clinic, or all children with rheumatoid arthritis under care at a specific hospital specializing in the treatment of autoimmune diseases.

Then a sampling plan or a protocol for actually selecting the sample from the accessible population is formulated. The researcher makes decisions about how participants will be approached, how the study will be explained, and who—the researcher or a research assistant—will select the sample. Regardless of who implements the sampling plan, consistency in how it is done is of paramount importance. In reading a research report, you want to find a description of the sample, as well as the sampling procedure, in the study. On the basis of the appropriateness of what has been reported, you can make judgements about the soundness of the sampling protocol, which of course will affect the interpretations of the findings.

Finally, once the accessible population and sampling plan have been established, permission is obtained from the institution's research board, which is commonly referred to as the *research ethics board*. This permission provides free access to the desired population.

When an appropriate sample size and sampling strategy have been used, the researcher can feel more confident that the sample is representative of the accessible population; however, it is more difficult to feel confident that the accessible population is representative of the target population. Are nurse practitioners in New Brunswick representative of all nurse practitioners in Canada? It is impossible to know for sure. Researchers must exercise judgement when assessing typicality. Unfortunately, no guidelines for making such judgements exist, and critiquers have even less basis on which to make such decisions. The best rule to use when evaluating the representativeness of a sample and its generalizability to the target population is to be realistic and conservative about making sweeping claims in relation to the findings.

Research Hint

Remember to evaluate the appropriateness of the generalizations made about the findings of a quantitative study in view of the target population, the accessible population, the type of sampling strategy, and the sample size. In qualitative research, evaluate the transferability of the findings on the basis of the research design and its sampling strategy and size.

APPRAISING THE EVIDENCE

Sample

The criteria for critiquing the sampling technique of a study are presented in the Critiquing Criteria box. You (the reader) and the researcher approach the "Sample" section of a research report with different perspectives. You need to raise the following two questions:

1. If this study were to be replicated, is enough information available about the nature of the population, the sample, the sampling strategy, and the sample size for another investigator to carry out the study?
2. Are the previously mentioned factors appropriate for the particular research design, and, if not, which factors require modification, especially if the study is to be replicated?

Sampling is considered to be one important aspect of the methodology of a research study. Thus, data pertaining to the sample usually appear in the "Methodology" section of the research report. The sampling content presented should reflect the outcome of a series of decisions based on sampling criteria appropriate to the design of the study, as well as the options and limitations inherent in the context of the investigation. The following discussion highlights several sampling criteria that you should

APPRAISING THE EVIDENCE—cont'd

Sample

consider when you evaluate the merit of a sampling strategy in relation to a specific research study.

Initially, the parameters or attributes of the study population should clearly specify to what population the findings may be generalized. In general, the target population of the study is not specifically identified by the researcher, but the nature of it is implied in the description of the accessible population, the sample, or both. For example, if a researcher states that 100 participants were randomly selected from a population of men and women older than 65 and with a diagnosis of COPD who were treated in a respiratory rehabilitation program at a particular hospital during 2011, you can specifically evaluate the parameters of the population. The demographic characteristics of the sample (e.g., age, gender, diagnosis, ethnicity, religion, and marital status) should also be presented in either a tabular or a narrative summary because they provide further explication about the nature of the sample and enable you to evaluate the sampling procedure more accurately. For example, in their study on predictors of workplace integration for internationally educated nurses (IENs) in Canada, Covell et al. (2017) presented detailed data summarizing demographic variables of importance. These data are reproduced as follows:

The participants were mostly middle-aged (M = 47 years, SD = 11), female (85.2%), and self-identified as a visible minority (57.5%). About half of the IENs received their basic nursing education in a developing country, mostly Philippines and India (54.4%). Most respondents were RNs (89.2%), and the remaining were Licensed Practical Nurses (LPNs) (9.6%) or Registered Practical/Psychiatric Nurses (RPNs) (1.1%) (p. 6).

This example illustrates how a detailed description of the sample both provides a frame of reference for the study population and sample and generates questions to be raised. When this demographic sample information is available, you are able to evaluate the sampling strategy and the impact on the findings. Also helpful is the researcher's rationale for having elected to study one type of population versus another. For example, Covell et al. (2017) wrote that in the last decade, there has been a dramatic increase in IENS, and they would like to find

out how IENs can be facilitated into the Canadian nursing workforce.

In a research study in which a nonprobability sampling strategy is used, it is particularly important to fully describe the population and the sample in terms of who the study participants were, how they were chosen, and the reason they were chosen. If these criteria are adhered to, the degree of heterogeneity or homogeneity of the sample can be determined. The use of a homogeneous sample minimizes the amount of sampling error introduced, a problem particularly common in nonprobability sampling.

Next, the defined representativeness of the population should be examined. Probability sampling is clearly the ideal sampling procedure for ensuring the representativeness of a study population. Use of random selection procedures (e.g., simple random, stratified random, cluster, or systematic sampling strategies) minimizes the occurrence of conscious and unconscious biases that affect the researcher's ability to generalize about the findings from the sample to the population. You should be able to identify the type of probability strategy used and determine whether the researcher adhered to the criteria for a particular sampling plan. In experimental and quasiexperimental studies, you must also know whether or how the participants were assigned to groups. If the criteria have not been followed, you have a valid reason for being skeptical about the proposed conclusions of the study.

Random selection is the ideal in establishing the representativeness of a study population; more often, however, realistic barriers (e.g., institutional policy, inaccessibility of participants, lack of time or money, and current state of knowledge in the field) necessitate the use of nonprobability sampling strategies. Many important research problems that are of interest to nurses do not lend themselves to experimental design and probability sampling, particularly qualitative research designs. A well-designed, carefully controlled study with a nonprobability sampling strategy can yield accurate and meaningful findings that make a significant contribution to nursing's scientific body of knowledge. As the critiquer, you must ask a philosophical question: "If it is not possible or appropriate to conduct an experimental or quasiexperimental investigation

Continued

APPRAISING THE EVIDENCE—*cont'd*

Sample

with the use of probability sampling, should the study be abandoned?" The answer usually suggests that it is better to perform the investigation and be fully aware of the limitations of the methodology than not to acquire the potential knowledge. The researcher is always able to move on to subsequent studies that either replicate the initial study or entail the use of more stringent design and sampling strategies to refine the knowledge derived from a nonexperimental study.

The greatest difficulty in nonprobability sampling stems from the fact that not every element in the population has an equal chance of being represented in the sample. Therefore, some segment of the population will probably be systematically underrepresented. If the population is homogeneous with regard to critical characteristics, systematic bias will not be an important problem. Few of the attributes that researchers are interested in, however, are sufficiently homogeneous to render sampling bias an irrelevant consideration.

Next, the sampling plan's suitability to the research design should be evaluated. In experimental and quasiexperimental designs, some form of random selection or random assignment of participants to groups is used (see Chapter 11). In critiquing the report, you evaluate whether the researcher adhered to the principles of random selection and assignment. Lack of adherence to such principles compromises the representativeness of the sample and the external validity of the study. The following are questions that you might pose in relation to this issue:

- Has a random selection procedure (e.g., a table of random numbers) been identified?
- Has the appropriate random sampling plan been selected? In other words, has a proportional stratified sampling plan been selected instead of a simple random sampling plan in a study in which three distinct occupational levels appear to be critical variables for stratification?
- Has the particular random sampling plan been carried out appropriately? In other words, if a cluster sampling strategy was used, did the sampling units logically progress from the largest to the smallest?

Random sampling should not be regarded as a perfect method of obtaining a representative sample. Sometimes,

bias is inadvertently introduced even when random selection is used. In many nonexperimental designs, nonprobability sampling strategies are used. For such studies, you can ask whether a nonexperimental design and a related nonprobability sampling plan were most appropriate. Sometimes, if the researchers had used another type of design or sampling plan, they could have constructed a stronger study that would have produced findings that were more generalizable and more reliable. In critiquing, however, you are rarely in a position to know what factors entered into the decision to plan one type of study rather than another.

You should then determine whether the sample size is appropriate and its size justifiable. The researcher usually indicates in a research article how the sample size was determined; a similar indication is also seen commonly in doctoral dissertations. The method of arriving at the sample size and the rationale should be briefly mentioned. For example, a researcher may state the following:

A power analysis was performed to calculate the number of participants required in this study exploring mindfulness and anxiety in pregnant women. Previous 8-week mindfulness interventions in pregnant women showed medium-to-large effect sizes for anxiety (Cohen's d, 0.48–0.66) and depression (Cohen's d, 0.42–0.75). Thus, at an effect size of d = 0.58, and allowing for a 25% attrition rate, the total number of participants required was 125 for a power of 0.8 (Yang et al., 2019, p. 69).

Kim and De Gagne (2018) did a power analysis to determine that the required sample size should be 26 participants in each group for an effect size of 0.8 at a significance level of 0.05. (p. 35). Their study compared the effects of two debriefing methods (instructor-led vs. peer-led) on nursing skills, knowledge, self-confidence, and quality of debriefing among undergraduate students (p. 34).

The importance of such examples lies in understanding that this type of statement meets the criteria stated at the beginning of the paragraph and should be evident in the research report. Other considerations with regard to sample size, especially when the sample size appears to be small or inadequate and no rationale is stated for the size, are as follows:

APPRAISING THE EVIDENCE—cont'd

Sample

- How will the sample size affect the accuracy of the results?
- Are any subsets or cells of the sample overrepresented or underrepresented?
- Are any of the subsets so small as to limit meaningful comparisons?
- Has the researcher examined the effect of attrition on the results?
- Has the researcher recognized and identified any limitations posed by the size of the sample?

Essentially, these criteria necessitate that you carefully scrutinize several important elements pertaining to sample size that have implications for the generalizability of the findings. Keep in mind that in reports of qualitative studies, neither the predetermining nor the method of determining the sample size will be discussed. Rather, the sample size depends on the methodology used and is a function of data saturation (see Chapter 8).

With qualitative research designs, you apply criteria related to sampling strategies that are relevant for a particular type of qualitative study. In general, sampling strategies are purposive because the study of specific phenomena in their natural setting is emphasized; any participant belonging to a specified group is considered to represent that group. For example, in the qualitative study by Udod and associates (2020), the specified group was nurse managers implementing the lean management system in Saskatchewan. The researchers' goal was to explore the perceptions and experiences of nurse managers involved in implementing the Lean management system in a Western Canadian province.

Finally, the "Sample" section of the research report should provide evidence that the rights of human participants have been protected. You will evaluate whether permission was obtained from an institutional research ethics board that reviewed the study with regard to maintaining ethical research standards (see Chapter 6). For example, the research ethics board examines the research proposal to determine whether the introduction of an experimental procedure may be potentially harmful and therefore undesirable. You also need to examine the report for evidence of the participants' informed consent, as well as protection of their confidentiality or anonymity. Research studies that do not demonstrate evidence of having met these criteria are highly unusual. Nevertheless, you will want to be certain that ethical standards that protect sample participants have been maintained.

Many factors must be considered when you critique the "Sample" section of a research report. The type and appropriateness of the sampling strategy become crucial elements in the analysis and interpretation of data, in the conclusions derived from the findings, and in the generalizability of the findings from the sample to the population. As stated earlier in this chapter, the major purpose of sampling is to increase the efficacy of a research study by representing the particular population so that not every element need be studied, while producing the findings that can be generalized from the sample to the population. You must demonstrate that the sampling strategy used provided a valid basis for the findings and their generalizability.

CRITIQUING CRITERIA

1. Have the sample characteristics been completely described?
2. Can the parameters of the study population be inferred from the description of the sample?
3. To what extent is the sample representative of the population as defined?
4. Are criteria for eligibility in the sample specifically identified?
5. Have sample delimitations been established?
6. Would it be possible to replicate the study population?
7. How was the sample selected? Is the method of sample selection appropriate?
8. What kind of bias, if any, is introduced by this method?
9. Is the sample size appropriate? How is it substantiated?
10. Does the researcher indicate that the rights of participants have been ensured?
11. Does the researcher identify the limitations in generalizability of the findings from the sample to the population?
12. Is the sampling strategy appropriate for the design of the study and level of evidence provided by the design?
13. Does the researcher indicate how replication of the study with other samples would provide increased support for the findings?

Are those limitations appropriate?

CRITICAL THINKING CHALLENGES

- A research classmate asks the instructor the following question: "Why isn't it better to study an entire population of patients with lung cancer instead of using the research technique of sampling?" How would you answer this question? Include examples that will help the student see your point of view.

- In the report of a quasiexperimental study, the researchers indicated that they used a convenience sample with random assignment. How is this possible? Would they have used a nonprobability or a probability sample? If you agree that this is a legitimate sampling technique, present both the advantages and the disadvantages; if you disagree, indicate your rationale.

- Your research class is having a debate on probability sampling versus nonprobability sampling with regard to desirability and feasibility. You are assigned to present the advantages of nonprobability sampling in nursing research. What arguments would you use?

- Discuss the principle of "larger is better" and its relationship to network sampling and the sample size of qualitative studies. Include in your discussion the concept of data saturation and the use of computer technology.

- Your research classmate is arguing that a random sample is always better, even if it is small and represents only one site. Another student is arguing that a very large convenience sample representing multiple sites can be very significant. Which classmate would you defend, and why?

CRITICAL JUDGEMENT QUESTIONS

1. Why should a researcher avoid drawing conclusions or making generalizations based on the experience of a small number of participants?
   a. Small samples invalidate hypotheses
   b. The researcher may be unable to eliminate his or her bias
   c. Data obtained from a small number may inadequately represent the phenomenon
   d. Small numbers of participants increase the threat to internal validity influenced by history

2. What is the difference between an "accessible population" and a "target population"?
   a. The accessible population meets the inclusion criteria, and the target population meets the exclusion criteria
   b. The target population meets the inclusion criteria, and the accessible population meets the exclusion criteria
   c. The accessible population represents the entire set of cases the researcher wishes to study, and the target population represents that part of the accessible population that could feasibly be included in the study
   d. The target population represents the entire set of cases the researcher wishes to study, and the accessible population represents that part of the target population that could feasibly be included in the study

3. What is the appropriate sampling interval for drawing a systematic sample of 25 subjects who had breast enhancement surgery from 200 people who had that surgery during 1 year at a specific medical centre?
   a. Every 4th patient
   b. Every 5th patient
   c. Every 8th patient
   d. Every 10th patient

KEY POINTS

- Sampling is a process in which representative units of a population are selected for study. Researchers select representative segments of the population because selecting entire populations of interest to obtain accurate and meaningful information is rarely feasible or necessary.
- Researchers establish eligibility criteria; these are descriptors of the population and provide the basis for inclusion into a sample. Eligibility criteria can include age, gender, socioeconomic status, level of education, religion, and ethnicity.

- The researcher must identify the target population (i.e., the entire set of cases about which the researcher would like to make generalizations). Because of pragmatic constraints, however, the researcher usually uses an accessible population (i.e., one that meets the population criteria and is available).
- A sample is a set of elements that make up the population.
- A sampling unit is the element or set of elements used for selecting the sample. The foremost criterion in evaluating a sample is the representativeness or congruence of characteristics with the population.
- Sampling strategies consist of nonprobability and probability sampling.
- In nonprobability sampling, the elements are chosen by nonrandom methods. Types of nonprobability sampling include convenience, quota, and purposive sampling.
- Probability sampling is characterized by the random selection of elements from the population. In random selection, each element in the population has an equal and independent chance of being included in the sample. Types of probability sampling include simple random, stratified random, cluster, and systematic sampling.
- Sample size is a function of the type of sampling procedure being used, the degree of precision required, the type of sample estimation formula being used, the heterogeneity of the study attributes, the relative frequency of occurrence of the phenomena under consideration, and the cost.
- Criteria for selecting a sample vary according to the sampling strategy. Systematic organization of the sampling procedure minimizes bias. The target population is identified, the accessible portion of the target population is delineated, permission to conduct the research study is obtained, and a sampling plan is formulated.
- In critiquing a research report, you evaluate the sampling plan for its appropriateness in relation to the particular research design.

- The completeness of the sampling plan is examined with regard to the potential replicability of the study. In critiquing, you evaluate whether the sampling strategy is the strongest plan for the particular study under consideration.
- An appropriate systematic sampling plan will maximize the efficiency of a research study. It will increase the accuracy and meaningfulness of the findings and enhance the generalizability of the findings from the sample to the population.

FOR FURTHER STUDY

Go to Evolve at http://evolve.elsevier.com/Canada/LoBiondo/Research for the Audio Glossary.

REFERENCES

Balneaves, L. G., & Alraja, A. A. (2019). Guarding their practice": A descriptive study of Canadian nursing policies and education related to medical cannabis. *BMC Nursing, 8*, 66. https://doi.org/10.1186/s12912-0190390-7.

Benbow, S., Forchuk, C., Berman, H., Gorlick, C., & Ward-Griffin, C. (2019). Spaces of Exclusion: Safety, Stigma, and Surveillance of Mothers Experiencing Homelessness. *The Canadian Journal of Nursing Research = Revue Canadienne de Recherche En Sciences Infirmieres, 51*(3), 202–213. https://doi.org/10.1177/0844562119859138.

Billingham, S. A., Whitehead, A. L., & Julious, S. A. (2013). An audit of sample sizes for pilot and feasibility trials being undertaken in the United Kingdom registered in the United Kingdom Clinical Research Network database. *BMC Medical Research Methodology, 13*, 104. https://doi.org/10.1186/1471-2288-13-104.

Buck-McFadyen, E., & MacDonnell, J. (2017). Contested practice: political activism in nursing and implications for nursing education. *International Journal of Nursing Education and Scholarship, 14*(1). https://doi.org/10.1515/ijnes-2016-0026.

Chan, R., Booth, R., Strudwick, G., & Sinclair, B. (2019). Nursing students' perceived self-efficacy and the generation of medication errors with the use of an electronic medication administration record (eMAR) in clinical simulation. *International Journal of Nursing Education Scholarship, 16*(1). https://doi.org/10.1515/ijnes-2019-0014.

Covell, C. L., Primeau, M.-D., Kilpatrick, K., & St-Pierre, I. (2017). Internationally educated nurses in Canada: Predictors of workforce integration. *Human Resources for Health, 15*(1), 1–16. https://doi.org/10.1186/s12960-017-0201-8.

Creswell, J. W. (1998). *Qualitative inquiry and research design: Choosing among five traditions.* Thousand Oaks, CA: Sage Publications.

Currie, G., & Szabo, J. (2020). Social isolation and exclusion: the parents' experience of caring for children with rare neurodevelopmental disorders. *International Journal of Qualitative Studies on Health and Well-Being, 15*, (1). https://doi.org/10.1080/17482631.2020.1725362.

Dennis, C., Merry, L., & Gagnon, A. (2017). Postpartum depression risk factors among recent refugee, asylum-seeking, non-refugee immigrant, and Canadian-born women: results from a prospective cohort study. *Social Psychiatry and Psychiatric Epidemiology, 52*(4), 411–422. https://doi.org/10.1007/s00127-017-1353-5.

Donnelly, M. B., Horsley, T. L., Adams, W. H., Gallagher, P., & Zibricky, C. D. (2017). Effect of simulation on undergraduate nursing students' knowledge of nursing ethics principles. *Canadian Journal of Nursing Research, 49*(4), 153–159. https://doi.org/10.1177/0844562117731975.

Dosani, A., Hemraj, J., Premji, S. S., Currie, G., Reilly, S. M., Lodha, A. K., Young, M., & Hall, M. (2017). Breastfeeding the late preterm infant: Experiences of mothers and perceptions of public health nurses. *International Breastfeeding Journal, 12*, 23. https://doi.org/10.1186/s13006-017-0114-0.

Fox, M. T., Sidani, S., & Brooks, D. (2010). Differences in sleep complaints in adults with varying levels of bed days residing in extended care facilities for chronic disease management. *Clinical Nursing Research, 19*(2), 181–202. https://doi.org/10.1177/1054773810365957.

Ganann, R., Sword, W., Newbold, K. B., Thabane, L., Armour, L., & Kint, B. (2019). Provider perspectives on facilitators and barriers to accessible service provision for immigrant women with postpartum depression: A qualitative study. *Canadian Journal of Nursing Research, 51*(3), 191–201. https://doi.org/10.1177/0844562119852868.

Graziotti, A. L., Hammond, J., Messinger, D. S., et al. (2012). Maintaining participation and momentum in longitudinal research involving high-risk families. *Journal of Nursing Scholarship, 44*(2), 120–126.

Guruge, S., Sidani, S., Wang, L., Sethi, B., Spitzer, D., Walton-Roberts, M., & Hyman, I. (2019). Understanding social network and support for older immigrants in Ontario, Canada: Protocol for a mixed-methods study. *JMIR Aging, 2*(1), e12616. https://doi.org/10.2196/12616.

Havaei, F., MacPhee, M., & Susan Dahinten, V. (2016). RNs and LPNs: Emotional exhaustion and intention to leave. *Journal of Nursing Management, 24*, 393–399. https://doi-org.ezproxy.library.yorku.ca/10.1111/jonm.12334.

Henrique, A. J., Gabrielloni, M. C., Rodney, P., & Barbieri, M. (2018). Non-pharmacological interventions during childbirth for pain relief, anxiety, and neuroendocrine stress parameters: A randomized controlled trial. *International Journal of Nursing Practice, 24*(3), e12642. https://doi.org/10.1111/ijn.12642.

Hertzog, M. A. (2008). Consideration in determining sample sizes for pilot studies. *Research in Nursing & Health, 32*, 180–191.

Im, E. O., Chang, S. J., Ko, Y., Chee, W., Stuifbergen, A., & Walker, L. (2012). A national internet survey on midlife women's attitudes toward physical activity. *Nursing Research, 61*(5), 342–352. https://doi.org/10.1097/NNR.0b013e31825da85a.

Jackson, K. T., & Dennis, C. L. (2017). Lanolin for the treatment of nipple pain in breastfeeding women: A randomized controlled trial. *Maternal and Child Nutrition, 13*(3), 1–10. https://doi.org/10.1111/mcn.12357.

Kim, S. S., & De Gagne, J. C. (2018). Instructor-led vs. peer-led debriefing in preoperative care simulation using standardized patients. *Nurse Education Today, 71*, 34–39. https://doi.org/10.1016/j.nedt.2018.09.001.

King-Shier, K. M., Dhaliwal, K. K., Puri, R., LeBlanc, P., & Johal, J. (2019). South Asians' experience of managing hypertension: A grounded theory study. *Patient Preference and Adherence, 13*, 321–329. https://doi.org/10.2147/PPA.S196224.

Koopman, W. J., LeBlanc, N., Fowler, S., et al. (2016). Hope, coping, and quality of life in adults with myasthenia gravis. *Canadian Journal of Neuroscience Nursing, 38*(1), 56–64.

Laschinger, H. K. S., Read, E., Wilk, P., et al. (2014). The influence of nursing unit empowerment and social capital on unit effectiveness and nurse perceptions of patient care quality. *Journal of Nursing Administration, 44*(6), 347–352.

Morse, J. M. (1994). Designing funded qualitative research. In N. K. Denzin, & Y. S. Lincoln (Eds.), *Handbook of qualitative research* (pp. 220–235). Thousand Oaks, CA: Sage.

Newman, K., Doran, D., & Nagle, L. M. (2014). The relation of critical care nurses' information-seeking behavior with perception of personal control, training, and non-routineness of the task. *Dynamics, 25*(1), 13–18.

O'Byrne, P., Bryan, A., Hendriks, A., et al. (2014). Social marginalization and internal exclusion: Gay men's understandings and experiences of community. *Canadian Journal of Nursing Research, 46*(2), 57–79.

Palys, T. (2008). Purposive sampling. In L. M. Given (Ed.). *The Sage encyclopedia of qualitative research methods* (Vol. 2, pp. 697–698). Los Angeles: Sage.

Paul-Savoie, E., Bourgault, P., Potvin, S., Gosselin, E., & Lafrenaye, S. (2018). The impact of pain invisibility on patient-centered care and empathetic attitude in chronic pain management. *Pain Research & Management*. https://doi.org/10.1155/2018/6375713.

Penz, K. L., Stewart, N. J., Karunanayake, C. P., Kosteniuk, J. G., & MacLeod, M. L. P. (2018). Competence and confidence in rural and remote nursing practice: A structural equation modelling analysis of national data. *Journal of Clinical Nursing, 28*, 1664–1679. https://doi.org/10.1111/jocn.14772.

Pesut, B., Thorne, S., Stager, M. L., Schiller, C. J., Penney, C., Hoffman, C., Greig, M., & Roussel, J. (2019). Medical assistance in dying: A review of Canadian nursing regulatory documents. *Policy, Politics & Nursing Practice, 20*(3), 113–130. https://doi.org/10.1177/1527154419845407.

Ridout, J., Aucoin, J., Browning, A., et al. (2014). Does perioperative documentation transfer reliability? *Computers, Informatics, Nursing, 32*, 37–42.

Rostad, H. M., Utne, I., Grov, E. K., Småstuen, M. C., Puts, M., & Halvorsrud, L. (2018). The impact of a pain assessment intervention on pain score and analgesic use in older nursing home residents with severe dementia: A cluster randomised controlled trial. *International Journal of Nursing Studies, 84*, 52–60. https://doi.org/10.1016/j.ijnurstu.2018.04.017.

Sandelowski, M. (1995). Sample size in qualitative research. *Research in Nursing & Health, 18*, 179–183.

Santiago, C., Roza, D., Porretta, K., & Smith, O. (2019). The use of tablet and communication app for patients with endotracheal or tracheostomy tubes in the medical surgical intensive care unit: A pilot, feasibility study. *Canadian Journal of Neuroscience Nursing, 30*(1), 17–23. https://doi.org/10.13140/RG.2.2.19835.57125.

Sawatzky, R., Roberts, D., Russell, L., Bitschy, A., Ho, S., Desbiens, F-F., Chan, E. K. H., Tayler, C., & Stajduhar, K. (2019). Self-perceived competence of nurses and care aides providing a palliative approach in home, hospital, and residential care settings: A cross-sectional survey. *Canadian Journal of Nursing Research, 53*(1), 64–77. https://doi.org/10.1177/0844562119881043.

Sim, J., Saunders, B., Waterfield, J., & Kingstone, T. (2018). Can sample size in qualitative research be determined a priori? *International Journal of Social Research Methodology, 21*(5), 619–634. https://doi.org/10.1080/13645579.2018.1454643.

Tryphonopoulos, P. D., & Letourneau, N. (2020). Promising results from a video-feedback interaction guidance intervention for improving maternal–infant interaction quality of depressed mothers: A feasibility pilot study. *Canadian Journal of Nursing Research, 52*(2), 74–87. https://doi.org/10.1177/0844562119892769.

Turner-Bowker, D., Lamoureux, R. E, Stokes, J., Litcher-Kelly, L., Galipeau, N., Yaworsky, A., Solomon, J., & Shields, A. L. (2018). Informing a priori sample size estimation in qualitative concept elicitation interview studies for clinical outcome assessment instrument development. *Value in Health, 21*(7), 839–842. https://doi.org/10.1016/j.jval.2017.11.014.

Udod, S. A., Duchscher, J. B., Goodridge, D., Rotter, T., McGrath, P., & Hewitt, A. D. (2020). Nurse managers implementing the lean management system: A qualitative study in Western Canada. *Journal of Nursing Management, 28*, 221–228. https://doi-org.ezproxy.library.yorku.ca/10.1111/jonm.12898.

Viechtbauer, W., Smits, L., Kotz, D., Budé, L., Spigt, M., Serroyen, J., & Crutzen, R. (2015). A simple formula for the calculation of sample size in pilot studies. *Journal of Clinical Epidemiology, 68*(11), 1375–1379. https://doi.org/10.1016/j.jclinepi.2015.04.014.

Yang, M., Jia, G., Sun, S., Ye, C., Zhang, R., & Yu, X. (2019). Effects of an online mindfulness intervention focusing on attention monitoring and acceptance in pregnant women: A randomized controlled trial. *Journal of Midwifery & Women's Health, 64*, 68–77. https://doi.org/10.1111/jmwh.12944.

CHAPTER 14

Data-Collection Methods

Mina D. Singh | Ramesh Venkatesa Perumal

LEARNING OUTCOMES

After reading this chapter, you will be able to do the following:

- Define the types of data-collection methods used in nursing research.
- List the advantages and disadvantages of each of these methods.
- Compare how specific data-collection methods contribute to the strength of evidence in a research study.
- Critically evaluate the data-collection methods used in published nursing research studies.

KEY TERMS

biological measurement	intervention fidelity	physiological measurement
closed-ended item	interview	questionnaire
concealment	Likert-type scale	reactivity
consistency	measurement	records or available data
debriefing	objective	scale
external criticism	open-ended item	scientific observation
internal criticism	operational definition	social desirability
intervention	operationalization	systematic

STUDY RESOURCES

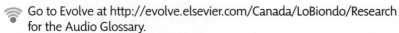 Go to Evolve at http://evolve.elsevier.com/Canada/LoBiondo/Research for the Audio Glossary.

QUANTITATIVE DATA COLLECTION

NURSES USE ALL OF THEIR SENSES when collecting data from the patients to whom they provide care. Nurse researchers also have many ways to collect information about their research participants. Both the data collected when they perform patient care and the data collected for the purpose of research are objective and systematic. Objective means that the data must not be influenced by the person who collects the information, and systematic means that the data must be collected in the same methodical way by each person involved in the collection procedure. The methods that researchers use to collect information about participants are the identifiable and repeatable operations that define the major variables being studied.

Operationalization is the process of translating the concepts of interest to a researcher into observable and measurable phenomena. For example, in their study on the nursing students' perceived self-efficacy and generation of medication errors with the use of an electronic medication administration (eMAR) in clinical simulation, Chan et al. (2019) used Bandura's (1997) definition of self-efficacy, in that it refers to an individual's psychological conviction that he or she can successfully execute the behaviour required to produce the desired outcome. They also used the term *confidence* interchangeably with *self-efficacy* in the study.

This purpose of this chapter is to familiarize you with the various ways in which researchers collect information from and about participants. The chapter provides nurse readers with the tools for evaluating the selection, use, and practicality of the various ways to collect data.

MEASURING VARIABLES OF INTEREST

To a large extent, the success of a study depends on the quality of the data-collection methods chosen and employed. Researchers have many types of methods available for collecting information from participants in research studies. *Measurement* is a term used in quantitative research and is the assignment of numbers to objects or events according to rules; determining which measurement to use in a particular investigation may be the most difficult and time-consuming step in the study design. In addition, nurse researchers have an array of quality instruments with adequate reliability and validity (see Chapter 15). This aspect of the research process necessitates painstaking effort from the researcher. Thus, the process of evaluating and selecting the available tools to measure variables of interest is crucial for the potential success of the study. In this section, the selection of measures and the implementation of the data-collection process are discussed. An algorithm that influences a researcher's choice of data-collection methods is diagrammed in the Critical Thinking Decision Path.

Information about phenomena of interest to nurses can be collected in many different ways. Nurses are interested in the biological and physical indicators of health (e.g., blood pressure and heart rate), but they are also interested in complex psychosocial questions presented by patients. Psychosocial variables, such as anxiety, hope, social support, and self-concept, may be measured by several different techniques, such as observation of behaviour, self-reports of feelings, or self-reports about attitudes in interviews or questionnaires. To study variables of interest, researchers also may use data that have already been collected for another purpose, such as records, diaries, or other media.

Selection of the data-collection method begins during the literature review. As noted in Chapter 5, one purpose of the literature review is to provide clues about instrumentation. As the literature review is conducted, the researcher begins to explore how previous investigators defined and operationalized variables similar to those of interest in the current study. The researcher uses this information to define conceptually the variables to be studied. Once a variable has been defined conceptually, the researcher returns to the literature to define the variable operationally—that is, describe how a concept is measured and what instruments are used to capture the essence of the variable. This operational definition translates the conceptual definition into behaviours or verbalizations that can be measured for the study. In this second literature review, the researcher searches for measurement instruments that might be used "as is" or adapted for use in the study. If instruments are available, the researcher must obtain the author's permission for their use.

The following examples illustrate the relationship of conceptual and operational definitions. Stress research is of interest to researchers from many disciplines, including nursing. Definitions of stressors may be psychological, social, or physiological. If researchers are interested in studying stressors, they must first define

CRITICAL THINKING DECISION PATH

Data-Collection Methods

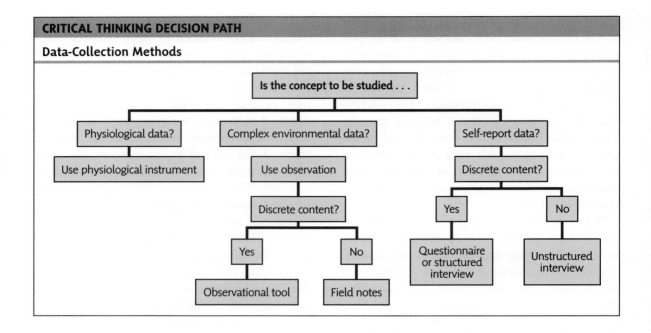

what they mean by the concept of "stressor," both conceptually and operationally. Quality-of-life or health-related quality-of-life research is popular with researchers from many disciplines, including nursing.

Quality of life or health-related quality of life may also be interpreted in a general way (well-being) or be related specifically to a type of illness. Therefore, if researchers are interested in studying quality of life, they need first to define what they mean by the concept of "quality of life." For example, Oviedo et al. (2019) indicated that health-related quality of life is a subjective, multidimensional, integrative construct that includes individual physical and mental well-being (p. 988). If another researcher disagreed with this definition or was more interested in the quality of life of people with another specific illness or the quality of life of children, a different instrument might be more appropriate.

Sometimes no suitable measuring device exists, and so the researcher must then decide how important the variable is to the study and whether a new device should be constructed. The construction of new instruments for data collection that have reasonable reliability and validity (see Chapter 15) is a difficult task. If no suitable measuring device exists, the researcher may decide not to study a variable, or the researcher may decide to invest time and energy in instrument development. Either decision is acceptable, depending on the goals of the study and the goals of the researcher.

Research Hint

Remember that the researcher may not always present complete information about the way the data were collected, especially when established tools were used. To learn about the tool that was used, the reader may need to consult the original article that described the use or development of the tool.

Whether the researcher uses available methods or creates new ones, once the variables have been operationally defined in a manner consistent with the aims of the study, the population to be studied, and the setting, the researcher decides how the data-collection phase of the study will be implemented. This decision concerns how the instruments for data collection will be given to the participants. Consistency is the most important issue in this phase.

Consistency in data collection means that the method used to collect data from each participant in the study is exactly the same or as close to the same as possible. Consistency can minimize the bias introduced when more than one person collects the data. Data collectors must be carefully trained and supervised. To ensure consistency in data collection, sometimes referred to as intervention fidelity, researchers must train data collectors in the methods to be used in the study so that each data collector acquires the information in the same way. Information about how to observe, ask questions, and collect data often is included in a kind of "cookbook" protocol or manual for the research project. A researcher needs to spend time developing the protocol and training data collectors to gather data systematically and reliably. Comments about their training and the consistency with which they collected data for the study should be provided by the researcher. An index of agreement called the *kappa statistic* is used to measure interrater agreement, where researchers will indicate the range of agreement expressed as a percentage of agreement among raters or observers or as a coefficient of agreement that considers the element of chance (coefficient kappa).

An example of intervention fidelity is given in the study by Boitor et al. (2019), in which they designed an intervention to evaluate the effects of hand massage on the pain intensity and pain-related interference in cardiac surgery patients. One interventionist delivered all hand massages and hand holdings except for one that was given by the research coordinator. The interventions were standardized across participants. The interventionist was a registered nurse trained in massage therapy through an accredited workshop of 6 hours by a professional therapist (p. 574).

Another example of the importance of training data collectors appears in the study by Arnstein et al. (2019) where they were validating a new

pain scale on hospitalized adults. Data collectors completed initial training that included a full discussion of the study and research questions, ethical responsibilities in data collection, and the data-collection protocol. The principle investigator or one of the co-investigators met with the data collectors each month during data collection to determine if retraining is necessary.

 Evidence-Informed Practice Tip ____

It is difficult to place confidence in a study's findings if the data-collection methods are not consistent.

TYPES OF DATA-COLLECTION METHODS

In general, data-collection methods can be divided into the following five types: *physiological measurements, observational methods, interviews* and *questionnaires,* and *records or available data.* Each method has a specific purpose, as well as certain advantages and disadvantages inherent in its use. In the following sections, these data-collection methods are discussed, along with their respective uses and problems.

Physiological or Biological Measurements

In everyday practice, nurses collect physiological data about patients, such as their temperature, pulse rate, blood pressure, blood glucose level, urine specific gravity, and pH of bodily fluids. Such data are frequently useful to nurse researchers. Because physiological variables, such as cardiac output and blood pressure, can be measured in several different ways, researchers need to measure these outcomes at similar intervals and in similar ways for all participants of the study. An example of a study using a physiological variable is that by Wang et al. (2018) who used HbA1c and blood glucose levels in their study on a nurse-led smartphone-based self-management programme for poorly controlled type 2 diabetes.

Physiological measurement and biological measurement involve the use of specialized equipment to determine the physical and biological status of participants. Frequently, such measurements also require specialized training. These measurements can be *physical*, such as weight or temperature; *chemical*, such as blood glucose level; *microbiological*, as with cultures; or *anatomical*, as in radiological examinations. What distinguishes these measurements from others used in research is that special equipment is needed to make the observation. A researcher can say, "This participant feels warm," but to determine how warm the participant is requires the use of a sensitive instrument: a thermometer.

The advantages of using physiological data-collection methods include their objectivity, precision, and sensitivity. Such methods are generally considered to yield objective findings because unless a technical malfunction occurs, two readings of the same instrument taken at the same time by two different nurses are likely to yield the same result. Because such instruments are intended to measure the variable being studied, they offer the advantage of being precise and sensitive enough to pick up subtle variations in the variable of interest. Also, the deliberate distortion of physiological information by a participant in a study is highly unlikely to occur.

Physiological measurements are not without inherent disadvantages, however. Some instruments, if not available through a hospital, may be quite expensive to obtain and use. In addition, the accurate use of such instruments often necessitates specialized knowledge and training. Another problem with physiological measurements is that simply by using them, the variable of interest may be changed. Although some researchers think of these instruments as being nonintrusive, the presence of some types of devices might change the measurement. For example, the presence of a heart rate monitoring device might make some patients anxious and thereby increase their heart rate. In addition, nearly all types of measuring devices are affected in some way by the environment. Even a simple thermometer can be affected

by the participant's drinking something hot or cold immediately before the temperature is taken. Thus, when assessing studies that use physiological measurements you need to consider whether the researcher controlled such environmental variables in the study. Finally, a physiological way to measure the variable of interest may not exist. On occasion, researchers try to force a physiological parameter into a study in an effort to increase the precision of measurement. If the device does not measure the variable of interest, however, the validity of the device's use is suspect.

Observational Methods

Although observing the environment is a normal part of living, scientific observation places a great deal of emphasis on the objective and systematic nature of the observation. The researcher is not merely watching what is happening but is watching with a trained eye for certain specific events. Scientific observation fulfills the following four conditions:

1. The observations undertaken are consistent with the study's specific objectives.
2. A standardized and systematic plan exists for the observation and the recording of data.
3. All of the observations are checked and controlled.
4. The observations are related to scientific concepts and theories.

Observation is particularly suitable as a data-collection method in complex research situations that are best viewed as total entities and that are difficult to measure in parts, such as studies dealing with the nursing process, parent–child interactions, or group processes (see Practical Application box for an example). In addition, observational methods can be the best way to operationalize some variables of interest in nursing research studies, particularly individual characteristics and conditions, such as traits and symptoms; verbal and nonverbal communication behaviours, activities, and skill attainment; and environmental characteristics.

Practical Application

Coker et al. (2017) conducted an observational study related to oral care interventions by nurses to hospitalized older people. Nurses were shadowed (one per evening) during their evening care encounters with their assigned patients. In addition to being observed, nurses were engaged in conversation during the observations. The research observer did not use a structured observation checklist but rather described the interventions that were provided.

Observational methods can also be distinguished by the role of the observer. This role is determined by the amount of interaction between the observer and the people being observed. Each of the following four basic types of observational roles is distinguishable by the amount of concealment or intervention implemented by the observer:

1. Concealment without intervention
2. Concealment with intervention
3. No concealment without intervention
4. No concealment with intervention

These methods are illustrated in Figure 14.1; examples are given later. Concealment refers to a study method in which participants do not know that they are being observed; through intervention, the observer provokes actions from those who are being observed.

Observational studies commonly involve no concealment and no intervention. In this case, the researcher obtains informed consent from the participant to be observed and then simply observes the participant's behaviour.

When a researcher is concerned that the participants' behaviour will change as a result of being observed (reactivity), the type of observation most commonly employed is that of concealment without intervention. In this case, the researcher watches the participants without their knowledge of the observation and does not provoke them into action. Often, such concealed observations involve the use of hidden television cameras, audio recordings, or one-way mirrors. Concealment without intervention is often used in observational studies of children. You may be familiar with rooms with one-way mirrors through which a researcher can observe the behaviour of the occupants of the room without being observed by them. Such studies allow the observation of children's natural behaviour and are often used in developmental research. Observing participants without their knowledge may violate assumptions of informed consent; therefore, researchers face ethical problems with this type of approach. However, researchers sometimes have no other way to collect such data, and the data collected are unlikely to have negative consequences for the participant. In these cases, the disadvantages of the study are outweighed by the advantages. Furthermore, the problem of consent is often handled by informing participants after the observation and allowing them the opportunity to refuse to have their data included in the study and to discuss any questions they might have. This process is called debriefing.

		Concealment	
		Yes	No
Intervention	Yes	Researcher hidden / An intervention	Researcher open / An intervention
	No	Researcher hidden / No intervention	Researcher open / No intervention

FIG. 14.1 Types of observational roles in research.

When the observer is neither concealed nor intervening, the ethical question is not a problem. Here, the observer makes no attempt to change the participants' behaviour and informs them that they are to be observed. Because the observer is present, this type of observation allows a greater depth of material to be studied than if the observer is separated from the participants by an artificial barrier, such as a one-way mirror. In a commonly used observational technique, the researcher functions as part of a social group to observe the participants. For example, in their study, Coker et al. (2017) used unconcealed observation, with the nurses and patients giving full consent for participation in the study. The problem with this type of observation, however, is reactivity (also referred to as the Hawthorne effect; see Chapter 10), or the distortion created when the participants change behaviour because they know they are being observed.

No concealment with intervention is used when the researcher is observing the effects of an intervention introduced for scientific purposes. Because the participants know they are participating in a research study, few problems with ethical concerns occur, but reactivity is a problem with this type of study.

Concealed observation with intervention involves staging a situation and observing the behaviours that are evoked in the participants as a result of the intervention. Because the participants are unaware of their participation in a research study, this type of observation has fallen into disfavour and is rarely used in nursing research.

Observational methods may be structured or unstructured. Unstructured observational methods are not characterized by a total absence of structure but rather usually involve collecting descriptive information about the topic of interest. In unstructured observations, the observer keeps field notes that record the activities, as well as the observer's interpretations of these activities. Field notes are usually not restricted to any particular type of action or behaviour; rather, they are intended to depict a social situation in a more general sense.

Another type of unstructured observation is the use of stories or anecdotes, which usually focus on the behaviours of interest and frequently add to the richness of research reports by illustrating a particular point.

The use of structured observations without a standardized tool involves specifying in advance what behaviours or events are to be observed and preparing forms for record keeping, such as categorization systems, checklists, and rating scales. Whichever system is employed, the observer watches the participant and then marks on the recording form what was seen. In both cases, the observations must be similar among the observers (see the earlier discussion and Chapter 15 for an explanation of interrater reliability). Thus, observers need to be trained to be consistent in their observations and ratings of behaviour.

Evidence-Informed Practice Tip

When you read a research report that uses observation as a data-collection method, you will want to note evidence of consistency across data collectors through use of internal consistency reliability data in quantitative research and credibility in qualitative research. When that evidence is present, you can have greater confidence in the results.

Scientific observation has several advantages as a data-collection method. The main advantage is that observation may be the only way for the researcher to study the variable of interest. For example, what people say they do is often not what they really do. Therefore, if the study is designed to obtain substantive findings about human behaviour, observation may be the only way to ensure the validity of the findings. In addition, no other data-collection method can match the depth and variety of information that can be collected with the techniques of scientific observation. Such techniques are also flexible in that they may be used in both experimental and nonexperimental designs and in laboratory and field studies.

Research Hint _____

Sometimes researchers carefully train observers or data collectors, but the research report does not address this training. The limitations on length of research reports often prevent the inclusion of certain information. Readers can often assume that if reliability data are provided, then appropriate training occurred.

As with all data-collection methods, observation also has its disadvantages. Earlier in this chapter, the problems of reactivity and ethical concerns were mentioned with regard to concealment and intervention. In addition to these problems, data obtained by observational techniques are vulnerable to the bias of the observer. Emotions, prejudices, and values can influence the way that behaviours and events are observed. In general, the more the observer needs to make inferences and judgements about what is being observed, the more likely it is that distortion will occur. Thus, in judging the adequacy of observational methods, you will need to consider how observational tools were constructed and how observers were trained and evaluated.

Interviews, Surveys, and Questionnaires

Participants in a research study often have information that is important to the study and that can be obtained only by asking the participants. Such questions may be asked through the use of interviews, surveys, and questionnaires. For both, the purpose is to ask participants to report data for themselves, but each method has unique advantages and disadvantages. The interview is a method of data collection in which a data collector questions a participant verbally. Interviews may be face to face or performed over the telephone, e-mail, video-conferencing, or other electronic means and may consist of open-ended or closed-ended questions. In contrast, both surveys and questionnaires are instruments designed to gather data from individuals about knowledge, attitudes, beliefs, and feelings. Surveys and questionnaires are used interchangeably, but there is a difference.

A survey can include both a questionnaire and/or an interview, whereas a questionnaire is a written set of questions within the survey aimed at getting specific information about individuals. Surveys are also thought of being inclusive of both the questionnaire and the process of collecting, and analyzing and forecasting of a problem, attitude, or opinion. Survey research relies almost entirely on questioning participants with either interviews or questionnaires, but these methods of data collection can also be used in other types of research (see also Chapter 12).

No matter what type of study is conducted, the purpose of questioning participants is to seek information. This information may be of either direct interest, such as the participant's age, or indirect interest, such as when the researcher uses a combination of items to estimate the degree to which the respondent has a particular trait or characteristic. An intelligence test is an example of how individual items are combined with several others to develop an overall scale of intelligence. When items of indirect interest on a survey or questionnaire are combined to obtain an overall score, the measurement tool is called a scale.

The investigator determines the content of an interview or questionnaire from the literature review (see Chapter 5). When evaluating interviews and questionnaires, you should consider the content of the scale, the individual items, and the order of the items. The basic standard for evaluating the individual items in an interview or questionnaire is that the item must be clearly written so that the intention of the question and the nature of the information sought are clear to the respondent. The only way to know whether the questions are understandable to the respondents is to pilot test them in a similar population. It is also critical not to rely on only the instrument developer's reports of reliability and validity (see Chapter 15). A pilot test allows researchers to test the reliability and validity for their unique sample rather than relying only on previously reported results.

Although each questionnaire item must consist of only one question or concept, be free of suggestions, and be worded with correct grammar, such items may be either open-ended or closed-ended. An open-ended item is used when the researcher wants the participants to respond in their own words or when the researcher does not know all of the possible alternative responses. A closed-ended item is a question that the respondent may answer with only one of a fixed number of alternative responses. Many scales use a fixed-response format called a Likert-type scale. A Likert-type scale is a list of statements for which responses are varying degrees of agreement or opinion—for example, whether respondents "strongly agree," "agree," "disagree," or "strongly disagree." Sometimes finer distinctions are given, or a neutral category (e.g., "no opinion") may be provided. The use of the neutral category, however, sometimes creates problems because it is often the most frequent response and is difficult to interpret. Fixed-response items also can be used for questions requiring a "yes" or "no" response or when the interview or questionnaire has categories, as with income.

Evidence-Informed Practice Tip

Scales used in nursing research should have evidence of adequate reliability and validity so that readers feel confident that the findings reflect what the researcher intended to measure (see Chapter 15).

Figure 14.2 shows a few items from a fictional survey of pediatric nurse practitioners. The first items are taken from a list of similar items, and they are both closed-ended and of a Likert-type format. Note that respondents are asked to choose how strongly they agree with each item. In using these questions in the survey, respondents are forced to choose from only these answers because it is thought that these will be the only responses. The only possible alternative response is to skip the item, leaving it blank.

Sometimes researchers have no idea or only a limited idea of what the respondent will say, or researchers want the answer in the respondent's

own words, as with the second (open-ended) set of items. In this situation, respondents may also leave the item blank but are not forced to make a particular response.

Interviews and questionnaires are commonly used in nursing research. Both are strong approaches to gathering information for research because they enable the researcher to approach the task directly. In addition, both can elicit certain kinds of information, such as the participants' attitudes and beliefs, that would be difficult to obtain without asking the participant directly.

All methods that involve verbal reports, however, share a problem with accuracy. Often, it is impossible to know whether what the researcher is told is indeed true. For example, people are known to respond to questions in a way that makes a favourable impression. This response style is known as social desirability, which can be regarded as resulting from two factors: self-deception and other-deception.

Neyerhof (2006) has discussed the two main modes of coping with social desirability bias. The first mode is aimed at the detection and measurement of social desirability bias and is represented by two methods: the use of social desirability scales and the rating of item desirability. The second mode is aimed at preventing or reducing social desirability bias and is represented by the following methods: forced-choice items, the randomized response technique, the bogus pipeline, self-administration of the questionnaire, the selection of interviewers, and the use of proxy participants. Neyerhof found that no one method excelled completely and suggested that a combination of prevention and detection methods is the best strategy to reduce social desirability bias. Recent trends have led to the use of social desirability scales, as variables, within studies to determine the extent of social desirability. The most popular of these scales used to be the Marlowe-Crowne Social Desirability scale (MCSDS) but now the current gold standard is the Balanced Inventory of Desirable Responding (BIDR),

Closed-Ended (Likert-Type Scale)
A. How satisfied are you with your current position?
    1. Very satisfied
    2. Moderately satisfied
    3. Undecided
    4. Moderately dissatisfied
    5. Very dissatisfied
B. To what extent do the following factors contribute to your current level of positive satisfaction?

	Not at all	Very little	Somewhat	Moderate amount	A great deal
1. % of time in patient care	1	2	3	4	5
2. Type of patients	1	2	3	4	5
3. % of time in educational activity	1	2	3	4	5
4. % of time in administration	1	2	3	4	5

Closed-Ended
A. On average, how many patients do you see in one day?
    1. 1 to 3
    2. 4 to 6
    3. 7 to 9
    4. 10 to 12
    5. 13 to 15
    6. 16 to 18
    7. 19 to 20
    8. More than 20
B. How would you characterize your practice?
    1. Too slow
    2. Slow
    3. About right
    4. Busy
    5. Too busy

Open-Ended
A. Are there incentives that the Canadian Nurses Association ought to provide for members that are not currently being provided?

FIG. 14.2   Examples of closed-ended and open-ended questions.

which is considered more sensitive because its development incorporated newer theoretical and empirical of Social Desirability Responding (SDR) and more sophisticated multivariate techniques (Lambert et al., 2016).

Questionnaires and interviews also have some specific purposes, advantages, and disadvantages. Questionnaires are useful tools when the purpose is to collect information. If questionnaires are too long, however, respondents are not likely to complete them. Questionnaires are most useful when the set of questions to be asked is finite and the researcher can be assured of the clarity and specificity of the items. Face-to-face techniques or interviews are most appropriate when the researcher may need to clarify the task for the respondent or is interested in obtaining more personal information from the respondent. Telephone interviews allow the researcher to reach more respondents than face-to-face interviews and provide more clarity than questionnaires.

Research Hint _____

Remember that sometimes researchers make trade-offs when determining the measures to be used. For example, if a researcher wants to learn about an individual's attitudes regarding practice, and practicalities preclude using an interview, a questionnaire may be used instead.

Pauly and colleagues (2015) used both unconcealed observations and in-depth interviews to understand what constitutes culturally safe care for people who use illicit drugs. Both the nurses and patients were asked questions about their experiences in giving and receiving care, their understanding of comfort and safety, and their experiences of health care settings and any barriers and enablers in providing and receiving care (p. 124). Two researchers conducted 275 hours of unconcealed observations to gain an understanding of the various contexts under which nurses provide care to persons who use illicit drugs. This use of multiple measures provides a more complete picture than the use of just one measure.

When determining whether to use interviews or questionnaires, researchers often face difficult choices. The final decision is based on the instruments available and their relative costs and benefits.

Both face-to-face and telephone interviews have some advantages over questionnaires. The rate of response to interviews is almost always better than that to questionnaires, which helps eliminate bias in the sample (see Chapter 13). Respondents seem to be less likely to hang up the telephone or to close the door in an interviewer's face than to throw away a questionnaire. Another advantage of the interview is that some people—such as young children, people with visual impairments, and people who are illiterate—cannot fill out a questionnaire but can participate in an interview. With an interview, the data collector knows who is giving the answers. When questionnaires are mailed, for example, anyone in the household could be the person who supplies the answers.

Interviews also allow for some safeguards to be built into the interview situation. Interviewers can clarify misunderstood questions and observe the level of the respondent's understanding and cooperativeness. In addition, the researcher has strict control over the order of the questions. With questionnaires, the respondent can answer questions in any order. Changing the order of the questions can sometimes change the response.

Finally, interviews allow for richer and more complex data to be collected. The interview questioning can be open-ended or closed-ended; in either case, interviewers can probe to understand why a respondent answered in a particular way. In the qualitative study by Woodgate et al. (2020), open-ended, face-to-face interviews were conducted to gather the experiences of youth living with anxiety. Two interview sessions were carried out. The first interview session opened with the question, "Can you please tell me a little bit about yourself?" This was followed up with questions to get at the youth's story (p. 4). Semi-structured interviews were used by Currie and Szabo (2020) in their study to explore the parents' experience of caring for medical and social care needs for children with rare neurodevelopmental disorders.

Interviews can also be conducted in a group setting, sometimes called a *focus group approach or focus group interview*, which may include about six to eight participants. Bottorff, Haines-Saah, Oliffe, and colleagues (2014) used a semi-structured interview schedule to guide focus group discussions to engage youth in discussing the merits and limitations of a variety of sample messages related to smoking and breast cancer and in generating ideas to guide youth-friendly message development and delivery media. Eight semi-structured focus groups were held outside school hours in community locations over a period of four months. Two focus groups were held with each of the following groups: First Nations and Métis girls, non-Indigenous girls, First Nations and Métis boys, and non-Indigenous boys. The aim was to capture diversity of opinion within each subgroup and to meet target participant numbers. These small-group interviews allowed the participants to freely explain and share information individually and collectively. Agreement and disagreement among participants may be elicited, which allows the researchers to obtain specific information from a number of participants efficiently and simultaneously.

Questionnaires are much less expensive to administer than interviews because interviews may require the hiring and training of interviewers. Thus, if a researcher has a fixed amount of time and money, a larger and more diverse sample can be obtained with questionnaires. Questionnaires also provide complete anonymity, which may be important if the study deals with sensitive issues. Finally, the fact that no interviewer is present assures the researcher and the reader that no interviewer bias will occur. Interviewer bias occurs when the interviewer unwittingly leads the respondent to answer in a certain way. This problem is especially pronounced in studies with unstructured interview formats. A subtle nod of the head, for example, could lead a respondent to

change an answer to correspond with what he or she perceives that the researcher wants to hear.

For instance, McDonald et al. (2018) converted their questionnaire, Student Adaptation to College Questionnaire, to an online format for easier access for both the participants for completion and the researchers for data analysis.

In another study, Covell et al. (2017) mailed an invitation letter to participate in their study with the questionnaire to 13,748 internationally educated nurses. There were three reminders to increase response rate. Participants could complete the questionnaire anonymously online or by postal mail (p. 4).

Records or Available Data

All of the data-collection methods discussed thus far concern the ways that nurse researchers gather new data to study phenomena of interest. Not all studies, however, require a researcher to acquire new information. Existing information can sometimes be examined in a new way to study a problem. The use of records and available data is sometimes considered to be primarily the concern of historical research, but hospital records, care plans, and existing data sources (e.g., the census) are frequently used for collecting information. What sets these studies apart from a literature review is that these available data are examined in a new way and not merely summarized; they also answer specific research questions.

Records or available data, then, are forms of information that are collected from existing materials, such as hospital records, historical documents, or audio or video recordings, and are used to answer research questions in a new manner. For example, Kaasalainen et al. (2019) conducted a chart audit to examine current rates of resident deaths, emergency department use within the last year of life, and hospital deaths for long-term care residents. Because the data-collection step of the research process is often the most difficult and time consuming, the use of available records often produces a significant saving of time. If the records have been kept in a similar manner over time, analysis of these records allows examination of trends over time. In addition, the use of available data decreases problems of reactivity and response set bias. The researcher also does not have to ask individuals to participate in the study.

However, institutions are sometimes reluctant to allow researchers access to their records. If the records are kept so that an individual cannot be identified, access for research purposes is usually not a problem. Also, the Privacy Act, a federal law, protects the rights of individuals who may be identified in records, which would be a violation of anonymity.

One problem that affects the quality of available data concerns survival of records. If the records available are not representative of all of the possible records, the researcher may have a problem with bias. Often, because researchers have no way to tell whether the records have been saved in a biased manner, they need to make an intelligent guess as to their accuracy. For example, a researcher might be interested in studying socioeconomic factors associated with the suicide rate. These data frequently are underreported because of the stigma attached to suicide, and so the records would be biased. Recent interest in computerization of health records has led to an increase in the discussion about the desirability of access to such records for research. At this time, how much of such data will continue to be readily available for research without consent is unclear.

Another problem is related to the authenticity of the records. The distinction of primary and secondary sources is as relevant in this discussion as it was in the discussion of the literature review to determine the source of the work (see Chapter 5). A book, for example, may have been ghostwritten, but all credit was accorded to the known author. The researcher may have a difficult time ferreting out these subtle types of biases.

Lastly, existing records may be missing a significant amount of data. For example, years of education may be recorded on only a portion of the sample records. Nonetheless, records and available data constitute a rich source of data for study.

ONLINE AND COMPUTERIZED METHODS OF DATA COLLECTION

With the fast-paced progression of the Internet and computer technology, many researchers are using online data collection. The information obtained can be quantitative or qualitative, closed-ended or open-ended. This method of data collection can take the form of Web-based surveys or data input directly into microcomputers. For example, Corby et al. (2021) used an online survey hosted by Fluid Surveys in their study to investigate the predictors of prenatal breastfeeding self-efficacy.

Many online survey tools, such as SurveyMonkey or QuestionPro or Fluid Surveys, are available; a survey can be downloaded quickly and the results obtained for a small fee. The advantages of this method are that it is anonymous and inexpensive; respondents can fill out the survey in their own time; a large number of participants can be accessed; respondent time is reduced; data-collection time is reduced; duplicate responses can be identified; and, for the researcher, implementation is time efficient. The disadvantages are that not everyone has access to a computer or is computer literate, the response rates may be low, and a large amount of data may be missing. In addition, the researcher has to ensure that the cloud where the data is collected and stored is in Canada and follow the guidelines for Personal Health Information Protection Act PHIPA) (Information and Privacy Commissioner of Ontario, 2015).

Computerized data collection can be accomplished through the use of laptop computers or electronic tablets or smartphones. Researchers can input their data directly into these handheld microcomputers. The data can then be transferred to a larger computer for analysis.

Evidence-Informed Practice Tip

A critical evaluation of any data-collection method includes evaluating the appropriateness, objectivity, consistency, and credibility of the method employed.

CONSTRUCTION OF NEW INSTRUMENTS

As already mentioned in this chapter, researchers sometimes cannot locate an existing instrument or method with acceptable reliability and validity to measure the variable of interest. This situation is often the case when part of a nursing theory is tested or when the effect of a clinical intervention is evaluated. For example, Vincelette et al. (2019) developed, validated, and assessed the psychometric properties of a survey related to cardiopulmonary resuscitation among intensive care nurses (see Chapter 15).

Instrument development is complex and time consuming, however. It consists of the following steps:

- Defining the construct to be measured
- Formulating the items (questions)
- Assessing the items for content validity
- Developing instructions for respondents and users
- Pretesting and pilot testing the items
- Estimating reliability and validity

Defining the construct (concepts at a higher level of abstraction) to be measured requires that the researcher develop an expertise in the construct, which necessitates an extensive review of the literature and of all tests and measurements that deal with related constructs. The researcher uses all this information to synthesize the available knowledge so that the construct can be defined.

Once the construct is defined, the individual items for measuring the construct can be developed. The researcher will develop many more items than are needed to address each aspect of the construct or subconstruct. A panel of experts in the field evaluates the items so that the researcher is assured that the items measure what they are intended to measure (content validity; see Chapter 15).

Eventually, the number of items is decreased because some items will not elicit the intended information and will be dropped. In this phase, the researcher needs to ensure consistency both among the items and in testing and scoring procedures.

Finally, the researcher administers or pilot tests the new instrument by applying it to a group of people who are similar to those who will be studied in the larger investigation. The purpose of this analysis is to determine the quality of the instrument as a whole (reliability and validity) and the ability of each item to discriminate individual respondents (variance in item response). The researcher also may administer a related instrument to see whether the new instrument is sufficiently different from the older one.

It is important that researchers who invest significant time in tool development publish their results. For example, Hart et al. (2019) were interested in understanding the surgical neonatal nursing workload. From their literature review, they determined that there was no tool that adequately describes the nursing workload associated with neonates. They decided to modify a validated NICU nursing tool to better meet the needs of the surgical NICU patients. This type of research serves not only to introduce other researchers to the tool but also to ultimately enhance the field, inasmuch as the ability to conduct meaningful research is limited only by the ability to measure important phenomena.

Research Hint

Determine whether a newly developed survey or questionnaire was pilot tested to obtain preliminary evidence of reliability and validity.

QUALITATIVE DATA COLLECTION

In qualitative research, data collection is more flexible and may evolve over the course of the study. Some of the data-collection methods outlined previously are also used in qualitative research, such as observations and semi-structured interviews. For example, Pesut et al. (2020) used semi-structured interviews in the qualitative study to better understand nursing practice within the legislative approaches to medically assisted dying. In addition, other methods, such as focus groups and photovoice, are used, or textual data is gathered from media or policy documents.

Focus Groups

A focus group is a type of interview of about five to eight people on the topic of interest. The interviewer has predetermined questions with probes, in the event that the group is not forthcoming with information. The setting for this interview is usually a neutral one. Most qualitative researchers use voice recorders so that they can be sure that they have captured what the participant says. This reduces the need to write things down and frees up the researchers to listen fully. Interview recordings are usually transcribed verbatim and then listened to for accuracy. In a research report, investigators describe their procedures for collecting the data, such as obtaining informed consent, all the steps from initial contact to the end of the study visit, and how long each interview or focus group lasted or how much time the researcher spent "in the field" collecting data. For example, in the qualitative portion of their mixed method study, Verkuyl and Hughes (2019) used focus groups to explore students' experiences and outcomes using virtual gaming simulation as well

as to describe and expand on the findings from the quantitative data (p. 11).

Photovoice

Photography has been used in research since the 1950s, as photographs provide a permanent record of events and activities. In the early 1990s, Dr. Caroline Wang developed *photovoice*, an innovative approach used in participatory action research (Wang, 1999) in which interviews are stimulated and guided by photographs. These photographs empower members of marginalized groups to work together to "identify, represent and enhance their community through a specific photographic technique" (Wang & Burris, 1997). They also aid in breaking down barriers between researchers and participants. Participants use photographs, which act as prompts, to help others to see their world, and stories are told while discussing the photographs; this can be empowering to the individual. Photovoice requires that community members take on multiple roles, such as photographer, key informant, and co-researcher.

Scruby et al. (2019) used photovoice to explore social support, sport participation, and rural women's health. Participants were asked to photograph images they felt represented health in the context of the curling rink; these images were analyzed thematically.

APPRAISING THE EVIDENCE

Data-Collection Methods

Evaluating the adequacy of data-collection methods from written research reports is often problematic for new nursing research readers. Because the tool itself is not available for inspection, you may not feel comfortable judging the adequacy of the method without seeing it. However, you can ask questions to judge the method chosen by the researcher. These questions are listed in the Critiquing Criteria box.

In all studies, data-collection methods should be clearly identified. The conceptual and operational definitions of each important variable should be present in the report. Sometimes it is useful for the researcher to explain why a particular method was chosen. For example, if the study dealt with young children, the researcher may explain that a questionnaire was deemed to be an unreasonable task, and so an interview was chosen.

APPRAISING THE EVIDENCE—cont'd

Data-Collection Methods

Once you have identified the method chosen to measure each variable of interest, you should decide whether the method used was the best way to measure the variable. For example, if a questionnaire was used, you might wonder why the researcher decided not to use an interview. Also consider whether the method was appropriate to the clinical situation. Does it make sense to interview patients in the recovery room, for example?

Once you have decided whether all relevant variables are operationalized appropriately, you can begin to determine how well the method was carried out. For studies involving physiological measurement, determine whether the instrument was appropriate to the problem and not forced to fit it. The rationale for selecting a particular instrument should be given. For example, it may be important to know that the study was conducted under the auspices of a manufacturing firm that provided the measuring instrument. In addition, the researcher should have made provisions to evaluate the accuracy of the instrument and the skill level of the people who used it.

Several considerations are important when you read studies that involve observational methods. Who were the observers, and how were they trained? Is there any reason to believe that different observers perceived events or behaviours differently? Remember that the more inferences the observers are required to make, the more likely it is that observations will be biased. Also, consider the problem of reactivity: In any observational situation, it is possible that the mere presence of the observer will cause the participant to change the behaviour in question. Of importance is not that reactivity could occur but the extent to which reactivity could affect the data. Finally, consider whether the observational procedure was ethical.

You need to consider whether the participants were informed that they were being observed, whether any intervention was performed, and whether the participants had agreed to be observed.

Interviews and questionnaires should be clearly described to allow the reader to decide whether the variables were adequately operationalized. Sometimes the researcher will reference the original report about the tool, and you may wish to read this study before deciding whether the method was appropriate for the current study. Also, the respondents' task should be clear. Thus, the researcher should have made provisions for the participants to understand both their overall responsibilities and the individual items of the interview or questionnaire. The following questions must be considered: Who were the interviewers in the interview situation? Does the researcher explain how they were trained to decrease any interviewer bias?

Available data, such as medical records, are subject to internal and external criticism. Internal criticism concerns the evaluation of the worth of the records and refers primarily to the accuracy of the data. The researcher should present evidence that the records are genuine. External criticism is concerned with the authenticity of the records. Are the records really written by the first author? The researcher may have a biased sample of all of the possible records in the problem area, which may have a profound effect on the validity of the results.

Once you have decided that the data-collection method used was appropriate for the problem and the procedures were appropriate for the population studied, the reliability and validity of the instruments themselves need to be considered. These characteristics are discussed in Chapter 15.

CRITIQUING CRITERIA

1. Is the framework for research clearly identified?

DATA-COLLECTION METHODS

1. Are all of the data-collection instruments clearly identified and described?

2. Is the rationale for their selection given?
3. Is the method used appropriate for the problem being studied?
4. Were the methods used appropriate for the clinical situation?

5. Are the data-collection procedures similar for all participants?
6. Were efforts made to ensure intervention fidelity through the data-collection protocol?

Continued

PHYSIOLOGICAL MEASUREMENT

1. Is the instrument used appropriate for the research problem and not forced to fit it?
2. Is a rationale given for why a particular instrument was selected?
3. Is there a provision for evaluating the accuracy of the instrument and the skill of the people who used it?

OBSERVATIONAL METHODS

1. Who conducted the observation?
2. Were the observers trained to minimize any bias?
3. Was an observational guide provided?
4. Were the observers required to make inferences about what they saw?

5. Is there any reason to believe that the presence of the observers affected the behaviour of the participants?
6. Were the observations performed according to the principles of informed consent?

INTERVIEWS/FOCUS GROUPS

1. Is the interview schedule described adequately enough for you to know whether it covers the purpose of the study?
2. Is it clear that the participants understood the task and the questions?
3. Who were the interviewers, and how were they trained?
4. Is any interviewer bias evident?

QUESTIONNAIRES

1. Is the questionnaire described well enough for you to know whether it covers the purpose of the study? Is evidence provided that participants were able to perform the task?
2. Is it clear that the participants understood the questionnaire?
3. Are the majority of the items appropriately closed- or open-ended?

AVAILABLE DATA AND RECORDS

1. Are the records used appropriate for the problem being studied?
2. Are the data examined in such a way as to provide new information and not summarize the records?
3. Has the author addressed questions of internal and external criticism?
4. Is there any indication of selection bias in the available records?

CRITICAL THINKING CHALLENGES

- Physiological measurements are objective, precise, and sensitive. Discuss factors that might influence their validity and feasibility.

- A student in research class asks why nurses who participate in a clinical research study in the role of a data collector or who perform a "treatment intervention" need to be trained. What important factors or rationale would you offer to support the establishment of interrater reliability?

- Observation is a data-collection method used frequently in nursing research. Discuss the factors that make nurses perfect potential candidates for this role and the disadvantages of using this method.

- Studies often use a survey to collect data. How can researchers increase their return rate for the survey, and how do they determine whether the survey return is adequate?

CRITICAL JUDGEMENT QUESTIONS

1. In a study conducted at a large long-term care facility, two data collectors examined the correct use of personal protective equipment (PPE) on 100 nurses. The examinations were independently performed on the same day. A comparison of the results indicated that the data collectors scored 90 of the 100 nurses following the correct protocol for wearing and removing PPE. What can be determined from this finding?

   a. Interrater reliability between the two data collectors was high.
   b. Interrater reliability between the two data collectors was low.
   c. The data-collection method was inappropriate for the phenomenon under investigation.
   d. In order to establish interrater reliability, the two data collectors should have examined each nurse's behaviour at the same time.

2. Which of the following is an example of a physiological measurement?

   a. Definition of a type "A" behaviour pattern
   b. Description of self-care behaviour abilities in patients with dementia.
   c. HbA1C blood levels
   d. Adjusted scores on the State-Trait Anxiety Scale

3. Which data-collection method is most appropriate for measuring postpartum depression?
   a. Assessment of estrogen levels
   b. Unstructured interview
   c. Visual analog pain scale
   d. Edinburgh Postnatal Depression Scale

KEY POINTS

- Data-collection methods are described as being both objective and systematic. The data-collection methods of a study provide the operational definitions of the relevant variables.
- Types of data-collection methods include physiological measurements, observational methods, interviews, questionnaires, and records or available data. Each method has advantages and disadvantages.
- Physiological measurements are the methods in which technical instruments are used to collect data about patients' physical, chemical, microbiological, or anatomical status. These methods are suited to studying how to improve the effectiveness of nursing care. Physiological measurements are objective, precise, and sensitive, but they may be very expensive and may distort the variable of interest.
- Observational methods are used in nursing research when the variables of interest deal with events or behaviours. Scientific observation requires preplanning, systematic recording, controlling the observations, and determining the relationship to scientific theory. This method is best suited to research problems that are difficult to view as part of a whole. Observers may be required to perform or not perform interventions, and their activity may be concealed or obvious.
- Observational methods have several advantages: (1) they provide flexibility to measure many types of situations, and (2) they enable a great depth and breadth of information to be collected.

- Observation has disadvantages as well: (1) data may be distorted as a result of the observer's presence (reactivity), (2) concealment requires the consideration of ethical issues, and (3) data from observations may be biased by the person who is doing the observing.
- Interviews are data-collection methods commonly used in nursing research. Items on interview schedules may be of direct or indirect interest. Participants may be asked either open-ended or closed-ended questions. The form of the question should be clear to the respondent, free of suggestion, and grammatically correct.
- Questionnaires, or surveys, are useful when the number of questions to be asked is finite. The questions need to be clear and specific. Questionnaires are less costly and less time consuming to administer to large groups of participants, particularly if the participants are geographically widespread. Questionnaires also can be completely anonymous and prevent interviewer bias.
- Interviews are most appropriate when a large response rate and an unbiased sample are important because the refusal rate for interviews is much lower than that for questionnaires. Interviews enable the participation of people who cannot use a questionnaire, such as children and people who are illiterate. An interviewer can clarify and maintain the order of the questions for all participants.
- Records or available data are also an important source of research data. The use of available data may save the researcher considerable time and money in conducting a study. This method reduces problems with both reactivity and ethical concerns. However, records and available data are subject to problems of availability, authenticity, and accuracy.
- A critical evaluation of data-collection methods should emphasize the appropriateness, objectivity, and consistency of the method employed.

🛜 FOR FURTHER STUDY

Go to Evolve at http://evolve.elsevier.com/Canada/
LoBiondo/Research for the Audio Glossary.

REFERENCES

Arnstein, P., Gentile, D., & Wilson, M. (2019). Validating the functional pain scale for hospitalized adults. *Pain Management Nursing, 20*(5), 418–424. https://doi.org/10.1016/j.pmn.2019.03.006.

Bandura, A. (1997). *Self-efficacy: The exercise of control*. New York: W. H. Freeman.

Bottorff, J. L., Haines-saah, R., Oliffe, J. L., Struik, L. L., Bissell, L. J. L., Richardson, C. P., Gotay, C., Johnson, K. C., Hutchinson, P., Bottorff, J. L., Haines-saah, R., Oliffe, J. L., Struik, L. L., Bissell, L. J. L., Richardson, C. P., Gotay, C., Johnson, K. C., & Hutchinson, P. (2014). Designing tailored messages about smoking and breast cancer : A focus group study with youth. *Canadian Journal of Nursing Research, 46,* 66–86.

Chan, R., Booth, R., Strudwick, G., & Sinclair, B. (2019). Nursing students' perceived self-efficacy and the generation of medication errors with the use of an electronic medication administration record (eMAR) in clinical simulation. *International Journal of Nursing Education Scholarship, 16*(1). https://doi .org/10.1515/ijnes-2019-0014.

Coker, E., Ploeg, J., Kaasalainen, S., & Carter, N. (2017). Observations of oral hygiene care interventions provided by nurses to hospitalized older people. *Geriatric Nursing, 8*(1), 17–21. https://doi.org/10.1016/j .gerinurse.2016.06.018.

Corby, K., Kane, D., & Dayus, D. (2021). Investigating predictors of prenatal breastfeeding self-efficacy. *Canadian Journal of Nursing Research, 53*(1), 56–63. https://doi.org/10.1177/0844562119888363.

Covell, C. L., Primeau, M.-D., Kilpatrick, K., & St-Pierre, I. (2017). Internationally educated nurses in Canada: Predictors of workforce integration. *Human Resources for Health, 15*(1), 1–16. https://doi .org/10.1186/s12960-017-0201-8.

Currie, G., & Szabo, J. (2020). Social isolation and exclusion: the parents' experience of caring for children with rare neurodevelopmental disorders. *International Journal of Qualitative Studies on Health and Well-being, 15*(1), Article 1725362. https://doi.org/10.1080 /17482631.2020.1725362.

Hart, K., Marchuk, A., Walsh, J. L., & Howlett, A. (2019). Validation of a surgical neonatal nursing workload tool. *Journal of Neonatal Nursing, 25*(6), 293–297. https://doi.org/10.1016/j.jnn.2019.06.002.

Information and Privacy Commissioner of Ontario. IPC. (2015). https://www.ipc.on.ca/.

Kaasalainen, S., Sussman, T., Durepos, P., McCleary, L., Ploeg, J., Thompson, G., & Team, SPA-LTC (2019). What are staff perceptions about their current use of emergency departments for long-term care residents at end of life. *Clinical Nursing Research, 28*(6), 692–707. https://doi.org/10.1177/1054773817749125.

Lambert, C. E., Arbuckle, S. A., & Holden, R. R. (2016). The Marlowe-Crowne Social Desirability Scale outperforms the BIDR Impression Management Scale for identifying fakers. *Journal of Research in Personality, 61,* 80–86. https://doi.org/10.1016/j.jrp.2016.02.004.

McDonald, M., Brown, J., & Knihnitski, C. (2018). Student perception of initial transition into a nursing program: A mixed methods research study. *Nurse Education Today, 64,* 85–92. https://doi.org/10.1016/j.nedt.2018.01.028.

Neyerhof, A. J. (2006). Methods of coping with social desirability bias: A review. *European Journal of Psychology, 15,* 263–280.

Oviedo, G. R., Tamulevicius, N., Onagbiye, S. O., Phidza, M., Sedumedi, C. M., Cameron, M., & Moss, S. J. (2019). Quality of life, physical activity and cardiorespiratory fitness in black African women: B-Healthy project. *Quality of Life Research, 29,* 987–997.

Pauly, B., McCall, J., Browne, A. J., Parker, J., & Mollison, A. (2015). Toward cultural safety: Nurse and patient perceptions of illicit substance use in a hospitalized setting. *Advances in Nursing Science, 38*(2), 121–135. https://doi.org/10.1097/ ANS.0000000000000070.

Pesut, B., Thorne, S., Schiller, C., Greig, M., Roussel, J., & Tishelman, C. (2020). Constructing good nursing practice for medical assistance in dying in Canada: An interpretive descriptive study. *Global Qualitative Nursing Research, 7.* https://doi .org/10.1177/2333393620938686.

Scruby, L. S., Rona, H. A., Leipert, B. D., Mair, H. L., & Snow, W. M. (2019). Exploring social support, sport participation and rural women's health using Photovoice: The Manitoba Experience. *Canadian Journal of Nursing Research, 51*(4), 233–244. https:// doi.org/10.1177/0844562119832395.

Verkuyl, M., & Hughes, M. (2019). Virtual gaming simulation in nursing education: A mixed-methods study. *Clinical Simulation in Nursing, 29,* 9–14. https://doi .org/10.1016/j.ecns.2019.02.001.

Vincelette, C., Quiroz-Martinez, H., Fortin, O., & Lavoie, S. (2019). Preliminary development and validation of the Nurse Cardiopulmonary Resuscitation Survey (NCRS) among intensive care unit nurses. *Official Journal of the Canadian Association of Critical Care Nurses, 30*, 24–31.

Wang, C. (1999). Photovoice: A participatory action research strategy applied to women's health. *Journal of Women's Health, 8*(2), 185–192.

Wang, C., & Burris., M. A (1997). Photovoice: Concept, methodology, and use for participatory needs assessment. *Health Education and Behaviour, 24*(3), 369–387.

Wang, W., Seah, B., Jiang, Y., Lopez, V., Tan, C., Lim, S. T., Ren, H., & Khoo, Y. H. (2018). A randomized controlled trial on a nurse-led smartphone-based self-management programme for people with poorly controlled type 2 diabetes: A study protocol. *Journal of Advanced Nursing, 74*(1), 190–200. https://doi .org/10.1111/jan.13394.

Woodgate, R. L., Tailor, K., Tennent, P., Wener, P., & Altman, G. (2020). The experience of the self in Canadian youth living with anxiety: A qualitative study. *PLoS ONE, 15*(1), Article e0228193. https://doi .org/10.1371/journal.pone.0228193.

CHAPTER 15

Rigour in Research

Mina D. Singh | Lorraine Thirsk

LEARNING OUTCOMES

After reading this chapter, you will be able to do the following:

- Discuss the purposes of reliability and validity.
- Define reliability.
- Discuss the concepts of stability, equivalence, and homogeneity as they relate to reliability.
- Compare the estimates of reliability.
- Define validity.
- Compare content validity, criterion-related validity, and construct validity.
- Discuss how measurement error can affect the outcomes of a research study.
- Identify the criteria for critiquing the reliability and validity of measurement tools.
- Use the critiquing criteria to evaluate the reliability and validity of measurement tools.
- Understand how to evaluate the quality of qualitative research
- Discuss the purpose of credibility, auditability, and fittingness.
- Apply the critiquing criteria to evaluate the rigour in a qualitative report.
- Discuss how evidence related to research rigour contributes to clinical decision-making.

KEY TERMS

alpha coefficient
alternate-form reliability
auditability
chance error
Cohen's kappa
concurrent validity
constant error
construct validity
content validity
contrasted-groups approach
convergent validity
credibility
criterion-related validity
Cronbach's alpha
divergent validity
equivalence

error variance
face validity
factor analysis
fittingness
homogeneity
hypothesis-testing
    approach
internal consistency
interrater reliability
item-to-total correlation
known-groups approach
Kuder-Richardson (KR-20)
    coefficient
methodological coherence
multitrait-multimethod
    approach

observed test score
parallel-form reliability
predictive validity
random error
reflexivity
reliability
reliability coefficient
rigour
split-half reliability
stability
systematic error
test-retest reliability
trustworthiness
validation sample
validity

STUDY RESOURCES

Go to Evolve at http://evolve.elsevier.com/Canada/LoBiondo/Research for the Audio Glossary.

IN BOTH QUANTITATIVE AND QUALITATIVE RESEARCH, the purpose is to collect trustworthy data that can be used for analyses to make generalizations about the population and that are transferable to other groups. Because findings need to be generalizable and transferable, measurement of nursing phenomena is a major concern of nursing researchers, and rigour is strived for. Rigour refers to the strictness with which a study is conducted to enhance the quality, believability, or trustworthiness of the study findings. Rigour in quantitative research is determined by measurement instruments that validly and reliably reflect the concepts of the theory being tested, so that conclusions drawn from a study will be valid and will advance the development of nursing theory and evidence-informed practice. Thus, psychometric assessments are designed to obtain evidence of the quality of these instruments—that is, their reliability and validity.

Issues of reliability and validity are of central concern to the researcher, as well as to you as the critiquer of research. From either perspective, the measurement instruments that are used in a research study must be evaluated. Many new constructs are relevant to nursing theory, and a growing number of established measurement instruments are available to researchers. However, researchers often face the challenge of developing new instruments and, as part of that process, establishing the reliability and validity of those tools.

In qualitative research, rigour, often called trustworthiness, is ascertained by credibility, auditability, and fittingness. The growing importance of measurement issues, tool development, and related issues (e.g., reliability and validity, qualitative rigour) is evident in issues of the *Journal of Nursing Measurement, Canadian Journal of Nursing Research, International Journal of Qualitative Methods*, and other nursing research journals. In this chapter, concepts related to quantitative rigour are discussed first, followed by factors that contribute to the trustworthiness of qualitative research.

When you read quantitative research studies and reports, you must assess the reliability and validity of the instruments used in each study to determine the soundness of the selection of these instruments in relation to the concepts or variables under investigation. The appropriateness of the instruments and the extent to which reliability and validity are demonstrated have a profound influence on the findings and on the internal and external validity of the study. Invalid measures produce invalid estimates of the relationships between variables, thus affecting internal validity. The use of invalid measures also leads to inaccurate generalizations to the populations being studied, thus affecting external validity and the ability to apply or not apply research findings in clinical practice. Thus, the assessment of reliability and validity is an extremely important skill to develop for critiquing nursing research.

Regardless of whether a new or already developed measurement tool is used in a research study, evidence of reliability and validity is crucial. Box 15.1 identifies several Internet resources that you can use to access and evaluate the reliability and validity of the measurement instruments used in research studies.

RELIABILITY

People are considered reliable when their behaviour is consistent and predictable. Likewise, the **reliability** of a research instrument is the extent to which the instrument yields the same results on

INTERNET RESOURCES FOR ACCESSING AND EVALUATING THE VALIDITY AND RELIABILITY OF MEASUREMENT INSTRUMENTS*

- **Mental Measurements Yearbook—Test Reviews Online**
  - To subscribe, visit https://marketplace.unl.edu/buros/
  - Contains online abstracts of 3,500 commercially available tests, of which more than 2,800 have been critically appraised by the Buros Institute. These reviews also appear in the print version of the Mental Measurements Yearbook series. Searches can be conducted by author or by using the 18 search categories.
- **WORLDviews on Evidence-Based Nursing**
  - To subscribe, visit https://sigmapubs.onlinelibrary.wiley.com/journal/17416787
  - Provides full-text articles and searches, hypertext navigation, links to Cumulative Index to Nursing and Allied Health Literature (CINAHL) and MEDLINE, and tables and figures.
- **the Sigma Repository (formerly the Virginia Henderson Global Nursing e-Repository)**
  - To subscribe, visit https://www.sigmarepository.org/
  - Includes the following databases: Registry of Nurse Researchers, Registry of Research Projects, and Registry of Research Results. This repository also has printed materials such as: Directory of Unpublished Experimental Mental Measures, Instruments for Clinical Health-Care Research, The Instruments of Psychiatric Research, Measuring Health: A Guide to Rating Scales and Questionnaires, and The Mental Measurements Yearbook.
- **Sigma Theta Tau International Honor Society of Nursing**
  - 550 West North Street Indianapolis, IN 46202; 317-634-8171; https://www.sigmanursing.org/
  - Supports the learning, knowledge, and professional development of nurses. Also promotes resources to bridge research and clinical practice.
- **PROQOLID: Patient-Reported Outcome and Quality of Life Instruments Database**
  - https://www.webcitation.org/getfile?fileid=b3447074665f3736126b320f83ff98304e2f43dcIdentifies and describes quality-of-life instruments.

*See Chapter 5 for detailed information about Internet resources.

repeated measures. Reliability, then, is concerned with consistency, accuracy, precision, stability, equivalence, and homogeneity. Concurrent with questions of validity, or after these questions are answered, the researcher and you, as the critiquer, ask how reliable the instrument is.

A reliable measure can produce the same results if the behaviour is measured again by the same scale. Reliability, then, refers to the proportion of accuracy to inaccuracy in measurement. In other words, if researchers use the same or comparable instruments on more than one occasion to measure behaviours that ordinarily remain relatively constant, the researchers would expect similar results if the tools are reliable.

The three main attributes of a reliable scale are **stability**, homogeneity, and equivalence. The stability of an instrument refers to the instrument's ability to produce the same results with repeated testing. The **homogeneity**, or **internal consistency**, of an instrument means that all of the items in a tool measure the same concept or characteristic. An instrument is said to exhibit equivalence if the tool produces the same results when equivalent or parallel instruments or procedures are used. Each of these attributes and the means to estimate them are discussed here. Before these are discussed, however, an understanding of how to interpret reliability is essential.

Interpretation of the Reliability Coefficient

Because all of the attributes of reliability are concerned with the degree of consistency between scores that are obtained at two or more independent times of testing, these attributes often are expressed in terms of a correlation coefficient. The **reliability coefficient**, or **alpha coefficient**, expresses the relationship between the error variance, true variance, and the observed score, and it ranges from 0 to 1. A correlation of 0 indicates no relationship, and thus the error variance is high. When the error variance in a measurement instrument is low, the reliability coefficient is closer to 1. The closer to 1 the coefficient is, the more reliable the tool is. For example, suppose that a reliability coefficient of a tool is reported to be .89. This number indicates that the error variance is small and the tool has little measurement error.

But if the reliability coefficient of a measure is reported to be .49, the error variance is high, and the tool has a problem with measurement error. For a tool to be considered reliable, a level of .70 or higher should be reported, although the intended purpose of the instrument needs to be considered if lower levels are accepted.

The interpretation of the reliability coefficient depends on the proposed purpose of the measure. Seven major tests of reliability can be used to calculate a reliability coefficient, depending on the nature of the tool: *test-retest reliability, parallel- or alternate-form reliability, item-to-total correlation, split-half reliability, Kuder-Richardson coefficient, Cronbach's alpha, and interrater reliability.* These tests are discussed as they relate to the attributes of stability, homogeneity, and equivalence (Box 15.2). In critiquing research reports, you should be aware that no single best way exists to assess reliability in relation to these attributes and that the researcher's method should be consistent with the aim of the research.

Stability

An instrument is thought to be stable or to exhibit stability when repeated administration of the instrument yields the same results. Researchers are concerned with an instrument's stability because they expect the instrument to measure a concept consistently over a period of time. Measurement over time is important in a longitudinal study because in that type of research, an instrument is used on several occasions. Stability is also a consideration when a researcher is conducting an intervention study that is designed to effect a change in a specific variable. In this case, the instrument is administered once and then again after the alteration or change intervention has been completed. The tests that are used to estimate stability are test-retest reliability and parallel- or alternate-form reliability.

Test-Retest Reliability

Test-retest reliability is the stability of the scores of an instrument when it is administered more than once to the same participants under similar conditions. Scores from repeated testing are compared. This comparison is expressed by a correlation coefficient, usually a Pearson *r* (see Chapter 17). The interval between repeated administrations varies and depends on the concept or variable being measured. For example, if the variable that the test measures is related to developmental stages in children, the interval between test administrations should be short. The amount of time over which the variable was measured should also be recorded in the report.

An example of an instrument that was assessed for test-retest reliability is O'Keefe-McCarthy, McGillion, Nelson, and associates' (2014) Prodromal-Symptoms Screening Scale. Test-retest reliability was assessed at approximately a 2-week interval, and a high test-retest reliability coefficient ($r = .81$, $p < .01$) was obtained. The interval was adequate (2 weeks between testing), and coefficients exceeded .80 and were thus very good (Nunnally & Bernstein, 1994).

Parallel- or Alternate-Form Reliability

Parallel-form reliability is applicable and can be tested only if two comparable forms of the same instrument exist. **Parallel-form reliability**, or

---

BOX 15.2

MEASURES USED TO TEST RELIABILITY

STABILITY
Test-retest reliability
Parallel- or alternate-form reliability

HOMOGENEITY
Item-to-total correlation
Split-half reliability
Kuder-Richardson (KR-20) coefficient
Cronbach's alpha

EQUIVALENCE
Parallel- or alternate-form reliability
Interrater reliability

alternate-form reliability, is like test-retest reliability in that the same individuals are tested more than once within a specific interval, but in the assessment of parallel-form reliability, a different form of the same test is given to the participants on the second testing. Parallel forms or tests contain the same types of items that are based on the same domain or concept, but the wording of the items is different. The development of parallel forms is desired if the instrument is intended to measure a variable for which a researcher believes that "testwiseness" will be a problem; that is, respondents might recognize the test items and try to answer them in the same way as previously, instead of spontaneously.

Practically speaking, developing alternative forms of an instrument is difficult because of the many issues of reliability and validity. If alternative forms of a test exist, they should be highly correlated if they are to be considered reliable.

Research Hint

When a longitudinal design with multiple data-collection points is being conducted, look for evidence of test-retest reliability or parallel-form reliability.

Homogeneity, or Internal Consistency

Another attribute related to reliability of an instrument is the homogeneity with which the items within the scale reflect or measure the same concept. In other words, the items within the scale are correlated with, or complementary to, each other, and the scale is *unidimensional*. A unidimensional scale measures one concept, such as exercise self-efficacy. A total score is then used in the analysis of data.

Corby et al. (2019) tested the reliability of the scales they used in their study to investigate predictors of prenatal breastfeeding self-efficacy. They found that the Cronbach's alpha for the Breastfeeding Self-Efficacy Scale-short form was .94, the perceived Stress Scale was .895, and the State-Trait Anxiety Inventory was .927. These reliability coefficients provided sufficient evidence of the internal consistency of these instruments

for the sample. Another example is provided by Kennedy et al. (2015) where the estimated Cronbach's alpha for the revised 22-item NCSES (Nursing Competence Self-Efficacy Scale) with the study population was high .919 (Kennedy, et al., 2015, p. 554). Homogeneity can be assessed with one of four methods: item-to-total correlation, split-half reliability, Kuder-Richardson coefficient, or Cronbach's alpha.

Research Hint

When the characteristics of a study sample differ significantly from those of the sample in the original study, check to see whether the researcher has re-established the reliability of the instrument with the current sample.

Item-to-Total Correlation

The **item-to-total correlation** is a measure of the relationship between each scale item and the total scale. When item-to-total correlations are calculated, a correlation for each item on the scale is generated (Table 15.1). Items that do not achieve a high correlation may be deleted from the instrument. In a research study, the lowest and highest item-to-total correlations are typically reported; the other correlations are usually not reported unless the study is a methodological investigation. An example of an item-to-total correlation report is illustrated in the study by Sidani et al. (2017), who tested the reliability and validity of

TABLE **15.1**

EXAMPLES OF ITEM-TO-TOTAL CORRELATIONS FROM COMPUTER-GENERATED DATA

ITEM	ITEM-TO-TOTAL CORRELATION
1	.5069
2	.4355
3	.4479
4	.4369
5	.4213
6	.4216

the Multi-Dimensional Treatment Satisfaction Measure (MDTSM). In that study, the item-to-total correlations were greater than .30 (p. 9). According to Nunnally and Bernstein (1994), these results are acceptable because the minimal mandatory correlation should be greater than .30.

Split-Half Reliability

Split-half reliability involves dividing a scale into halves and making a comparison. The halves may be, for example, odd-numbered and even-numbered items or a simple division of the first from the second half, or items may be randomly grouped into halves that will be analyzed opposite one another. Split-half reliability provides a measure of consistency in terms of sampling the content. The two halves of the test or the contents in both halves are assumed to be comparable, and a reliability coefficient is calculated. If the scores for the two halves are approximately equal, the test may be considered reliable.

The Spearman-Brown formula is one method of calculating the reliability coefficient. In a study to evaluate the reliability and validity of the Cancer Loneliness Scale (CLS) and the Cancer-related Negative Social Expectations Scale (CRNSES), Kara and Cinar (2020) used the split-half reliability method by means of Item Total Score Correlation, Cronbach's Alpha Coefficient, and Spearman-Brown Coefficient Value. There are seven items in the Cancer Loneliness Scale and five items in the Cancer-related Negative Social Expectations Scale. They found that for the CLS, the Cronbach's alpha coefficente was 0.88 and the Spearman-Brown correlation value was r = 0.81. For the CRNSES, the Cronbach's alpha coefficente was 0.82 and the Spearman-Brown correlation value was r = 0.86. For both scales, the correlation coefficient between the split-half of the scale was above 0.70, and thus the internal consistency is high (Boyle, Saklofske, & Matthews, 2015).

Kuder-Richardson Coefficient

The **Kuder-Richardson (KR-20) coefficient** is the estimate of homogeneity used for instruments that have a dichotomous response format. A *dichotomous response format* is one in which the answer to a question should be either "yes" or "no" or either "true" or "false." The technique yields a correlation that is based on the consistency of responses to all items of a single form of a test that is administered once.

Because the scale was a binary format (true/false), the Kuder-Richardson reliability for the entire scale was calculated at .75, which is acceptable, having exceeded the minimum acceptable score of .70; however, the magnitude of the correlation is not robust.

Cronbach's Alpha

The fourth and most commonly used test of internal consistency is Cronbach's alpha. Cronbach's alpha is a test of internal consistency in which each item in the scale is simultaneously compared with the others, and a total score is then used to analyze the data. Many tools used to measure psychosocial variables and attitudes have a Likert-type scale response format (Figure 15.1), which is very suitable for testing internal consistency. In a Likert-type scale format, the participant responds to a question on a scale of varying degrees of intensity between two extremes. The two extremes are anchored by responses ranging from, for example, "strongly agree" to "strongly disagree" or from "most like me" to "least like me." The points between the two extremes may range from 1 to 5 or 1 to 7. Participants are asked to circle the response that most closely represents what they believe. Examples of reported Cronbach's alpha for various studies are given in Box 15.3.

Figure 15.1 displays examples of items from a tool in which a Likert-type scale format was used to develop a nurses' perception of clinical reasoning instrument (Liou, Liu, Tsai et al., 2015). Boscart et al. (2018) tested the psychometric properties of Team Member Perspectives of Person-Centered (TM-PCC) survey. The testing revealed that there were

Directions: Please read each item and circle the number that best describes your current performance. There is no right or wrong answer.
5 = Strongly agree, 4 = Agree, 3 = Neutral, 2 = Disagree, 1 = Strongly disagree

1. I know how to collect an admitted patient's health information quickly.	5	4	3	2	1
2. I can apply proper assessment skills to collect a patient's current health information.	5	4	3	2	1
3. I can identify abnormalities from the collected patient information.	5	4	3	2	1
4. I can identify a patient's health problems from the abnormal information collected.	5	4	3	2	1
5. I can recognize possible early signs or symptoms when a patient's health deteriorates.	5	4	3	2	1
6. I can explain the mechanism and development associated with the early signs or symptoms when a patient's health deteriorates.	5	4	3	2	1
7. I can accurately prioritize and manage any identifiable patient problems.	5	4	3	2	1
8. I can correctly explain the mechanism behind a patient's problems.	5	4	3	2	1
9. I can set nursing goals properly for the identified patient problems.	5	4	3	2	1
10. I can provide appropriate nursing intervention for the identified patient problems.	5	4	3	2	1
11. I am knowledgeable of each nursing intervention provided.	5	4	3	2	1
12. I can identify and communicate vital information clearly to the doctors based on the patient's current condition.	5	4	3	2	1
13. I can anticipate the prescription ordered by the doctor according to the patient information provided.	5	4	3	2	1
14. I can accurately evaluate and identify whether a patient's condition is improved.	5	4	3	2	1
15. I know the follow-up steps to take if the patient's condition does not improve.	5	4	3	2	1

FIG. 15.1 Example of a Likert-type scale response format. From Liou, S. R., Liu, H. C., Tsai, H. M., et al. (2015). The development and psychometric testing of a theory-based instrument to evaluate nurses' perception of clinical reasoning competence. *Journal of Advanced Nursing, 72*(3), 707–717. Copyright © 2015 John Wiley & Sons Ltd.

BOX 15.3

EXAMPLES OF REPORTED CRONBACH'S ALPHA

"Inter-item correlation coefficients were reviewed for redundancy (r > .85) among items. Item-to-total correlation coefficients > .30 and alpha coefficient ≥ .70 supported the TSC (Therapeutic Self-Care) measure's internal consistency reliability" (Sidani & Doran, 2014, p. 20).
"For the ETBQ-S [Empowering Teaching Behaviours Questionnaire], Cronbach's alpha reliability coefficients for subscales ranged from .74 to .96 with an overall reliability of .89" (Babenko-Mould et al., 2012, p. 7).
"Internal consistency for survey responses in hospital using Cronbach's alpha was 0.95" (McQueen et al., 2013, p. 66).
"The estimated Cronbach's alpha for the revised 22-item NCSES [Nursing Competence Self-Efficacy Scale] with the study population was high (.919)" (Kennedy et al., 2015, p. 554).

TABLE 15.2

CRONBACH'S ALPHA SCORES FOR THE FOUR DOMAINS OF THE NURSING COMPETENCE SELF-EFFICACY SCALE

OPTIONS	CRONBACH'S ALPHA
Supporting Social Relationships	.83
Familiarity with Residents' Preferences	.71
Meaningful Resident–Staff Relationships	.62

Adapted from Boscart, V. M., Davey, M., Ploeg, J., Heckman, G., Dupuis, S., Sheiban, L., Luh Kim, J., Brown, P., & Sidani, S. (2018). Psychometric evaluation of the Team Member Perspectives of Person-Centered Care (TM-PCC) survey for long-term care homes. *Healthcare, 6*(2), 59. https://doi.org/10.3390/healthcare6020059.

---

three separate domains: supporting social relationships, familiarity with residents' preferences, and meaningful resident-staff relationships, as illustrated in Table 15.2. Cronbach's alpha ranged from .62 to .83, and the overall Cronbach's alpha was .82, thereby providing sufficient evidence of the internal consistency of the instrument.

Research Hint

If a research article provides information about the reliability of a measurement instrument but does not specify the type of reliability, it is probably safe to assume that internal consistency reliability was assessed with Cronbach's alpha.

Equivalence

Equivalence is either the consistency or agreement among observers who use the same measurement tool or the consistency or agreement between alternative forms of a tool. An instrument is thought to demonstrate equivalence when two or more observers have a high percentage of agreement about a certain behaviour or when alternative forms of a test yield a high correlation. Two methods to test equivalence are interrater reliability and alternate- or parallel-form reliability.

Interrater Reliability

Some measurement instruments are not self-administered questionnaires but instead are direct measurements of observed behaviour that must be systematically recorded. Such instruments must be tested for **interrater reliability** (the consistency of observations between two or more observers with the same tool). To accomplish interrater reliability, either two or more individuals should make an observation or one observer should observe the same behaviour on several occasions. The observers should score their observations with regard to the definition and operationalization of the behaviour to be observed.

When the research method of direct observation of a behaviour is required, consistency (or reliability) of the observations among all observers is extremely important. Interrater reliability concerns the reliability (or consistency) of the observer, not the reliability of the instrument. Interrater reliability is expressed either as a percentage of agreement between scorers or as a correlation coefficient of the scores assigned to the observed behaviours.

One method of calculating interrater reliability is Cohen's kappa, a coefficient of agreement between two raters that is considered to be a more precise estimate of interrater reliability. **Cohen's kappa** expresses the level of agreement that is observed beyond the level that would be expected by chance alone. A Cohen's kappa of .80 or better is generally assumed to indicate good interrater reliability. A

Cohen's kappa of .68 allows tentative conclusions to be drawn when lower levels of reliability are acceptable (McDowell & Newell, 1996). In their study describing the validation of a surgical neonatal nursing workload tool, Hart et al. (2019) checked for interrater reliability. To determine the validity of the Winnipeg Assessment of Neonatal Nursing Needs Tool-Surgical Complex (WANNNT-SC), the charge nurse on each shift was asked how many nurses, based off professional judgement were asked to meet unit staffing needs. Another senior nurse (rater) was asked to complete the blinded surgical tool within 1 hour of the charge nurse (p. 295). The overall interrater Kappa was .73, with a confidence interval ranging from .60–.87.

 Evidence-Informed Practice Tip _____
Interrater reliability is important for minimizing bias.

Parallel- or Alternate-Form Reliability

Parallel- or alternate-form reliability was described in the discussion of stability (see pp. 331–332). Use of parallel forms is thus a measure of stability and equivalence. The procedures for assessing equivalence through the use of parallel forms are the same.

VALIDITY

Validity refers to whether a measurement instrument accurately measures what it is intended to measure. To be valid, an instrument must first be reliable; without reliability, the instrument cannot have validity. However, reliability, although necessary, is not a sufficient condition for validity. Internal and external validity of a study are discussed in Chapter 10.

For example, a valid instrument that is intended to measure anxiety does so; it does not measure another construct, such as stress. A reliable measure can consistently rank participants on a given construct (e.g., anxiety), but a valid measure correctly measures the construct of interest. A measure can be reliable but not valid. Suppose that a researcher wanted to measure anxiety in patients by measuring their body temperatures. The researcher could obtain highly accurate, consistent, and precise temperature recordings, but such a measure would not be a valid indicator of anxiety. Thus, the high reliability of an instrument is not necessarily congruent with evidence of validity. A valid instrument, however, is reliable. If an instrument is erratic, inconsistent, and inaccurate, it cannot validly measure the attribute of interest.

The three major kinds of validity—content, criterion-related, and construct validity—vary according to the kind of information provided and the investigator's purpose. In critiquing research articles, you will want to evaluate whether sufficient evidence of validity is present and whether the type of validity is appropriate to the design of the study and instruments used in the study. The sample that provides the initial data for determining the reliability and validity of a measurement tool is termed a **validation sample**.

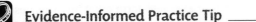

Evidence-Informed Practice Tip

Selecting measurement instruments that have strong evidence of validity increases the reader's confidence in the study findings—that the researchers actually measured what they intended to measure.

Content Validity

Content validity is the degree to which the content of the measure represents the universe of content—that is, the domain of a given construct. The universe of content provides the framework and basis for formulating the items that will adequately represent the content. When an investigator is developing a tool and issues of content validity arise, the concern is whether the measurement tool and the items it contains are representative of the universe of content that the researcher intends to measure. The researcher begins by defining the concept and identifying the dimensions that are the components of the concept. The items that reflect the concept and its dimensions are formulated (see Practical Application box for an example).

When the researcher has completed this task, the items are submitted to a panel of judges considered to be experts on this concept. Researchers typically request that the judges indicate their level of agreement with the scope of the items and the extent to which the items reflect the concept under consideration. The formula for evaluating agreement among experts on individual items is the number agreeing with an item divided by the number of experts. When the concept being rated is relevance, there are two standard methods for computing content validity. The first method is an item-level content validity index (I-CVI), which is computed as the number of experts giving a rating 3 or 4 to the relevancy of each item, divided by the total number of experts. This is usually the first round of rating content validity. In some validation research, there is a second round of agreement where an overall scale content validity is calculated. Oetker-Black and Davis (2019) in the development of the Mock Code Self-Efficacy scale established content validity by using two experts who actively teach cardiopulmonary resuscitation (CPR). The experts assessed if the items included accurately represented CPR skills. Each item was evaluated for relevance, clarity in representing the skills, and sufficiency. The experts were asked to assess the relevance and content of items. A content validity index was used to rate relevance of each item using a 4-point scale. All items received a rating of 3 or 4 by the experts, indicating that all items had content validity (p. 37).

Practical Application

Vincelette et al. (2019) reported on the preliminary development and validation of the nurse cardiopulmonary resuscitation survey (NCRS) among intensive care unit nurses. They first reviewed the literature and found that there was a gap in this area. Items for the scale were generated by one of the authors, based on the 2015 guidelines for advanced cardiovascular life support (ACLS). Two items were deemed repetitive and removed before submitting the instrument to face validity experts. The assessment of face validity led to the adjustment of the word choice of three items that were perceived as unclear. This step led to a final version that was submitted to an independent expert panel to assess content validity.

A subtype of content validity is **face validity**, which is a rudimentary type of validity in which the instrument intuitively gives the appearance of measuring the concept. To establish face validity, colleagues or participants are asked to read the instrument and evaluate the content in terms of whether it appears to reflect the concept that the researcher intends to measure. This procedure may be useful in the tool development process in terms of determining the readability and clarity of the content. Face validity, however, should in no way be considered a satisfactory alternative to other types of validity. In the development of the Mock Code Self-Efficacy Scale for nursing students, Oetker-Black and Davis (2019) established face validity by using five senior undergraduate nursing students to review the questions and the reading level.

Evidence-Informed Practice Tip

When face validity and content validity, the most basic types of validity, are the only types of validity reported in a research article, you, as a research consumer, cannot appraise the measurement tools as having strong psychometric properties; thus, you would lack confidence in the usefulness of the study findings.

Criterion-Related Validity

Criterion-related validity is the degree of relationship between the participant's performance on the measurement tool and the participant's actual behaviour. The criterion is usually the second measure, which is used to assess the same concept being studied.

Two types of criterion-related validity are concurrent and predictive. Concurrent validity is the degree of correlation of two measures of the same construct administered at the same time. A high correlation coefficient indicates agreement between the two measures. **Predictive validity** is the degree of correlation between the measure of the concept and a future measure of the same concept. Because of the passage of time, the correlation coefficients are likely to be lower for predictive validity studies.

For example, in a study by Ford-Gilboe et al. (2016) describing the development and validation of Composite Abuse Scale (Revised)—Short Form (CASR-SF), they examined concurrent validity through measures of depression, symptoms of PTSD and coercive control. As expected, CASR-SF total scores were moderately correlated with each validation measure, providing support for concurrent validity of the instrument construct validity.

Construct Validity

Construct validity is the extent to which a test measures a theoretical construct or trait. To establish this type of validity, the researcher attempts to validate a body of theory underlying the measurement and testing of the hypothesized relationships. Empirical testing confirms or fails to confirm the relationships that would be predicted among concepts and, as such, provides more or less support for the construct validity of the instruments measuring those concepts. Establishing construct validity is a complex process, often involving several studies and approaches. The following approaches are discussed in this section: hypothesis-testing, convergent and divergent, contrasted-groups, and factor-analytical.

In their study, Sidani et al. (2017) assessed construct validity of the MDTSM discussed in Item-to-Total Correlation section earlier, by factor analysis and relationships between the variables. They found that there was a positive relationship between the MDTSM subscales and self-reported adherence to therapy, which means that high levels of satisfaction were associated with high levels of adherence (p. 9).

Hypothesis-Testing Approach

When the **hypothesis-testing approach** is used, the investigator uses the theory or concept underlying the measurement instrument to validate the instrument. The investigator accomplishes this task first by developing hypotheses about the behaviour of individuals with varying scores on the measure; then by gathering data to test the hypotheses; and, finally, on the basis of the findings, by making inferences about whether the rationale underlying the instrument's construction is adequate to explain the findings. Hypothesis-testing approaches include convergent validity, divergent validity, and known-groups validity.

For example, Lambert et al. (2015) used a hypothesis-testing approach to establish the Appraisal of Caregiving Scale. This scale was designed to evaluate stress associated with caregiving for someone with advanced cancer. Construct validity was tested positively on the basis of two hypotheses: (1) that depressed caregivers had higher stress scores than non-depressed caregivers and (2) younger caregivers reported significantly higher scores on the General Stress subscale than older caregivers.

CONVERGENT AND DIVERGENT APPROACHES. Two strategies for assessing construct validity are convergent and divergent approaches.

Convergent validity exists when two or more tools that are intended to measure the same construct are administered to participants and are found to be positively correlated. A correlational analysis (i.e., a test of relationship; see Chapters 12 and 17) determines whether the measures are positively correlated, in which case convergent validity is said to be supported.

In contrast to convergent validity, the calculation of **divergent validity** requires measurement approaches that differentiate one construct from others that may be similar. Sometimes researchers search for instruments that measure the opposite of the construct. If the divergent measure is negatively related to other measures, the measure's validity is strengthened.

As an example, Melnyk, Oswalt, and Sidora-Arcoleo (2014) assessed the psychometric properties of scores on the Neonatal Intensive Care Unit Parental Beliefs Scale (NICU PBS) in a sample of mothers and fathers of preterm infants receiving intensive care. The NICU PBS is a rating instrument designed to assess parental beliefs about their premature infant and their role during hospitalization. For convergent and divergent (discriminant) validity assessment, correlation analysis of the Time 1 data was used for assessment of the NICU PBS with maternal demographic

characteristics (age, education, employment status), mental health, stress, pregnancy history variables (gravidity, high-risk status, subsequent pregnancy in 12 months), and baby outcome variables (Clinical Risk Index for Babies [CRIB] scores, birth weight, NICU length of stay). Higher total PBS scores were associated with younger maternal age, lower education, lower income, receipt of Medicaid, minority status, mothers' employment, no biological father in the study, higher gravidity, having had another child in the past 12 months, shorter NICU length of stay, and lower stress, anxiety, and depression.

A specific method of assessing convergent and divergent validity is the **multitrait-multimethod approach**. Similar to the divergent validity approach just described, this method, proposed by Campbell and Fiske (1959), also involves examining the relationships between instruments that are intended to measure the same construct and between those that are intended to measure different constructs. A variety of measurement strategies, however, are used. In other words, this approach is a type of validation in which more than one method is used to assess the accuracy of an instrument. For example, anxiety could be measured by the following:

- Administering the State-Trait Anxiety Inventory
- Recording blood pressure readings
- Asking the participant about anxious feelings
- Observing the participant's behaviour

The results of one of these measures should then be correlated with the results of each of the others in a multitrait-multimethod matrix (Waltz, Strickland, & Lenz, 1991).

The use of multiple measures of a concept decreases systematic error. The use of a variety of data-collection methods (e.g., self-report, observation, interview, and collection of physiological data) also diminishes the effect of systematic error.

Contrasted-Groups Approach

In the **contrasted-groups approach** (sometimes called the **known-groups approach**) to the development of construct validity, the researcher identifies two groups of individuals expected to score extremely high or extremely low in the characteristic being measured by the instrument. The instrument is administered to both groups, and the differences in scores are examined. If the instrument is sensitive to individual differences in the trait being measured, the mean performance of these two groups should differ significantly, and evidence of construct validity would be supported. A t test or analysis of variance is used to statistically measure the difference between the two groups.

Factor-Analytical Approach

A final approach to assessing construct validity is **factor analysis**. This procedure gives the researcher information about the extent to which a set of items measures the same underlying construct or the same dimension of a construct. In factor analysis, the researcher assesses the degree to which the individual items on a scale truly cluster around one or more dimensions. Items designed to measure the same dimension should load on the same factor; those designed to measure differing dimensions should load on different factors (Nunnally & Bernstein, 1994).

A factor analysis also indicates whether the items in the instrument reflect a single construct or several constructs. Several factors may be identified in a set of data. The study must have a large sample size in order to conduct a factor analysis. Nunnally and Bernstein (1994) recommended 10 observations for each variable. Thus, to develop the factor structure and reliability of the Nursing

Competence Self-Efficacy Scale, Kennedy and associates (2015) used 252 students to test 22 items.

 Research Hint _____

When validity data about a study's measurement instruments are not included in a research article, you cannot determine whether the intended concept is being captured by the measurement tool. Before you use the results, check the instrument's validity by reviewing the original source.

 Evidence-Informed Practice Tip _____

When the tools used in a study are presented, note whether the sample used to develop the measurement instruments is similar to your patient population.

The Critical Thinking Decision Path will help you assess the appropriateness of the type of validity and reliability selected for use in a particular research study.

Researchers may be concerned about whether the scores that were obtained for a sample of participants were consistent, true measures of the behaviours, and thus an accurate reflection of the differences between individuals. The extent of variability in test scores that is attributable to error rather than a true measure of the behaviours is the error variance.

An **observed test score** that is derived from a set of items consists of the true score plus error (Figure 15.2). The error may be either chance (random) error or systematic error.

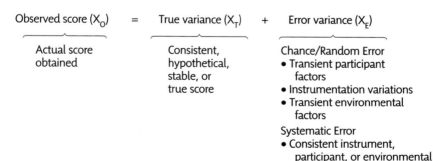

FIG. 15.2 Components of observed scores.

A chance error or a random error is an error that is difficult to control (e.g., a respondent's anxiety at the time of testing). These errors are unsystematic and are not predictable; thus, they cannot be corrected. However, awareness of the sources of these errors may help the researcher minimize their effect on measurement accuracy. These sources are as follows:

1. Transient human conditions, such as hunger, fatigue, health, lack of motivation, and anxiety, which are often beyond the awareness and control of the examiner.

2. Variations in the measurement procedure, such as misplacement of the blood pressure cuff, not waiting for a specific time period before taking the blood pressure, or placing the arm randomly in relation to the heart while measuring blood pressure; changing the wording of interview questions between administrations; or environmental factors, such as the presence of others while data are being obtained, a cold room, or discomfort with the researcher (who is part of the environment).

3. Errors in data processing, such as coding errors and incorrect inputting into the computer.

Chance errors affect an individual's observed score, so that the person's observed score may be higher than his or her true score, whereas another person's observed score may be lower than his or her true score. Instruments that are free of chance errors are considered reliable. A **systematic error** or a **constant error** is a measurement error that is attributable to relatively stable characteristics of the study population that may bias their behaviour, cause incorrect instrument calibration, or both. Such error has a systematic biasing influence on the participants' responses and thereby influences the validity of the instruments. Level of education, socioeconomic status, social desirability, response pattern, or other characteristics may influence the validity of the instrument by altering the measurement of the "true" responses in a systematic way. For example, a participant who wants to please the investigator may constantly answer items in a socially desirable way, thus making the estimate of validity inaccurate.

Systematic error also occurs when an instrument is improperly calibrated. Consider a scale that consistently gives a person's weight at 1 kg less than the actual body weight. The scale could be quite reliable (i.e., capable of reproducing the precise measurement), but the result is consistently invalid. Systematic error is considered part of the true score. The multimethod-multitrait approach is one method of decreasing systematic error. The validity of an instrument is the extent to which it is free of both chance errors and systematic errors.

The amount of detail about reliability and validity varies considerably among research articles. When the focus of a study is tool development, psychometric evaluation—including extensive reliability and validity data—is carefully documented and appears throughout the article rather than briefly in the "Instruments" section, as in other research studies.

RIGOUR IN QUALITATIVE RESEARCH

It is important to keep in mind that qualitative research is an umbrella term that covers a variety of research methods. While there are general principles when evaluating rigour or trustworthiness in qualitative studies, there are also differences across methods that will influence criteria for evaluating. Although there is still debate amongst researchers about how to best evaluate qualitative research, there is consensus that given its increasing prevalence and use in evidence-informed practice, there should be some evaluation of quality (Williams et al., 2020).

As in quantitative research, the basic approach to ensure rigour in qualitative research is employing methodical research design, data collection, interpretation, and communication. Qualitative researchers seek to achieve two goals: (1) to account for the method and the data, which must be independent so that another researcher can analyze the same data in the same way and make the same conclusions; and (2) to produce a credible

CRITICAL THINKING DECISION PATH

Determining the Appropriate Type of Validity and Reliability Selected for a Study

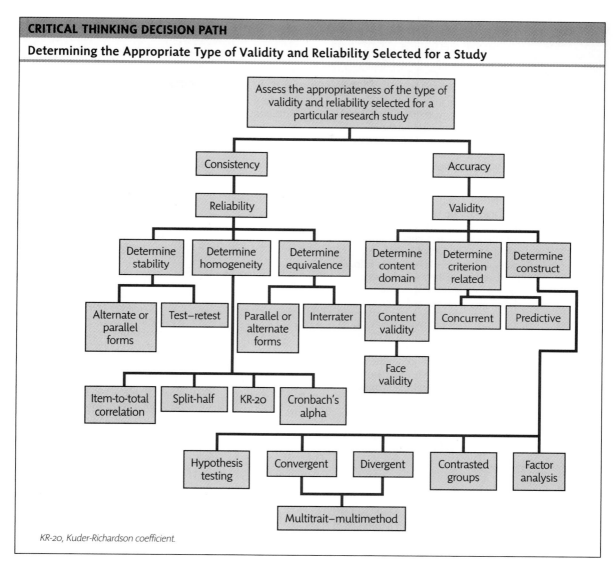

KR-20, Kuder-Richardson coefficient.

and reasoned explanation of the phenomenon under study. Thus, the rigour in qualitative methodology is judged by unique criteria appropriate for the research approach and is often called trustworthiness. Credibility, auditability, and fittingness are some of the scientific criteria for *trustworthiness* proposed for qualitative research studies by Lincoln and Guba (1985), along with authenticity (Guba & Lincoln, 1994). The meaning of credibility, auditability, and fittingness are briefly explained in Table 15.3.

Morse et al. (2002) offered a different viewpoint and terminology to describe rigour in qualitative research. They argued that ensuring rigour is part of the process of the research, rather than a post hoc evaluation of the presented research study, and that reliability and validity are useful terms in qualitative research. In qualitative research, reliability means showing consistent support for the findings across participants; validity means the data are appropriate and provide an accurate account of participants (Spiers et al., 2018). Verification refers to the

TABLE 15.3	
CRITERIA FOR JUDGING SCIENTIFIC RIGOUR: CREDIBILITY, AUDITABILITY, FITTINGNESS	
CRITERIA	**CHARACTERISTICS**
Credibility	Truth of findings as judged by participants and others within the discipline. For example, you may find the researcher returning to the participants to share interpretation of findings and query accuracy from the perspective of the persons living the experience.
Auditability	Accountability as judged by the adequacy of information leading the reader from the research question and raw data through various steps of analysis to the interpretation of findings. For example, you should be able to follow the reasoning of the researcher step by step through explicit examples of data, interpretations, and syntheses.
Fittingness	Faithfulness to the everyday reality of the participants, described in enough detail so that others in the discipline can evaluate importance for their own practice, research, and theory development. For example, you will know enough about the human experience being reported that you can decide whether it "rings true" and is useful for guiding your practice.

TABLE 15.4	
VERIFICATION STRATEGIES IN QUALITATIVE RESEARCH	
STRATEGY	**DESCRIPTION**
Investigator responsiveness	-ongoing analysis forces purposive sampling-ensure analysis holds together; be open to new ideas, giving up those that are not supported by the data
Methodological coherence	-coherence between the research question and the methods-question should match the method, which matches the data collection and analysis procedures
Appropriate sampling	-participants should be appropriate; those who have knowledge of the research topic-adequate number to account for different aspects of phenomenon
Concurrent data collection and analysis	-analysis begins as data collection begins-ensures mutual interaction between "what is known and what one needs to know" (p. 18)
Thinking theoretically	-building a solid foundation, in incremental steps-emerging ideas are reconfirmed in new data
Theory development	-move between a micro perspective of data to a macro conceptual/theoretical understanding

Adapted from: Morse et al. (2002). Verification strategies for establishing reliability and validity in qualitative research. *International Journal of Qualitative Methods*, 1(2), 13–22. https://sites.ualberta.ca/~iiqm/backissues/1_2Final/pdf/morseetal.pdf.

process of evaluating the multiple decisions made during the research, which contribute to the validity and reliability of the qualitative study (Morse et al., 2002). Verification strategies proposed by Morse et al. (2002) are found in Table 15.4. Other terms you may encounter are transparency, reflexivity, dependability, and transferability.

Research Hint

Different qualitative methods will use different processes to ensure rigour. Understanding the different qualitative methods, as presented in Chapter 8, is an important part of assessing a qualitative research report. Evaluating adherence to the stated method is an important aspect of rigour in qualitative research; this is called *methodological coherence*. There should be enough description of the research process in the "Methods" section that you can evaluate this coherence.

Credibility

Credibility is a characteristic of qualitative research that refers to the accuracy, validity, and soundness of data. It is similar to internal validity in qualitative research. The methods to ensure credibility are prolonged engagement, persistent observation, peer debriefing, and member checks (Lincoln, 1995). In prolonged engagement and persistent observation, the researchers spend sufficient time with the study's participants to check for discrepancies in responses. Peer debriefing is conducted with experts in the field, whose probing questions and review about the research can assist the researchers in improving trustworthiness in the data. Member checking verifies the accuracy of participants' responses by asking the study participants to review the themes and narratives to determine whether the researchers accurately described their experiences (Lincoln & Guba, 1985). Member checking is not an appropriate strategy for all qualitative methods (Morse et al., 2002).

Triangulation, crystallization, and searching for disconfirming evidence through negative case analyses are also used to ensure credibility and confirmability. In Chapter 7, triangulation—the cross-checking and verification of data through the use of different information sources, such as a variety of data sources, investigators, theoretical models, and research methods—and crystallization in both qualitative and mixed method research are discussed. Triangulation is viewed as offering completeness to naturalistic inquiry (Tobin & Begley, 2004), but may not be appropriate for all methods.

Auditability and Fittingness

Engaging in an inquiry audit establishes both the auditability and the fittingness of the data. **Auditability** is the characteristic of a qualitative study, developed by the investigator's research process, that allows another researcher or a reader to follow the thinking or conclusions of the investigator. Auditability means the researcher presents a decision trail to the reader, and this allows the reader of the research to better judge its quality or trustworthiness (Sandelowski, 1986). Fittingness is the degree to which study findings are applicable or transferable outside the study situation and the degree to which the results are meaningful to individuals not involved in the research. The audit trail was proposed by Guba (1981) to allow external auditors to follow the trail of qualitative data gathering and has been described by Lincoln and Guba (1985) as "the most important trustworthiness technique available" (p. 283). The audit trail involves reviewing all documents relating to the study, such as the research protocol, memos and correspondences, research tools, and field notes.

An example of how transferability was enhanced in a grounded theory study is provided by King-Shier et al. (2019). They were able to develop rich descriptions of the management of hypertension within a group of South Asians. Careful sampling to ensure representation, rigourous data analysis procedures, and data saturation contributed to the ability of others to see utility of the results in other contexts (p. 323).

Authenticity

Authenticity refers to fairness in the presentation in that all value conflicts, differences, and views of the participants are noted in the analysis. The reader can understand the moods and experiences of the participants while reading the thematic analyses (Guba & Lincoln, 1994). A variety of viewpoints should be offered, and not only those that align with the researchers' previously held views and opinions (Tobin & Begley, 2004).

Reflexivity. Reflexivity refers to the researcher's process of reflection and critical thinking during the research process. In particular, the researcher should reflect on whether or how they have influenced sampling, data collection, analysis, and presentation of the findings (Williams et al., 2020). This is often supported by a skeptical peer review during the research process or during the publication process (Buetow, 2019). Another technique to promote reflexivity is the keeping of field notes or reflective journals during the research process. Ethnographers, for example, will routinely document changes in their ideas, beliefs, and values as they are engaged in the research.

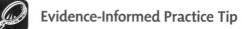 **Evidence-Informed Practice Tip** ___

The narrative or visual formats used by qualitative researchers can be an artistic as well as a scholarly endeavour (Sandelowski, 2015). As a reader, it is important to be critical about the presentation of the research, and how that might affect what you take away from it. Can good writing cover up bad research? Or can good research be overlooked because of poor writing?

Tools for Appraising Qualitative Research. Critical appraisal checklists and frameworks to assess qualitative research can be found from numerous sources. It is important to keep in mind that there are two types of tools: those intended to provide guidance in appraisal of quality, and those that provide guidance and criteria for researchers and reviewers in terms of how to report a qualitative research project (Williams et al., 2020). Meyrick (2006) offered a useful model for evaluating qualitative research based on guiding principles of transparency and conducting research systematically (Figure 15.3). This model captures many of the suggestions described previously regarding rigour in qualitative research.

Practical Application

Benbow et al. (2019) incorporated several strategies to ascertain rigour in their study to better understand the unique narratives of social exclusion for mothers experiencing homelessness. In terms of credibility, the researcher ensured prolonged engagement in community agencies, which involved opportunities for follow-up interviews with participants and e-mail/telephone/face-to-face follow-up with service providers and community agencies to discuss study results. The follow-up interviews were not for member checking, but to share and co-construct current understandings and provide an opportunity for participants to review their transcripts. An audit trail was used to make clear all decision-making throughout the analysis process. Each decision was tracked and supported with raw data, while being grounded in the study purpose and the theoretical lens of the study. Fittingness was achieved during follow-up interviews where the researcher gained insight and special attention was paid to convergent and divergent perspectives within and across participants. Because the criteria of credibility, fittingness/transferability, and auditability were met, trustworthiness was achieved.

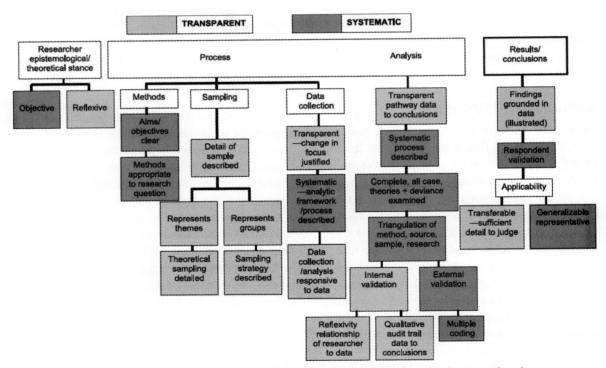

FIG. 15.3 Quality framework for qualitative research. From Meyrick, J. (2006). What is good qualitative research: A first step towards a comprehensive approach to judging rigour/quality. *Journal of Health Psychology*, 11(5), 799–808. https://doi.10.1177/1359105306066643.

APPRAISING THE EVIDENCE

Reliability and Validity

Reliability and validity are two crucial aspects in the critical appraisal of a measurement instrument. The reviewer evaluates an instrument's level of reliability and validity, as well as how they were established. In a research report, the reliability and validity for each measure should be presented. If these data have not been presented, the reviewer must seriously question the merit and use of the tool and the study's results. Criteria for critiquing reliability and validity are presented in the Critiquing Criteria box.

If reliable and valid questionnaires are not used in a study, the results cannot be credible. As a critiquer, you have an ethical responsibility to question the reliability and validity of instruments used in research studies and to examine the findings in view of the quality of the instruments used and the data presented. The following discussion highlights key areas related to reliability and validity that should be evident in a research article.

Appropriate reliability tests should have been performed by the developer of the measurement tool and should then have been included by the current user in the research report. If the initial standardization sample and the current sample have different characteristics, the reader would find either (1) that a pilot study for the present sample would have been conducted to determine whether the reliability was maintained or (2) that a reliability estimate was calculated for the current sample. For example, if the standardization sample for a tool that measures "satisfaction in an intimate heterosexual relationship" comprises undergraduate college students and if an investigator plans to use the tool with married couples, the reliability of the tool should be established with the latter group.

The investigator determines which type of reliability procedure is used in the study, depending on the nature of the measurement tool and how it will be used. For example, if the instrument is to be administered twice, you might determine that test-retest reliability should have been used to establish the stability of the tool. If an alternate form of the instrument has been developed for use in a repeated-measures design, evidence of alternate-form reliability should be presented to determine the equivalence of the parallel forms.

If the degree of internal consistency among the items is relevant, an appropriate test of internal consistency should be presented. In some instances, more than one type of reliability is presented, but you should determine whether all are appropriate. For example, the Kuder-Richardson formula implies that a single right or wrong answer exists, which makes use of the coefficient inappropriate with scales that provide a format of three or more possible responses. In such cases, another formula is applied, such as Cronbach's alpha.

Another important consideration is the acceptable level of reliability, which varies according to the type of test. Coefficients with reliability of .70 or higher are desirable. The validity of an instrument is limited by its reliability; in other words, less confidence can be placed in scores from tests with low-reliability coefficients.

Satisfactory evidence of validity is probably the most difficult determination for you as reviewer. This aspect of measurement is most likely to fall short of meeting the required criteria. Validity studies are time consuming and complex, and researchers sometimes settle for presenting minimal validity data.

Therefore, you should closely examine the item content of a tool when you evaluate its strengths and weaknesses and try to find conclusive evidence of content validity. In the body of a research article, however, it is unusual to have more than a few sample items available for review. Thus, you should determine whether the appropriate assessment of content validity was used to meet the researcher's goal.

Such procedures provide assurance that the tool is psychometrically sound and that the content of the items is consistent with the conceptual framework and the construct definitions. Construct validity and criterion-related validity are two of the more precise statistical tests of whether the tool measures what it is intended to measure. Ideally, an instrument should provide evidence of content validity, as well as criterion-related or construct validity, before a reviewer invests a high level of confidence in the tool.

You should also expect to see the strengths and weaknesses of instrument reliability and validity presented in the "Discussion," "Limitations," or

Continued

┌───┐
APPRAISING THE EVIDENCE—*cont'd*
Reliability and Validity

"Recommendations" section, or in all of these sections, of a research article. In this context, the reliability and validity might be discussed in relation to other tools devised to measure the same variable. The relationship of the study's findings to the strengths and weaknesses in instrument reliability and validity is another important discussion point.

Finally, the researcher should propose recommendations for improving future studies in relation to instrument reliability and validity. For example, in the "Implications for Future Research and Practice" section of a report about developing and validating the Nursing Competence Self-Efficacy Scale, Kennedy and associates (2015) noted

that they will be conducting a replication of this initial psychometric assessment with a larger sample to support the factor structure in the study.

Collegial dialogue is also an approach to evaluating the merits and shortcomings of an existing instrument, as well as a newly developed one, that is reported in the nursing literature. Such an exchange promotes the understanding of methodologies and techniques of reliability and validity, stimulates the acquisition of a basic knowledge of psychometrics, and encourages the exploration of alternative methods of observation and the use of reliable and valid tools in clinical practice.
└───┘

CRITIQUING CRITERIA

QUANTITATIVE STUDIES

1. Was an appropriate method used to test the reliability of the tool?
2. Is the reliability of the tool adequate?
3. Was an appropriate method used to test the validity of the instrument?
4. Is the validity of the measurement tool adequate?
5. If the sample from the developmental stage of the tool was different from the current sample, were the reliability and validity recalculated to determine whether the tool is still adequate?

6. Have the strengths and weaknesses of the reliability and validity of each instrument been presented?
7. Are the strengths and weaknesses of the research appropriately addressed in the "Discussion," "Limitations," or "Recommendations" sections of the report?

QUALITATIVE STUDIES

1. Do the authors explain the process of the research, including the specific qualitative method used?
2. Is evidence provided that the researcher's interpretation is supported by the data?

3. Can the reader follow the researcher's thinking?
4. Does the study follow the principles and processes of the stated research method?
5. Can the findings be applicable to outside the study situation?
6. Are the results meaningful to individuals not involved in the research?
7. Do the conclusions, implications, and recommendations give the reader a context in which to use the findings?
8. Do the conclusions reflect the study's findings?
9. Is there evidence of researcher reflexivity?

CRITICAL THINKING CHALLENGES

- Discuss the three types of validity that must be established before a reviewer invests a high level of confidence in the tool. Include examples of each type of validity.
- What are the major tests of reliability? Is it necessary to establish more than one measure of reliability for each instrument used in a study? Which do you think is the most essential

measure of reliability? Include examples in your answer.
- Is it possible to have a valid instrument that is not reliable? Is the reverse possible? Support your answer with instruments you might use in the clinical setting with your patients.
- What are some ways in which credibility, auditability, and fittingness can be evaluated?
- How do you think the concept of evidence-informed practice has changed research utilization

models? Is the review of the literature the same when a research proposal is developed as it is when the steps of research utilization or an evidence-informed practice protocol is implemented? Support your position.

CRITICAL JUDGEMENT QUESTIONS

1. In testing a new scale to measure nursing students' clinical competency in simulation, the researchers administered repeatedly and obtained the same results, this is called?

   a. Validity
   b. Reliability
   c. Consistency
   d. Predictability

2. A newly developed instrument is found to have a Cronbach's alpha of .82. What is the correct interpretation of this finding?

   a. The instrument has no internal consistency
   b. The instrument has a low degree of internal consistency
   c. The instrument has a moderate degree of internal consistency
   d. The instrument has a relatively high degree of internal consistency

3. What is the formal term for rigour in qualitative research?

   a. Identifying metaphors from data
   b. Describing the insiders' view of data
   c. Bracketing
   d. Trustworthiness

KEY POINTS

- Reliability and validity are crucial aspects of conducting and critiquing research.
- Validity refers to whether an instrument measures what it is purported to measure. It is a crucial aspect of evaluating a tool.
- Three types of validity are content validity, criterion-related validity, and construct validity.

- The choice of a validation method is important and is made by the researcher on the basis of the characteristics of the measurement device in question and its use.
- Reliability refers to the ratio between accuracy and inaccuracy in a measurement device.
- The major tests of reliability are test-retest reliability, parallel- or alternate-form reliability, split-half reliability, item-to-total correlation, the Kuder-Richardson coefficient, Cronbach's alpha, and interrater reliability.
- The selection of a method for establishing reliability depends on the characteristics of the tool, the testing method that is used for collecting data from the standardization sample, and the kinds of data that are obtained.
- Credibility, auditability, and fittingness are criteria for judging the scientific rigour of a qualitative research study.

 FOR FURTHER STUDY

Go to Evolve at http://evolve.elsevier.com/Canada/LoBiondo/Research for the Audio Glossary.

REFERENCES

Benbow, S., Forchuk, C., Berman, H., Gorlick, C., & Ward-Griffin, C. (2019). Spaces of exclusion: Safety, stigma, and surveillance of mothers experiencing homelessness. *Canadian Journal of Nursing Research, 51*(3), 202–213. https://doi.org/10.1177/0844562119859138.

Boscart, V. M., Davey, M., Ploeg, J., Heckman, G., Dupuis, S., Sheiban, L., Luh Kim, J., Brown, P., & Sidani, S. (2018). Psychometric evaluation of the team member perspectives of person-centered care (TM-PCC) survey for long-term care homes. *Healthcare (Basel, Switzerland), 6*(2), 59. https://doi.org/10.3390/healthcare6020059.

Boyle, G. J., Saklofske, D. H., & Matthews, G. (2015). Criteria for selection and evaluation of scales and measures. In G. J. Boyle, D. H. Saklofske, & G. Matthews (Eds.), *Measures of personality and social psychological constructs* (pp. 3–15). Philadelphia: Elsevier Academic Press. https://doi.org/10.1016/B978-0-12-386915-9.00001-2.

Buetow, S. (2019). Apophenia, unconscious bias and re-flexivity in nursing qualitative research. *International Journal of Nursing Studies, 89*, 8–13. https://doi.org/10.1016/j.ijnurstu.2018.09.013.

Campbell, D., & Fiske, D. (1959). Convergent and discriminant validation by the matrix. *Psychological Bulletin, 53*, 273–302.

Corby, K., Kane, D., & Dayus, D. (2019). Investigating predictors of prenatal breastfeeding self-efficacy. *Canadian Journal of Nursing Research, 53*(1), 56–63. https://doi.org/10.1177/0844562119888363.

Ford-Gilboe, M., Wathen, C. N., Varcoe, C., MacMillan, H. L, Scott-Storey, K., Mantler, T., Hegarty, K., & Perrin, N. (2016). Development of a brief mea-sure of intimate partner violence experiences: the Composite Abuse Scale (Revised)-Short Form (CASR-SF). *BMJ Open, 6*, 12. https://doi.org/10.1136/bmjopen-2016-012824.

Guba, E. G. (1981). Criteria for assessing the trust-worthiness of naturalistic enquiries. *Educational Communication and Technology Journal, 29*, 75–91.

Guba, E., & Lincoln, Y (1994). Competing paradigms in qualitative research. In N. Denzin, & Y. Lincoln (Eds.), *Handbook of qualitative research* (pp. 105–117). Thousand Oaks, CA: Sage.

Hart, K., Marchuk, A., Walsh, J.-L., & Howlett, A. (2019). Validation of a surgical neonatal nurs-ing workload tool. *Journal of Neonatal Nursing, 25*(6), 293–297. https://doi.org/10.1016/j.jnn.2019.06.002.

Kara, E., & Cinar, I.O. (2020). Validity and reliability of The Cancer Loneliness and The Cancer-Related Negative Social Expectations Scale. *International Journal of Assessment Tools in Education, 7* (3), 392–403. https://doi.org/10.21449/ijate.711073.

Kennedy, E., Tomblin-Murphy, G., Martin-Misener, R., et al. (2015). Development and psychometric assess-ment of the Nursing Competence Self-Efficacy Scale. *Journal of Nursing Education, 54*(10), 550–558.

King-Shier, K. M., Dhaliwal, K. K., Puri, R., LeBlanc, P., & Johal, J. (2019). South Asians' experience of managing hypertension: A grounded theory study. *Patient Preference and Adherence, 13*, 321–329. https://doi.org/10.2147/PPA.S196224.

Lambert, S.D., Yoon, H., Ellis, K.R., & Northouse, L. (2015). Measuring appraisal during advanced cancer: psychometrica testing of the appraisal of caregiv-ing scale. *Patient Education and Counselling, 98*(5), 633–639.

Lincoln, Y. S. (1995). Emerging criteria for qualita-tive and interpretive research. *Qualitative Inquiry, 3*, 275–289.

Lincoln, Y. S., & Guba, E. G. (1985). *Naturalistic in-quiry*. New York: Sage.

Liou, S. R., Liu, H. C., Tsai, H. M., et al. (2015). The de-velopment and psychometric testing of a theory-based instrument to evaluate nurses' perception of clinical reasoning competence. *Journal of Advanced Nursing, 72*(3), 707–717.

McDowell, I., & Newell, C. (1996). *Measuring health: A guide to rating scales and questionnaires*. New York: Oxford University Press.

Melnyk, B. M., Oswalt, K. L., & Sidora-Arcoleo, K. (2014). Validation and psychometric properties of the Neonatal Intensive Care Unit Parental Beliefs Scale. *Nursing Research, 63*(2), 279–289.

Meyrick, J. (2006). What is good qualitative research? A first step towards a comprehensive approach to judging rigour/quality. *Journal of Health Psychology, 11*(5), 799–808. https://doi.org/10.1177/1359105306066643.

Morse, J. M., Barrett, M., Mayan, M., Olson, K., & Spiers, J. (2002). Verification strategies for establish-ing reliability and validity in qualitative research. *International Journal of Qualitative Methods, 1*(2), 13–22. https://doi.org/10.1177/160940690200100202.

Nunnally, J. C., & Bernstein, I. H. (1994). *Psychometric theory* (3rd ed.). New York: McGraw-Hill.

Oetker-Black, S. L., & Davis, T. (2019). Psychometric evaluation of the Mock Code Self-Efficacy Scale. *Nursing Education Perspectives, 40*(1), 35–40. https://doi.org/10.1097/01.NEP.0000000000000341.

O'Keefe-McCarthy, S., McGillion, M., Nelson, S., et al. (2014). Content validity of the Toronto Pain Management Inventory–Acute Coronary Syndrome Version. *Canadian Journal of Cardiovascular Nurses, 24*(2), 11–18.

Sandelowski, M. (1986). The problem of rigor in qualita-tive research. *Advances in Nursing Science, 8*(3), 27–37. https://doi.org/10.1097/00012272-198604000-00005.

Sandelowski, M. (2015). A matter of taste: Evaluating the quality of qualitative research. *Nursing Inquiry, 22*(2), 86–94. https://doi.org/10.1111/nin.12080.

Sidani, S., Epstein, D. R., & Fox, M. (2017). Psychometric evaluation of a multi-dimensional measure of satisfaction with behavioral interven-tions. *Research in Nursing & Health, 40*(5), 459–469. https://doi.org/10.1002/nur.21808.

Spiers, J., Morse, J. M., Olson, K., Mayan, M., & Barrett, M. (2018). Reflection/commentary on a past article: Verification strategies for establishing reliability and validity in qualitative research. *International Journal of Qualitative Methods, 17*(1-2). https://doi.org/10.1177/1609406918788237.

Tobin, G. A., & Begley, C. M. (2004). Methodological rigour within a qualitative framework. *Journal of Advanced Nursing, 48*, 388–396.

Vincelette, C., Quiroz-Martinez, H., Fortin, O., & Lavoie, S. (2019). Preliminary development and validation of the Nurse Cardiopulmonary Resuscitation Survey (NCRS) among intensive care unit nurses. *Official Journal of the Canadian Association of Critical Care Nurses, 30*, 24–31.

Waltz, C., Strickland, O., & Lenz, E. (1991). *Measurement in nursing research* (3rd ed.). Philadelphia: F.A. Davis.

Williams, V., Boylan, A. M., & Nunan, D. (2020). Critical appraisal of qualitative research: necessity, partialities and the issue of bias. *BMJ Evidence-Based Medicine, 25*(1), 9–11. https://dx.doi.org/10.1136/bmjebm-2018-111132.

CHAPTER 16

Qualitative Data Analysis

Lorraine Thirsk | Sarah Stahlke

LEARNING OUTCOMES

After reading this chapter, you will be able to do the following:

- Examine the processes of qualitative data analysis.
- Outline the steps common to qualitative data analysis.
- Describe how data are interpreted to form meaningful units (themes).
- Summarize the process of identifying themes and categories and the relationships between them.
- Compare the process of creating and presenting interpretations from select qualitative methods.
- Assess the integrity of data analysis from a qualitative study.

KEY TERMS

codes	data analysis	thematic analysis
coding	data display	themes
constant comparative method	data reduction	
	member checking	

STUDY RESOURCES

 Go to Evolve at http://evolve.elsevier.com/Canada/LoBiondo/Research for the Audio Glossary.

QUALITATIVE DATA ANALYSIS is a multifaceted, complex, and systematic process. The data generated through a qualitative research project can include transcripts of interviews, narratives, documents, photographs, media such as newspapers and movies, and field notes. Qualitative researchers collect enormous amounts of data, which must be managed carefully; several hundred pages of transcript can result from 25 interviews. To add to the complexity of qualitative data analysis, many researchers take different approaches to analysis, based on the purpose of the study and the conceptual framework or methodology used. This chapter expands on the discussion in Chapter 9, in which the analysis of data was introduced in the context of several qualitative research traditions, such as phenomenology, grounded theory, ethnography, and qualitative description. General principles and common types of analysis are reviewed, along with specific examples of some common analytical processes and considerations.

DATA MANAGEMENT

The open nature of qualitative inquiry typically results in the collection of more data than required. Glesne (2011) refers to the sheer volume of the data collected as "fat data." Consequently, researchers must be methodical in their organization and management of the data. Some researchers will organize all of these data by hand, but computer software can also be used to simplify the storage and retrieval of data. In addition, researchers are also required to develop a decision or audit trail, which necessitates the tracking of the participants, the original audio recordings, and original and photocopied documents. Moreover, all the data must be kept secure to maintain confidentiality.

Audio Recording Interviews

As discussed in Chapter 8, qualitative researchers gather data from a variety of sources, including interviews, observations, narratives, and focus groups (Merriam & Tisdell, 2016). Interviews are the most common source and serve as the primary source of data for many qualitative research projects. Typically, interviews are audio-recorded and transcribed to facilitate analysis. For example, Pauly et al. (2015) interviewed 34 people in a private setting and audio recorded the meeting. Although some researchers believe that a recording device inhibits the free flow of discussion, Seidman (2013) and other authors have found that most participants and interviewers forget about the presence of the device. Consequently, most researchers record interviews and then transcribe them verbatim into written text. Some researchers may consider summarizing or paraphrasing the spoken words (Seidman, 2013), but this is not commonly practised. Most researchers wish to use the original words from the participants so that the researcher's recall of the interview dialogue and their own interpretations do not become intertwined with the participant's thoughts. The presence of the original words

allows the reader to check the authenticity of the data. New researchers may transcribe the recording into text themselves; however, most researchers use a transcriptionist. It is recommended that the researcher spot-check interviews to ensure accuracy of the transcription.

Electronic Data Management and Software

Regardless of the type of qualitative data collected, it is usually converted to an electronic format (Averill, 2015) to facilitate analysis and sharing with collaborators. Computer software to organize and retrieve data is referred to as computer-assisted qualitative data analysis software (CAQDAS). There are many computer programs to choose from, such as ATLAS.ti, Ethnograph, HyperRESEARCH, Inspiration, QSR NVivo, QSR XSight, and C-I-SAID.

Unlike computer programs used with quantitative data, these programs do not analyze data. Data analysis and interpretation remain largely the task of the researcher. In other words, CAQDAS cannot "think for the researcher" (Glesne, 2011, p. 207). However, using computer programs for orderly organization and grouping of data facilitates the researcher's job of analysis and interpretation.

💡 Research Hint

There have been advances in text analysis software, called natural language processing (NLP), that may assist in the analysis of large volumes of textual data. Renz et al. (2018) suggested this might be helpful to analyze text from larger data sets and can also be used for triangulation purposes along with conventional analysis. NLP can examine the arrangement, frequency, and types of words used but does have limits. As in all research, it is important that the method fits with answering the research question and that there is methodological coherence.

All data must be backed up and stored in multiple places, such as a cloud storage site, while ensuring security of the data to protect participant confidentiality. Lost data cannot be replaced easily.

There have been some concerns raised about the use of CAQDAS and the effect on the quality of analysis. Maher et al. (2018) compared analysis techniques for a grounded theory study using traditional, manual methods (i.e., paper, highlighters, sticky notes, large display boards) with digital coding using CAQDAS. They argued that deep and insightful interaction with data is necessary for qualitative analysis and that interacting with data in a physical way allows for different perceptions of the material. Digital tools support a more sequential or mathematical mode of cognition, whereas manual methods support more relational and contextual modes of cognition (Maher et al., 2018). This slower and more kinetic mode of interacting with the data was found to be preferential in terms of developing interpretive insights; digital analysis resulted in a smaller and more fragmented view of the data that also made it more difficult to discuss and reflect on interpretations with colleagues (Maher et al., 2018).

Data Repositories and Sharing Data

Data repositories can be used to securely store research data and facilitate sharing of data. Research funding agencies as well as editors of academic journals encourage researchers to make their data available to other researchers for either replicability studies or systematic reviews (Chauvette et al., 2019). Field notes are also an important source of data in qualitative research and may also be useful in secondary data analyses, such as meta-synthesis (Phillippi & Lauderdale, 2018). There are some ethical, methodological, and legal concerns to keep in mind when considering making original qualitative data available to others (Chauvette et al., 2019), and often there is compelling ethical rationale to keep it private (Guishard, 2018). This is particularly important in research with Indigenous communities, where it may be the community and not the researcher who controls the data.

OVERVIEW OF DATA ANALYSIS

The purpose of **data analysis** is to answer the research question (Merriam & Tisdell, 2016). Although analysis among different qualitative approaches differ, there are a few general processes: preparing and organizing the data, reading (and rereading) the database, organizing or reducing the data through coding or themes, representing the findings in figures, narratives, or tables, and forming interpretations (Creswell & Poth, 2018). When does data collection end and data analysis begin? Most commonly in qualitative research, data collection and analysis are done concurrently, although obviously at least some data needs to be collected prior to analysis. Many researchers believe that the stages of data collection and data analysis should be integrated (Denzin & Lincoln, 2000; Merriam & Tisdell, 2016; Miles et al., 2014; Streubert & Carpenter, 2011), whereas others believe that these stages should be separate (Seidman, 2013). This will be largely dependent on the method of qualitative research, and the researcher should explain this process in the study.

Many researchers begin a preliminary analysis as the material accumulates. Typically, the qualitative researcher transcribes all of the interviews, field notes, and observations as they are collected. As each piece of data is transcribed, researchers begin a preliminary analysis during which they determine what additional data need to be collected.

Qualitative researchers look for "insight, meaning, understanding, and larger patterns of knowledge, intent, and action" in the data (Averill, 2015, p. 1). Patton (2002) encouraged researchers to do their "very best with . . . full intellectual capacity to fairly represent the data and communicate what the data reveal given the purpose of study" (p. 433). Recall from previous chapters that qualitative research is often an inductive process—where specific details are examined to generate theory or overarching explanations. As described earlier, qualitative analysis is not a linear process; rather, it is cyclical, transformative, reciprocal, and iterative. Miles et al. (2014, p. 10) have identified some common features among different approaches to qualitative data analysis:

1. Affixing codes or themes to a set of field notes, interview transcripts, or documents
2. Sorting and shifting though these coded materials to identify similar phrases, relationships between variables, patterns, themes, distinct differences between subgroups, and common sequences
3. Isolating these patterns and processes, and commonalities and differences, and taking them out to the field in the next wave of data collection
4. Noting reflections of other remarks in the margins
5. Gradually elaborating a small set of assertions, propositions, and generalizations that cover the consistencies discerned in the database
6. Confronting those generalizations with a formalized body of knowledge in the form of constructs or theories

Guidelines such as these are useful, but they serve only as recommendations. Each qualitative study is unique and is reliant on the creativity, intellect, style, and experience of the researcher. Another example of the steps of qualitative analysis is presented in Figure 16.1.

During the data analysis phase, all researchers fully immerse themselves in the data over a period of weeks to months. This process requires constant reading and rereading of the text until an understanding is reached about what the data convey (Polit & Beck, 2017). Many researchers also listen to the recorded interviews several times to increase their understanding and to align the emotive component. For example, during the interviews in the study by Pesut et al. (2020; Appendix A), the transcripts included the emotions, such as crying, that were evident in the interviews. In addition, the principal researcher listened to the audio recordings. Observations written by the researcher during the interviews can capture these important elements as well. An important part of the data analysis is the interplay between data gathering or questioning and verifying what is heard and understood. Researchers continue to ask whether what they understood before is still relevant after subsequent interviews, observations, and reading of related documents. This "cyclic nature of questioning and verifying is an important aspect of data collection and analysis" (Streubert & Carpenter, 2011, p. 46).

Miles et al. (2014) refer to three discrete stages of data analysis: data reduction, data display, and conclusion drawing and verification (Figure 16.2). Many of the common methods used in nursing research fit into this general view of qualitative analysis.

Data Reduction

According to Miles et al. (2014), **data reduction** is "the process of selecting, focusing, simplifying, abstracting, and transforming the data that appear in written-up field notes or transcriptions" (p. 10). This process is ongoing as data are collected. Glesne (2011) suggested three steps to help researchers analyze qualitative data. The first step is to write memos during the data-collection stage,

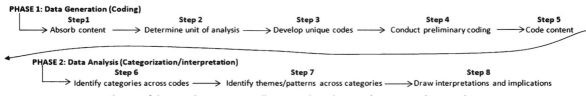

PHASE 1: Data Generation (Coding)

Step1	Step 2	Step 3	Step 4	Step 5
→ Absorb content	→ Determine unit of analysis	→ Develop unique codes	→ Conduct preliminary coding	→ Code content

PHASE 2: Data Analysis (Categorization/interpretation)

Step 6	Step 7	Step 8
→ Identify categories across codes	→ Identify themes/patterns across categories	→ Draw interpretations and implications

FIG. 16.1   Phases of data analysis. From: Roller, M. R. (2019). A quality approach to qualitative content analysis: Similarities and differences compared to other qualitative methods. *Forum: Qualitative Social Research, 20*(3), 1–21. https://o-doi-org.aupac.lib.athabascau.ca/10.17169/fqs-20.3.3385.

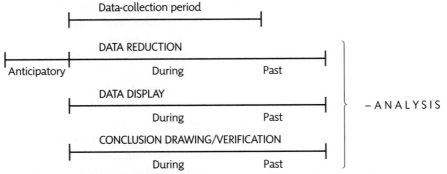

FIG. 16.2   Components of data analysis: Interactive model. From Miles, M. B., Huberman, A. M., & Saldaña, J. (2014). *Qualitative data analysis: A methods sourcebook* (3rd ed.). Thousand Oaks, CA: Sage (Display 1.1, p. 14).

which allows researchers to record thoughts about the data as these thoughts occur. Analytical files are developed to sort data into general categories, such as interview questions, people, and places, as well as useful quotations from the interviews and relevant quotations from the literature. These files help organize researchers' thoughts and those of others. This is sometimes referred to as reflective journaling and can be helpful to track decision-making, reflect on emotions, and note thoughts about what is happening in the research (Polit & Beck, 2017).

Next, Glesne (2011) recommends the development of rudimentary coding schemes. **Coding** is a progressive marking, sorting, resorting, and defining and redefining of the collected data. Coding allows researchers to transform the "unstructured and messy data to ideas about what is going on in the data" (Richards & Morse, 2007, p. 133). The data can then be organized into meaningful clusters of data by grouping related or similar data. Often, these clusters or groups of data are labelled as **themes**, or structured meaning units of data that occur frequently in the text. **Thematic analysis**—the process of recognizing and recovering the emergent themes—is an important aspect of organizing data. Coding is a large part of qualitative data analysis and will be described further in the next section.

Evidence-Informed Practice Tip _____

"Coding is nothing more than assigning some sort of shorthand designation to various aspects of your data so you can easily retrieve specific pieces of data" (Merriam & Tisdell, 2016, p. 199).

Lastly, Glesne (2011) recommends that researchers write themselves monthly field reports as a way of systematically reviewing the progress and determining the next steps. Aside from helping researchers keep track of their progress and communicate progress with other members of the research team, monthly summaries often result in new insights and new ways of approaching the research. This also helps to develop the audit trail and track decision-making, which is an important part of rigour in qualitative research (see Chapter 15).

Coding

There is considerable variety in the process of coding, depending on the method, disciplinary orientation, and philosophical basis for the research. Denzin and Lincoln (2000) describe the fundamental steps in coding of data as sampling, identifying themes, building code-books, and marking texts. Richards and Morse (2007) describe three types of coding: descriptive, topic, and analytic. Researchers use some, or all, of these types of coding. *Descriptive coding* helps the researcher keep track of factual knowledge (e.g., gender). In *topic coding*, used most commonly, the data are grouped together by topic "to reflect on all the different ways people discuss particular topics, to seek patterns in their responses, or to develop dimensions of that experience" (Richards & Morse, 2007, p. 134). As the categories become more complicated, the topic coding becomes analytic. *Analytic coding* is more theoretical and leads to the development of themes. Although coding may sound complicated to you, remember that this process is evolutional, and it varies from project to project and from researcher to researcher. For example, many researchers conducting narrative inquiry do not use coding, data reduction, and some of the other commonly used methods of data analysis.

Miles et al. (2014) described the process of coding taking place in two steps. The first is described as *first cycle coding*, in which the data are assigned to data chunks. While there are many types of coding, Saldaña (2013) suggests three foundational types of coding in this first step:

- Descriptive coding: labels are assigned, composed as a short phrase or word
- In vivo coding: short phrases or words are drawn from the participants' own language
- Process coding: "ing" is used to describe observations or actions (e.g., knowing)

The second step, finding themes, occurs during and after data collection. These themes or basic units of analysis can be entire texts (e.g., interview transcripts, responses to surveys), grammatical segments (words, phrases, sentences, paragraphs), formatting units (rows, pages), or clusters of texts that reflect a single theme. Most researchers try to divide data into units of analysis that do not overlap with others. Researchers approach this step in a variety of ways; for example, experts in grounded theory recommend that the researcher read the text line by line. Miles et al. (2014) describe this second phase of coding as pattern codes. While the first cycle summarized chunks of data, in this second cycle the first-cycle codes are organized into a smaller number of categories, themes, or constructs.

The coding process itself is analysis (Miles et al., 2014). **Codes** are simply tags or labels that are assigned to the themes; often, the code itself is only one to four words long. Major codes may exist along with subcodes. Codes evolve during the analysis; more may be added, and others may be blended. They mean something to the researcher and are not typically included in the research report. As the coding and themes are fine-tuned and finalized, much of the analysis is completed.

Richards and Morse (2007) described two primary steps to data analysis: categorizing and conceptualizing: "Categorizing is how we understand and come to terms with the complexity of data in everyday life" (p. 155). Coding is one method for categorizing the data: however, other researchers in qualitative studies can think about data without coding. Conceptualizing moves up the ladder of abstraction (see Chapter 2) to build frameworks of concepts or theory. It is a process of forming theoretical definitions to "make sense" or organize the data. Phenomenology, ethnography, and grounded theory are all methods that necessitate conceptualization.

In Table 16.1, the differences in the methods of abstraction are described by means of the following questions:

- When does abstraction occur?
- Where does abstraction come from?
- How is abstraction done?
- What analytical outcome is being sought?

While not all qualitative methods are concerned with identifying themes, thematic analysis is common across several qualitative approaches. Thorne (2020) argued that finding themes is only an initial step in data analysis and that further analysis and interpretation are needed in order for the research to make a useful contribution to nursing, although it may not always be necessary to generate a new theory. Braun and

TABLE **16.1**

DOING ABSTRACTION IN THREE DIFFERENT METHODS

METHOD	WHEN DOES ABSTRACTION OCCUR?	WHERE DOES ABSTRACTION COME FROM?	HOW IS ABSTRACTION DONE?	WHAT ANALYTICAL OUTCOME IS BEING SOUGHT?
Phenomenology	Not until one has the data: previous ideas and knowledge may be bracketed	Themes and meanings in accounts, texts	Deep immersion, focus, thorough reading	To describe the essence of a phenomenon
Ethnography	Prior knowledge of site, situation; understanding develops during field research	Knowledge of social and economic setting; observation and learning from the setting	Rich description; combination of qualitative and quantitative patterning, coding, comparing, reviewing field notes	To identify themes and patterns; to explain and account for a social and cultural situation
Grounded theory	Abstraction is from the data but can be informed by previously derived theories	Categories derived from data (observations or line-by-line analysis of texts); constant comparison with other situations or settings	Theoretical sensitivity; seeking concepts and their dimensions; open coding, dimensionalizing, memo writing, diagramming	To identify a core category and theory grounded in data

From Morse, Janice M.; Richards, Lyn. (2007). *Read me first for a user's guide to qualitative methods.* Thousand Oaks, CA: SAGE Publications Inc.

Clark (2006) described two levels of thematic analysis: semantic and latent. In semantic analysis, there is little beyond what the participant said, although the interpretation may also include theorizing about the significance of patterns that were selected from the data. In latent analysis, the goal is to "identify or examine underlying ideas, assumptions, and conceptualizations—and ideologies—that are theorized as shaping or informing the semantic content" (Braun & Clarke, 2006, p. 84). When reading qualitative research, notice the level of analysis that has been conducted. Do the findings reflect themes that are still close to the description provided by participants, or is there a significant amount of interpretation? Do the researchers focus on understanding the hidden assumptions behind what is said, or is the data taken at face value? Understanding this will help you to determine the process and level of analysis.

Evidence-Informed Practice Hint____

Thematic analysis may lend itself to track repeated patterns and frequency or prevalence of concepts found in qualitative data (Braun & Clark, 2006). These may be described in the findings as common themes, or that several participants reported a similar idea. In some qualitative research methods, such as hermeneutics, ideas and concepts that are unique to one participant may be the foundation of analysis. This is called the "fecundity of the individual case" (Jardine, 1992).

Rigour in Data Reduction and Abstraction

Increasingly, there is an expectation that researchers explicitly describe the process of data analysis. For example, Bourque Bearskin et al. (2016; Appendix C) wrote about her own experiences and background, to position herself in context of the research. Indigenous research methodologies were explained and referenced in the section titled "Research Framework." The "Data

Analysis" section described the iterative process of analysis, as well as the use of member checking and peer debriefing. The focus of the research study presented in Appendix C was the finding of *Ontological Beginnings and Epistemological Openings*. This included two subthemes of *Early roots of Indigenous knowledge* as well as *Integrating roots of knowledge into nursing practices*. In the presentation of the analysis, Bourque Bearskin et al. included participant quotes as well as referencing other published information to help explain and expand the analysis.

In the study by Pesut et al. (2020; Appendix A), the authors stated they followed interpretive description in their analysis. They further described how the audio recordings were handled, who developed initial codes, and how subsequent analysis refined these codes. They found three themes in their data: *Systems, Teams,* and *Processes.* The results section presents their analysis according to these themes and includes several participant quotes that help to further explain and explore the findings. All of the participant quotes are coded so that the participants' confidentiality is maintained, and the reader gets a sense of the numerous perspectives represented.

In their focused ethnography of managers' roles in supporting teamwork, Stahlke and Dahlke (2020) followed line-by-line coding, found persistent words and phrases, and grouped these ideas into themes. These themes, along with exemplary quotes from participants, can be found in Table 16.2.

One of the major pitfalls in qualitative and, particularly, thematic analysis is the use of interview questions to organize the analysis (Braun & Clark, 2006). Braun and Clark (2006) claim that this represents a failure to do *any* analysis. They described three types of questions that are used in qualitative research:

1. The main research question that guides the inquiry.
2. The questions asked of participants during the interviews.
3. The questions asked of the data during the analysis.

Thorne (2020) suggested that this third set of questions should include things like "Why have we noticed these patterns?" and not just a reporting of the patterns. Our cognitive processes are attuned to find patterns and meaning in events and experiences, and whether these are significant,

TABLE 16.2	
EXAMPLES OF THEMES FROM FOCUSED ETHNOGRAPHY	
THEME	**ILLUSTRATIVE QUOTES**
Manager visibility	"I just really think [name of supervisor] is amazing. I truly do. She is our manager, but I have seen her in the kitchen, cooking food, preparing things...She doesn't have to; she could stay in her office. I think that helps the team. It's like that [idea of] walk a mile in my shoes." (Activity Aide)"The willingness is there, which is amazing...It definitely motivates staff; I think even frontline staff see it as 'Oh they don't just sit in their office.'" (Recreation Therapist)"The entire leadership team is continually trying to figure out how we can be more approachable." (Nurse Educator)
Conflict management	"So, when you start sweeping things underneath the carpet, you're going to get a great big bump and someone's going to trip...We need strong management that says 'this is the way it is.'" (HCA)
Organizational values	"What interferes with teamwork? Being totally frustrated with the system. Seeing the business side of it...having the business side run over the care side." (HCA)"The policy here, even my director of care will say, is residents first...before any paperwork or any doctor's order, residents first." (LPN)

Source: From Stahlke, S., & Dahlke, S. (2020). The relational role of managers in support of teamwork. *Nursing Leadership, 33*(1), 112–121.

or exist, needs careful reflection and attention (Buetow, 2019).

Research Hint

Qualitative researchers will often include their interview guide in the publication of the research report. Review the interview guide and see how it compares to the results section of the research study. Did the authors use their interview questions to organize their themes, or did they move beyond this analysis, asking different questions of the data and presenting new information?

Data Display

The next major step in data analysis is the data display. Miles et al. (2014) define data display as "a visual format that presents information systematically so the user can draw conclusions and take needed action" (p. 108). This display helps the researcher understand the data and can be in the form of graphs, flowcharts, matrices, or any other visual representation. Like the rest of

the analysis, the data display changes as more is known about the phenomenon under study. For example, Thirsk et al. (2021) developed a taxonomy from their data examining supports and barriers to family-centered care in adult critical care areas. Two broad domains were identified (people and structure), and each of these domains included four concepts and numerous subconcepts. This framework evolved as more data were collected and analyzed and through many discussions with the research team. The final data representation can be seen in Figure 16.3.

Although many researchers use figures and charts as part of their data display, profiles or vignettes can also display what is to be learned from the participant's experience. Vignettes of the participant's experience can summarize what was learned from each participant and can then be shared with each participant for validation (Seidman, 2013). This narrative form transforms the text into a story—a compelling way of sharing meaning.

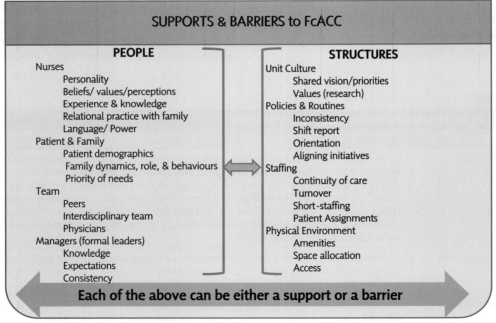

FIG. 16.3   Taxonomy of supports and barriers. From Thirsk, L.M., Vandall-Walker, V., Rasiah, J., & Keyko, K. (2021). A taxonomy of supports and barriers to family-centered adult critical care: A qualitative descriptive study. *Journal of Family Nursing*. https://doi.org/10.1177/1074840721999372.

For example, Smith et al. (2018) studied the experiences of mothers whose children were in long-term treatment for substance use disorders. This narrative inquiry engaged four women to understand their experiences and explore the "dominant and competing stories of motherhood, family, and substance abuse" (p. 512). Vignettes were developed with each of the four participants as a way of introducing the reader to the participants and their story. An example of one vignette is as follows:

> Mary's son was 7 months into treatment when we first met. Substance abuse entered Mary's life in an unexpected way. Mary grew up living the story of a happy child in a loving carefree family. She explained, "I thought this is how all families were supposed to be—happy, loving, supportive, and carefree—I didn't know addiction as a child." Life changed for Mary when she married a man who later became dependent on drugs. Mary described feeling confused and rejected. She told of a painful journey of a wife and mother who struggled to understand her husband's and later her son's substance abuse. Mary did not know how to make sense of her identity as a wife and mother amid growing family troubles. Mary began treatment embarrassed by her inability to "fix the problem," and she felt too ashamed to ask for help. In treatment, Mary became more aware of substance abuse and of herself as she connected with support. She said, "I was given permission to stop trying to fix, to change, or control my son. I am now focused on what I feel." Mary left treatment looking ahead to the ongoing emotional work of living amid substance abuse in her family context. (Smith et al., 2018, pp. 514–515)

Rich descriptions, such as those found in narratives or direct quotations, enliven the data and give meaning to people's experiences. Most qualitative research includes selected quotations to illustrate the themes and to provide readers with the opportunity to understand and validate the themes chosen by the researcher. For example, Thirsk et al. (2021) selected the following quotes to demonstrate how the relationship between the nurse and the family influences family-centered care and that not all nurses make connections with all families.

I-5: You'll see certain family members not want to leave the patient's side when certain nurses are working with them. And then, if you have a comfortable dynamic, they'll go home to sleep or have a shower...they feel comfortable [enough] to leave.

I-5: I find that families will find a nurse that they connect with. And then, although that might not be the nurse assigned that particular day, they'll seek them out to ask questions.

As another example of rich description, Table 16.3 includes selected quotations from participants to support the themes emerging from Burns et al.'s (2019) study examining Mi'kmaq women's access to prenatal care.

When the data are presented, the most important consideration for the research is to ensure that the presentation supports the findings and relays what needs to be known (Streubert & Carpenter, 2011). The analysis and presentation need to be convincing to the reader, who has not read the entire data set (Braun & Clark, 2006). The purpose of the study determines how the story is told. If the method is descriptive phenomenology, the focus is on the description of the lived experiences, whereas in a grounded theory study, the focus is on a more careful description of how the narrative gives rise to the analysis and interpretation, which results in theory development.

CONCLUSION DRAWING AND VERIFICATION

Conclusion drawing starts at the beginning of data collection but is not finalized until the project is completed. Although qualitative research is inductive, it is tempting to draw conclusions prematurely. The challenge for the researcher is to remain amenable to new ideas, themes, and concepts as they appear.

Conclusion drawing is essentially the description of the relationship between the themes. Richards and Morse (2007) describe this process

TABLE **16.3**

EXAMPLES OF SELECTED QUOTATIONS TO SUPPORT THE THEMES

THEMES	SUBTHEME	EXAMPLE OF A QUOTATION
Closing the gaps in prenatal care	Traveling the distance	*This is her first baby. Yeah, so she's going into it blind* (referring to the lack of prenatal classes in the community).
Social support networks during pregnancy	Family support	*So we talk a lot about our own experiences and what we did, and what happened to us, and what we would suggest for other women.*
	Professional support	*If I had any concerns about my pregnancy, I would go to the Health Centre first because we have a Community Health Nurse and the Family Support Worker. They're really accommodating. If you need them, they're there.*
Cultural beliefs and preferences	Importance of traditions	*Prenatal care means taking care of your body, but also your mind and your spirit when you're pregnant.* *It is an honour to sweat with a pregnant woman because she is bringing life into the world.*
	Providing culturally safe care	*I found at the hospital here they're very open and embrace our differences. There was no limit to how many people in the room when I was in labour. Which I know, you know, they don't allow for everyone but it's important for us. Just very respectful.*

From Burns, L., Whitty-Rogers, J., & MacDonald, C. (2019). Understanding Mi'kmaq women's experiences accessing prenatal care in rural Nova Scotia. *Advances in Nursing Science*, 2, 139. https://doi.org/10.1097/ANS.0000000000000248.

as "doing abstraction" (p. 158), in which data are moved from categories (codes and themes) to concepts and constructs. As discussed earlier and shown in Table 16.1, the ways of abstracting vary with the type of method. Grounded theory formalizes this stage through the development of models, which lead to theory. Verification occurs as the data are collected; this process can vary from questioning one's own conclusion through the rechecking of the text to verification by colleagues and to finding new cases and applying the model to them. In grounded theory and many other qualitative methods, researchers use the **constant comparative method**, in which new data are compared as they emerge with data previously analyzed.

Miles et al. (2014) have stated that this process of making sense of the data is a skill that all nurses have. People make sense of the world around them by organizing and interpreting it; this skill is applied to drawing and verifying conclusions. Miles et al. (2014) list the following 13 tactics for analyzing the data (pp. 277–278):

1. Noting patterns and themes (repetitive or recurring patterns among many separate pieces of data)
2. Clustering (grouping together things that seem to share characteristics)
3. Making metaphors (using a literary device in which different things are compared to make sense of the experience)
4. Counting (noting that something is happening a number of times)
5. Making contrasts or comparisons (comparing sets of things)
6. Partitioning variables (breaking down the themes into smaller units)

7. Subsuming particulars into the general (using a higher level of abstraction)
8. Factoring (generating words [factors] to express common findings)
9. Noting relationships between variables (depicting the relationships between the findings)
10. Finding intervening variables (discerning other variables that may link findings together)
11. Building a logical chain of evidence (validating each of the relationships identified)
12. Making conceptual or theoretical coherence (linking the findings into an overarching "how" and "why" of the phenomenon under study)

Refer to Miles et al. (2014) for more detail about these tactics. Merriam and Tisdell's (2016) text on qualitative research also described the step-by-step process.

To verify their findings, Thirsk et al. (2021) moved back and forth between the emerging categories of the taxonomy and the interview transcripts. This involved rereading transcripts and revising the taxonomy through numerous discussions with the research team until all of the reported barriers and supports were documented. Other researchers can use different methods to validate their themes. Pesut et al. (2020) drew on information gathered from a systematic review and analysis of policy documents to help situate their qualitative findings and explain the consequences of legislative decisions. Stahlke and Dahlke (2020) built variation into their sample, created thick descriptions of their participants' experiences, documented their decision-making during analysis, and discussed emerging ideas with each other.

No matter what method is used, researchers ask themselves, "What have I learned? How do I understand this, make sense of it and see the connections in it?" (Seidman, 2013). The conclusions drawn are simply to "describe, make contributions and contribute to greater understanding, or at least, more informed questioning" (Glesne, 2011, p. 210). As discussed in Chapter 7, through the processes of reflexivity, researchers constantly compare their findings with their own personal beliefs

and knowledge to ensure that the analysis reflects the participants' beliefs rather than their own.

SPECIFIC ANALYTICAL PROCEDURES

The processes of data analysis vary according to the type of qualitative research. Table 16.4 summarizes the methods of analysis in qualitative methods, including phenomenology, ethnography, grounded theory, and qualitative description. Excerpts from Canadian studies are included to exemplify the methods.

Research Hint

In participatory action research the participants, or collaborators, in the project are often involved in the process of data analysis. For example, Doré et al. (2018) involved hemodialysis nurses in their PAR on nursing burnout. After phase one focus groups, two nurses from the advisory team were included in the initial discussion to strengthen the analysis and interpretations. This first round of analysis was then presented in subsequent focus groups for further discussion, and the final analysis resulting from these discussions was also confirmed with the advisory team. Engaging participants in this manner means the participants have some control of the analysis, rather than this lying solely with the research team.

TRUSTWORTHINESS

As described in Chapter 15, rigour in qualitative research is determined by credibility, auditability, and fittingness as the criteria for evaluation, although there is still a debate about the most appropriate terminology (see Morse et al., 2015). Trustworthiness is important for determining the integrity, or soundness, of the data interpretation or analysis. To ensure the trustworthiness of their findings, qualitative researchers must ask themselves the following questions (Hollway & Jefferson, 2000):

- What do you notice? The researcher has captured some impressions about the data; however, information may be missing. Detailed or thick descriptions of the phenomenon also allow the reader to assess whether the account "rings true."
- Why do you notice what you notice? Researchers must consider their own biases and

TABLE **16.4**

METHODS OF ANALYSIS AND EXEMPLARS

TRADITION	METHOD OF ANALYSIS	EXAMPLE
Phenomenology: includes a variety of traditions	• Immersion in the data: listen to recordings, read and reread transcripts • Identify and extract significant statements • Determine relationships among the extracted statements (themes) • Prepare exhaustive description of the phenomenon and the relationships among the themes • Synthesize the themes into a consistent description or statement of the phenomenon under study (essence)	Lamb et al. (2019) "Conscientious objection and nurses: Results of an interpretive phenomenological study. "These authors explored nurses' experiences of making a conscientious objection to further understand the moral choices and encounters with ethical issues. In this phenomenological approach, analysis is continuous and builds off previous interpretation. They organized the data into six themes: encountering the problem, knowing oneself, taking a stand, alone and uncertain, caring for others, perceptions of support. The authors offer an example of a quote that supports the theme of knowing oneself: *"Adding the word objection to it I feel like it has so much more power . . . you know, kind of doing what is wrong and questioning what's right, but I feel like this has more positive connotation to it, like you have a choice, you're not feeling this residual distress and you just have to accept that's the way it is. I think it almost, it's a little empowering.*
Ethnography	• Immersion in the data • Identify patterns and themes • Complete a cultural inventory • Interpret the findings • Compare the findings with those in the literature	Sutherland et al. (2017) "Structural impact on gendered expectations and exemptions for family caregivers in hospice palliative home care" Pauly et al. (2015) collected data through interviews, observations, and document reviews. Initial codes were developed through multiple readings of the data, and codes were compared to develop themes. All of the co-authors were involved in every aspect of the data analysis, which resulted in the development of three themes.
Grounded theory	• Examine data carefully line by line • Divide data into discrete parts • Compare data for similarities and differences • Compare data with other data continuously in a process: constant comparative method • Cluster codes to form categories • Expand and develop categories or collapse them into one another • Determine relationships between categories	King-Shier et al. (2019) "South Asians' experience of managing hypertension: a grounded theory study. "The authors implemented the main features of grounded theory such as theoretical sampling, continual comparison of data and codes, which influenced questions asked of participants, line-by-line reading, axial and selective coding. The results were modelled in a diagram showing the process of managing hypertension.
Qualitative Description	• Identify themes, primarily from textual data from interviews • Create a description that would be meaningful to others. • Provide representative quotes to explore complexity of phenomenon.	Stahlke Wall (2018) "The impact of regulatory perspectives and practices on professional innovation in nursing". The author analyzed interviews and categorized findings into several themes: problematic regulatory processes; specific process issues; and impacts of conservative regulation. In addition, a negative case was included in the analysis because one participant's experience with the nursing regulator was different than the other participants. This exploration of a negative case helps to recognize the variance in and complexity with the phenomenon.

predispositions as they interpret the data to produce trustworthy interpretations. Many researchers use a journal to document their reflections to monitor their own developing interpretations.

- How can you interpret what you notice? Credibility stems from prolonged engagement and persistent observation. To be able to complete a full interpretation, the researcher must spend a sufficient amount of time in the field to build sound relationships with the participants.

- How can you know that your interpretation is the "right" one? In some qualitative methods, researchers will use **member checking.** Member checking is the collaborative process of involving participants in data analysis by verifying and refining data and research findings for congruency with their experiences and meanings (Gillis & Jackson, 2002, p. 216). It is used more in descriptive qualitative research, where the analysis stays "close" to the participants language, and is often

important in research with Indigenous peoples and communities. The further the abstraction, the less useful member checking is. The researcher is also checking whether the connections between the categories or themes are logical. Inviting other experts to review the data analysis is another option for many researchers. This occurs primarily in research teams when collaborators review, discuss, and make decisions about the analysis. Reviewing the data and checking the interpretations also occurs during the publication process as peers review the presented research study. In addition, some researchers analyze their data from several different frameworks (a form of triangulation) to increase the trustworthiness of the data analysis.

Finally, it is important to consider the limitations of the study. Many researchers describe the issues they faced so that readers will understand the research in the proper context (Glesne, 2006).

APPRAISING THE EVIDENCE

Qualitative Data Analysis

The general criteria for critiquing qualitative data analysis are proposed in the Critiquing Criteria box; however, remember that many different approaches to data analysis exist. The data analysis is consistent with the research methodology, the question, and the design. For example, researchers using grounded theory build a case for substantive theory, explaining the phenomenon under study, whereas a researcher in phenomenological studies is interested in expressing the meaning of the phenomenon itself.

Regardless of the study's research method, several commonalities exist among methods used in qualitative data analysis. For example, analysis is conducted alongside the data collection, and in most cases the two processes are interrelated. Researchers become immersed in

the data; they listen over and over to the interviews, read and reread the transcripts, and spend substantial time in the field. Although the methods may differ, the text is coded to search for themes and categories through a process of data reduction. As themes emerge, logical connections and relationships between the themes are identified to form a whole picture. The results are displayed in such a manner that the reader can understand and validate the conclusions that the researcher has drawn through the use of diagrams, tables, charts, direct quotations from the participants, and rich descriptions of the findings. In summary, qualitative data analysis involves much disparate data and transforms them into a coherent whole or story to provide and explanation of human experience.

CRITIQUING CRITERIA

1. The method of data analysis should be clearly stated.
2. The strategy of data analysis should be appropriate for the methodology of the study.
3. The steps of analysis should be listed for readers to follow.
4. The researcher should provide evidence that his or her interpretation captures
   the phenomenon under study.
5. The researcher should address the credibility, auditability, and fittingness of the data.

CRITICAL THINKING CHALLENGES

▨ Is it important for the researcher to personally transcribe the interviews?

▨ Why do some researchers reread the literature as themes emerge from the data?

▨ Often, data analysis takes place as data are collected. How can analysis of the data change the data collection?

▨ Some researchers validate their interpretation of the data through a process of member checking. What happens if the participants indicate that the analysis does not reflect their experience?

CRITICAL JUDGEMENT QUESTIONS

1. Why is it important for qualitative researchers to listen to the recorded interviews?
   a. It validates the participants' stories
   b. It allows for the addition of paraverbal data
   c. It is required by research ethics boards
   d. It improves triangulation of data

2. Which of the following is NOT part of qualitative data analysis?
   a. Concurrent data collection and data analysis
   b. Coding systems
   c. Immersive reading of data
   d. Testing hypotheses

3. How do researchers determine that data analysis is complete?
   a. When sufficient participants have been interviewed
   b. When the researcher is saturated
   c. When substantial analysis has been created
   d. When the research grant has been spent

KEY POINTS

- Qualitative data are text derived from transcripts of interviews, narratives, documents, media such as newspapers and movies, and field notes.
- Computer software can be used to simplify the storage and retrieval of data.
- Qualitative research data can be managed through the use of computers, but the researcher must interpret the data.
- Data analysis and data collection are parallel processes.
- Qualitative analysis is not a linear process; rather, it is a cyclical and iterative process.
- The three discrete stages of data analysis are data reduction, data display, and conclusion drawing and verification.
- Data are organized into meaningful chunks of data through a clustering of related or similar data and are labelled as themes.
- Coding is the process of progressively marking, sorting, resorting, and defining and redefining the collected data.
- Data display involves the use of graphs, flowcharts, matrices, or any other visual representation to assemble data and to allow for conclusion drawing.
- Grounded theorists use the constant comparative method, in which new data are compared with data previously analyzed.
- Member checking, used in some qualitative methods, is the process of sharing findings with the participants in order to check whether the interpretation of the findings is accurate.

📶 FOR FURTHER STUDY

Go to Evolve at http://evolve.elsevier.com/Canada/LoBiondo/Research for the Audio Glossary.

REFERENCES

Averill, J. (2015). Qualitative data analysis. In M. De Chesnay (Ed.), *Nursing research using data analysis: Qualitative designs and methods in nursing.* New York: Springer Publishing Company.

Bourque Bearskin, L., Cameron, B. L., King, M., & Pillwax, C. W. (2016). Mâmawoh Kamâtowin, "Coming together to help each other in wellness": Honouring Indigenous nursing knowledge. *International Journal of Indigenous Health, 11*(1), 18–33. https://doi.org/10.18357/ijih111201615024.

Braun, V., & Clarke, V. (2006). Using thematic analysis in psychology. *Qualitative Research in Psychology, 3*(2), 77–101. http://dx.doi.org/10.1191/1478088706qp063oa.

Buetow, S. (2019). Apophenia, unconscious bias and reflexivity in nursing qualitative research. *International journal of nursing studies, 89*, 8–13. https://doi.org/10.1016/j.ijnurstu.2018.09.013.

Burns, L., Whitty-Rogers, J., & MacDonald, C. (2019). Understanding Mi'kmaq women's experiences accessing prenatal care in Rural Nova Scotia. *Advances in Nursing Science, 2*, 139. https://doi.org/10.1097/ANS.0000000000000248.

Chauvette, A., Schick-Makaroff, K., & Molzahn, A. E. (2019). Open data in qualitative research. *International Journal of Qualitative Methods, 18*. https://doi.org/10.1177/2F1609406918823863.

Creswell, J. W., & Poth, C. N. (2018). *Qualitative inquiry and research design: Choosing among five approaches.* Thousand Oaks, CA: Sage Publications.

Denzin, N., & Lincoln, Y. (2000). *Handbook of qualitative research* (2nd ed.). Thousand Oaks, CA: Sage.

Doré, C., Duggett-Leger, L., McKenna, M., Salsberg, J., & Breau, M. (2018). Participatory action research to empower hemodialysis nurses and reduce risk of burnout. *The CANNT Journal, 28*(3), 40–53. https://cannt-acitn.ca/cannt-journal/.

Gillis, A., & Jackson, W. (2002). *Research for nurses: Methods and interpretation.* Philadelphia: F.A. Davis.

Glesne, C. (2006). *Becoming qualitative researchers: An introduction* (3rd ed.). Don Mills, ON: Longman.

Glesne, C. (2011). *Becoming qualitative researchers: An introduction* (4th ed.). Toronto: Pearson.

Guishard, M. A. (2018). Now's not the time! Qualitative data repositories on tricky ground: Comment on Dubois et al. (2018). *Qualitative Pyschology, 5*(3), 402–408. http://dx.doi.org/10.1037/qup0000085.

Hollway, W., & Jefferson, T. (2000). *Doing qualitative research differently: Free association, narrative and the interview method.* Thousand Oaks, CA: Sage.

Jardine, D. W. (1992). The fecundity of the individual case: Considerations of the pedagogic heart of interpretive work. *Journal of Philosophy of Education, 26*(1), 51–61. https://doi.org/10.1111/j.1467-9752.1992.tb00264.x.

King-Shier, K. M., Dhaliwal, K. K., Puri, R., LeBlanc, P., & Johal, J. (2019). South Asians' experience of managing hypertension: A grounded theory study. *Patient Preference and Adherence, 13*, 321. https://doi.org/10.2147/PPA.S196224.

Lamb, C., Babenko-Mould, Y., Evans, M., Wong, C. A., & Kirkwood, K. W. (2019). Conscientious objection

and nurses: Results of an interpretive phenomenological study. *Nursing Ethics, 26*(5), 1337–1349. https://doi.org/10.1177/F0969733018763996.

Maher, C., Hadfield, M., Hutchings, M., & de Eyto, A. (2018). Ensuring rigor in qualitative data analysis: A design research approach to coding combining NVivo with traditional material methods. *International Journal of Qualitative Methods, 17*, 1–13. https://doi.org/10.1177/1609406918786362.

Merriam, S. B., & Tisdell, E. J. (2016). *Qualitative research: A guide to design and implementation.* San Francisco: Jossey-Bass.

Miles, M. B., Huberman, A. M., & Saldaña, J. (2014). *Qualitative data analysis: Methods source book* (3rd ed.). Thousand Oaks, CA: Sage.

Morse, J. M. (2015). Critical analysis of strategies for determining rigor in qualitative inquiry. *Qualitative Health Research, 25*(9), 1212–1222. https://doi.org/10.1177/1049732315588501.

Patton, M. (2002). *Qualitative research & evaluation methods* (3rd ed.). Thousand Oaks, CA: Sage.

Pauly, B., McCall, J., Browne, A. J., et al. (2015). Toward cultural safety: Nurse and patient perceptions of illicit substance use in a hospitalized setting. *Advances in Nursing Science, 38*(2), 121–135.

Pesut, B., Thorne, S., Schiller, C. J., Greig, M., & Roussel, J. (2020). The rocks and hard places of MAiD: A qualitative study of nursing practice in the context of legislated assisted death. *BMC Nursing, 19*(1), 1–14. https://doi.org/10.1186/s12912-020-0404-5.

Phillippi, J., & Lauderdale, J. (2018). A guide to field notes for qualitative research: Context and conversation. *Qualitative Health Research, 28*(3), 381–388. https://doi.org/10.1177/1049732317697102.

Polit, D. F., & Beck, C. T. (2017). *Nursing research: Generating and assessing evidence for nursing practice* (10th ed.). Philadelphia: Wolters Kluwer.

Renz, S. M., Carrington, J. M., & Badger, T. A. (2018). Two strategies for qualitative content analysis: An intramethod approach to triangulation. *Qualitative Health Research, 28*(5), 824–831. https://doi.org/10.1177/1049732317753586.

Richards, L., & Morse, J. M. (2007). *Read me first for a user's guide to qualitative methods* (2nd ed.). Thousand Oaks, CA: Sage.

Roller, M. R. (2019). A quality approach to qualitative content analysis: Similarities and differences compared to other qualitative methods. *Forum: Qualitative Social Research, 20*(3), 1–21. https://0-doi-org.aupac.lib.athabascau.ca/10.17169/fqs-20.3.3385.

Saldaña, J. (2013). *The coding manual for qualitative researchers* (2nd ed.). New York: Oxford University Press.

Seidman, I. (2013). *Interviewing as qualitative research: A guide for researchers in education and the social sciences* (4th ed.). New York: Teachers College Press.

Smith, J. M., Estefan, A., & Caine, V. (2018). Mothers' experiences of supporting adolescent children through long-term treatment for substance use disorder. *Qualitative Health Research, 28*(4), 511–522. https://doi.org/10.1177/1049732317747554.

Stahlke, S., & Dahlke, S. (2020). The relational role of managers in support of teamwork. *Nursing Research, 33*(1), 112–121.

Stahlke Wall, S. (2018). The impact of regulatory perspectives and practices on professional innovation in nursing. *Nursing Inquiry, 25*(1), e12212. https://doi.org/10.1111/nin.12212.

Streubert, H. J., & Carpenter, D. (2011). *Qualitative research in nursing: Advancing the humanistic imperative* (5th ed.). Philadelphia: Wolters Kluwer.

Sutherland, N., Ward-Griffin, C., McWilliam, C., & Stajduhar, K. (2017). Structural impact on gendered expectations and exemptions for family caregivers in hospice palliative home care. *Nursing Inquiry, 24*(1), e12157. https://doi.org/10.1111/nin.12157.

Thirsk, L. M., Vandall-Walker, V., Rasiah, J., & Keyko, K. (2021). A taxonomy of supports and barriers to family-centered adult critical care: A qualitative descriptive study. *Journal of Family Nursing.* https://doi.org/10.1177/1074840721999372.

Thorne, S. (2020). Beyond theming: Making qualitative studies matter. *Nursing Inquiry, 27*(1), e12343. https://doi.org/10.1111/nin.12343.

CHAPTER 17

Quantitative Data Analysis

Mina D. Singh

LEARNING OUTCOMES

After reading this chapter, you will be able to do the following:

- Differentiate between descriptive and inferential statistics.
- State the purposes of descriptive statistics.
- Identify the levels of measurement in a research study.
- Describe a frequency distribution.
- List measures of central tendency and their use.
- List measures of variability and their use.
- Identify the purpose of inferential statistics.
- Distinguish between a parameter and a statistic.
- Explain the concept of probability as it applies to the analysis of sample data.
- Distinguish between type I and type II errors and their effects on a study's outcome.
- Distinguish between parametric and nonparametric tests.
- List the commonly used statistical tests and their purposes.
- Critically analyze the statistics used in published research studies.

KEY TERMS

alpha
analysis of covariance (ANCOVA)
analysis of variance (ANOVA)
chi-square (χ^2)
confidence interval
correlation
degree of freedom
descriptive statistics
Fisher's exact probability test
frequency distribution
inferential statistics
interval measurement

kurtosis
level of significance (alpha level)
levels of measurement
mean (M)
measurement
measures of central tendency
measures of variability
median
modality
mode
multiple regression
nominal measurement
nonparametric statistics

nonparametric tests of significance
normal curve
null hypothesis
odds ratio
ordinal measurement
p value
parameter
parametric statistics
Pearson correlation coefficient (Pearson r)
percentile
population
post hoc analysis
power

probability	semiquartile range (semi-interquartile range)	statistic
range		t statistic
ratio measurement	skew	type I error
sampling error	standard deviation	type II error
scatter plots	standard error of the mean	Z score
scientific hypothesis		

STUDY RESOURCES

 Go to Evolve at http://evolve.elsevier.com/Canada/LoBiondo/Research for the Audio Glossary.

STATISTICS ARE USED EXTENSIVELY IN health care research literature. Descriptive and inferential statistics are described in the "Methods" section, the "Results" section, or both sections of a research article.

As a reader, you do not analyze the data yourself, but it is important to understand the researcher's challenge in analyzing the data. After carefully collecting data, the researcher is faced with the task of organizing and analyzing the individual pieces of information so that the meaning of study results is clear. The researcher must choose methods of organizing and analyzing the raw data on the basis of the design, the type of data collected, and the hypothesis or question that was tested. Statistical procedures are used to organize and give meaning to the data.

The "Results" section of a research article contains the data generated from the testing of the hypothesis or research questions. These data are the result of analysis with both *descriptive* and *inferential statistics*. An example of what may be found is as follows: "Overall, the majority (n = 41, 53%) of women in the lanolin group were 'very satisfied' with the effects of lanolin in treating their nipple pain…This difference in maternal satisfaction between the groups was statistically significant," (Jackson and Dennis, 2017: see Appendix B). The data in Table 2 of Appendix B (Jackson and Dennis) are known as descriptive statistics, which are usually the first set of statistical results in a report or published article.

Descriptive statistics are used to summarize and organize data. The techniques used allow researchers to arrange data visually to display meaning and to help in understanding the sample characteristics and variables before the researchers engage in inferential data analyses. In some studies, descriptive statistics may be the only results sought from statistical analysis. Descriptive statistical techniques include measures of central tendency, which describe the average member of a sample, such as mode, median, and mean; measures of variability, such as range and standard deviation (SD); and some correlation techniques, such as a scatter plots, which are a visual representation of the strength and magnitude of the relationship between two variables.

In contrast to descriptive statistics, inferential statistics allow researchers to estimate how reliably they can make predictions and generalize findings on the basis of the data. Inferential statistics are statistical details that combine mathematical processes and logic to test hypotheses about a population with the help of sample data. Through the use of inferential statistics, researchers can draw conclusions that extend beyond the immediate data of the study. An example of inferential statistics is in the study by Havaie et al. (2016): The LPNS [Licensed Practical Nurses] who were likely or very likely to leave had higher emotional exhaustion levels (mean = 33.9,

SD = 11.5) than LPNs who were unlikely or very likely to leave (mean = 27.0, SD = 13.9). This difference was statistically significant [t(132) = −3.0, p < 0.01] (p. 396).

The purpose of this chapter is to demonstrate how researchers use descriptive and inferential statistics in nursing research studies so that you, as a reader, will be better able to determine the appropriateness of the statistics used and to interpret the strength and quality of the reported findings, their clinical significance, and their applicability to practice. Basic concepts and terminology common in evidence-informed practice publications are presented in Chapter 21. The information in this chapter will help you begin to make sense of the statistics used in research papers.

DESCRIPTIVE STATISTICS

Levels of Measurement

Measurement is the assignment of numbers to variables or events according to rules. Every variable in a research study that is assigned a specific number must be similar to every other variable assigned that number. For example, male participants may be assigned the number 1 and female participants the number 2. The measurement level is determined by the nature of the object or event being measured. Levels of measurement—categorization of the precision with which an event can be measured—from low to high are nominal, ordinal, interval, and ratio (Table 17.1). The levels of measurement help determine the type of statistics to be used in analyzing data. The higher the level of measurement, the greater the flexibility the researcher has in choosing statistical procedures. Every attempt should be made to use the highest level of measurement possible so that the maximum amount of information will be obtained from the data. The Critical Thinking Decision Path illustrates the relationship between levels of measurement and appropriate choice of specific descriptive statistics.

In nominal measurement, variables or events are classified into categories (see Table 17.1). The

TABLE **17.1**

SCALES OF MEASUREMENT		
MEASUREMENT LEVEL	**DESCRIPTION**	**EXAMPLE**
Nominal (may be dichotomous or categorical)	Variables or events are classified into categories; the categories are mutually exclusive, there is no ranking. Dichotomous variables are mutually exclusive and have two true values: e.g., true/false, male/female. Categorical variables are mutually exclusive and have more than two true values: e.g., marital status may be single, married, divorced, separated, widowed.	Gender Hair colour Marital status Religious affiliation
Ordinal	Sorting on relative rankings of variables or events	High school education and less/more than high school education
Ordinal Scale treated as Interval	Rank ordering on an attribute and specifies the difference between the ranks, then a value is assigned to each category	Highly disagree -1, disagree-2, neutral (neither agree or disagree)-3, agree-4, highly agree-5
Interval	Rank ordering on an attribute and specifies the difference between the ranks, assume equivalent distance between the ranks	Body temperature - the distance between 95 C and 100 C is the same as 101 C and 106 C
Ratio	Highest level of measurementAbsolute zero, so can divide, multiply	A person weighing 100 kg is twice as heavy as one who weighs 50 kg

categories are mutually exclusive; a variable or an event either has or does not have the characteristic of a particular category. The numbers assigned to each category are nothing more than labels; such numbers do not indicate more or less of a characteristic. Nominal measurement can be used to categorize a sample with regard to such information as gender, hair colour, marital status, or religious affiliation.

Hisel's (2019) study examining the level of work engagement among four groups of nurses: Veteran-aged, Baby Boomer, Generation X, and Millennial registered nurses—involved nominal measurement. The nominal level of measurement allows the least amount of mathematical manipulation. Most commonly, the frequency of each event is counted, as is the percentage of the total that each category represents.

A variable at the nominal level can also be considered a *dichotomous* or a *categorical* variable.

A dichotomous nominal variable has only two true values, such as true/false or gender (male/female) (see Table 17.1). Nominal variables that are categorical still have mutually exclusive categories but have more than two true values, such as marital status (single, married, divorced, separated, or widowed). In both cases, the nominal variables are mutually exclusive. The gender variable of the undergraduate nurses in the study by Goldsworthy et al. (2019) in Appendix D would be considered a dichotomous nominal variable (male/female).

Ordinal measurement reveals relative rankings of variables or events. The numbers assigned to each category can be compared, and the members of a higher ranked category can be said to have more of an attribute than members of a lower ranked category. The intervals between numbers on the scale are not necessarily equal, and zero is not absolute but arbitrary. For example, ordinal

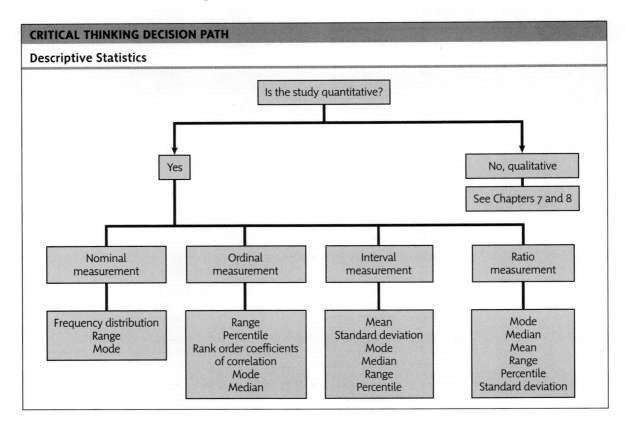

CRITICAL THINKING DECISION PATH

Descriptive Statistics

Is the study quantitative?

Yes

No, qualitative

See Chapters 7 and 8

Nominal measurement	Ordinal measurement	Interval measurement	Ratio measurement
Frequency distribution Range Mode	Range Percentile Rank order coefficients of correlation Mode Median	Mean Standard deviation Mode Median Range Percentile	Mode Median Mean Range Percentile Standard deviation

measurement is used to formulate class rankings, in which one student can be ranked higher or lower than another. However, the actual grade point averages of students may differ widely. Another example is ranking individuals by their level of education, as in the study by Brown et al. (2018) with the variable "age," with categories < 25, 25–35, 36–45, 46–55, and > 55 years of age. Age in categories is an example of an ordinal variable.

The New York Heart Association's classification of cardiac failure adopted by the Canadian Cardiovascular Society (Ezekowitz et al., 2017) consists of four classifications. Classification I represents no symptoms, whereas classification IV represents symptoms at rest with any minimal activity; however, an individual in class IV cannot be said to be four times sicker than an individual in class I. Lauck and colleagues (2016) used this classification in their study to explore factors influencing patients' decision making to undergo TAVI (transcatheter aortic valve implantation) eligibility assessment to inform practice, programme development, health policy, and future research.

With ordinal-level data, the amount of mathematical manipulation possible is limited. In addition to what is possible with nominal-level data, medians, percentiles, and rank-order coefficients of correlation can be calculated (Table 17.2). In most cases, ordinal variables in a scale are treated

as interval measurements when converted to numerical codes. For example, when patients are asked to rate their level of satisfaction with life as "not satisfied," "satisfied," or "very satisfied," their responses are an ordinal measurement. When their ratings are treated numerically and coded as 1, 2, and 3, respectively, their ordinal responses are treated as interval measurement. For example, Doktorchik et al. (2018) investigated whether the patterns of change in anxiety and depression during pregnancy can predict preterm birth. State anxiety was measured on the Spielberger State Anxiety Scale, which is a self-report questionnaire including 20 questions on a 4-point scale, with higher numbers corresponding to higher anxiety, the highest score being 80.

In interval measurement, events or variables are ranked on a scale with equal intervals between the numbers. The zero point remains arbitrary and not absolute. For example, interval measurements are used in measuring temperatures on the Fahrenheit scale. The distances between degrees are equal, but the zero point is arbitrary and does not represent the absence of temperature. Test scores also represent interval-level data. The differences between test scores represent equal intervals, but a score of zero does not represent the total absence of knowledge.

In many areas in the social sciences, including nursing, the classification of the level of

TABLE **17.2**

LEVEL OF MEASUREMENT SUMMARY TABLE

MEASUREMENT	DESCRIPTION	MEASURES OF CENTRAL TENDENCY	MEASURES OF VARIABILITY
Nominal	Classification	Mode	Modal percentage, range, frequency distribution
Ordinal	Relative rankings	Mode, median	Modal percentage, range, frequency, percentile, semiquartile range, frequency distribution
Interval	Rank ordering with equal intervals	Mode, median, mean	Modal percentage, range, percentile, semiquartile range, standard deviation
Ratio	Rank ordering with equal intervals and absolute zero	Mode, median, mean	All

measurement of intelligence, aptitude, and personality tests is controversial; some researchers regard these measurements as ordinal and others as interval. You need to be aware of this controversy and to examine each study individually in terms of how the data are analyzed. Interval-level data allow more manipulation of data, including the addition and subtraction of numbers and the calculation of means. Because of this additional manipulation, many authorities argue for the higher classification level. The Clinical Self-Efficacy Scale used by Goldsworthy et al. (2019) is an example of ordinal measurements but is used as an interval measurement (see Appendix D).

In ratio measurement, events or variables are ranked on scales with equal intervals and absolute zeros (see Table 17.2). The number represents the actual amount of the property the object possesses. Ratio measurement is the highest level of measurement but is usually achieved only in the physical sciences. Examples of ratio-level data are height, weight, pulse, and blood pressure. All mathematical procedures can be performed with data from ratio scales. Therefore, the use of any statistical procedure is possible as long as it is appropriate for the design of the study.

Research Hint

Descriptive statistics assist in summarizing the data. The descriptive statistics calculated must be appropriate for both the purpose of the study and the level of measurement.

Frequency Distribution

One of the most basic ways of organizing data is in a frequency distribution. In a frequency distribution, the number of times each event occurs is counted, or the data are grouped and the frequency of each group is reported. For example, an instructor reporting the results of an examination could report the number of students receiving each individual grade or could group the grades in ranges and report the number of students who received each group of grades. When reviewing a

frequency distribution, symmetry and kurtosis are noted. A distribution can be symmetrical (shaped like a bell) or asymmetrical, where most of the information is to one side, either to the left or the right. Kurtosis is the peakedness of the distribution. Table 17.3 shows the results of an examination given to a class of 51 students. The results are reported in two ways. The columns on the left give the raw data tally and the frequency for each grade, whereas the columns on the right give the grouped data tally and grouped frequencies. In research studies, the results are grouped rather than reported individually for each participant.

When data are grouped, the researcher needs to define the size of the group or the interval width so that no score is categorized into two groups and all groups are mutually exclusive. The groupings of the data in Table 17.3 prevent overlap; each score is categorized into only one group. If the grouping had been 70 to 80 and 80 to 90, scores of 80 would have been categorized into two categories. The grouping should allow for a precise presentation of the data without serious loss of information. Very large interval widths lead to loss of data information and may obscure patterns in the data. If the test scores in Table 17.3 had been grouped as 40 to 69 and 70 to 99, the pattern of the scores would have been obscured.

Information about frequency distributions may be presented in the form of a table, such as Table 17.3, or in the form of a graph. Figure 17.1 illustrates the most common graph forms: the histogram and the frequency polygon. These two methods are similar in that in both, scores or percentages of occurrence are plotted against frequency. The greater the number of points plotted, the smoother is the resulting graph. The shape of the resulting graph allows for observations that further describe the data.

Bar graphs present categorical data (nominal and ordinal variables) with rectangular bars with heights or lengths proportional to the values that they represent. The bars can be plotted vertically or horizontally. The bars do not touch each other;

TABLE **17.3**					
FREQUENCY DISTRIBUTION					
INDIVIDUAL			**GROUP**		
SCORE	TALLY	FREQUENCY	SCORE	TALLY	FREQUENCY
90	I	1	>89	I	1
88	I	1	80–89		15
86	I	1			
84	I	6			
82	II	2			
80		5			
78		5	70–79	III	23
76	I	1			
74	II	7			
72	IIII	9			
70	I	1			
68	III	3	60–69		10
66	II	2			
64	IIII	4			
62	I	1			
60		0			
58	I	1	<59	II	2
56		0			
54	I	1			
52		0			
50		0			
Total		51	Total		51

Mean, 74.51; standard deviation, +12.1; median, 74; mode, 72; range, 36 (54–90).

this illustrates that the variables are continuous as in a histogram.

Measures of Central Tendency

Measures of central tendency answer questions such as "What does the average nurse think?" and "What is the average temperature of patients on a unit?" These measures yield a single number that describes the middle of the group and summarizes the members of a sample. In statistics, the three measures of central tendency are the mode, the median, and the mean. Depending on the distribution, these measures may not all give the same answer to the question "What is the average?" Each measure of central tendency has a specific use and is most appropriate for specific kinds of measurement and types of distributions. Of the measures of central tendency, the mean is the most stable and the median the most typical. If the distribution of a sample is symmetrical and unimodal, the mean, median, and mode coincide.

 Research Hint _____

Measures of central tendency are descriptive statistics that describe the characteristics of a sample.

MODE. The mode is the most frequent score or result and can be obtained by inspection of the frequency distribution table or graph. Note that a sample distribution can have more than one mode. The number of modes, or peaks, contained in a distribution is called the modality of the distribution. The mode is the type of descriptive statistic most appropriately used with nominal-level data but can be used with all levels of measurement (see Table 17.2). The mode cannot be used for any subsequent calculations and is unstable; in other words, the mode can fluctuate widely from sample to sample from the same population. A change in just one score in Table 17.3 would change the mode from 72.

MEDIAN. The median is the middle score: of the other scores, 50% are higher and 50% are lower. The median is not sensitive to extremes in high and low scores; thus, it is a more accurate estimator of central tendency in non-normal distributions. In the series of scores in Table 17.3, the twenty-sixth score is always the median, regardless of how much the high and low scores change. The median is best used when the data are skewed (see the "Normal Distribution" section) and the

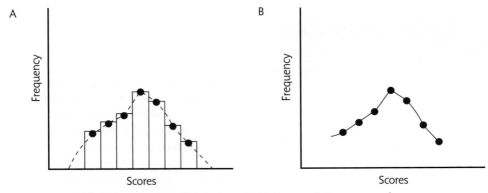

FIG. 17.1 Frequency distributions. **A,** Histogram. **B,** Frequency polygon.

researcher is interested in the "typical" score. For example, if age is a variable, and if a wide range with extreme scores may affect the mean, it would be appropriate to also report the median. The median is easy to find either by inspection or by calculation and can be used with ordinal or higher data, as shown in Table 17.2.

MEAN. The mean (M) is the arithmetical average of all scores and is used with interval- or ratio-level data (see Table 17.2). Most statistical tests of significance refer to the mean, the most widely used measure of central tendency, which is referred to in general conversations as the average. Because the mean is affected by every score, it is affected by extreme scores; however, the larger the sample size, the less effect a single extreme score will have on the mean. For normally distributed populations, the mean is an appropriate measure of central tendency and is generally considered the single best point for summarizing data.

Research Hint

Of the three measures of central tendency, the mean is the most stable, the least affected by extremes, and the most useful for other calculations. The mean can be calculated only with interval- and ratio-level data.

Héon and associates (2016) used a table to describe the sample characteristics in their study that they used to rule out confounding variables.

The summary statistics in Appendix D about the sample, comparing the experimental group with the control group, were reported in narrative form; for example, "mothers had an average age of 29.3 years (SD = 5.4; EG: mean = 28.6 ± 5.7; CG; mean = 30.0 ± 5.1)" (p. 575). They did inferential statistics to determine whether there was a difference in ages and found no statistical difference: $p = .419$ (p. 575).

Normal Distribution

The theoretical concept of normal distribution is based on the observation that data from repeated interval or ratio measurements will gather at a midpoint in a distribution, approximating the normal curve illustrated in Figure 17.2. In addition, if the means of a large number of samples of the same interval- or ratio-level data are calculated and plotted on a graph, that curve also approximates the normal curve. This tendency of the means to approximate the normal curve is termed the *sampling distribution of the means*. The mean of the sampling distribution of the means is the mean of the population.

In visual representations of statistics, the normal curve is unimodal and symmetrical about the mean. The mean, median, and mode are equal. An additional characteristic of the normal curve is that a fixed percentage of the scores is located within a given distance of the mean. As shown in Figure 17.2, about 68% of the scores or means

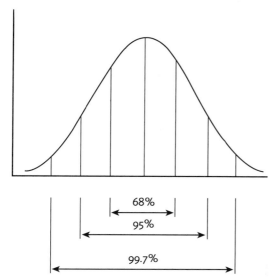

FIG. 17.2 The normal distribution and associated standard deviations.

are within 1 standard deviation of the mean, 95% within 2 standard deviations of the mean, and 99.7% within 3 standard deviations of the mean.

SKEWNESS. Skew is a measure of the asymmetry of a set of scores. Not all samples of data approximate the normal curve. Some samples are nonsymmetrical, and the peak is off centre. For example, worldwide individual income has a positive skew: Most individuals have incomes in the low-to-moderate range and few in the upper range. In a positive skew, the peak of the distribution curve

would be to the left of a normal curve, and the mean is to the right of the median. In contrast, age at death in Canada has a negative skew because most deaths occur at older ages. In a negative skew, the peak of the distribution curve would be to the right of a normal curve, and the mean is to the left of the median. Figure 17.3 illustrates positive and negative skew. In each diagram, the peak is off centre, and one "tail" of the curve is longer.

If the distribution is skewed, the mean will be pulled in the direction of the long tail of the distribution. With a skewed distribution, all three statistics should be reported.

 Evidence-Informed Practice Tip ____
The descriptive statistics for a sample indicate whether the sample data are skewed.

Interpreting Measures of Variability

Variability or dispersion is concerned with the spread of data. Measures of variability—statistical procedures that describe the level of dispersion in sample data—answer questions such as "Is the sample homogeneous or heterogeneous?" and "Is the sample similar or different?" If a researcher measures oral temperatures in two samples, one sample drawn from a healthy population and one sample from a hospitalized population, it is possible that the two samples will have the same mean. However, a wider range of temperatures is

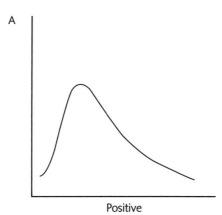

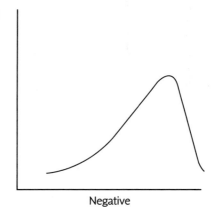

Positive   Negative

FIG. 17.3 Positive and negative skew. A, Positive skew. B, Negative skew.

more likely to be found in the hospitalized sample than in the healthy sample. Measures of variability are used to describe these differences in the dispersion of data. As with measures of central tendency, the various measures of variability are appropriate to specific kinds of measurement and types of distributions.

Research Hint

Descriptive statistics related to variability enable you to evaluate the homogeneity or heterogeneity of a sample.

RANGE. The range is the simplest but most unstable measure of variability. Range is the distance between the highest and lowest scores. A change in either of these two scores would change the range. The range should always be reported with other measures of variability. For example, Castonguay et al. (2017) tested body-related shame and guilt as predictors of breast cancer survivors' (BCS') moderate to vigorous intensity physical activity (MVPA) during six months. They found that there was quite a spread in of ages in their sample, from 30 years old to 79 years old (Table 17.4). Range affects the standard deviation, as discussed later. The range in Table 17.4 could easily change with an increase or decrease in the high scores or the low scores with a different sample.

SEMIQUARTILE RANGE. The semiquartile range (semi-interquartile range) is the range of the middle 50% of the scores. It is more stable than the overall range because it is less likely to be changed by a single extreme score. The semiquartile range lies between the upper and lower quartiles; the upper quartile consists of the top 25% of scores, and the lower quartile consists of the lowest 25% of the scores. In Table 17.3, the middle 50% of the scores are between 68 and 78, and the semiquartile range is 10.

PERCENTILE. A percentile represents the percentage of scores that a given score exceeds. The median

TABLE 17.4

DESCRIPTIVE STATISTICS AND SCORE RANGES OF STUDY VARIABLES (N = 149)

VARIABLE	X-BAR	SD	RANGE
Age (years)	55.34	10.5	30–79
Body mass index (kg/m-sq)	25.86	5.33	18–43
Depression	1.48	0.7	0–3
Months since diagnosis	16.46	9.46	2–26
Months since treatment	9.48	8.41	0–13
Body-related shame	2.64	0.91	1–5
External regulation	0.39	0.58	0–4
Introjected regulation	1.17	1.07	0–4
Autonomous regulation	2.61	0.98	0–4
Identified regulation	2.62	0.85	0–4
Intrinsic regulation	2.54	1.07	0–4
MVPA at T1	1.08	1.51	0–7
MVPA at T2	0.81	1.22	0–5

Variable	n	%
Current smoker	9	6
Education		
Some high school	7	5
High school diploma	20	13
Some college	12	8
College or technical diploma	29	20
Undergraduate degree	41	28
Graduate degree	40	27
Stage of cancer		
I	62	42
II	63	42
III	24	16

MVPA - moderate to vigorous physical activity; T1- time 1 (baseline); T2 - time 2 (six months later)

Adapted from Castonguay, A., Wrosch, C., Pila, E., & Sabiston, C. (2017). Body-related shame and guilt predict physical activity in breast cancer survivors over time. *Oncology Nursing Forum, 44*(4), 465–475. https://doi.org/10.1188/17.ONF.465-475.

is the fiftieth percentile, and in Table 17.3, it is a score of 74. A score in the ninetieth percentile is exceeded by only 10% of the scores. The zero percentile and the hundredth percentile are usually not used.

STANDARD DEVIATION. The standard deviation is the most frequently used measure of variability and is based on the concept of the normal curve (see Figure 17.2). The standard deviation is a measure of average deviation of the scores from the mean and, as such, should always be reported with the mean. The standard deviation accounts for all scores and can be used to interpret individual scores. For the examination in Table 17.3, the mean was 74.51 and the standard deviation was 12.1; thus, a student should know that 68% of the grades were between 86.61 and 62.41. If the student received a grade of 88, he or she would know that this grade was better than those of most of the class, whereas a grade of 58 would indicate that the student did not do as well as most of the class. Table 2 in Appendix D from the study by Goldsworthy and colleagues (2019) reports the mean and standard deviation of the study variables' on the Clinical Self-Efficacy Scale within- and between-group pre-post intervention in the treatment and control groups. As illustrated in this table, the mean difference between the pre and post scores, for the treatment group on "recognizing a patient with no pulse" was 8.04 (SD = 12.41), whereas the mean difference score for the control group was 2.45 (SD = 10.44). This means that 68% of the of the change in the treatment group was between a score of 3.37 and 20.45 on self-efficacy and 68% of the control group was between 7.99 and 12.89. This table allows the reader to inspect the data and see the variation in the data, and these data shows that the self-efficacy of treatment group after the intervention. In assessing SD, it is also important to note the size of the SD, a small standard deviation indicates that the data points tend to be very close to the mean; a large standard deviation indicates that the data points are spread out over a large range of values. If two samples had a mean equal to 2, but one had a SD of 8.0 and the other had a SD of 3.0, the first sample would be more heterogeneous.

The standard deviation is used in the calculation of many inferential statistics. One limitation of the standard deviation is that it is expressed in terms of the units used in the measurement and cannot be used to compare means that have different units. If researchers were interested in the relationship between height measured in centimetres and weight measured in kilograms, it would be necessary to convert the height and weight measurements to standard units, or Z scores. The Z score is used to compare measurements in standard units. Each of the scores is converted to a Z score, and then the Z scores are used to examine the relative distance of the scores from the mean. A Z score of 1.5 means that the observation is 1.5 standard deviations above the mean, whereas a score of −2 means that the observation is 2 standard deviations below the mean. By using Z scores, a researcher can compare results from scales that use different measurement units, such as height and weight.

Research Hint
Many measures of variability exist. The standard deviation is the most stable and useful because it provides a visual image of how the scores are dispersed around the mean.

INFERENTIAL STATISTICS

Inferential statistics combine mathematical processes with logic and allow researchers to test hypotheses about a population by using data obtained from probability samples. Statistical inference is generally used for two purposes: to estimate the probability that statistics found in the sample accurately reflect the population parameter and to test hypotheses about a population.

In the first purpose, a parameter is a characteristic of a population—a well-defined set that has certain specified properties—whereas a statistic is a characteristic of a sample. Statistics are used to estimate population parameters. Suppose that a researcher randomly selects 100 people with chronic lung disease and uses an interval-level scale to study their knowledge of the disease. A mean score of 65 for these participants represents the sample statistic. If the researcher were able to study every participant with chronic lung disease, he or she also could calculate an average knowledge score, and that score would be the parameter for the population. Researchers are rarely

able to study an entire population, but inferential statistics provide evidence that allow them to make statements about the larger population from studying the sample.

Both parametric and nonparametric inferential tests can be used in data analyses (Tables 17.5 and 17.6). Parametric statistical models are based on assumptions about the distributions of sample values and parameters; thus, in these models, means and variances are used to test significance. Nonparametric tests are used when populations have non-normal distributions or when

TABLE **17.5**

TESTS OF DIFFERENCES BETWEEN MEANS

| LEVEL OF MEASUREMENT | ONE GROUP | TWO GROUPS | | MORE THAN TWO GROUPS |
		RELATED	INDEPENDENT	
NONPARAMETRIC				
Nominal	Chi-square	Chi-square Fisher's exact probability test	Chi-square	Chi-square
Ordinal	Kolmogorov-Smirnov test	Sign test Wilcoxon matched-pairs test	Chi-square	Chi-square
PARAMETRIC				
Interval or ratio	Correlated t test ANOVA (repeated measures)	Correlated t test	Independent t test	ANOVA
			ANOVA	ANCOVA MANOVA

ANCOVA, analysis of covariance; ANOVA, analysis of variance; MANOVA, multivariate analysis of variance.

TABLE **17.6**

TESTS OF ASSOCIATION

LEVEL OF MEASUREMENT	TWO VARIABLES	MORE THAN TWO VARIABLES
NONPARAMETRIC		
Nominal	Phi coefficient Point-biserial correlation	Contingency coefficient
Ordinal	Kendall's tau Spearman's rho	Discriminant function analysis
PARAMETRIC		
Interval or ratio	Pearson r	Multiple regression Path analysis Canonical correlation

researchers wish to explore associations among variables. In these tests, no assumptions about the distribution of the data are made.

The example of the study of patients with lung disease alludes to two important qualifications of how a study must be conducted so that inferential statistics may be used. First, the sample was selected randomly—that is, through the use of probability methods (see Chapter 13). Because you are already familiar with the advantages of probability sampling, you know that in order to make generalizations about a population from a sample, that sample must be representative. All procedures for inferential statistics are based on the assumption that the sample was drawn with a known probability. Second, the scale had to reflect the interval level of measurement. The mathematical operations involved in inferential statistics require this level of measurement. Note that researchers who use nonprobability methods of sampling also use inferential statistics. To compensate for the use of nonprobability sampling

methods, researchers use techniques such as sample size estimation through power analysis. The following two Critical Thinking Decision Paths provide algorithms that reflect inferential statistics and that researchers use for statistical decision making.

Evidence-Informed Practice Tip

Try to determine whether the statistical test chosen was appropriate for the design, the type of data collected, and the level of measurement.

Hypothesis Testing

The second and most commonly used purpose of inferential statistics is hypothesis testing. Statistical hypothesis testing allows researchers to make objective decisions about the outcome of their study and to answer questions such as "How much of this effect is a result of chance?"; "How strongly are these two variables associated with each other?"; and "What is the effect of the intervention?"

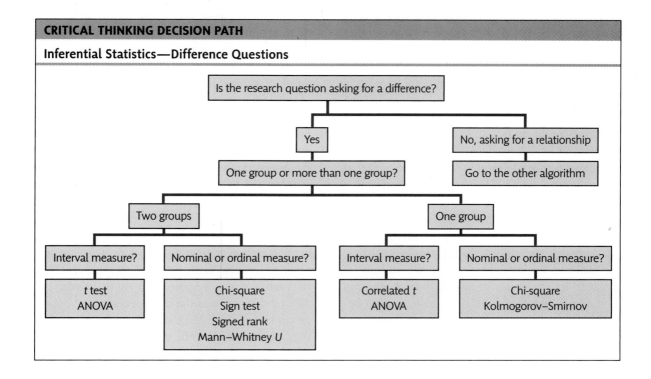

CRITICAL THINKING DECISION PATH

Inferential Statistics—Difference Questions

- Is the research question asking for a difference?
  - Yes
    - One group or more than one group?
      - Two groups
        - Interval measure? → t test / ANOVA
        - Nominal or ordinal measure? → Chi-square / Sign test / Signed rank / Mann–Whitney U
      - One group
        - Interval measure? → Correlated t / ANOVA
        - Nominal or ordinal measure? → Chi-square / Kolmogorov–Smirnov
  - No, asking for a relationship
    - Go to the other algorithm

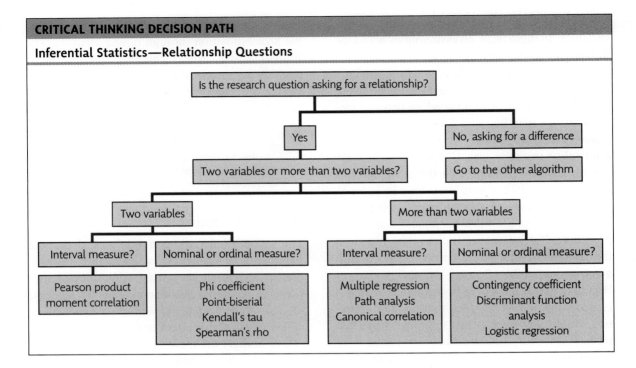

CRITICAL THINKING DECISION PATH

Inferential Statistics—Relationship Questions

The procedures used to make inferences are based on principles of negative inference. For example, to study the effect of a new educational program for patients with chronic lung disease, the researcher would actually have two hypotheses: the scientific hypothesis and the null hypothesis. The research or scientific hypothesis (H1) is what the researcher believes the outcome of the study will be. In this example, the scientific hypothesis would be that the educational intervention would have a marked effect on the outcome in the experimental group in comparison with that in the control group. The null hypothesis (also called the *statistical hypothesis* or H_0), which is the hypothesis that actually can be tested by statistical methods, would be that no difference exists between the groups. In inferential statistics, the null hypothesis is used to test the validity of a scientific hypothesis in sample data. According to the null hypothesis, no relationship exists between the variables, and any observed relationship or difference is merely a function of chance fluctuations in sampling.

The concept of the null hypothesis is often confusing. An example may help clarify this concept. Sherrard, Duchesne, Wells, and colleagues (2015) used an interactive voice response to follow patients with acute coronary syndrome best practice guidelines and compared this to the usual care offered by the best practice guidelines. On the basis of this hypothesis, Sherrard and colleagues wanted to determine whether the differences found in the dependent variables of medication adherence and adverse effects differed significantly between the intervention group and the control group. The authors had to use the null hypothesis—that no difference would exist between the intervention and control groups—to test the scientific hypothesis. They found a significant improvement in medication adherence and a decrease in unplanned medical visits by the group that received interactive voice response. In other words, the differences between the control and intervention group scores were large enough to conclude that they were unlikely to be caused by chance. Thus, the null hypothesis was rejected.

In another example, Bilik et al. (2020) examined the effects of web-based concept mapping education on nursing students' concept mapping and critical thinking skills. Their research hypotheses were: 1) there is a difference in mean scores for concept evaluation keys between students receiving web-based concept mapping education and those not receiving this education, and 2) there is a difference in mean scores on the Critical Thinking Motivational Scale (CTMS) between students receiving web-based concept mapping education and those receiving this education (p. 2). They reported significant differences between the groups (p = 0.00) for hypothesis 1, thus the null hypothesis was rejected. In regards to hypothesis 2, the experimental and control groups differed significantly in their scores for the subscales of CTMS expectancy (p = 0.037), attainment (p = 0.015), and utility (p = 0.015), but they did not differ significantly in terms of the subscales value (p = 0.225) and cost (p = 0.070) (p. 4); thus, hypothesis 2 was partially met. See information on the interpretation of p values in the "Level of Significance" section.

All statistical hypothesis testing is a process of disproof or rejection. It is impossible to prove that a scientific hypothesis is true, but it is possible to demonstrate that the null hypothesis has a high probability of being incorrect. To reject the null hypothesis, therefore, is to show support for the scientific hypothesis, which is the desired outcome of most reports of inferential statistics.

Research Hint

Remember that most samples used in clinical research are samples of convenience, but most researchers use inferential statistics. Although such use violates one of the assumptions of such tests, the tests are robust enough to not seriously affect the results unless the data are skewed in unknown ways.

Probability

The researcher can never *prove* the scientific hypothesis but can show support for it by rejecting the null hypothesis—that is, by showing that the null hypothesis has a high probability of being incorrect. The theory underlying all of the procedures discussed in this chapter is probability theory. Probability is a concept that people talk about all the time, such as the chance of rain, but have a difficult time defining. The probability of an event is the event's long-run relative frequency in repeated trials under similar conditions. In other words, the statistician does not think of the probability of obtaining a single result from a single study but rather of the chances of obtaining the same result from an idealized study that can be carried out many times under identical conditions. The notion of repeated trials allows researchers to use probability to test hypotheses.

Statistical probability is based on the concept of sampling error. The use of inferential statistics is based on random sampling. However, even when samples are randomly selected, the possibility of errors in sampling always exists. Therefore, the characteristics of any given sample may be different from those of the entire population.

Suppose that a large group of patients with decubitus ulcers is available for study and that researchers wish to learn the average length of time for such ulcers to heal with the usual nursing care. If the researchers studied the entire population, they might obtain an average healing time of 50 days, with a standard deviation of 10 days. Now, suppose that the researchers did not have the money necessary to study all the patients but wished to conduct several consecutive studies of this condition. For this study, the researchers would first select a sample of 25 patients, calculate the mean and standard deviation, and then select the next sample. If this process is repeated many times in different samples, a different mean for each sample would probably result. For example, the researchers might find that one sample's mean might be 50.5 days, the next 47.5, and the next 62.5. The tendency for statistics to fluctuate from one sample to another is known as sampling error.

Sampling distributions are theoretical. In practice, researchers do not routinely draw consecutive samples from the same population; they usually compute statistics and make inferences on the basis of data from one sample. However, the knowledge of the properties of the sampling distribution—if these repeated samples are hypothetically obtained—enables the researcher to draw a conclusion on the basis of data from one sample. Such a conclusion is possible because the sampling distribution of the means has certain known properties.

The sampling distribution of the means is shaped like a normal curve, and the mean of the sampling distribution is the mean of the population. As discussed in the earlier "Normal Distribution" section, because the sampling distribution of the means is normal, several other important characteristics are revealed. When scores are normally distributed, 68% of them are between +1 standard deviation and −1 standard deviation, or the probability is 68 per 100 that any one randomly drawn sample mean is within the range of values between +1 standard deviation and −1 standard deviation (see Figure 17.2). In the example described earlier, if only one sample were selected, the chance of finding a sample mean between 40 and 60 would be 68%. The standard deviation of a theoretical distribution of sample means is called the standard error of the mean. The word *error* is used because the various means that make up the distribution contain an error in their estimates of the population mean. The error is considered to be standard because it implies the magnitude of the average error, just as a standard deviation implies the average variation from one mean. The *smaller* the standard error, the *less* variable are the sample means and the *more accurate* are those means as estimates of the population value.

Although researchers rarely construct sampling distributions, standard error can be estimated because it bears a systematic relationship to the sample standard deviation and the size of the sample. Thus, increasing the size of the sample will increase the accuracy of estimates of population parameters. It is intuitive that an increase in the size of a sample will decrease the likelihood that one outlying score will dramatically affect the sample mean (see Chapter 13). The other reason that the sampling distribution is so important is that all statistics have sampling distributions. Researchers consult these distributions when making determinations about rejecting the null hypothesis.

Evidence-Informed Practice Tip

Remember that the strength and quality of evidence are enhanced by repeated trials that have consistent findings, thereby increasing the generalizability of the findings and applicability to clinical practice.

Type I and Type II Errors

The researcher's decision to accept or fail to accept (reject) the null hypothesis is based on a consideration of the probability that the observed differences are a result of chance alone. Because data on the entire population are not available, the researcher cannot flatly assert that the null hypothesis is or is not true. Thus, statistical inference is always based on incomplete information about a population, and errors can occur when such inferences are made. These errors are classified as type I and type II.

A type I error is the researcher's incorrect decision to reject the null hypothesis (Kline, 2005); that is, the researcher has found that results are statistically significant, but in fact they are not, and has accepted the alternate hypothesis. If, however, the researcher had found that the groups did not differ perhaps because only a few patients had been studied or the design of the study was poor for determining differences, a type II error might occur. In a type II error—also known as beta (β)—the results from the sample data lead to the failure to reject the null hypothesis when it is actually false; that is, no statistically significant differences between groups were found but there are indeed real differences. Power is the conditional prior probability that the researcher will decide correctly to reject the null hypothesis when it is actually false (Kline, 2005). A standard value of power of .8 is used to conduct power analyses in studies to determine sample size before the study begins; this means that the researcher is accepting 20% risk of Type II error. Power and beta are complementary and sum to 1.00. When power is increased, type II error is decreased, and vice versa.

In Campbell-Yeo, Johnston, Joseph, and colleagues' (2015) study on cobedding and recovery time after heel lance in preterm twins, one null hypothesis of the study was that there would be no differences in pain response and time to return to physiological measures between the experimental and control groups. Campbell-Yeo and colleagues reported a significant difference in recovery time; that is, the time was shorter in the cobedding group, mean = 75.6 seconds (SD, 70.0), compared with the usual care group, mean = 142.1 seconds (SD, 138.1, $p = .001$). If the differences found were truly a function of chance (because this group of participants was unusual in some way) and if the number of participants was too small, a type II error would occur. Thus, the simplest way of reducing Type II error is to increase the sample size.

The relationship of the two types of errors is shown in Figure 17.4. When you critique a study to determine whether a type I error has occurred (rejecting the null hypothesis when it is actually true), you should consider the reliability and

validity of the instruments used. For example, if the instruments did not accurately and precisely measure the intervention variables, the conclusion could be that the intervention made a difference, but, in reality, it did not. It is critical to consider the reliability and validity of all of the measurement instruments reported (see Chapter 15). In a practice discipline, type I errors usually are considered more serious because if a researcher declares that differences exist where none are present, then patient care can potentially be affected adversely. Type II errors (accepting the null hypothesis when it is false) may occur if the sample in the study is too small, thereby limiting the opportunity to measure the *treatment effect*, a true difference between two groups. A larger sample size improves the ability to *detect the treatment effect*—that is, the differences between two groups. If no significant difference is found between two groups with a large sample, this finding provides stronger evidence (than with a small sample) not to reject the null hypothesis.

Level of Significance

The researcher does not know when an error in statistical decision making has occurred. It is possible to know only that the null hypothesis is indeed true or false if data from the total population are available. However, the researcher can control the risk of making type I errors by setting the level of significance before the study begins (a priori). The level of significance (alpha level) is the probability of making a type I error—in other words, the conditional probability of rejecting the

Conclusion of test of significance	REALITY	
	Null hypothesis is true	Null hypothesis is not true
Not statistically significant	Correct conclusion	Type II error
Statistically significant	Type I error	Correct conclusion

FIG. 17.4 Outcome of statistical decision making.

null hypothesis when it is actually true. Alpha, or the level of significance, is considered an a priori probability because it is set before the data are collected, and it is a conditional probability because the null hypothesis is assumed to be true. The minimum level of significance acceptable for nursing research is .05. If the researcher sets alpha at .05, the researcher is willing to accept the fact that if the study were done 100 times, the decision to reject the null hypothesis would be wrong in 5 of those 100 trials, only if the null hypothesis is true.

Sometimes the researcher wants to have a smaller risk of rejecting a true null hypothesis; in that case, the level of significance may be set at .01. In this case, the researcher is willing to make the wrong decision only once in 100 trials. The decision as to how strictly the alpha level should be set depends on how important it is not to make an error. For example, if the results of a study are to be used to determine whether a great deal of money should be spent in an area of nursing care, the researcher may decide that the accuracy of the results is so important that an alpha level of .01 is chosen. In most studies, however, alpha is set at .05.

Another concept, the p value, is needed to interpret the alpha value. The p value, or probability value, is the probability of obtaining, from the study data, a test statistic, such as the mean, a result equal to or "more extreme" than what was actually observed, when the null hypothesis is true. The p value is different from alpha because it is calculated from the sample data and is considered the *exact level of significance*. Thus, if this exact level of significance is less than the conditional a priori probability of making a type I error ($p <$ alpha), then the null hypothesis is rejected, and the result is considered statistically significant at that alpha level. For example, if the alpha is set at .05 and the p value is found to be .04, then the results are considered statistically significant.

Whatever level of significance is set, the researcher either rejects or accepts the null hypothesis when comparing the statistical results with the preset alpha. For example, in Ingram et al.'s (2016) study, the hypothetical null hypothesis regarding no change in level of knowledge about care of delirious clients after participating in an education session was rejected, as the researchers found statistical significance, because the variables of the hypothesis were significant at the .05 level or lower; in other words, the p values were less than alpha. Jackson and Dennis (2017), however, failed to reject the null hypothesis and found that pain scores were not significantly different between the experimental and control groups (Appendix B).

Perhaps you are thinking that researchers should always use the lowest alpha level possible because it makes sense that they would like to keep the risk of both types of errors at a minimum. Unfortunately, decreasing the risk of making a type I error increases the risk of making a type II error; that is, the stricter the researcher is in preventing the rejection of a true null hypothesis, the more likely the researcher is to accept a false null hypothesis. Therefore, researchers always have to accept more of a risk of one type of error when setting the alpha level.

Another method of determining the level of significance and whether to accept or reject the null hypothesis is called the *critical values method*. In this method, by calculating the estimates of population mean and standard deviation, a range of values is determined from which the researcher can compare the sample mean findings and decide whether to reject the null hypothesis.

Suppose researchers want to know the importance of support groups for caregivers of older adults. They ask 100 caregivers to rate the importance of support groups to them by using an instrument that ranges from 0 (not important at all) to 100 (very important). If Figure 17.2 represents the theoretical distribution for this study (a normal distribution with a mean of 50), 68% of the population would score between 40 and 60, and 95% would score between 30 and 70. Thus, the null hypothesis would be that the mean score for the population of caregivers would be 50, and the scientific hypothesis would be greater or less than 50. After measurements with this sample are completed, the researchers find that the sample mean score is 75. This mean is consistent with the scientific hypothesis, and the researchers can be 95% sure that, most of the time, the sample mean score would fall under this cut-off; thus, they would have confidence in rejecting the null hypothesis. In other words, only 5 of 100 times would they obtain this result by chance alone.

 Research Hint _____

Decreasing the alpha level acceptable for a study increases the chance that a type II error will occur. When a researcher is conducting many statistical tests, the probability that some of the test results will be significant increases as the number of tests increases. Therefore, when a large number of tests are being conducted, many researchers decrease the alpha level to .01.

Practical and Statistical Significance

Statistical significance and practical significance are not the same. When a researcher finds a hypothesis statistically significant, this finding is unlikely to have happened by chance. In other words, if the level of significance has been set at .05, the odds are 95% that the researcher will make the correct conclusion on the basis of the results of the statistical test performed on sample data. The researcher would reach the wrong conclusion only 5 times in 100.

Suppose that a researcher is interested in the effect of loud rock music on the behaviour of laboratory mice. The researcher could design an experiment to study this question and find that loud music makes the mice act strangely. A statistical test suggests that this finding is not the result of chance. However, such a finding may or may not have practical significance, even though the finding has statistical significance. Whereas some authorities would argue that this study might have relevance to understanding the behaviour of teenagers, others would argue that the study has no practical value. Thus, the findings of a study may have statistical significance, but they may have no practical value or significance.

Although researchers should consider the practicality of a problem in the early stages of a research project (see Chapter 3), a distinction between the statistical and practical significance of the findings also should be made in the discussion of the results of a study. Some authorities believe that if the findings are not statistically significant, they have no practical value. In Jackson and Dennis' (2017) study, in Appendix D, the research hypothesis was not statistically supported, but nonsupported hypotheses provide as much information about the intervention as do the supported hypotheses. They found that application of lanolin to painful/damaged nipples in the immediate postpartum period does not significantly decrease nipple pain or improve breastfeeding outcomes when compared with usual care. The data allowed the researchers to return to the previous literature in the area and discern from those findings both statistical and practical significance.

Evidence-Informed Practice Tip ____

You study the results to determine the effectiveness of the new treatment and the size and clinical importance of the effect.

Tests of Statistical Significance

Tests of statistical significance may be parametric or nonparametric. In most studies in nursing research literature, investigators use parametric tests that have the following three attributes:
1. The estimation of at least one population parameter
2. Measurement at the interval level or higher
3. Assumptions about the variables being studied
   One assumption is usually that the variable is normally distributed in the overall population.

In contrast to parametric tests, nonparametric tests of significance are not based on the estimation of population parameters, so their assumptions about the underlying distribution are less restrictive. Nonparametric tests are usually applied when the variables have been measured on a nominal or ordinal scale.

Some debate surrounds the relative merits of the two types of statistical tests. The moderate position taken by most researchers and statisticians is that nonparametric statistics—also called *distribution-free tests*—are best used when the data cannot be assumed to be at the interval level of measurement or when the sample is small and the normality of the underlying distribution cannot be inferred. If these assumptions can be made, however, most researchers prefer to use parametric statistics, which are more powerful and more flexible than nonparametric statistics. Because stringent assumptions for parametric tests makes them more powerful than nonparametric tests, researchers are able to formulate simple sample statistics, such as the mean and the standard deviation, which enables them to accurately estimate population parameters with standard sampling distributions to obtain probabilities regarding the null hypotheses.

Researchers use many different statistical tests of significance to test hypotheses; however, the procedure and the rationale for their use are similar from test to test. Once the researcher has chosen a significance level and collected the data, the data are used to compute the appropriate test statistic. Each test has a related theoretical distribution that shows the probable and improbable values for that statistic. On the basis of the statistical result and the values in the distribution, the researcher either accepts or rejects the null hypothesis and then reports both the statistical result and its probability. Thus, a researcher may perform a t test, obtain a value of 8.98, and report that it is statistically significant at the $p < .05$ level. This means that in 100 tests, the researcher had five chances to conclude wrongly that this result could not have been obtained by chance.

The likelihood of finding a statistic that is high enough to be statistically significant is increased as the sample size increases. This likelihood is indicated by the degrees of freedom, which are

often reported with the statistic and the probability value. Usually abbreviated as *df*, the degree of freedom is the freedom of a score's value to vary depending on the other scores and the sum of these scores; thus, $df = N - 1$. For example, imagine you have four numbers represented by letters (*a, b, c,* and *d*) that must add up to a total of *x*; you are free to randomly choose the first three numbers, but the fourth must be chosen to make the total equal to *x*, and thus your degree of freedom is 3.

To make statistical inferences from data, many types of tests can be conducted. Tables 17.5 and 17.6 list the tests most commonly used for inferential statistics. The test used depends on the level of the measurement of the variables in question and the type of hypothesis being studied. These statistics test two types of hypotheses: that difference exists between groups (see Table 17.5) and that a relationship exists between two or more variables (see Table 17.6). In addition, many types of regression analyses are available to predict the dependent variable. Simple regression analyses (one independent variable) and multiple regression analyses (several independent variables) are used when the dependent variable is at the interval level or higher.

Research Hint

The use of nonparametric statistics in a study does not mean that the study is useless. The use of nonparametric statistics is appropriate when measurements are not made at the interval level or the variable under study is not normally distributed.

Evidence-Informed Practice Tip

Try to discern whether the test for analyzing the data was chosen because it gave a significant p value. A statistical test should be chosen on the basis of its appropriateness for the type of data collected, not because it gives the answer that the researcher hoped to obtain.

Tests of Differences

The type of test used for any particular study depends primarily on whether the researcher examines differences in one, two, or three or more groups and whether the data to be analyzed are nominal, ordinal, or interval (see Table 17.5). Suppose that a researcher constructs an experimental study with an after-only design (see Chapter 11). What the researcher hopes to determine is that the two randomly assigned groups are different after the introduction of the experimental treatment. If the measurements taken are at the interval level, the researcher would use the t test to analyze the data. If the t statistic was found to be high enough to be unlikely to have occurred by chance, the researcher would reject the null hypothesis and conclude that the two groups were indeed more different than would have been expected on the basis of chance alone. In other words, the researcher would conclude that the experimental treatment had the desired effect.

Osahor et al.'s (2019) study on the relationship between math personality, math anxiety, test preparation strategy, and medication dose calculations in first-year nursing students illustrated the use of the t statistic. In this study, the t test was used to determine differences in math anxiety between collaborative students and students in the compressed program. The results showed that students in the collaborative program were more anxious (t (161) $= -2.67$, $p = .008$) and used more test preparation strategies (t (161) $= -2.67$, $p = .008$) than students in the compressed program.

Evidence-Informed Practice Tip

Tests of difference are most commonly used in experimental and quasiexperimental designs that provide level II and level III evidence.

PARAMETRIC TESTS. The t statistic is commonly used in nursing research. This statistic reflects whether two group means are different. Thus, the t statistic is used when the researcher has two groups, and the question is whether the mean scores on some measure are more different than would be expected by chance. To use this test, the variables must have been measured at the interval or ratio level, and the two groups must be independent, meaning that nothing in one group helps determine what is in the other group. If the groups are related in some way, as when samples are matched (see Chapter 13), and the researcher also wants to determine differences between the two groups, a paired, or correlated, t test would be used.

The t statistic illustrates one of the major purposes of research in nursing: to demonstrate that differences exist between groups. Groups may be naturally occurring collections, such as age groups, or they may be experimentally created, such as treatment and control groups. Sometimes a study has more than two groups, or measurements are taken more than once.

ANALYSIS OF VARIANCE (ANOVA). Analysis of variance (ANOVA) is a test similar to the t test, but the procedure is testing for differences when there are three or more groups. For example, Subedi et al. (2019) used five levels of education—illiterate, literate, primary, secondary, and college—to determine how general well-being is affected by Bhutanese refugees. They found a statistical difference (F (4,103) $= 3.02$, $p = .02$). Tukey's honestly significant difference post hoc test indicated that there was a minimal significant difference between "college" and "literate" ($p = .05$) and "college" and "illiterate" ($p = .05$) (p. 172). These researchers used analysis of variance (ANOVA), because there were five groups. Like the t statistic, the ANOVA statistic is used to test whether group means differ, but instead of testing each pair of means separately, ANOVA accounts for the variation between groups and within groups. The ANOVA is usually performed with two or more groups by an F test rather than multiple pairs of t tests (see Practical Application box). If multiple pairs of t tests are done, the type I error rate would increase.

There are many ANOVA tests; for example, a one-way ANOVA, as in the Subedi et al. (2019) study, is used to test the relationship between one categorical independent variable (levels f education) and one continuous variable (well-being). A two-way ANOVA is used to test the relationship between two categorical independent variables, each with more than one level such as gender (male and female) and level of education (illiterate, literate, primary, secondary, and college) and one continuous variable (well-being).

Practical Application

Dahlke et al. (2019) conducted a study to explore student nurses' perceptions about older people. Nursing students' perceptions about working with older people was measured by Burbank's Perceptions of Caring for Older People's scale. There was statistical difference at the $p = 0.05$ level in the Burbank scores for the six different clinical rotation groups ($F (5,364) = 2.6$, $p = 0.024$.

In another example, Hroch et al. (2019) examined preregistration nursing students' knowledge and attitudes about the assessment and management of pain in four education sites from two post-secondary institutions. They used the Knowledge and Attitudes Survey Regarding Pain (KASRP) instrument. One of their analyses consisted of examining institution and program on KASRP scores. The ANOVA results, F test$= 20.5$, $p = .011$, indicated that there were differences in knowledge and attitudes regarding pain based on two variables, type of program and institution; thus, this is a two-way ANOVA.

When more than two groups are compared over time, a repeated-measures ANOVA is used, because this variation of the ANOVA takes into account the fact that multiple measures at several times affect the potential range of scores. As an example, Murray et al. (2019) explored new graduate registered nurses' (NGRNs) knowledge and attitudes concerning medical error and patient safety, at three time points (commencement, three months, six months) during their first 6 months of professional practice. A one-way repeated measures ANOVA was used to investigate the effect of time on self-reported knowledge and attitudes regarding medical errors and patient safety in NGRNs.

POST HOC ANALYSIS. When the decision according to the ANOVA is to reject the null hypothesis, this indicates that at least one of the means

is not the same as the other means, as in Rajacich and associates' (2014) study. To determine where the difference in means lies, a post hoc analysis is conducted; in this analysis, pairs of means in the main effects and interaction effects are compared to determine whether they are statistically different. Many post hoc analyses are available; the most common include Tukey's Honestly Significant Difference (HSD), the Scheffé analysis, and the Bonferroni analysis. This type of post hoc analysis is also known as paired comparisons. In the Hroch et al. study (2019), post hoc comparisons (Tukey's HSD) revealed that the statistically significant difference was between the B.SC.N. program in situation A and both programs in institution b-the B.Sc.N and Practical Nursing (P.N.). There was no statistically significant difference in KASRP scores between the B.Sc.N. and P.N. programs in institution B.

In the study by Dahlke et al. (2019), post hoc comparisons using Tukey HSD test that the mean Burbank score for students in their fourth clinical rotation was significantly different from students who had not had a clinical rotation and from students who had one clinical rotation.

Research Hint

A research report may not always refer to the test that was done. The reader can find this information by looking at the tables. For example, a table with t statistics contains a column for t values, and an ANOVA table lists F values.

In Premji et al.'s (2018) study examining what it means to be a mother of late preterm infant, including a mother's level of confidence in caring for her late preterm infant over time (3–4 weeks and 6–8 weeks) , and the effect of maternal depression of this experience, several paired t-tests were done on maternal confidence. There was a significant decrease in confidence between Time 1 and Time 2, on such the knowledge subscale in relation to "*I know when my baby wants me to play with him/her,*" "*when my baby is cranky, I know the reason,*" and "*I can tell when my baby is tired and needs to sleep.*" In other cases, particularly in experimental work, researchers use t tests or ANOVA to determine whether random assignment to groups was effective in creating groups that are equivalent before the experimental treatment is introduced. In this case, a researcher wants to show that no difference exists among the groups.

In many cases, researchers check whether groups are different at the beginning of a study or baseline by using the technique of analysis of covariance (ANCOVA). ANCOVA also entails measuring differences among group means and helps researchers equate the groups under study on an important variable, to answer the question: are the observed mean differences real or are they false? This false difference is called spurious. ANCOVA allows researchers to control for confounding variables statistically. For example, Tryphonopoulos and Letourneau (2020) tested a video-feedback interaction guidance intervention designed to improve maternal–infant interaction, depressive symptoms, and cortisol patterns of depressed mothers and their infants. They used the ANCOVA to control for pre-test scores on each of the outcome variables (maternal and infant cortisol, maternal depression, Nursing Child Assessment Teaching Scale (NCATS), and CARE-Index (p. 6). Results supported two of the three proposed hypotheses, where maternal and infant cortisol and maternal depression decreased due to the intervention. In the unsupportive hypothesis related to the NCATS scale, the researchers found that there were significant differences favouring the intervention group in scores for *Sensitivity to Cues*, *Cognitive Growth Fostering*, and *Caregiver Total Contingency* subscales (p. 8).

NONPARAMETRIC TESTS. When data are at the nominal or ordinal level and the researcher wants to determine whether groups are different, the chi-square, another commonly used statistic, is helpful. The chi-square (X^2) is a nonparametric statistic used to determine whether the frequency

in each category is different from what would be expected by chance. Adhikari et al. (2017) studied whether neighbourhood socioeconomic status predicts the risk of preterm birth. They conducted several chi-square tests to explore maternal characteristics across preterm birth status. One such test was to explore the association between the categorical variable "parity" (primiparous and multiparous) and another categorical variable "type of birth" (preterm or term birth); therefore the chi-square test was performed and the results were statistically significant. Another example is Benzies et al. (2019), who determined the effect of an enhanced parenting kit given at birth on a) early parenting experiences and (b) use of educational resources and community services; again, these two variables are categorical. They performed a chi-square test between the intervention and comparison group and found that parents in the intervention group were more likely to be aware of the Healthy Parents Healthy Children (HPHC) books than parents in the comparison group (X^2 (1, N = 367) = 5.78, p = .016).

As with the t test and ANOVA, if the calculated chi-square is high enough, the researcher would conclude that the frequencies found would not be expected on the basis of chance alone, and the null hypothesis would be rejected. Although this test is robust and can be used in many different situations, it cannot be used to compare frequencies when samples are small and expected frequencies are less than six in each cell. In those instances, Fisher's exact probability test is used.

When the data are ranks, or are at the ordinal level, several other nonparametric tests may be used: the Kolmogorov-Smirnov test, the sign test, the Wilcoxon matched-pairs test, the signed-rank test for related groups, the median test, and the Mann-Whitney *U* test for independent groups. Explanation of these tests is beyond the scope of this chapter; readers who desire further information should consult a general statistics book.

In nursing research studies, several different statistical tests are often used. Pike et al.'s (2019) study illustrated the use of several of these statistical tests. They examined the relationship between candidate variables (e.g., academic performance, demographics) on their NCLEX-RN outcome (pass/fail). Data measured at the nominal level were gender, program type (regular vs, fast-track); continuous level variables were age and high school and nursing GPA. For data measured at the interval level, such as age and high school and nursing GPA, the t test was used. Finally, to test the differences between the two groups, the chi-square method was used for nominal variables, such as gender and NCLEX-RN outcome.

Tests of Relationships

Researchers often are interested in exploring the *relationship* between two or more variables. In such studies, they use statistics that determine the correlation, or the degree of association, between two or more variables. Tests of the relationships between variables are sometimes considered to be descriptive statistics when they are used to describe the magnitude and direction of a relationship of two variables in a sample and when the researcher does not wish to make statements about the larger population. Such statistics also can be inferential when they are used to test hypotheses about the correlations that exist in the target population.

In tests of the null hypothesis, no relationship is assumed to exist between the variables. Thus, when a researcher rejects this type of null hypothesis, the conclusion is that the variables are, in fact, related. Suppose that a researcher is interested in the relationship between the age of patients and the length of time it takes them to recover from surgery. As with other statistics discussed, the researcher would design a study to collect the appropriate data and then analyze the data by using measures of association. In this example, age and length of time until recovery can be considered interval measurements. The researcher would use the Pearson correlation coefficient (Pearson *r*; also called the *Pearson*

product-moment correlation coefficient) in which the calculation reflects the degree of relationship between two interval variables. The distribution of the Pearson r enables the researcher to determine whether the value obtained is likely to have occurred by chance. Again, the research reports both the value of the correlation and its probability of occurring by chance.

Correlation coefficients can range in value from −1.0 to +1.0 and also can be zero. A zero coefficient means that no relationship exists between the variables. *A perfect positive correlation* is indicated by a coefficient of +1.0 and *a perfect negative correlation by a coefficient* of −1.0. The meaning of these coefficients is illustrated by the example from the previous paragraph. If no relationship exists between the age of the patient and the time required for the patient to recover from surgery, the correlation would be zero. However, a correlation of +1.0 would mean that the older the patient is, the longer the recovery time is. A negative coefficient would imply that the younger the patient is, the longer the recovery time is. Figure 17.5 illustrates a perfect positive correlation, a perfect negative correlation, and a zero correlation. A correlation value of 0 to .2 is considered extremely weak, a value of .2 to .4 is weak, a value of .4 to .6 is moderate, a value of .6 to .8 is strong, and a value of .8 to 1.0 is very strong (Bluman, 2014).

Of course, relationships are rarely perfect. The magnitude of the relationship is indicated by how close correlation is to the absolute value of 1 (see Practical Application box). Thus, a correlation of −.76 is just as strong as a correlation of +.76, but the direction of the relationship is opposite. In addition, a correlation of .76 is stronger than a correlation of .32. In testing hypotheses about the relationships between two variables, the researcher considers whether the magnitude of the correlation is large enough not to have occurred by chance. This is the meaning of the probability value, or the *p* value, reported with correlation coefficients. As with other statistical tests of

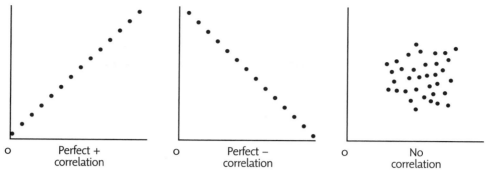

FIG. 17.5   Scatter plots illustrating the different types of correlations.

significance, the larger the sample is, the greater the likelihood of finding a significant correlation. Therefore, researchers also report the degrees of freedom associated with the test performed.

> ### Practical Application
> An example of a descriptive, correlational study is that of Levya-Moral et al. (2019), describing nursing faculty attitudes and beliefs about persons living with HIV. There were correlations between stereotype and prejudice ($r = .73$, $p < .001$), stereotype and discrimination ($r = .91$, $p < .001$), and discrimination and prejudice ($r = .83$, $p < .001$).
> Winsett et al. (2016) conducted correlations between two interval variables and found that as perception of staff adequacy declined, reasons for missed care increased in importance: communication ($r = -.272$, $p = .006$), material resource ($r = -.240$, $p = .006$); and the labor resource ($r = -.255$, $p = .001$). All of these variables were measured with validated scales.

Nominal- and ordinal-level data also can be tested for relationships by nonparametric statistics. When two variables being tested are only dichotomous (e.g., male/female; yes/no), the phi coefficient can be used to express relationships. When the researcher is interested in the relationship between a nominal variable and an interval variable, the point-biserial correlation is used. Spearman's rho is used to determine the degree of association between two sets of ranks, as is Kendall's tau. All of these correlation coefficients may range in value from -1.0 to $+1.0$. These tests are listed in Table 17.6.

Nursing problems are rarely so simple that they can be explained by only two variables. When researchers are interested in studying complex relationships among more than two variables, they use techniques other than those discussed thus far. When researchers are interested in understanding more about a problem than just the relationship between variables and in making predictions they often use regression. There are several types of regression including simple, multiple and logistic regression. Simple regression is looking at the relationship of two continuous variables, with one predicting the other, while multiple regression is conducted when the researcher is exploring the relationship between one dependent variable at the interval level and several independent variables is measured. Multiple regression is the expansion of correlation to include more than two variables and is used when the researcher wants to determine what variables contribute to the explanation of the dependent variable and to what degree. Researchers also use logistic and ordinal regression for prediction when variables are binary/ordinal, but these statistical tests are outside the scope of this textbook.

An example of multiple regression is a researcher may be interested in determining what factors help women decide to breastfeed their infants. A number of variables—such as the mother's age, previous experience with breastfeeding, number of other children, and knowledge of the advantages of breastfeeding—might be measured and then analyzed to determine whether they, separately and together, are predictive of the length of breastfeeding. The results of such a study might help nurses know that a younger mother with only one other child might be more likely to benefit from a teaching program about breastfeeding than would an older mother with several other children.

In reading research reports, you will often see multiple regression techniques described as *forward solution, backward solution, or stepwise solution*. These techniques are used in multiple regression to find the smallest group of variables that will account for the greatest proportion of variance in the dependent variable. In the forward solution, the independent variable that has the highest correlation with the dependent variables is entered first, and the next variable is the one that will increase the explained variance the most. In the backward solution, all variables are entered into the solution, and each variable is deleted to determine whether the explained variance drops significantly. The stepwise solution is a combination of the two approaches. In general, all of the approaches yield similar, although not identical, results.

Using multiple regression, Corby et al. (2021) investigated the predictors of prenatal breastfeeding self-efficacy. The following variables predicted breastfeeding self-efficacy among primiparous women: feeling prepared for labor and birth ($\beta = 0.244$), income ($\beta = -0.184$), anxiety ($\beta = -0.291$), length of plan to exclusively breastfeed ($\beta = 0.212$), maternal education ($\beta = 0.159$), and marital status ($\beta = 0.152$). The predictors among multiparous women were: breastfeeding knowledge ($\beta = 0.188$), anxiety ($\beta = -0.285$), length of prior exclusive breastfeeding experience ($\beta = 0.309$), and plan to exclusively breastfeed ($\beta = -0.153$). These data allowed them to build on the past research that they had reviewed and to suggest both future descriptive and intervention research, thus moving the data toward evidence-informed practice.

 Evidence-Informed Practice Tip ____

Tests of relationship are usually associated with nonexperimental designs that provide level IV evidence. A strong, statistically significant relationship between variables often provides support for replicating the study, in order to increase the consistency of the findings and provide a foundation for developing an intervention study.

The Use of Confidence Intervals

A confidence interval is a range of values, based on a random sample, that is often described with measures of central tendency and measures of association and provides the nurse with a measure of precision or uncertainty about the sample findings. In other words, the confidence interval is an estimated range of values, which is likely to include an unknown population parameter calculated from a given set of sample data. Interval estimation is useful as it provides a range of values within which a parameter (e.g., mean) has a specific probability of lying. Determining a confidence interval around a sample mean sets a range of values for the population mean as well as the probability of being right, that is, the estimate is made with a certain degree of confidence.

Typically, investigators record their confidence interval results as a 95% degree of certainty; sometimes, the degree of certainty is recorded as 99%. Today, professional journals often require investigators to report confidence intervals as one of the statistical methods used to interpret study findings. Even when confidence intervals are not reported, they can be easily calculated from study data. The method for performing these calculations is widely available in statistical texts. The 95% confidence interval is a set of values that you can be 95% certain contains the true mean of the population. As the sample size increases, this range of interval values will narrow, indicating that the mean is more accurate compared with a smaller sample. In addition to the parameters, confidence intervals can be established around other measures such odds ratios (OR).

Odds ratio is a very effective way of determining the association between two variables, mostly the influence of one factor on the outcome of interest. In nursing, <u>odds ratio is becoming an increasingly reported statistic in published papers.</u> The derivation of odds ratios is outside the scope of this textbook, but interpreting it is very simple. If the odds ratio is 1.24, the likelihood of having the outcome is 24% higher ($1.24 - 1 = B$ 0.24 i.e. 24%) than the comparison group.

An example is in the Adhikari Dahal et al. (2017) study that explored paediatric and perinatal epidemiology variation in maternal co-morbidities. The results were that OR 2.5 (95%, CI 1.8, 3.5), HIV OR 3.3 (95% CI 1.5, 8.3), pre-existing diabetes OR 1.7 (95% CI 1.1, 2.6), and prolonged stay OR 1.5 (95% CI 1.4, 1.6) were significantly more likely to occur in the most deprived areas than in the least deprived areas (p. 277). An example of interpretation is that prolonged stay in the OR will occur 25% more in women in deprived areas. The confidence level of the odds ratios is the probability that the confidence interval contains the true odds ratio. If the study was repeated and the range calculated each time, you would expect the true value to lie within these ranges 95% of the time. The confidence interval helps place the results in context for all patients in the study.

Research Hint

When evaluating whether you should spend time reviewing an article, examine the article's tables. The information you need to answer your clinical question should be contained in one or more of the tables.

Evidence-Informed Practice Tip

A basic understanding of statistics will improve your ability to assess the effect of the independent variable on the dependent variable and related patient outcomes for your patient population and practice setting.

APPRAISING THE EVIDENCE

Descriptive and Inferential Statistics

Many students who have not had a course in statistics think they cannot critique the statistics of research. However, students should be able to critically analyze the use of statistics even if they do not understand how the numbers presented were derived. What is most important in critiquing this aspect of a research study is that the procedures for summarizing and analyzing the data make sense in view of the purpose of the study (see the Critiquing Criteria box).

Before you decide whether the statistics used make sense, return to the beginning of the study and determine the purpose. Although descriptive statistics are used in all studies to summarize the data obtained, many investigators use inferential statistics to test specific hypotheses. In a report of an exploratory study, it is possible that only descriptive statistics are presented because the purpose is to describe the characteristics of a population.

Just as the hypotheses or research questions should follow from the purpose of a study, so should the hypotheses or research questions suggest the type of analysis that follows. The hypotheses or the research questions should indicate the major variables that are expected to be presented in summary form. Each of the variables in the hypotheses or research questions should be presented in the "Results" section along with appropriate descriptive information.

After you study the hypotheses or research questions, proceed to the "Methods" section. Using the operational definition provided, identify the levels of measurement used to measure each of the variables listed in the hypotheses or research questions. From this information, you should be able to determine the measures of central tendency and variability that should be used to summarize the data. For example, you would not expect to see a mean used as a summary statistic for the nominal variable of gender; gender would probably be reported as a frequency distribution. The means and standard deviations should be provided for measurements performed

Continued

APPRAISING THE EVIDENCE—cont'd

Descriptive and Inferential Statistics

at the interval level. The sample size is another feature described in the "Methods" section that is helpful for evaluating the researcher's use of descriptive statistics. The larger the sample is, the less chance there is that one outlying score will affect the summary statistics.

If tables or graphs are used, they should agree with the information presented in the text. The tables and charts should be clearly and completely labelled. If the researcher presents grouped frequency data, the groups should be logical and mutually exclusive. The size of the interval in grouped data should not obscure the pattern of the data, nor should it create an artificial pattern. Each table and chart should be referred to in the text, but each should add to the text, not merely repeat it. Each table or graph should have an obvious connection to the study.

In reading a table such as Table 17.4, first look at the table title. The title should give an indication of the information in the table. Next, review the column headings. Do these headings follow from the title? Is each heading clear, and are any nonstandard abbreviations explained? Are the statistics contained in the table appropriate to the level of measurement used? In Table 17.4, the column headings follow from the title. Each study variable is listed, along with its mean and standard deviation. Mean and standard deviation are appropriate statistics because these data were regarded as interval-level data.

After you evaluate the descriptive statistics, evaluate the inferential statistical analysis of a research report, beginning with the hypothesis or research question. If the hypothesis or research question indicates that a relationship will be found, you should expect to find indices of correlation. If the study is experimental or quasiexperimental, the hypothesis should indicate that the author is looking for differences between the groups studied, and you would expect to find statistical tests of differences between means that test the effect of the intervention.

As you read the "Methods" section of the article, again consider the level of measurement used to measure the important variables. If the level of measurement is interval or ratio, the statistics will probably be parametric. If the variables are measured at the nominal or ordinal level, however, the statistics used should be nonparametric. Also, consider the sample size and remember that samples need to be large enough to enable the assumption of normality. If the sample is quite small—for example, 5 to 10 participants—the researcher may have violated the assumptions necessary for inferential statistics to be used (see Chapter 13). Thus, the important question is whether the researcher has provided enough justification to use the statistics presented.

Finally, consider the results as they are presented. Enough data should be presented for each hypothesis or research question for you to determine whether the researcher actually examined each one. The tables should accurately reflect the procedure performed and be in harmony with the text. For example, the text should not say that a test result reached statistical significance, but the tables show that the probability value of the test was higher than .05. If the researcher used analyses that are not discussed in this text, you may want to refer to a statistics text to decide whether the analysis was appropriate for the hypothesis or research question and the level of measurement.

You should critique two other aspects of the data analysis. The study should not read as if it were a statistical textbook. The results should be presented clearly enough that the reader can determine what was done and what the results were. In addition, the author should distinguish between the practical and the statistical significance of the evidence in relation to the findings. Some results may be statistically significant, but their practical importance may be doubtful in terms of applicability to a patient population or clinical setting. In this case, the author should note the deficiency. Alternatively, a research report may be elegantly presented, but the findings do not impress you. Such a feeling may indicate that the practical significance of the study and its findings have not been adequately explained in the report. From an evidence-informed practice perspective, a significant hypothesis or research question should contribute to improving patient care and clinical outcomes.

Note that the critical analysis of a research article's statistical analysis is not conducted in a vacuum. The adequacy of the analysis can only be judged in relation to

APPRAISING THE EVIDENCE—cont'd

Descriptive and Inferential Statistics

the other important aspects of the article: the problem, the hypotheses, the research question, the design, the data-collection methods, and the sample. If these aspects of the research process are not considered, the statistics themselves have very little meaning. Statistics can be misleading; thus, the researcher must use the appropriate statistic for the problem. For example, a researcher may use a nonparametric statistic when a parametric statistic is appropriate. Because parametric statistics are more powerful than nonparametric statistics, the result of the parametric analysis may not have been what the researcher expected. However, the nonparametric result might be in the expected direction, and so the researcher reports only that result.

CRITIQUING CRITERIA

1. Were appropriate descriptive statistics used?
2. What level of measurement is used for each major variable?
3. Is the sample size large enough to prevent one extreme score from affecting the summary statistics used?
4. What descriptive statistics are reported?
5. Were these descriptive statistics appropriate to the level of measurement for each variable?
6. Are appropriate summary statistics provided for each major variable?
7. Does the hypothesis indicate that the researcher tested for differences between groups or tested for relationships? What is the level of significance?
8. Does the level of measurement enable the use of parametric statistics?
9. Is the sample size large enough to use parametric statistics?
10. Has the researcher provided enough information for you to decide whether the appropriate statistics were used?
11. Are the statistics used appropriate for the problem, the hypothesis, the method, the sample, and the level of measurement?
12. Are the results for each of the hypotheses presented clearly and appropriately?
13. If tables and graphs are used, do they agree with the text and extend it, or do they merely repeat it?
14. Are the results clear?
15. Is a distinction made between practical significance and statistical significance? How is it made?

CRITICAL THINKING CHALLENGES

- Discuss the ways a researcher might use a computer to analyze data and present the descriptive statistical results of a study.
- What is the relationship between the level of measurement used and the choice of a statistical procedure? How is the level of measurement related to the level of evidence in the study design?
- What type of visual depiction can be used to show the use of correlations? Use examples from clinical practice to illustrate the difference between positive and negative correlations.
- A classmate states that it is ridiculous for the instructor to have students critique the descriptive statistics used in a study when none of the students has taken a statistics course. Would you agree or disagree? Defend your position.
- What assumptions are violated when a clinical research study uses a convenience sample and applies inferential statistics?
- What are the advantages and disadvantages of decreasing the alpha level for a study? What is the relationship between setting an alpha level and type I and type II errors?
- Discuss the parameters for using nonparametric statistics in a study and their effect on the usefulness of applying the evidence provided by the findings in practice.
- A research study's findings are not considered significant at the .05 level; are they deemed to provide evidence that is applicable to practice? Justify your answer.

CRITICAL JUDGEMENT QUESTIONS

1. What level of measurement would a type of nursing degree be considered?
   a. Nominal
   b. Ordinal
   c. Interval
   d. Ratio

2. In a study of nurses' willingness to care for patients choosing Medical Assistance in Dying (MAID), it was found that the greater the nurses' spirituality, the lower the willingness to provide care. Which type of correlation does this finding represent?
   a. No correlation
   b. Perfect correlation
   c. Positive correlation
   d. Negative correlation

3. Which of the following research questions may be answered through statistical hypothesis testing?
   a. What is the relationship between perceived social support and psychological adjustment to breast cancer in unmarried women?
   b. What percentage of women who smoke marijuana during pregnancy have low-birth-weight babies?
   c. What is the degree of compliance in adolescents who take oral contraceptives?
   d. What is the experience of living with AIDS?

KEY POINTS

- Descriptive statistics are a means of describing and organizing data gathered in research.
- The four levels of measurement are nominal, ordinal, interval, and ratio. Measurement at each level is performed with appropriate descriptive techniques.
- Measures of central tendency describe the average member of a sample. The mode is the score that occurs most frequently, the median is the middle score, and the mean is the arithmetical average of the scores. The mean is the most stable and useful of the measures of central tendency and, with the standard deviation, forms the basis for many inferential statistics.
- The frequency distribution is depicted in tabular or graphic form and allows calculation or observation of characteristics of the data distribution, including skewness, symmetry, modality, and kurtosis.
- In nonsymmetrical distributions, the degree and direction of the pull of the off-centre peak are described in terms of skew.
- The ranges reflect differences between high and low scores.
- The standard deviation is the most stable and most useful measure of variability. It is derived from the concept of the normal curve. In the normal curve, sample scores and the means of large numbers of samples cluster around the midpoint in the distribution, and a fixed percentage of the scores is within given distances of the mean. This tendency of means to approximate the normal curve is called the *sampling distribution of the means*. A Z score is the standard deviation converted to standard units.
- Because the sampling distribution of the means follows a normal curve, researchers are able to estimate the probability that a certain sample will have the same properties as the total population of interest. Sampling distributions provide the basis for all inferential statistics.
- Inferential statistics allow researchers to estimate population parameters and to test hypotheses about populations from sample data. The use of these statistics allows researchers to make objective decisions about the outcome of the study. Such decisions are based on the rejection or acceptance of the null hypothesis, which is that no relationship exists between the variables.
- If the null hypothesis is supported, then the findings are likely to have occurred by chance. If the null hypothesis is rejected, then a

relationship does exist between the variables and is unlikely to have occurred by chance.

- Statistical hypothesis testing is subject to two types of errors: type I and type II.
- A type I error is the researchers' incorrect decision to reject the null hypothesis.
- A type II error occurs when the results from the sample data lead to the acceptance of the null hypothesis when it is actually false; this error is also known as beta (β).
- The researcher controls the risk of making a type I error by setting the alpha level, or level of significance. Unfortunately, reducing the risk of a type I error by reducing the level of significance increases the risk of making a type II error.
- The results of statistical tests are reported to be significant or nonsignificant. For a result to be statistically significant, the probability of occurring must be less than .05 or .01, depending on the level of significance set by the researcher.
- Commonly used parametric and nonparametric statistical tests include tests for differences between means, such as the t test and ANOVA, and tests for differences in proportions, such as the chi-square test.
- Tests in which data are examined for the presence of relationships include the Pearson r, the sign test, the Wilcoxon matched-pairs test, the signed-rank test, and multiple regression.
- The most important aspect of critiquing statistical analyses is the relationship between the statistics used and the problem, design, and method used in the study. Clues to the appropriate statistical test to be used by the researcher should stem from the researcher's hypotheses. You also should determine whether all of the hypotheses have been presented in the article.
- A basic understanding of statistics will improve your ability to think about the level of evidence provided by the study design and findings and their relevance to patient outcomes for your patient population and practice setting.

🛜 FOR FURTHER STUDY

Go to Evolve at http://evolve.elsevier.com/Canada/LoBiondo/Research for the Audio Glossary.

REFERENCES

Adhikari Dahal, K., Premji, S., Patel, A. B., Williamson, T., Peng, M., & Metcalfe, A (2017). Variation in maternal co-morbidities and obstetric interventions across area-level socio-economic status: A cross-sectional study. *Paediatric Perinatal Epidemiology, 31*, 274–283. https://doi.org/10.1111/ppe.12370.

Benzies, K., Horn, S., Barker, L., Johnston, C., Berci, D., & Kurilova, J. (2019). Enhanced information package given at birth: Effects on early parenting experiences and use of educational resources and community services at age 3 Months. *Maternal and Child Health Journal,23*(3), 377–385. https://doi.org/10.1007/s10995-018-2670-3.

Bilik, Ö., Kankaya, E. A., & Deveci, Z. (2020). Effects of web-based concept mapping education on students' concept mapping and critical thinking skills: A double blind, randomized, controlled study. *Nurse Education Today, 86*, Article 104312. https://doi.org/10.1016/j.nedt.2019.104312.

Bluman, A. J. (2014). *A brief version elementary statistics: A step by step approach.* New York: McGraw-Hill.

Brown, R., Wey, H., & Foland, K. (2018). The relationship among change fatigue, resilience, and job satisfaction of hospital staff nurses. *Journal of Nursing Scholarship, 50*, 306–313. https://doi.org/10.1111/jnu.12373.

Campbell-Yeo, M., Johnston, C. C., Joseph, K. S., et al. (2015). Cobedding and recovery time after heel lance in preterm twins: Results of a randomized trial. *Pediatrics, 130*(3), 500–506.

Castonguay, A., Wrosch, C., Pila, E., & Sabiston, C. (2017). Body-related shame and guilt predict physical activity in breast cancer survivors over time. *Oncology Nursing Forum, 44*(4), 465–475. https://doi.org/10.1188/17.ONF.465-475.

Corby, K., Kane, D., & Dayus, D. (2021). Investigating predictors of prenatal breastfeeding self-efficacy. *Canadian Journal of Nursing Research, 53*(1), 56–63. https://doi.org/10.1177/0844562119888363.

Dahlke, S., Davidson, S., Duarte Wisnesky, U., Kalogirou, M. R., Salyers, V., Pollard, C., Fox, M. T., Hunter, K. F., & Baumbusch, J. (2019). Student nurses' perceptions about older people. *International*

Journal of Nursing Education Scholarship, 16(1). https://doi.org/10.1515/ijnes-2019-0051.

Doktorchik, C., Premji, S., Slater, D., Williamson, T., Tough, S., & Patten, S. (2018). Patterns of change in anxiety and depression during pregnancy predict preterm birth. *Journal of Affective Disorders, 227*, 71–78. https://doi.org/10.1016/j.jad.2017.10.001.

Ezekowitz, J. A., O'Meara, E., McDonald, M. A., et al. (2017). 2017 comprehensive update of the Canadian Cardiovascular Society guidelines for the management of heart failure. *The Canadian Journal of Cardiology, 33*(11), 1342–1433. https://doi.org/10.1016/j.cjca.2017.08.022.

Héon, M., Goulet, C., Garofalo, C., et al. (2016). An intervention to promote breast milk production in mothers of preterm infants. *Western Journal of Nursing Research, 38*(5), 529–552.

Hisel, M. E. (2019). Measuring work engagement in a multigenerational nursing workforce. *Journal of Nursing Management, 10*, 1–12. https://doi-org.ezproxy.library.yorku.ca/10.1111/jonm.12921.

Goldsworthy, S., Patterson, J. D., Dobbs, M., Afzal, A., & Deboer, S. (2019). How does simulation impact building competency and confidence in recognition and response to the adult and paediatric deteriorating patient among undergraduate nursing students? *Clinical Simulation in Nursing, 28*, 25–32. https://doi.org/10.1016/j.ecns.2018.12.001.

Havaei, F., MacPhee, M., & Susan Dahinten, V. (2016). RNs and LPNs: emotional exhaustion and intention to leave. *Journal of Nursing Management, 24*, 393–399. https://doi-org.ezproxy.library.yorku.ca/10.1111/jonm.12334.

Hroch, J., VanDenKerkhof, E. G., Sawhney, M., Sears, N., & Gedcke-Kerr, L. (2019). Knowledge and attitudes about pain management among Canadian nursing students. *Pain Management in Nursing, 20*(4), 382–389. https://doi.org/10.1016/j.pmn.2018.12.005.

Ingram, S., Babenko-Mould, Y., & Booth, R. (2016). Developing capacity to care for clients at risk for delirium and for acutely delirious clients. *Journal of Nursing Education and Practice, 6*(3). http://dx.doi.org/10.5430/jnep.v6n3p122.

Jackson, K. T., & Dennis, C. L. (2017). Lanolin for the treatment of nipple pain in breastfeeding women: a randomized controlled trial. *Maternal and Child Nutrition, 13*(3), 1–10. https://doi.org/10.1111/mcn.12357.

Kline, R. B. (2005). *Beyond significance testing: Reforming data analysis methods in behavioural research.* Washington, DC: American Psychological Association.

Lauck, S. B., Baumbusch, J., Achtem, L., et al. (2016). Factors influencing the decision of older adults to be assessed for transcatheter aortic valve implantation: An exploratory study. *European Journal of Cardiovascular Nursing, 15*(7), 486–494. https://doi.org/10.1177/1474515115612927.

Leyva-Moral, J. M., Dominguez-Cancino, K. A., Guevara-Vasquez, G. M., Edwards, J. E., & Palmieri, P. A. (2019). Faculty attitudes about caring for people living with HIV/AIDS: A comparative study. *The Journal of Nursing Education, 58*(12), 712–717. https://doi.org/10.3928/01484834-20191120-06.

Murray, M., Sundin, D., & Cope, V. (2019). New graduate nurses' clinical safety knowledge by the numbers. *Journal of Nursing Management, 27*(7), 1384–1390. https://doi.org/10.1111/jonm.12819.

Osahor, K., Woodend, K., & Mackie, J. (2019). The relationship between math personality, math anxiety, test preparation strategy and medication dose calculations in first year nursing students. *Journal of Nursing Education and Practice, 9*(8), 80. https://doi.org/10.5430/jnep.v9n8p80.

Pike, A. D., Lukewich, J., Wells, J., Kirkland, M. C., Manuel, M., & Watkins, K. (2019). Identifying indicators of National Council Licensure Examination for Registered Nurses (NCLEX-RN) success in nursing graduates in Newfoundland & Labrador. *International Journal of Nursing Education Scholarship, 16*(1). https://doi.org/10.1515/ijnes-2018-0060.

Premji, S. S., Pana, G., Currie, G., Dosani, A., Reilly, S., Young, M., Hall, M., Williamson, T., & Lodha, A. K. (2018). Mother's level of confidence in caring for her late preterm infant: A mixed method study. *Journal of Clinical Nursing, 27*(5-6), e1120–e1133.

Rajacich, D., Kane, D., Lafreniere, K., et al. (2014). Male RNs: Work factors influencing job satisfaction and intention to stay in the profession. *Canadian Journal of Nursing Research, 46*(3), 94–109.

Subedi, A., Edge, D. S., Goldie, C. L., & Sawhney, M. (2019). Resettled Bhutanese refugees in Ottawa: What coping strategies promote psychological well-being? *Canadian Journal of Nursing Research, 51*(3), 168–178. https://doi.org/10.1177/0844562119828905.

Tryphonopoulos, P. D., & Letourneau, N. (2020). Promising results from a video-feedback interaction guidance intervention for improving maternal–infant interaction quality of depressed mothers: A feasibility pilot study. *Canadian Journal of Nursing Research, 52*(2), 74–87. https://doi.org/10.1177/0844562119892769.

Winsett, R. P., Rottet, K., Schmitt, A., Wathen, E., & Wilson, D. Missed Nursing Care Collaborative Group. (2016). Medical surgical nurses describe missed nursing care tasks-Evaluating our work environment. *Applied Nursing Research, 32*, 128–133. https://doi .org/10.1016/j.apnr.2016.06.006.

Sherrard, H., Duchesne, L., Wells, G., et al. (2015). Using interactive voice response to improve disease management and compliance with acute coronary syndrome best practice guidelines: A randomized controlled trial. *Canadian Journal of Cardiovascular Nursing, 25*(1), 10–15.

CHAPTER 18

Presenting the Findings

Mina D. Singh

LEARNING OUTCOMES

After reading this chapter, you will be able to do the following:

- Discuss the difference between a study's "Results" section and the "Discussion" section.
- Identify the format of the "Results" section.
- Determine whether both statistically supported and statistically unsupported findings are discussed.
- Determine whether the results are objectively reported.
- Describe how tables and figures are used in a research report.
- List the criteria of a meaningful table.
- Identify the format and components of the "Discussion of the Results" section.
- Determine the purpose of the "Discussion" section.
- Discuss the importance of including the generalizations and limitations of a study in the report.
- Determine the purpose of including recommendations in the study report.
- Discuss how the strength, quality, and consistency of evidence provided by the findings are related to a study's limitations, generalizability, transferability, and applicability to practice.

KEY TERMS

confidence interval	generalizability	recommendations
findings	limitations	transferability

STUDY RESOURCES

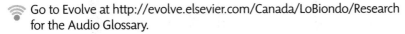 Go to Evolve at http://evolve.elsevier.com/Canada/LoBiondo/Research for the Audio Glossary.

THE ULTIMATE GOALS OF NURSING RESEARCH are to develop nursing knowledge and to promote evidence-informed nursing practice, thereby supporting the scientific basis of nursing. From the viewpoint of the research consumer, the analysis of the results, interpretations, and the conclusions that a researcher makes from a study becomes a highly important piece of the research report. After the analysis of the data, the researcher constructs an overall view of the findings, like putting the pieces of a jigsaw puzzle together to view the total picture. This process is analogous to evaluation, the last step in the nursing process. In the final sections of the report, after the statistical procedures have been applied, the statistical or numerical findings are described in relation to the theoretical framework, literature, methods, hypotheses, and problem statements. In qualitative research, after the content analyses have been concluded, the themes are discussed in relation to the literature, problem statements, and a theoretical framework, as appropriate.

The final sections of published research reports are generally titled "Results" and "Discussion," but other topics, such as limitations of findings, implications for future research and nursing practice, recommendations, and conclusions, may be addressed separately or subsumed within these sections. The format of the "Results" and "Discussion" is contingent on the stylistic considerations of the author and the journal. The function of these final sections is to depict all aspects of the research process, as well as to discuss, interpret, and identify the limitations, generalizations, and applicability relevant to the investigation, thereby furthering research-based practice.

The process that both the investigator and you as the research consumer use to assess the results of a study

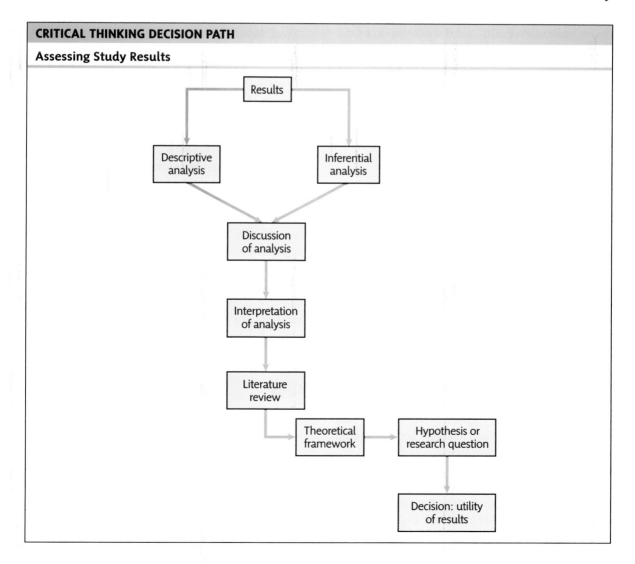

CRITICAL THINKING DECISION PATH

Assessing Study Results

is depicted in the Critical Thinking Decision Path. The goal of this chapter is to introduce the purpose and content of the final sections of a research investigation, in which the data are presented, interpreted, discussed, and generalized. An understanding of what an investigator presents in these sections will help you critically analyze the findings.

FINDINGS

The findings of a study are the results, conclusions, interpretations, recommendations, generalizations, and implications for future research and nursing practice, which are separated into two major areas: the results and the discussion of the results. The "Results" section focuses on the thematic results or statistical findings of a study, and the "Discussion" section focuses on the remaining topics. For both sections, as well as all other sections of a report, the same rule applies: The content must be presented clearly, concisely, and logically.

Evidence-Informed Practice Tip

Evidence-informed practice is an active process that requires you to consider how, and whether, research findings are applicable to your patient population and practice setting.

Presenting Quantitative Results

In the "Results" section of a research report, the researcher presents the quantitative data or numbers generated by the descriptive and inferential statistical tests or the themes from narratives generated from a content or coding analysis. The results of the data analysis are the foundation for the interpretations or "Discussion" section that follows the results. The "Results" section should then reflect the question being posed or hypothesis tested. The information from each hypothesis or research question should be presented sequentially. The tests used to analyze the data should be identified. If the author does not explicitly state the exact test that was used, then the values ob-

TABLE 18.1	
EXAMPLES OF REPORTED STATISTICAL RESULTS	
STATISTICAL TEST	**EXAMPLES OF REPORTED RESULTS**
Mean	$M = 118.28$
Standard deviation	$SD = 62.5$
Pearson correlation	$r = .39, p < .01$
Analysis of variance (ANOVA)	$F = 3.59; df = 2, 48; p < .05$
t test	$t = 2.65, p < .01$
Chi-square	$\chi^2 = 2.52, df = 1, p < .05$

df, degrees of freedom.

tained should be noted. The researcher typically provides the numerical values of the statistics and states the specific test value and probability level achieved (see Chapter 18). Examples of statistical tests and the corresponding statistical values can be found in Table 18.1. An example of a qualitative analysis with themes appears later in this chapter (see Table 18.4).

You should not be intimidated by numbers and symbols. Although these numbers are important, they are only one piece of the whole; the research process is much more important. Whether you superficially understand statistics or have an in-depth knowledge of statistics, you can expect to find the study results clearly stated. Thus, you should note the presence or absence of any statistically significant results. For the conceptual meanings of the numbers found in studies, refer to the discussion in Chapter 17.

Research Hint

In the "Results" section of a research report, the descriptive statistics are generally presented first, followed by the results of each hypothesis or research question tested.

The researcher must present the data for all of the hypotheses posed or research questions asked (e.g., whether the hypotheses were accepted or rejected, supported or not supported). If the data support the hypotheses, you might assume that the hypotheses were proven, but this is not necessarily true. It only means that the hypotheses were supported, and the results suggest that the relationships or differences tested, which were derived from the theoretical framework, were probably logical in that study's sample.

As a novice research consumer, you might also think that if a researcher's hypotheses are not supported statistically or are only partially supported, the study is irrelevant or possibly should not have been published. This is also not true. If the hypotheses are not supported, you should not expect the researcher to bury the work in a file. Reviewing and understanding unsupported hypotheses is as important for a research consumer as it is for the researcher. Information obtained from such studies can often be as useful as data obtained from supported studies.

Unsupported hypotheses can be used to suggest **limitations** (weaknesses) of particular aspects of a study's design and procedures. Data from such studies may suggest that current modes of practice or current theory in an area may not be supported by research and so should be reexamined and researched further. Data help generate new knowledge, as well as prevent knowledge stagnation.

In general, the results are interpreted in a separate section of the report. Sometimes the "Results" section contains not only the results but also the researcher's interpretations, which are more commonly found in the "Discussion" section. Integrating the results with the discussion in a report is the decision of the author or the journal editor. The two sections may be integrated when a study contains several segments that may be viewed as separate subproblems of a major overall problem.

When presenting the results, the investigator should show objectivity. The following quotation gives the appropriate way to express results:

Analysis of the effect of time was statistically significant for intensity and unpleasantness related to pain ($F = 160.395$, $p < 0.0001$).

Investigators would be accused of lacking objectivity if they stated the results as follows:

The results were not surprising, as we found a significant relationship between effect of time and intensity and unpleasantness, as we expected.

Opinions or reactionary statements to the data in the "Results" section are therefore avoided. Box 18.1 gives examples of objectively stated results.

You should consider the following points when you read a "Results" section:

- The investigators responded objectively to the results in the discussion of the results.
- In the discussion of the results, the investigators interpreted the results, with careful reflection on all aspects of the study that preceded the results.
- The data presented are summarized. Many data are generated, but only the critical summary numbers for each test are presented. Examples of summarized data are the means and standard deviations of age, education, and income. Including all data is too cumbersome. The "Results" section can be viewed as a summary.

BOX **18.1**

EXAMPLES OF OBJECTIVE STATEMENTS IN THE RESULTS SECTION

"Our findings indicate that age, education, and employment are significantly associated with Bhutanese refugee psychological well-being... younger people, aged 18 to 30 years, had better psychological well-being compared to those between 41 and 50 years (Subedi et al., 2019, p. 174)

Results suggest that most students found the [mentoring] programme either useful or very useful in easing their transition from student to new nurse. Students reported that the programme helped reduce their stress levels, gave them tools to deal with difficult situations, and increased their self-confidence as well as their motivation towards their nursing career (Lavoie-Tremblay, 2019, p. 72).

The results suggest that our sample of caregivers have moderate levels of self-reported PCC and empathy. In comparison with other studies, nurses and physicians who have participated in our study used more PCC than other groups of nurses and physicians with similar sociodemographic characteristics (Paul-Savoie et al., 2018, p. 4).

- The data are condensed both in the written text and through the use of tables and figures. Tables and figures facilitate the presentation of large amounts of data.
- Results for the descriptive and inferential statistics for each hypothesis or research question are presented. No data should be omitted even if insignificant.

In the study in Appendix B, Jackson and Dennis (2016) developed tables to present the results visually. Table 18.2 lists the demographic descriptive

<table>
<tr><td colspan="3">TABLE 18.2</td></tr>
<tr><td colspan="3">**DEMOGRAPHICS OF STUDY PARTICIPANTS**</td></tr>
<tr><td>**BASELINE CHARACTERISTICS (0–3 DAYS POSTPARTUM)**</td><td>**USUAL CARE (N = 93)**</td><td>**TREATMENT (N = 93)**</td></tr>
<tr><td>Age, mean (SD)</td><td></td><td></td></tr>
<tr><td>**Marital status**
Married/common-law
Single</td><td></td><td></td></tr>
<tr><td>**Ethnicity**
Caucasian
Non-caucasian</td><td></td><td></td></tr>
<tr><td>**Education**
Elementary
High school
College
University</td><td></td><td></td></tr>
<tr><td>**Annual household income**[a]
<$39,999
$40,000–99,999
>$100,000</td><td></td><td></td></tr>
<tr><td>**Breastfeeding level**
Exclusive
Almost exclusive
High
Partial</td><td></td><td></td></tr>
<tr><td>NRS, *mean* (SD)</td><td></td><td></td></tr>
<tr><td>SF-MPQ total, mean (SD)</td><td></td><td></td></tr>
<tr><td>BSES-SF, mean (SD)</td><td></td><td></td></tr>
</table>

[a]Participants did not wish to disclose their annual income (usual care group, *n* = 8; treatment group, *n* = 5). NRS, Numerical Rating Scale; SF-MPQ, Short-Form McGill Pain Questionnaire; BSES-SF, Breastfeeding Self-Efficacy Scale, Short Form.
Jackson, K. T., & Dennis, C. L. (2017). Lanolin for the treatment of nipple pain in breastfeeding women: a randomized controlled trial. *Maternal and Child Nutrition, 13*(3), 1–10. https://doi.org/10.1111/mcn.12357.

results about the study's participants; Table 18.3 lists the statistics of the variables measured in the study. Tables allow researchers to provide a more visually thorough explanation and discussion of the results. If tables and figures are used, they must be concise. Although the text is the major mode of communicating the results, the tables and figures serve a supplementary but independent role. The role of tables and figures is to report results with details that the investigator does not enter into the text. This does not mean that the content of tables and figures should not be mentioned in the text. The amount of detail that the author uses in the text to describe the specific tabular data varies with the needs of the researcher.

A good table meets the following criteria:
- It supplements and economizes the text.
- It has precise titles and headings.
- It does not repeat the text.

Table 18.4 is an example of a table that meets these criteria. This table, which is from the article by Benbow and associates (2019b), lists the study's themes from women who were homeless. Visualizing the findings of a study is easier if a table clearly summarizes the results, as this table does. Description of each messaging theme's preferences would have taken a lot of space, and the results would have been difficult to visualize. The table developed by the researchers allows you to not only visualize the concepts quickly but also assess the results.

Research Hint

A well-written "Results" section is systematic, logical, concise, and drawn from all of the analyzed data. All that is written in the "Results" section should be geared toward letting the data reflect the testing of the problems and hypotheses. The length of this section depends on the scope and breadth of the analysis.

Evidence-Informed Practice Tip

As you reflect on the results of a study, think about how the results fit with previous research on the topic and the strength and quality of available evidence on which to base clinical practice decisions.

BREASTFEEDING EXCLUSIVITY					
TIME	**INFANT FEEDING CATEGORY**	**USUAL CARE**	**TREATMENT**	**X² (DF)**	**P**
		(n = 84) N (%)	(n = 78) N (%)		
4 weeks postpartum	Exclusive or almost exclusive High or partial Token or bottle-feeding	52(61.9) 12 (14.3) 20 (23.8)	51(63.0) 18 (22.2) 12 (14.8)	3.2(2)	0.2
		Usual care	Treatment		
		n(%)	ᵃn(%)		
12 weeks postpartum	Exclusive or almost exclusive High or partial Token or bottle-feeding	42 (50.0) 11 (13.1) 31 (36.9)	43 (55.1) 13 (16.7) 22 (28.2)	1.5 (2)	

ᵃn = 81.

Jackson, K. T., & Dennis, C. L. (2017). Lanolin for the treatment of nipple pain in breastfeeding women: a randomized controlled trial. *Maternal and Child Nutrition, 13*(3), 1–10. https://doi.org/10.1111/mcn.12357.

THEMES RELATING TO HOMELESSNESS	
THEMES	**SUPPORTING QUOTES**
Until you hit rock bottom, there's no support	...it's unfortunate that it has to get to the point where you have to go to a shelter, instead of having a support system up before that...i did call a shelter..."we can't really do much for you unless you come in here"... If women have a place to go, a safe place to talk to somebody for that hour, they would probably make healthy choices before it got to the point where they had to come here [shelter].
It's just not enough: insufficient support	Anything is better than nothing and it beats having to sell yourself on the streets, but i need more money for Food and shelter...ask any mom on ow, food is an issue. We don't have enough money. I have to ask my mom to bring me food, but i'm still left without.
Help comes with a price: support with surveillance	...A couple of times we were in the shelter and [child protection services] was called and we weren't doing anything...they come to a person who has like two or three kids...and they are going to apprehend their kids, and i just think,...you have no clue what it is like to have to raise a child, and to go through struggles every day...how dare you look down your nose at me...from mothers who are so trying.
Every shelter is so different	Many mothers noticed a difference in how they were treated within and across various agencies, indicating how the autonomy and treatment of clients varied from agency to agency.

Benbow, S., Forchuk, C., & Gorlick, C., & Berman, H., & Ward-Griffin, C. (2019b). "Until you hit rock bottom there's no support": Contradictory sources and systems of support for mothers experiencing homelessness in southwestern Ontario. *Canadian Journal of Nursing Research, 51*(3), 179–190. https://doi.org/10.1177/0844562119840910.

Discussion of the Results

In the final section of the report, the investigator interprets and discusses the results of the study. In the discussion, a skilled researcher makes the data "come alive." The researcher interprets and gives meaning to the numbers in quantitative studies or the concepts in qualitative studies. You may ask how the investigator extracted the meaning that is applied in this section. If the researcher reports properly, the discussion will refer to the beginning of the study, in which a problem statement was identified and independent and dependent variables were related on the basis of a theoretical framework (see Chapter 2) and literature review (see Chapter 5). In this section, the researcher discusses the following:

- The supported and the nonsupported hypotheses
- The limitations, or weaknesses, of a study in view of the design and the sample or data-collection procedures
- How the theoretical framework was supported
- Additional or previously unrealized relationships suggested by the data

Even if the hypotheses are supported, the reviewer should not believe the conclusions to be the final word. Statistical significance is not the endpoint of a researcher's thinking, and low p values may not be indicative of research breakthroughs. Thus, statistical significance in a research study does not always mean that the results of a study are clinically significant. As the body of nursing research grows, so does the profession's ability to critically analyze beyond the test of significance and assess a research study's applicability to practice. Chapter 21 reviews methods for analyzing the usefulness of research findings. Within the nursing literature, discussion of clinical significance and evidence-informed practice has also emerged (Melnyk & Fineout-Overholt, 2018).

As indicated throughout this text, many important pieces in the research puzzle must fit together for a study to be evaluated as a well-done project. Therefore, researchers and reviewers should accept statistical significance with prudence. Statistically significant findings are not the sole means of establishing the study's merit. Remember that accepting statistical significance only means acceptance that the sample mean is the same as the population mean, which may not be true (see Chapter 18).

When the results do not statistically support the hypothesis, the researcher refers to the theoretical framework and analyzes the earlier thinking process. The results of nonsupported hypotheses do not require that the investigator find fault with each piece of the project. Such a course can become an overdone process. All research has weaknesses. This analysis is an attempt to identify the weaknesses and to suggest the possible or actual problems in the study. At times, the theoretical thinking is correct, but the researcher finds problems or limitations that could be attributed to the tools (see Chapter 16), the sampling methods (see Chapter 12), the design (see Chapters 11 and 12), or the analysis (see Chapters 17 and 18). Therefore, when the hypotheses are not supported, the investigator attempts to find facts rather than fault. The purpose of the discussion, then, is not to show humility or one's technical competence, but rather to enable reviewers to judge the validity of the interpretations drawn from the data and the general worth of the study.

In the "Discussion" section, the researcher summarizes all the aspects of the study and refers to the beginning to assess whether the findings support, extend, or counter the theoretical framework of the study. From this point, you can begin to think about clinical relevance, the need for replication, or the germination of an idea for further research study. Finally, you should find the results discussion either in a separate section or subsumed within the "Discussion" section, and it should include generalizability, applicability, and recommendations for future research, as well as a summary or a conclusion.

Generalizability is the extent to which data can be inferred to be representative of similar phenomena in a population beyond the study's sample. Reviewers of research are cautioned not to generalize beyond the population on which a study is based. Rarely, if ever, can one study be a recommendation for action. Beware of research studies that may overgeneralize. An example of making a sweeping generalization is concluding that all patients waiting for cardiac bypass surgery can benefit from preoperative teaching and support when the study sample consisted of only White men, 50 to 70 years of age. Attention must be paid to the "Limitations" section of an article to note what the researchers have considered to affect the generalizability of their study findings. Generalizations that draw conclusions and make inferences within a particular situation and at a particular time are appropriate.

An example of an appropriate generalization is from the study conducted by Coker et al. (2017), on the observations of oral hygiene care interventions provided by nurses to hospitalized older people. They concluded that the "the findings of this study cannot be generalized because the participants comprised a convenience sample of nurses from five hospitals in the same city" (p. 20). This type of statement is important for reviewers of research. It helps guide thinking in terms of a study's clinical relevance and suggests areas for further research (see Chapter 21).

In a mixed methods study, Dosani et al. (2017) indicated that "the findings of our study should be interpreted with caution given the limitations of our sample. Firstly, we used a convenience sample, therefore it is unclear how representative our quantitative descriptive data is of the general population of mother with LPIs [late preterm infants]. Secondly, our results likely do not reflect the experiences of less educated mothers or minority women. Finally, this study was limited to women who could read, write, and speak English fluently and therefore may impact the generalizability of our study findings" (p. 8).

Presenting Qualitative Results

Transferability is the extent to which findings from one qualitative research study have meaning in other studies with similar situations. Authors must note the issues of a qualitative study to prevent a sweeping transferability of findings, which would lead to misinterpretations of the results. In an example of how the limitations in a qualitative study can affect transferability,

Gauthier, Cossette, Ouimette, et al. (2016) conducted a study to pilot an intervention plan to support shared decision making when considering a vascular assist device for patients with advanced heart failure. The researchers noted multiple limitations of the study and that these may affect the transferability of findings. The study included only one cardiac centre. Also, only a few caregivers and patients were included in the study. Lastly, all the study participants were White. One study does not provide all of the answers, nor should it. The final steps of evaluation are critical links to the refinement of practice and the generation of future research. Evaluation of research, like evaluation of the nursing process, is not the last link in the chain but a connection between findings that may serve to improve nursing theory and nursing practice.

In another example regarding transferability, Dunwoody and colleagues (2018) conducted a qualitative study to explore the common meanings and shared practices of sedation assessment in the context of managing patients with an opioid. The researchers noted that an important limitation was that the geographical setting was limited to Ontario, a Canadian setting. They further stated that the knowledge gained "is not generalizable but may be transferable to other areas of nursing once explored as hermeutic methods dictate" (p. 113).

 Research Hint _____

It has been said that a good study is one that raises more questions than it answers. Thus, you should not view a study's limitations, generalizations, and implications of the findings for practice as an investigator's lack of research skills but as the beginning of the next step in the research process.

The final topic that the investigator integrates into the "Discussion" section is the recommendations. The recommendations are the investigator's suggestions for the study's application to practice, theory, and further research. These

BOX 18.2

EXAMPLES OF RESEARCH RECOMMENDATIONS AND PRACTICE IMPLICATIONS

RESEARCH RECOMMENDATIONS

- Other issues requiring further exploration include duration of video-feedback sessions, frequency of video-feedback sessions, optimal timing of the intervention (e.g., infant age in which intervention is likely to be most or least effective), the usefulness of longitudinal evaluation that may over time produce improvements in mothers' mental health as well as improvements in maternal–infant interaction (Woodgate et al., 2020, p. 10).
- "Studies with rigorous methodologies are needed to more fully understand how students are socialized as nurses and to determine how to enhance professionalism and prevent and intervene effectively in all forms of academic incivility. For instance, an ethnographic study could be conducted to understand the teaching–learning culture, including faculty role modeling, within current-day nursing education programs; and a grounded theory study could be conducted to understand how nursing students are taught nursing theories and philosophies that define what nursing is and how it ought to be practiced and the resultant impact of such teaching on students' demeanor" (Small et al., 2019, p. 142).
- "We particularly recommend prospective studies to examine the impact of supportive interventions to (a) enhance competence in a palliative approach, (b) enable identification of patients who would benefit from a palliative approach, (c) promote understanding of the benefits of a palliative approach, and (d) enhance workplace environments with the goal of improving care of people who have life-limiting illnesses" (Sawatzky et al., 2019, p. 12).
  "As none of the study participants in either community had children living in the home, this study could be replicated with a more diverse female population (e.g., young women and/or mothers with young children) that also includes the perspective of other under-represented groups (e.g., members of First Nations, Mennonite, Hutterite, newcomer refugee, and immigrant populations) to enrich knowledge and insights into the impacts of curling on rural women's health across various populations and life stages" (Scruby et al., 2019, p. 242).

PRACTICE IMPLICATIONS

"Few studies specifically focus on the body-related self-conscious emotional experiences of women who have recently been treated for breast cancer. Consequently, healthcare professionals may not be sensitive to the specific experience of body-related emotions in patients with cancer. In practice, healthcare professionals need to consider how emotions related to the body can affect health behaviours and associated mental and physical health" (Castonquay et al., 2016, p. 473).

- "In addition to licensed nurses, these study findings also point to the added benefit of the nurse practitioner role in LTC. For example, Site 1 provided an example that illustrated how they were able to keep a resident in LTC by using an external nurse practitioner to help "upskill" staff when needed in a timely manner, thereby allowing the resident to die "at home" (Kaasalainen et al., 2019, p. 703).
  "Nurse educators are increasing the amount of virtual experiences and distance learning in curriculum. These results provide a strong case for an immediate self-debrief after a virtual simulation experience to consolidate students learning, followed by a group debrief to deepen and extend knowledge" (Verkuyl et al., 2019, p. 37).
  "Findings from this study suggest the importance of assessing patients' receptiveness to telehealth and the factors influencing this receptiveness...Familiarizing older adults with telehealth care through opportunities to discuss its advantages/disadvantages, learn about others' experiences in using it, and to observe a telehealth encounter may enhance receptiveness" (Rush et al., 2019, p. 144).
  "Nurses are in unique positions to challenge existing systems of surveillance and promote access to safety and safe spaces for mothers experiencing homelessness. Nurses can begin this process by being aware of and sensitive to the complexity of social exclusion that shapes mothers' lives, as well as their experiences of discrimination and stigma from health and social professionals" (Benbow et al., 2019a, p. 209).

suggestions require the investigator to reflect on the question "What contribution to nursing does this study make?" Box 18.2 provides examples of recommendations for future research and implications for nursing practice. This evaluation places the study in the realm of what is known and what needs to be known before being used. Nursing has grown tremendously over the last century through the efforts of many nursing researchers and scholars.

APPRAISING THE EVIDENCE

Results and Discussion

The results and the discussion of the results are the researcher's opportunity to examine the logic of the hypothesis or question posed, the theoretical framework, the methods, and the analysis (see the Critiquing Criteria box). This final section requires as much logic, conciseness, and specificity as employed in the preceding steps of the research process.

For quantitative studies, the research consumer should be able to identify statements on the type of analysis that was used and whether the data statistically supported the hypothesis. These statements should be straightforward and not reflect bias. Auxiliary data or serendipitous findings also may be presented. If such auxiliary findings are presented, they should be stated as dispassionately as were the hypothesis data. The statistical test used also should be noted, as well as the numerical value of the data (see Tables 18.1, and 18.3). The presentation of the tests, the numerical values found, and the statements of support or nonsupport should be clear, concise, and systematically reported. For illustrative purposes that facilitate readability, the researchers should present extensive findings in tables rather than in the text.

For qualitative studies, the richness of the data should be described. The consumer must also have sufficient detail about the analysis, the coding, the categories of coding or themes, and the level of coding agreement.

The "Discussion" section should interpret the data, gaps, limitations, and conclusions of the study, as well as provide recommendations for further research. Drawing these aspects into the study should give the research consumer an understanding of the relationship between the findings and the theoretical framework. Statements reflecting the underlying theory are necessary, whether or not the hypotheses were supported.

If the findings were not supported, the consumer should—as the researcher did—attempt to identify, without fault finding, possible methodological problems. Finally, a concise presentation of the study's generalizability and the implications of the findings for practice and research should be evident. The last presentation can help the research consumer begin to rethink clinical practice, provoke discussion in clinical settings (see Chapter 21), and find similar studies that may support or refute the phenomena being studied to more fully understand the problem.

CRITIQUING CRITERIA

1. Are the results of each hypothesis presented?
2. Is the information regarding the results concisely and sequentially presented?
3. Are the tests that were used to analyze the data presented?
4. Are the results presented objectively?
5. If tables or figures are used, do they meet the following standards?
   - They supplement and economize the text.
   - They have precise titles and headings.
   - They do not repeat the text.
6. Are the results interpreted in light of the hypotheses and theoretical framework and all of the other steps that preceded the results?
7. If the data are supported, does the investigator provide a discussion of how the theoretical framework was supported?
8. If the data are not supported, does the investigator attempt to identify the study's weaknesses and strengths, as well as suggest possible solutions for the research area?
9. Does the researcher discuss the study's clinical relevance?
10. Are any generalizations made, and, if so, are they within the scope of the findings or beyond the findings?
11. Are any recommendations for future research stated or implied?
12. What is the study's strength of evidence?

CRITICAL THINKING CHALLENGES

■ Defend or refute the following statement: "All results should be reported and interpreted whether or not they support the hypothesis (hypotheses)."

■ What type of knowledge does the researcher draw on to interpret the results of a study?

■ What new knowledge is contributed from the research findings? Are they clinically significant and do they have practice implications?

■ Do you agree or disagree with the statement that a good study raises more questions than it answers? Support your view with examples.

■ How is it possible for readers of research to critique the findings and recommendations of a reported study? How could you use the Internet for critiquing the findings of a study?

■ Now that nursing students and nurses have access to reports of clinical problems (i.e., critiques of multiple studies available on a clinical topic) or critiques of individual studies of a clinical topic published in *Evidence-Based Nursing*, as well as published meta-analyses and meta-syntheses on clinical topics, why is it necessary for them to read and critique research studies on their own? Justify your response.

CRITICAL JUDGEMENT QUESTIONS

1. A researcher conducts a qualitative study that examines the lived experience of those being diagnosed with breast cancer. A reader critiquing the report would expect to find that the report:

   a. Presents the data in the form of narrative text
   b. Provides a detailed statistical analysis of study results
   c. Details independent and dependent variables
   d. Describes how the data related to tumour growth was analyzed

2. Which information is appropriate to exclude from the discussion section of a research publication?

   a. Detailed data presented in tables and figures
   b. The summary of the study's descriptive data
   c. Any results that were not statistically supported
   d. Inferential statistics for each hypothesis presented

3. Which research result is reported in an objective manner in the results section of a study?

   a. Surprisingly, the results showed a positive relationship between marital conflict and psychological adjustment in women with a childhood history of abuse
   b. A distressing result was found indicating a positive relationship between maternal smoking and respiratory distress in neonates
   c. The results indicated a positive relationship between death anxiety and adherence to medication regimens in gay men with HIV/AIDS
   d. Interestingly, a positive relationship was found between relapse to unsafe sex behaviors and an increase in teenage pregnancy

KEY POINTS

• The analysis of the findings is the final step of a research investigation. In this section, the research consumer will find the results presented in a straightforward manner.
• All results should be reported whether or not they support the hypothesis. Tables and figures may be used to illustrate and condense data for presentation.
• Once the results are reported, the researcher interprets the results. In this presentation, usually titled "Discussion," the consumer should be able to identify the key topics being discussed. The key topics, which include an interpretation of the results, are the limitations, generalizations, implications, and recommendations for future research.
• The researcher draws together the theoretical framework and makes interpretations based on the findings and theory in the section on the interpretation of the results. Both statistically supported and unsupported results

should be interpreted. If the results are not supported, the researcher should discuss the results reflecting on the theory, as well as possible problems with the methods, procedures, design, and analysis.

- The researcher should present the limitations or weaknesses of the study. This presentation is important because it affects the study's generalizability. The generalizations or inferences about similar findings in other samples also are presented in light of the findings.
- The research consumer should be alert for sweeping claims or overgeneralizations that a researcher may state. An overextension of the data can alert the consumer to possible researcher bias.
- The recommendations provide the consumer with suggestions regarding the study's application to practice, theory, and future research. These recommendations furnish the reader with a final perspective of the utility of the investigation's findings in practice.

📶 FOR FURTHER STUDY

Go to Evolve at http://evolve.elsevier.com/Canada/ LoBiondo/Research for the Audio Glossary.

REFERENCES

Benbow, S., Forchuk, C., Berman, H., Gorlick, C., & Ward-Griffin, C. (2019a). Spaces of exclusion: Safety, stigma, and surveillance of mothers experiencing homelessness. *Canadian Journal of Nursing Research, 51*(3), 202–213. https://doi .org/10.1177/0844562119859138.

Benbow, S., Forchuk, C., Gorlick, C., Berman, H., & Ward-Griffin, C. (2019b). "Until you hit rock bottom there's no support": Contradictory sources and systems of support for mothers experiencing homelessness in southwestern Ontario. *Canadian Journal of Nursing Research, 51*(3), 179–190. https://doi .org/10.1177/0844562119840910.

Castonquay, A., Wrosch, C., Pila, E., & Sabiston, C. (2017). Body-related shame and guilt predict physical activity in breast cancer survivors over time. *Oncology Nursing Forum, 44*(4), 465–475.

Coker, E., Ploeg, J., Kaasalainen, S., & Carter, N. (2017). Observations of oral hygiene care interventions provided by nurses to hospitalized older people. *Geriatric Nursing, 8*(1), 17–21. https://doi .org/10.1016/j.gerinurse.2016.06.018.

Dosani, A., Hemraj, J., Premji, S. S., Currie, G., Reilly, S. M., Lodha, A. K., Young, M., & Hall, M. (2017). Breastfeeding the late preterm infant: experiences of mothers and perceptions of public health nurses. *International Breastfeeding Journal, 12*, 23. https://doi .org/10.1186/s13006-017-0114-0.

Dunwoody, D. R., Jungquist, C. R., Chang, Y-P., & Dickerson, S. S. (2018). The common meanings and shared practices of sedation assessment in the context of managing patients with an opioid: A phenomenological study. *Journal of Clinical Nursing, 28*, 104–115. https://doi.org/10.1111/jocn.14672.

Gauthier, M. A., Cossette, S., Ouimette, M. F., & Harris, V. (2016). Intervention for advanced heart failure patients and their caregivers to support shared decision-making about implantation of a ventricular assist device. *Canadian Journal of Cardiovascular Nursing = Journal canadien en soins infirmiers cardio-vasculaires, 26*(2), 4–9.

Kaasalainen, S., Sussman, T., Durepos, P., McCleary, L., Ploeg, J., Thompson, G., & Team, SPA-LTC (2019). What are staff perceptions about their current use of emergency departments for long-term care residents at end of life? *Clinical Nursing Research, 28*(6), 692–707. https://doi.org/10.1177/1054773817749125.

Lavoie-Tremblay, M., Sanzone, L., Primeau, G., & Lavigne, G. L. (2019). Group mentorship programme for graduating nursing students to facilitate their transition: A pilot study. *Journal of Nursing Management, 27*(1), 66–74. https://doi.org/10.1111/jonm.12649.

Melnyk, B. M., & Fineout-Overholt, E. (2018). *Evidence-based practice in nursing and healthcare: A guide to best practice.* Philadelphia: Lippincott, Williams & Wilkins.

Paul-Savoie, E., Bourgault, P., Potvin, S., Gosselin, E., & Lafrenaye, S. (2018). The impact of pain invisibility on patient-centered care and empathetic attitude in chronic pain management. *Pain Research & Management, 2018*, 6375713. https://doi .org/10.1155/2018/6375713.

Rush, K. L., Hatt, L., Gorman, N., Janicki, L., Polasek, P., & Shay, M. (2019). Planning telehealth for older adults with atrial fibrillation in rural communities: Understanding stakeholder perspectives. *Clinical Nursing Research, 28*(2), 130–149. https://doi .org/10.1177/1054773818758170.

Sawatzky, R., Roberts, D., Russell, L., Bitschy, A., Ho, S., Desbiens, F-F., Chan, E. K. H., Tayler, C., & Stajduhar, K. (2019). Self-perceived competence of nurses and care aides providing a palliative approach in home, hospital, and residential care settings: A cross-sectional survey. *Canadian Journal of Nursing Research, 53*(1), 64–77. https://doi .org/10.1177/0844562119881043.

Scruby, L. S., Rona, H. A., Leipert, B. D., Mair, H. L., & Snow, W. M. (2019). Exploring social support, sport participation and rural women's health using Photovoice: The Manitoba Experience. *Canadian Journal of Nursing Research, 51*(4), 233–244. https:// doi.org/10.1177/0844562119832395.

Small, S. P., English, D., Moran, G., Grainger, P., & Cashin, G. (2019). "Mutual respect would be a good starting point:" Students' perspectives on incivility in nursing education. *Canadian Journal of*

Nursing Research, 51(3), 133–144. https://doi .org/10.1177/0844562118821573.

Subedi, A., Edge, D. S., Goldie, C. L., & Sawhney, M. (2019). Resettled Bhutanese refugees in Ottawa: What coping strategies promote psychological well-being? *Canadian Journal of Nursing Research, 51*(3), 168–178. https://doi.org/10.1177/0844562119828905.

Verkuyl, M., Hughes, M., Atack, L., McCulloch, T., Lapum, J., Romaniuk, D., & St-Amant, O. (2019). Comparison of self-debriefing alone or in combination with group debrief. *Clinical Simulation in Nursing, 37*, 32–39. https://doi.org/10.1016 /j.ecns.2019.08.005.

Woodgate, R. L., Tailor, K., Tennent, P., Wener, P., & Altman, G. (2020). The experience of the self in Canadian youth living with anxiety: A qualitative study. *PLoS ONE, 15*(1), e0228193. https://doi .org/10.1371/journal.pone.0228193.

Critiquing Research

RESEARCH **VIGNETTE**
Rural and Remote Nursing Research

Martha MacLeod

- Rural and remote nursing is complex, challenging, yet fulfilling. Nurses in rural areas depict their practice as "we're it" and describe themselves as "multi-specialist generalists."
- "Growing your own" nurses rather than recruiting nurses from outside rural and remote communities can be a highly successful strategy to retain nurses.
- Although incentives such as loan forgiveness help attract nurses to rural and remote communities, a myriad of other factors, including becoming engaged in the life of the community, along with having opportunities for advanced practice and career development, are useful in retaining nurses.
- Rural and remote nurses develop finely tuned skills in creating and sustaining effective working relationships in small communities where nurses and patients' relationships intersect in many places, as neighbours, fellow community members, and clients. These relationships give nurses unique insights into community needs.

When I began my nursing career in the 1970s, the voices of rural and remote nurses were seldom heard at policy and planning tables. Over the years, by participating in and drawing on research, rural and remote nurses' voices are increasingly heard, in advocating for changes in practice and policy, and in making a real difference in their communities.

My first insights about the difference research can make came as an undergraduate research assistant on a community health attitude survey in a rural Indigenous community. I was curious to learn how I could engage in research, and what this summer student experience on a research team could teach me. I lived and worked in the rural community and was immersed in the realities of conducting research with Indigenous people. I worked with community members to shape the study to fit with what was actually important to the people. The results from that study helped the community to establish a Community Health Centre. This experience laid the foundation of my collaborative, community-based, partnered approach and taught me how to listen and be responsive, rather than to impose an outside agenda.

In 1994, I undertook my first study of rural nursing practice, the *"We're It"* study. This qualitative (hermeneutic phenomenological) study articulated what rural nurses did in their everyday work. The study started when I asked a nurse manager at a 12-bed hospital, 220 km from the larger community, what was her most pressing issue. She said that it was really hard to communicate the realities of rural nursing, so that she could obtain the resources needed to support the nurses. I interviewed and shadowed 24 nurses in three small hospitals as they went about their work on all shifts and then analyzed and interpreted the findings with the nurses themselves. We were able to depict the complexity of rural nursing and convey what practice was like when they were the only staff present in the hospital and how they provided care that in urban settings would be handled by others. In one example, an urban intensive care nurse recommended the rural nurse call the respiratory therapist to help in an emergency, to which the rural nurse responded, "We *are* the respiratory therapist." This study gave nurses the opportunity to share what was important in their practice, as well as to identify changes that were needed to improve care for patients. As a result (MacLeod, 1999), two hospitals implemented clinical leader positions, rural nurses started to use the phrase "we're it" to communicate their practice, and the phrase was highlighted in a community nursing textbook.

In 2000, provincial and national policy makers said they needed information about the rural and remote nursing workforce to better plan for and support those nurses. *The Nature of Nursing Practice in Rural and Remote Canada (RRNI)* study (MacLeod et al., 2004) included a survey of 3933 registered nurses (RNs) and nurse practitioners (NPs) from all provinces and territories, in-depth interviews with 150 RNs, an analysis of documents, and an analysis of the Canadian Institute for Health Information (CIHI) Registered Nurses Database. In 2014, the *Nursing Practice in Rural and Remote Canada (RRNII)* study (MacLeod et al., 2017) surveyed 3822 regulated nurses (RNs, NPs, licensed or registered practical nurses, and registered psychiatric nurses) in all provinces and territories, updated the documentary analysis, and analyzed the CIHI Nurses Database. Both studies have had enduring provincial and national impacts. The *RRNI* study highlighted the importance and complexity of rural nursing, as well as the pressing need for rural nursing education. It resulted in the Rural Nursing Certificate Program, which continues at the University of Northern British Columbia. The findings have informed provincial and national recruitment and retention efforts.

Research has impacted direct nursing practice. Public health nurses in northern BC identified that a really challenging part of their practice was that they did not know whether their work with vulnerable families was actually making a difference for the families. Through interviews with nurses and families and shadowing of public health nurses in the *Working Relationship* study, we articulated how public health nurses were able to establish and maintain relationships that worked for both families and nurses (Moules et al., 2010). Through reflecting on the findings, the nurses implemented their practice differently and wove this information into orientations for new public health nurses. Several nurses received focused training in family interviewing, which prepared them to gather data for the study, and also extended their skills in working with vulnerable families.

Students were important research team members in each of these studies and fulfilled a variety of roles, including assisting with data collection, data analysis, and conducting guided research studies for graduate degrees. Seven students in the *We're It*, *RRNI,* and *Working Relationship* studies went on to become nursing faculty and continue to be engaged in research. Students across Canada have used the study results in their own research on rural nursing.

Research may seem to be a really long way away from caring for people, but it is not. When research arises from practice, directly addresses issues that really matter to clients and nurses, and is undertaken jointly by researchers and nurses, with the findings taken to workplaces and policy tables, change does happen. Nurses who take up research findings in practice are able to provide evidence-informed care. In undertaking rural research, I have learned:

- You can engage in research as a nursing student. You can learn about the realities of research and how you can use research in your practice.
- Relevant, responsive research begins with listening and focusing on what is important to nurses themselves.
- Rural and remote practice is often underappreciated and taken for granted. Nursing research helps to bring it out of the shadows and give nurses a way to advocate for themselves and their communities. ■

REFERENCES

See https://www.unbc.ca/rural-nursing for *RRNI* and *RRNII* publications.

MacLeod, M. (1999). "We're it": Issues and realities in rural nursing practice. In W. Ramp, J. Kulig, I. Townshend, & V. McGowan (Eds.), *Health in rural settings: Contexts for action* (pp. 165–178). Lethbridge, AB: University of Lethbridge Press.

MacLeod, M. L. P., Kulig, J. C., Stewart, N. J., Pitblado, J. R., & Knock, M. (2004). The nature of nursing practice in rural and remote Canada. *Canadian Nurse, 100*(6), 27–31.

MacLeod, M. L. P., Stewart, N. J., Kulig, J. C., Anguish., P., Andrews, M. E., Banner, D., Garraway, L., Hanlon, N., Karunanayake, C., Kilpatrick, K., Koren, I., Kosteniuk, J., Martin-Misener, R., Mix, N., Moffitt, P., Olynick, J., Penz, K., Sluggett, L., Van Pelt, L., Wilson, E., & Zimmer, L (2017). Nurses who work in rural and remote communities in Canada: A national survey. *Human Resources for Health, 15*(34). https://doi.org/10.1186/s12960-017-0209-0.

Moules, N. J., MacLeod, M. L. P., Hanlon, N., & Thirsk, L. (2010). "And then you'll see her in the grocery store": The working relationships of public health nurses and high priority families in rural and northern Canadian communities. *Journal of Pediatric Nursing, 25*, 327–334. https://doi.org/10.1016/j.pedn.2008.12.003.

CHAPTER 19

Critiquing Qualitative Research

Lorraine Thirsk

LEARNING OUTCOMES

After reading this chapter, you will be able to do the following:

- Identify the criteria for critiquing a qualitative research report.
- Evaluate the strengths and weaknesses of a qualitative research report.
- Describe the applicability of the findings of a qualitative research report.
- Construct a critique of a qualitative research report.

KEY TERMS

auditability	phenomena	transparency
credibility	reliability	trustworthiness
fittingness	rigour	
goodness	theoretical sampling	

STUDY RESOURCES

 Go to Evolve at http://evolve.elsevier.com/Canada/LoBiondo/Research
for the Audio Glossary.

THE RESEARCH USED TO SUPPORT EVIDENCE-INFORMED practice must be of good quality. Because the expansion in nursing research and related interventions affects increasing numbers of patients, the evaluation of this research is crucial to improving patients' outcomes.

The focus of this chapter is on assessing the quality of qualitative research studies. This chapter draws on content you have learned in previous chapters and provides two examples of critical appraisal. Nurses must fully understand how to assess the value of qualitative research, particularly in view of the requirement that nursing practice be evidence informed. Knowing that an article is peer-reviewed is insufficient to determine the application of the knowledge to nursing practice.

The essence of the successful critiquing of a research paper lies in achieving a balanced appraisal. The reader needs to look for the merits and demerits of the methods used as well as the applicability to the health care setting. A balanced appraisal also requires a degree of logic and objectivity in identifying the systematic course of enquiry which underpins the research. The ultimate aim of any critique undertaken by nurses is to consider the applicability to practice (Ingham-Broomfield, 2008, p. 103).

As a framework for understanding the appraisal of qualitative research as a basis for evidence-informed practice, a published research report, as well as critiquing criteria, are presented. The criteria are then used to demonstrate the process of appraising a qualitative research report.

STYLISTIC CONSIDERATIONS

Because the purpose of qualitative research is to describe, explore, or explain concepts and phenomena, the report is generally written in a narrative way that allows the researcher to convey the complexity of the phenomena being studied. One of the most common ways to convey the findings of qualitative research is to use quotations that reflect the participant's explanations of a phenomenon or topic. For this reason, the qualitative research report has a more conversational tone than a quantitative report. In addition, data are frequently articulated in concepts or phrases, which the researcher calls *themes* (see Chapter 9), as a way of describing large quantities of data in a condensed format.

The richness of the narrative provided in a qualitative research study cannot be shared in its entirety in a journal publication. Page requirements imposed by journals frequently limit the length of research reports. Despite this constraint, investigators in qualitative research need to illustrate the richness of the data and convey to the audience the relationship between the data collected and the analysis or findings. This is essential in order to document the rigour, or trustworthiness, of a qualitative research study. Conveying the entirety of the findings of a qualitative study is challenging in a published research report.

Guidelines for publication of research reports are generally listed in each nursing journal or are available from the journal editor. The primary goal of journal editors is to provide their readers with high-quality, informative, timely, and interesting articles. To meet this goal, regardless of the type of research report, editors prefer to publish manuscripts that have scientific merit, present new knowledge, support the current state of the science, and engage their readers. As stated earlier, the challenge in qualitative research is to meet these editorial requirements within the page limit imposed by the journal of interest.

Nursing journals may offer guidelines for evaluating qualitative and quantitative research reports, as discussed in Chapter 3. For example, the *International Journal of Nursing Studies* (IJNS), the journal where our first example article was published, encourages authors to use the Consolidated Criteria for Reporting Qualitative Research (COREQ; see Tong et al., 2007) checklist when submitting an article (IJNS, 2020). Often, peer reviewers are also encouraged to use this checklist in their review of the article. These checklists help to promote consistency in reporting of research but do not always capture quality of the research or significance of the contribution to nursing knowledge. Thus, importantly, the editors try to ensure that reviewers are knowledgeable in the method and subject matter of the study. This determination, however, is often based on the reviewer's self-identified area of interest. Research reports are often evaluated in accordance with the ideas or philosophical viewpoints held by the reviewer. The reviewer may have strong feelings about particular types of qualitative or quantitative research methods. Therefore, it is important to clearly state the qualitative approach used and, if appropriate, its philosophical base. When reading research, it is important to keep these perspectives and incentives in mind.

The principles for evaluating different qualitative research approaches are very similar fundamentally. While assessing the quality of research is important, there remains much debate in the literature about standards for assessing quality in qualitative research (Williams et al., 2020). Box 19.1 provides general guidelines

CRITIQUING GUIDELINES FOR QUALITATIVE RESEARCH

STATEMENT OF THE PHENOMENON OF INTEREST (CHAPTER 4)

1. What is the phenomenon of interest, and is it clearly stated for the reader?
2. What is the justification for using a qualitative method?
3. What are the philosophical underpinnings of the research method?

AUTHORS

1. What are the designations and roles of the authors? Are they credible people to do this research?
2. Do the authors position themselves in relation to the research and the participants? Do we know the background and potential influences or biases of the authors?

PURPOSE (CHAPTER 4)

1. What is the purpose of the study? Is it clearly stated and consistent throughout?
2. What is the projected significance of the work for nursing?

ETHICS (CHAPTER 6)

1. Is the protection of human subjects addressed?
2. Do the authors report procedures consistent with ethical principles of research?

METHOD (CHAPTER 9)

1. Is the method used to collect the data compatible with the purpose of the research?
2. Is the method adequate for addressing the phenomenon of interest?
3. If a particular approach is used to guide the inquiry, does the researcher complete the study according to the processes described? Is there methodological coherence?
4. Was this the most appropriate method to answer the research question?

SAMPLING (CHAPTER 13)

1. What type of sampling is used? Is it appropriate for the particular method?
2. Are the participants who were chosen appropriate for informing the research? Who might have been overlooked or excluded?

DATA COLLECTION (CHAPTERS 8, 9, AND 13)

1. Are the data to be collected focused on human experience?
2. Does the researcher describe the data-collection strategies (e.g., interview, observation, field notes)?
3. What are the procedures for collecting the data?
4. Is saturation of the data described?

DATA ANALYSIS (CHAPTERS 16)

1. What strategies are used to analyze the data?
2. Has the researcher reported the data truthfully?
3. Does the researcher describe the steps used for the data analysis?
4. Does the analysis move beyond the topics used in the interviews and offer further interpretation, conceptual framework or theory?

RIGOUR/TRUSTWORTHINESS (CHAPTER 15)

1. Do the researchers discuss how they promoted rigour, validity, or trustworthiness?

Credibility
- Do the participants recognize the experience as their own?
- Has adequate time been allowed to fully understand the phenomenon?
- Do the researchers offer a compelling explanation for their findings?

BOX 19.1

CRITIQUING GUIDELINES FOR QUALITATIVE RESEARCH—*cont'd*

Auditability
- Can the reader follow the researcher's thinking?
- Does the researcher document the research process?
- Are analytical decisions discussed with a team or peers and documented?

Fittingness
- Are the findings applicable outside of the study situation?
- Are the results meaningful to individuals not involved in the research?
- Is the strategy used for analysis compatible with the purpose of the study?

FINDINGS (CHAPTERS 8 AND 18)
1. Are the findings presented within a context?
2. Is the reader able to apprehend the essence of the experience from the report of the findings?
3. Do the researcher's conceptualizations accurately reflect the data?
4. Does the researcher place the report in the context of what is already known about the phenomenon? Was the existing literature on the topic related to the findings?

CONCLUSION, IMPLICATIONS, AND RECOMMENDATIONS (CHAPTER 18)
1. Do the conclusions, implications, and recommendations give the reader a context in which to use the findings?
2. Do the conclusions reflect the study findings?
3. What are the recommendations for future study? Do they reflect the findings?
4. How has the researcher made explicit the significance of the study for nursing theory, research, or practice?

for evaluating qualitative research. Figure 19.1 provides a common checklist that researchers, reviewers, and editors use to assess how the qualitative research was reported. The Joanna Briggs Institute in Australia, a research and development organization, lists a number of critical appraisal tools on its website, http://joannabriggs.org/research/critical-appraisal-tools.html, including a *Checklist for Qualitative Research*, useful for critiquing research articles. Other assessment tools to help in assessing research articles are available from the Critical Appraisal Skills Program (2020) at https://casp-uk.net/casp-tools-checklists/.

APPLICATION OF QUALITATIVE RESEARCH FINDINGS IN PRACTICE

As already stated, one of the purposes of qualitative research is to describe, understand, or explain phenomena. It is useful to add knowledge where quantitative approaches cannot, to understand patient perspectives and experiences, and

explain things that are puzzling (Thorne, 2020). In addition to clarifying phenomena, qualitative research can give voice to people who have been disenfranchised and whose experiences would have otherwise not been documented (Barbour & Barbour, 2003; Schepner-Hughes, 1992). Keeping the different purposes, or aims, of qualitative research in mind is necessary as you read research and think about how it might be applicable to your practice. Qualitative research will not tell you whether one treatment or intervention was more effective than another, but it may help you to understand some of the considerations for using the intervention with a specific population. If an intervention is not effective, qualitative research can help to explore why it was not effective or sustainable (Moore et al., 2015). Qualitative research may also help you to understand how other people experience a common health concern and attune you to the variety of experiences that patients may have (Thorne, 2020). It may also highlight issues that have been

COREQ (COnsolidated criteria for REporting Qualitative research) Checklist

A checklist of items that should be included in reports of qualitative research. You must report the page number in your manuscript where you consider each of the items listed in this checklist. If you have not included this information, either revise your manuscript accordingly before submitting or note N/A.

Topic	Item No.	Guide Questions/Description	Reported on Page No.
Domain 1: Research team and reflexivity			
Personal characteristics			
Interviewer/facilitator	1	Which author/s conducted the interview or focus group?	
Credentials	2	What were the researcher's credentials? E.g. PhD, MD	
Occupation	3	What was their occupation at the time of the study?	
Gender	4	Was the researcher male or female?	
Experience and training	5	What experience or training did the researcher have?	
Relationship with participants			
Relationship established	6	Was a relationship established prior to study commencement?	
Participant knowledge of the interviewer	7	What did the participants know about the researcher? e.g. personal goals, reasons for doing the research	
Interviewer characteristics	8	What characteristics were reported about the inter viewer/facilitator? e.g. Bias, assumptions, reasons and interests in the research topic	
Domain 2: S tudy design			
Theoretical framework			
Methodological orientation and Theory	9	What methodological orientation was stated to underpin the study? e.g. grounded theory, discourse analysis, ethnography, phenomenology, content analysis	
Participant selection			
Sampling	10	How were participants selected? e.g. purposive, convenience, consecutive, snowball	
Method of approach	11	How were participants approached? e.g. face-to-face, telephone, mail, email	
Sample size	12	How many participants were in the study?	
Non-participation	13	How many people refused to participate or dropped out? Reasons?	
Setting			
Setting of data collection	14	Where was the data collected? e.g. home, clinic, workplace	
Presence of non-participants	15	Was anyone else present besides the participants and researchers?	
Description of sample	16	What are the important characteristics of the sample? e.g. demographic data, date	
Data collection			
Interview guide	17	Were questions, prompts, guides provided by the authors? Was it pilot tested?	
Repeat interviews	18	Were repeat inter views carried out? If yes, how many?	
Audio/visual recording	19	Did the research use audio or visual recording to collect the data?	
Field notes	20	Were field notes made during and/or after the inter view or focus group?	
Duration	21	What was the duration of the inter views or focus group?	
Data saturation	22	Was data saturation discussed?	
Transcripts returned	23	Were transcripts returned to participants for comment and/or	

FIG. 19.1   COREQ Guidelines for reporting qualitative research.

Source: Tong, A., Sainsbury, P., & Craig, J. (2007). Consolidated criteria for reporting qualitative research (COREQ): A 32-item checklist for inter-views and focus groups. *International Journal for Quality in Healthcare, 19*(6), 349–357. https://doi.org/10.1093/intqhc/mzmo42.

Topic	Item No.	Guide Questions/Description	Reported on Page No.
		correction?	
Domain 3: analysis and findings			
Data analysis			
Number of data coders	24	How many data coders coded the data?	
Description of the coding tree	25	Did authors provide a description of the coding tree?	
Derivation of themes	26	Were themes identified in advance or derived from the data?	
Software	27	What software, if applicable, was used to manage the data?	
Participant checking	28	Did participants provide feedback on the findings?	
Reporting			
Quotations presented	29	Were participant quotations presented to illustrate the themes/findings? Was each quotation identified? e.g. participant number	
Data and findings consistent	30	Was there consistency between the data presented and the findings?	
Clarity of major themes	31	Were major themes clearly presented in the findings?	
Clarity of minor themes	32	Is there a description of diverse cases or discussion of minor themes?	

Developed from: Tong A, Sainsbury P, Craig J. Consolidated criteria for reporting qualitative research (COREQ): a 32-item checklist for interviews and focus groups. *International Journal for Quality in Health Care.* 2007. Volume 19, Number 6: pp. 349–357

Once you have completed this checklist, please save a copy and upload it as part of your submission. DO NOT include this checklist as part of the main manuscript document. It must be uploaded as a separate file.

FIG. 19.1 *cont'd*

previously overlooked or misunderstood. The second article by Robinson et al. (2020) is an example of using qualitative research to develop an intervention.

Another use of qualitative research is to initiate examination of important concepts in nursing practice, education, or administration. Stahlke Wall and Rawson (2016) used an interpretive description approach to understand the role of NPs in cancer care, including how NPs added value to patient care and how their role could be better supported. A qualitative approach to this question allowed for an in-depth exploration of the NP role in a specific clinical setting. Interpretive description is a qualitative method that has the specific aim of creating useful knowledge that is applicable to nursing practice (Thorne, 2008). Stahlke Wall and Rawson uncovered that there is still a lack of clarity in the NP role and that traditional professional hierarchies still seem to be impeding the success

of NPs in cancer care. The knowledge generated from this research would be useful for health care leaders and decision-makers when considering implementing and supporting NPs. Even though a different practice area may have different experiences, the authors found other studies, across many settings, to be very consistent with their findings (Stahlke Wall & Rawson, 2016). This study adds to the body of knowledge on NP role and health workforce by sensitizing leaders to possible issues.

Evidence-Informed Practice Tip _____

Qualitative research studies can be used to guide practice when they are applied within a context. The nurse should ask the following question: "Does this study provide me with a direction for caring for a particular patient group?" Keep in mind that nurse researchers examine topics related to clinical practice, but also leadership, education, administration, policy, and social processes and systems.

Finally, qualitative research can be used to discover information about phenomena of interest that can lead to instrument development. Usually, qualitative methods are used to direct the development of structured research instruments as part of a larger empirical research project. Instrument development from qualitative research studies is useful to practising nurses because it is grounded in the reality of human experience with a particular phenomenon. For example, after an initial qualitative exploration of the phenomenon, the researcher may develop a survey to collect the data related to specific variables.

CRITIQUE 1

The study "Mobilising evidence to improve nursing practice: A qualitative study of leadership roles and processes in four countries" by Harvey et al. (2019) is critiqued here. The narrative of the article is presented in its entirety and is followed by the critique on pp. 440–442.

Mobilising Evidence to Improve Nursing Practice: A Qualitative Study of Leadership Roles and Processes in Four Countries

Gill Harvey[a,*], Wendy Gifford[b], Greta Cummings[c], Janet Kelly[a], Roman Kislov[d], Alison Kitson[e], Lena Pettersson[f], Lars Wallin[g,h], Paul Wilson[d], Anna Ehrenberg[f]

ABSTRACT

BACKGROUND: The approach and style of leaders is known to be an important factor influencing the translation of research evidence into nursing practice. However, questions remain as to what types of roles are most effective and the specific mechanisms through which influence is achieved.

OBJECTIVES: The aim of the study was to enhance understanding of the mechanisms by which key nursing roles lead the implementation of evidence-based practice across different care settings and countries and the contextual factors that influence them.

DESIGN: The study employed a qualitative descriptive approach.

SETTINGS: Data collection was undertaken in acute care and primary/community health care settings in Australia, Canada, England and Sweden.

PARTICIPANTS: 55 individuals representing different levels of the nursing leadership structure (executive to frontline), roles (managers and facilitators), sectors (acute and primary/community) and countries.

METHODS: Individual semi-structured interviews were conducted with all participants exploring their roles and experiences of leading evidence-based practice. Data were analysed through a process of qualitative content analysis.

RESULTS: Different countries had varying structural arrangements and roles to support evidence-based nursing practice. At a cross-country level, three main themes were identified relating to different mechanisms for enacting evidence-based practice, contextual influences at a policy, organisational and service delivery level and challenges of leading evidence-based practice.

CONCLUSIONS: National policies around quality and performance shape priorities for evidence-based practice, which in

Harvey, G., Gifford, W., Cummings, G., Kelly, J., Kislov, R., Kitson, A., … & Ehrenberg, A. (2019). Mobilising evidence to improve nursing practice: A qualitative study of leadership roles and processes in four countries. *International journal of nursing studies*, *90*, 21–30. https://doi.org/10.1016/j.ijnurstu.2018.09.017

[a]Adelaide Nursing School, University of Adelaide, Australia
[b]School of Nursing, University of Ottawa, Canada
[c]Faculty of Nursing, University of Alberta, Canada
[d]Alliance Manchester Business School, University of Manchester, UK
[e]College of Nursing and Health Sciences, Flinders University, Adelaide, Australia
[f]School of Education, Health, and Social Studies, Dalarna University, Falun, Sweden
[g]Department of Neurobiology, Care Sciences and Society, Karolinska Institutet, Stockholm, Sweden
[h]Department of Health and Care Sciences, The Sahlgrenska Academy, University of Gothenburg, Sweden
*Corresponding author at: Adelaide Nursing School, University of Adelaide, Adelaide Health and Medical Sciences Building, North Terrace, Adelaide SA5005, Australia. E-mail address: gillian.harvey@adelaide.edu.au (G. Harvey).

turn influences the roles and mechanisms for implementation that are given prominence. There is a need to maintain a balance between the mechanisms of managing and monitoring performance and facilitating critical questioning and reflection in and on practice. This requires a careful blending of managerial and facilitative leadership. The findings have implications for theory, practice, education and research relating to implementation and evidence-based practice.

What is already known about the topic?
- Nursing leadership is an important factor influencing the implementation of evidence-based practice (EBP).
- Previous research has demonstrated that both formal and informal leaders – those with and without managerial responsibility- have a role to play in leading and enabling the delivery of EBP.
- Less is known about the specific types or combination of roles that are most effective or the mechanisms though which influence is achieved.

What this paper adds
- The national policy and regulatory environment influences the interpretation and operationalisation of EBP.
- Leadership for EBP is not role-specific; it requires a dynamic network which encompasses the range of skills required to optimise EBP.
- Insight into the mechanisms needed to enact EBP, ranging from managing and monitoring to facilitative, relationship-focused approaches, and the importance of achieving the right balance.

ARTICLE INFO

Article history:
Received 18 June 2018
Received in revised form 28 September 2018
Accepted 28 September 2018

KEYWORDS: Evidence-based practice, Facilitation, Knowledge translation, Implementation, Leadership, Managers, Facilitators

1 INTRODUCTION

Despite significant investments in health research within high-income countries, international evidence demonstrates that the implementation of research findings into improved practice, patient care and population health is often slow, incomplete and inconsistent (Schuster et al., 1998; Grol, 2001; Runciman et al., 2012). Reasons for this are multi-faceted and there is growing recognition that the traditional 'pipeline' model from knowledge production to implementation over-simplifies the complexities involved (Kitson et al., 2017; Braithwaite et al., 2018). As such, there is increased attention focused on how best to achieve implementation of research evidence in the most effective, efficient and timely ways possible. This links to broader debates about the concept of evidence-based practice (EBP) and how it has been interpreted since its initial iteration in the mid-1990s (Sackett et al., 1996). Critics have argued a need for a paradigm shift to prevent over-simplistic and overtly rational approaches to generating and applying evidence to inform clinical practice and patient care (Greenhalgh et al., 2014). In the context of this paper, we are particularly focusing on the implementation of EBP, which we define as the structures, roles and processes used to support the translation of evidence derived from multiple sources (research; clinical and patient experience; national, regional and local information) into nursing practice.

The challenges of implementing evidence into practice are of particular significance in nursing, given that it represents the largest professional workforce in healthcare. However, nursing and healthcare systems more generally are experiencing a time of significant change due to a combination of economic pressures, demographic shifts, technological advancement, problems with recruitment and retention, and changing public and political expectations. This is apparent across national and international health systems and presents an additional challenge in terms of delivering high quality, evidence-based care (Bodenheimer and Fernandez, 2005; Cosgrove et al., 2013; Cummings et al., 2008; Rudman et al., 2012). Furthermore, considerable variations exist within and across different countries in terms of how nursing is led, organised and managed at a strategic, organisational and operational level (Aiken et al., 2017).

Research into implementation highlights different factors that can influence whether and how research evidence is used in practice. These include factors relating to the evidence itself (for example, the extent to which research results are accepted or contested), the intended users of the evidence (for example, how motivated and capable nurses are to take on a practice change) and the context in which implementation is taking place (Kitson et al., 1998; Damschroder et al., 2009). The approach and style of leaders, both individually and collectively, can influence and potentially modify these factors. Leadership is known to be an important determinant of culture, which itself is a key characteristic of the context that shapes implementation and translation (McCormack et al., 2002; Gifford et al., 2014).

Several studies have examined the relationship between leadership and evidence implementation (Cummings et al., 2018). Aarons and colleagues developed a measure of unit level leadership for implementation that identifies four types of required leadership activity, termed proactive, knowledgeable, supportive and perseverant leadership (Aarons et al., 2014). The Ottawa Model of Implementation Leadership (O-MILe) presents a theoretical model for developing implementation leadership, focused around three categories of leadership behaviours, defined as relations, change and task oriented (Gifford et al., 2017). However, questions remain as to who is best placed to provide the type of leadership required to enhance implementation of evidence-based practice (EBP). For example, should leadership for EBP be provided by individuals with formal management authority or by people in roles with a specific remit for supporting implementation, education or practice development? Or is it a shared, collective responsibility within organisations? And how does the practice environment directly or indirectly impact what the assumed leaders do?

Some literature suggests that middle managers – those who supervise front-line employees, but are themselves supervised by senior managers – have an important, but as yet overlooked, role in implementing EBP (Birken et al., 2012). However, empirical studies testing interventions to build management capacity for implementing EBP have produced mixed results (Gifford et al., 2013; Tistad et al., 2016), linked to a view that the nurse manager's role in EBP is under-articulated, largely passive and limited by competing demands (Wilkinson et al., 2011) or that nurse managers lack the knowledge and skills needed to effectively support EBP (Gunning-berg et al., 2010; Ehrenberg et al., 2016).

Other studies have focused on individuals in designated roles for implementation-related activity (Harvey et al., 2002). A variety of different terms are used to describe these roles, which typically do not encompass formal management responsibility and can be broadly grouped together as 'facilitation'. Cranley and colleagues recently undertook a scoping review of facilitation roles and characteristics and identified nine types of roles, including opinion leaders, coaches, champions, knowledge brokers and clinical/practice facilitators. The different roles were seen to vary in terms of level of formality, position (internal or external to the organisation), main activities undertaken and key attributes and skills required (Cranley et al., 2017). Berta and colleagues (Berta et al., 2015) suggest that the mechanism through which facilitation influences implementation is one of building learning capacity, through stimulating higher-order (double and triple-loop) adaptive learning about how to apply research evidence to improve care processes. This is achieved through establishing internal and external meta-routines (selective processes) that empower front-line staff to change practice by identifying problems and seeking and applying appropriate solutions; by contrast, single-loop learning is more standardised and focuses on technical approaches to fix problems (Argyris and Schon, 1996).

Evidence on the effectiveness of facilitation as an implementation strategy is mixed. Studies in primary care and community settings that were not specifically focused on nursing practice, suggest evidence of impact, for example, in terms of improving the uptake of clinical guidelines in general practice (Baskerville et al., 2012) and significantly reducing neonatal mortality (Persson et al., 2013). By contrast, a cross-European study employing facilitation as an intervention to improve uptake of continence guideline recommendations in nursing home care showed no significant differences between intervention and control wards (Seers et al., 2018). This same study highlighted the importance of the relationship between facilitators and managers, the latter acting as key gatekeepers in terms of influencing whether and how effectively the facilitator could perform their intended role (van der Zijpp et al., 2016).

In summary, existing evidence provides a compelling case for the contribution of human agency – in the form of various leadership roles and processes – to enhance the implementation of evidence into practice. Managers and facilitators clearly have a potentially important contribution in terms of providing leader- ship for EBP. However, evidence of effectiveness is mixed and inconclusive. Questions remain as to what types of roles or combinations of roles are the most effective and through which mechanisms influence on practice is achieved. Context is recognized to be an important mediating factor in implementing EBP (Cummings et al., 2007), a fact that needs to be taken account of when considering roles, strategies and processes to enhance EBP. To date, studies of context have focused on the micro and meso levels of care whereas contextual factors at a macro level remain largely under-researched (Fitzgerald et al., 2002). Exploring these issues is key to developing capacity for delivering and supporting EBP. Moreover, knowledge about how to effectively leverage new and existing roles to implement EBP is transferable to support innovation and change more generally, an important requirement in the fast-changing environment of modern day healthcare. These questions form the backdrop of the study reported here.

1.1 Objectives

The primary objective of the study was to enhance understanding of the mechanisms by which key nursing roles lead the implementation of EBP across different care settings and countries and the contextual factors that influence them. In order to achieve this objective, the following research questions guided this study:

i   What roles do executive and clinical/frontline level leaders (managers and facilitators) play in supporting the implementation of EBP?
ii How are different roles enacted to promote and support implementation?
iii What contextual factors influence implementation roles and processes?

[Note: throughout the paper, we use the term 'leadership' to encompass managerial and facilitative roles]

2 METHODS

The study used a qualitative descriptive approach (Colorafi and Evans, 2016) based on individual interviews with identified nursing leaders, in managerial and facilitative roles, across healthcare settings in four countries. We opted for this as the most appropriate methodology as the aim was to develop a rich description of the phenomenon under study, namely leadership of EBP across four different countries.

2.1 Setting

Data collection was undertaken in acute care and primary/community health care settings in Australia, Canada, England and Sweden. These countries are comparable in broad terms of level of development (high-income countries), tax-based universal health care systems and national structures or systems for monitoring and/or regulating performance. Within each country, one or two organisations were selected using a combination of convenience and purposive sampling. From a convenience perspective, organisations were selected that were geographically close to the research team members responsible for data collection. Subsequently, the main criterion then used to select organisations was a self-declared commitment of the organisation's nursing leadership to EBP, including granting access to the research team to interview a range of staff involved in implementation (Table 19C1.1). Research team members in each country approached identified organisations directly with an invitation to participate in the research.

2.2 Sample Selection

The total study sample comprised 55 individuals who were purposefully recruited to represent different levels of the nursing structure (from executive to frontline), roles (managers and facilitators), sectors (acute and primary/community care) and countries. Most, but not all of the interviewees had a nursing qualification. Inclusion was based on the following criteria: those in managerial roles had a clearly defined responsibility for managing nurses and nursing care; facilitators were involved in providing and supporting education and practice development

for nursing staff. Initial contact was made with nursing executive leaders in each of the participating sites and these individuals were asked to make suggestions of other key people to contact within their organisation. These individuals were subsequently sent an email invitation with supporting information about the study. The majority of individuals approached agreed to participate; one person only (English sample) declined.

The breakdown of the sample by level, role and sector is detailed in Table 19C1.2. Participants were evenly spread across acute and primary/community care settings, in order to cover various healthcare contexts.

2.3 Procedure and Data Collection

Data collection took place between September 2015 and April 2016. After informed consent from the participants, semi-structured interviews were conducted. Interviews were carried out by a member of the research team (or a research assistant working with the research team member) in their own country (Australia: GH and JK;

TABLE **19C1.1**

CHARACTERISTICS OF THE STUDY SITES BY COUNTRY

	AUSTRALIA	CANADA	ENGLAND	SWEDEN
Organisations involved in the study	1 organisation providing acute care (2 hospitals) and primary and community care	2 organisations: • Western Canada; Province-wide provider of acute care (total of 106* hospitals) and community care • Eastern Canada; A publicly funded home care service provider *2 of the 106 hospitals were included in the study sample	1 integrated organisation providing acute care (1 hospital) and primary and community care	2 organisations: • County-wide provider of acute care (4 hospitals) and primary care • Municipality-wide provider of community care
National standards and/or accreditation of evidence-based practice	Australian Commission on Safety and Quality in Health Care	Accreditation Canada	The Care Quality Commission and National Institute for Care Excellence (NICE)	National Board of Health and Welfare

TABLE **19C1.2**

THE RESEARCH SAMPLE BY COUNTRY, LEVEL AND ROLE

	AUSTRALIA	CANADA	ENGLAND	SWEDEN	TOTAL
Executive/senior manager	1	6	2	2	11
Clinical/frontline manager	3	2	3	7	15
Executive/senior facilitator	2	1	3	4	10
Clinical/frontline facilitator	8	5	1	2	16
Hybrid (e.g. manager- facilitator)	-	-	3	-	3
Total	14	14	12	15	55

Canada: WG and a research assistant working with GC; England: RK and PW; Sweden: LP). All interviewers were working in academic positions (for example, Professors or senior researchers), were experienced in qualitative interviewing methods and employed a standard interview guide specific to the role of the participant, i.e. executive/senior manager, clinical/front-line manager or facilitator. Three separate study specific interview guides were developed for data collection, informed by a literature review and input from local stakeholder groups. The questions were related to these overall areas: Clarification of role and position in the organisation; Knowledge and decision-making; Experiences of EBP; Own role in EBP. Back translation was undertaken to verify congruence between the English and Swedish versions of the interview guide (Peterson, 2009).

Interviews were conducted on an individual basis, and mostly face-to-face at the workplace, although some took place by telephone (at the request of the interviewee). The interviews were conducted in English or Swedish and were typically 30–60 min duration. All interviews were digitally audio-recorded and transcribed verbatim; additional field notes were not routinely collected. Interviewees were offered the opportunity to have their transcription returned for verification purposes, although the majority did not accept this offer.

2.4 Data Analysis

Interview data were analysed by qualitative content analysis (Sandelowski, 2000) using QSR NVivo 10/11© software. This was initially undertaken at an individual country level by relevant members of the research team (3 each in Australia and Sweden; 2 in Canada and England). The analysis was guided by the research questions and participant responses to each question were grouped to form the unit of analysis. An iterative process was used to descriptively summarise the data involving: deductive coding of relevant passages using the words of participants; organising and grouping recurring ideas into response categories; inductively re-coding and condensing response categories to identify patterns, regularities and descriptive themes (Sandelowski, 2000). Throughout the analysis, preliminary codes and themes were discussed within the research team and reviewed for internal homogeneity (i.e. themes were consistent and fit together) and external heterogeneity (i.e. clear distinctions between each theme) and revised based on group discussion and further analysis. Cross-checking of transcripts occurred to enhance the trustworthiness of analysis, for example, by members of one country team analysing interview data from another country.

The majority of the research team were academics working in the field of knowledge translation and implementation science, with both theoretical and practical knowledge of the research topic. Regular project team meetings were organised to share insights and reflections on the data, in an open and critically constructive way. Analytical discussions took place via monthly Skype meetings. Additionally, three face-to-face meetings, each held over two days, took place at key points during study design, data analysis and interpretation of findings. Categories and themes were compared, initially at a country level and then at a cross-country level in order to find similarities and differences across different groups (i.e. managers and facilitators) and different settings (i.e. acute and primary/community care). In two countries (Australia and Sweden), feedback to local stakeholder groups was undertaken to sense-check and verify the emerging findings.

3 FINDINGS

At an organisational level, the different sites where data collection took place had varying structural arrangements and roles to support EBP, as evidenced by feedback from the senior managers interviewed and publicly available policy documents. These are summarised in Table 19C1.3.

Comparing findings at a cross-country level, three main themes emerged:

- Different mechanisms for EBP: Managing and monitoring versus connecting and enabling;
- Roles shaped by context: policy, organisational and service delivery level;
- Challenges of leading EBP.

In the presentation of the findings, direct quotes from interviewees are denoted according to country, role and setting: Country codes: A-Australia; CE-Canada East; CW-Canada West; E-England; S-Sweden; Roles: E-Executive/senior level manager; EF-Executive/senior level facilitator; M-Frontline manager; F-Front-line facilitator (numbers are used to differentiate interviewees in the same role); Setting: A-Acute; C-Community; A/C-Acute and Community

3.1 Different Mechanisms for EBP: Managing and Monitoring versus Connecting and Enabling

The data demonstrate two contrasting mechanisms by which nursing leaders sought to embed EBP, one more formalised and concerned with meeting expected performance standards, the other more enabling and relationship focused. Managers tended to emphasise the performance and monitoring aspects of their role, whilst facilitators highlighted a relationship-based approach, although overlaps between the two were apparent. Managers typically described their role in terms of providing direction, acting as role models, monitoring compliance against standards or guidelines, and maintaining overall oversight of evidence-based practice. At an executive level, this encompassed the provision of strategic leadership and high-level visionary direction, establishing an infrastructure and processes to enable and support EBP and collaborating with other relevant organisations and institutions at a local, regional and national level.

> I think from a nursing and midwifery point of view . . . . the concept of research and evidence based practice, ...is vitally important, one for the patients but also for the promotion and the organisation or stature within the broader health community. For me, I would think it was quite strategic . . . . . I knew I wanted an increased research profile . . . . So I think that in trying to raise the profile of research what you then do is you get people thinking about evidence based practice. [A-E-A/C]

At a clinical/unit level, the manager's role had a more operational focus and involved collecting and collating evidence to create policies, procedures and protocols, disseminating information to staff, undertaking audit and feedback to make sure that standards were followed and maintaining and supporting the professional development of staff. A manager working in the community described their role in governing quality and standards:

> We would go out with certain members of staff, we would go visiting patients, we do our documentation audit, we can check our home care assessment tools,

TABLE 19C1.3

STRUCTURES AND ROLES TO SUPPORT EBP AT AN ORGANISATIONAL LEVEL, BY COUNTRY

	AUSTRALIA	CANADA	ENGLAND	SWEDEN
Main structure/s leading and supporting evidence-based nursing practice	Centralized education function, underpinned by a commitment to Practice Development Participation in the Best Practice Spotlight Organisation (BPSO) Program (a Canadian initiative led by the Registered Nurses' Association of Ontario and involving partnership with international sites)	Acute care organisation Provincial level Knowledge Management Department, responsible for making evidence accessible and providing education to staff Community care organisation Virtual Resource Centre for online resources & advice Participation in BPSO Program	Centralized Quality Improvement Department coordinating multiple Quality Improvement Collaboratives Locally developed Nursing Assessment and Accreditation system, aiming to create sustainability of QI initiatives	Acute care organisation Central service units for EBP, providing QI support to department and unit managers Community care organisation Central resources for EBP
Roles	2 types of ward/unit (frontline) roles: • Nurse unit manager, operational focus; 'gatekeeper' role • Clinical practice consulant, clinical/educational focus Some evidence of role hybridity Nurse educators working from a central department with a (clinical) specialist focus	Acute care organisation Service level roles; Nurse Practitioners, Clinical Nurse Specialists, Clinical Nurse Educators, Clinical Implementation Managers, working with front-line staff to facilitate EBP Community care organisation Direct and indirect roles to support implementation; Advanced Practice Consultants, Clinical Improvement Coaches and Clinical Practice Resources Nurses	Acute and community focused roles with responsibility for coordinating the nursing accreditation system Front-line nurse managers with a strong patient safety and quality focus Hybrid roles – clinical specialist with some operational management responsibility – acting as a clinical expert for front-line staff	Acute care organisation Managers responsible for providing data to national quality registers Local facilitators working with front-line staff to implement EBP Community care organisation Relatively few facilitator roles to support local staff

our risk assessment tools . . . . And so there's a really robust structure in place regarding us monitoring who's working within the policies and procedures. [E-M5-C]

The nurse manager role was seen as a pivotal 'gatekeeper' in EBP that could act as either an enabler or an obstructer, as illustrated by the reflections of an executive nursing leader:

I think a lot of it has to do with the . . . . person who runs the ward, unit or service. To me, I think they're actually the most important people in the organisation, so to me they're the gatekeepers of the clinical care, the culture and how people conduct themselves . . . . Often I think the block's with the [nurse unit manager], not necessarily with the staff underneath. [A-EF1-A/C]

In contrast to the more direct strategic and operational influence of managers, facilitators tended to describe their role as supporting implementation through providing education and coaching, increasing staff awareness of evidence and EBP, enabling skills and capacity development amongst the nursing staff, addressing barriers to implementation and acting as a coordinator. This relied on 'softer' mechanisms, such as working alongside staff, having conversations and building communication networks

> It is about getting staff into this way of thinking. It should not go too fast. You need to be out there. I work a lot from here, in my office. What feels meaningful and valuable is to get out in practice and be there. And really translate evidence directly into everyday practice, so it becomes natural, and they understand what you are talking about. [S-F2-C]

The need for complementarity between roles was noted, particularly in the Canadian sites, which had a long history of creating structures and systems to support EBP. Here, managers recognised the importance of their role in terms of setting the tone, identifying priorities and advocating for resources, yet at the same time trusting and supporting others in terms of how to achieve the desired outcomes:

> I think all of us have our own, our roles . . . they should be complementary at the very least. . . . Dedicated facilitators, I just step aside and let them carry on 'cause that's what we hired them to do. And I appreciate the support. [CW-E1-C]

In a few instances, individuals exhibited roles that could be described as hybrid as they combined elements of both managerial and facilitative responsibility. This was particularly the case in the English sample where some nurse consultants also had formal management responsibility for more junior staff, which is not typically the case for nurse consultant roles. There were also examples where participants described enacting their role in away that melded aspects of facilitative and managerial leadership, as illustrated in this quote from a community-based nurse consultant in Australia:

> . . . the [middle] level role is that perfect balance between the management side and still really being on a practical level and being able to be engaged with my staff and encouraging them to do it as well. [A-F2-C]

3.2 Roles Shaped by Context: Policy, Organisational and Service Delivery Levels

Contextual influences on roles and processes supporting EBP were apparent at a policy, organisational and service level. Depending on the country, policy influences functioned mostly at a country (Australia and England) or a regional/provincial level (Sweden and Canada). In Australia and England, where there was a strong regulatory environment, an emphasis on national standards was apparent, accompanied by mandatory monitoring and accreditation systems. The influence of such formal regulatory arrangements on the interpretation and implementation of EBP was evident in the accounts of interviewees:

> . . . . I think there is a strong adherence to procedures and policies and following the national standards . . . . that sort of evidence is embedded into practice but the nurse or the midwife may not necessarily recognize that that's what they're doing . . . [A-EF2- A/C]

By contrast, in the less regulated systems in Sweden and Canada, external performance management appeared to be less of a concern or have a direct influence on EBP. For example, in Sweden, respondents talked about providing data to national quality registers but this was not the dominant narrative in their accounts of leading or supporting EBP in nursing

> . . . . we do quality assessments and audits according to the quality criteria the Board has set up. We also work on behalf of the MAS [medically responsible nurse] to follow up, for example, deviations and investigate more serious deviations. Through such work we can get feedback through data in the quality registers to be able to ensure that we are actually doing what we have decided to do. [S-F2-C]

At an organisational level, the strategic orientation of executive leaders appeared particularly important. In several of the organisations studied, there was an explicit philosophy and culture of continuous quality improvement, which clearly influenced the approach taken to implementing EBP. This was especially noticeable in the English site, which had a central Quality Improvement Department, responsible for coordinating initiatives such as quality improvement collaboratives, based on the Institute for Healthcare Improvement model (Institute for Healthcare Improvement, 2003). In terms of connecting with EBP, the approach used within nursing was to synthesise data generated by the improvement collaboratives into a set of nursing standards that were routinely monitored through an organisation-wide nursing accreditation system. In this way, local improvement data formed a key component of the evidence base that under- pinned nursing practice and ongoing accreditation was seen to fulfil the purpose of sustaining improvement. Two mid-level nursing roles existed within acute and community services to lead and coordinate the accreditation process.

> And then once we've got all the tests of change that do make a difference . . . then we formulate that into a change package with all the bundles in it and we publicize that [organisation] wide so that every ward should be doing that. And that's where I come in with the sustainability arm . . . because it's end up in the [nursing accreditation] document. So I will go onto the ward and I will ask staff, 'So, how do you detect a deteriorating patient? What are the seven elements of the bundle of care that we use in the acutely unwell change package?' [E-F1-A]

The two Canadian sites had a similar emphasis on quality improvement. However, there was not the same formalization of locally generated improvement data into an overarching accreditation or monitoring system. Both Canadian sites had a long history of implementing EBP. As a result, a substantial infrastructure for supporting EBP was evident at the provincial level:

> I think you have to have leadership at the top, and buy-in right at the top, and then you have to have an infrastructure . . . . to support staff access to the information, to, you know, have access to staff who may have the knowledge if we don't have it in writing somewhere, to, you know, the documentation tools,

the education, the orientation, all those things. You have to have champions. You've got to have people that are lined up with this that are carrying it on. You've got to have lots of cheerleaders . . . And then you have to have a system to measure it. [CE-E-C]

In Sweden, there was a unique feature that was not driven or organised around an external accreditation system, but involved combining local quality improvement work and benchmarking based on the national quality registers:

> . . . we have a business plan in which we have set up our own indicators to be able to follow our local results. From those indicators we set up targets that are different to those of the normal quality registers. They tell us how to measure, when, where and by whom. This gives us data from several sources. [S-F4-C]

Table 19C1.4 summarises the key findings in relation to policy/ organisational influences on EBP.

At a service level, differences were noted between acute and community/primary care services. This particularly related to contextual limitations experienced when delivering care in a person's home rather than in a clinical facility, both in terms of delivering EBP and undertaking audits. One example given related to difficulties of undertaking evidence-based wound care:

> . . . we're dealing with patients' own environments, which is challenging. For example, doing a simple dressing change, there might be a cat, there might be a dog, there might be a parrot. I'm trying to do a sterile procedure . . . . and we've got to try and be evidence-based practitioners, but also we need to be respectful of our patients and their wishes and how they live. [E-M4-C]

The community setting also presented challenges in terms of monitoring and evaluating the implementation of EBP as practitioners were typically working alone:

> . . . well I think that barriers [are] oversight and being able to monitor in the community - we don't have an electronic health record for nursing yet, and that's a draw back because there's so much that's happening that we're not able to capture yet. We would do chart audits and that kind of thing but it's paper based and because the charts go into the home - you know we're not always getting those charts back in fairly large numbers. [CE-M4- A]

TABLE 19C1.4

SUMMARY OF KEY FINDINGS BY COUNTRY

	AUSTRALIA	CANADA	ENGLAND	SWEDEN
Policy context	National healthcare accreditation scheme, based around 10 National Safety and Quality Health standards, developed by the Australian Commission on Safety and Quality in Healthcare	Primary responsibility for health system governance decentralized to provinces and territories Accreditation Canada – voluntary participation, but majority of organisations opt in	National performance management framework and systems (e.g. NICE standards and Care Quality Commission) Public healthcare system highly regulated	National practice guidelines and quality registers (> 100). Clinical settings report data to registers; these provide online feedback to local authorities and the public. Voluntary participation, not an accreditation system
Organisational context	Strong commitment to EBP at a strategic level Influence of external regulatory framework on policy and procedures guidance (PPG) and related auditing Complementary frontline roles, encompassing managerial and facilitative leadership Some evidence of hybrid manager/facilitator roles Difficult balance between embedding formalised PPG and encouraging and supporting critical thinking amongst clinical staff	Long history of supporting EBP Well-developed provincial and organisational infrastructure, including access to evidence-based resources and specialist roles to facilitate implementation Strong leadership support and strategic oversight from senior and middle-level managers Delegated responsibility and authority for implementation to facilitators Use of quality improvement (QI) methods and processes to guide implementation	Strong organisational emphasis on quality improvement; well-developed supporting infrastructure and culture QI the main vehicle for implementing EBP Improvement data feeding into a locally developed Nursing Assessment and Accreditation System to embed best practice Central QI Department, but few roles with a designated responsibility for facilitating implementation All leaders/managers involved in QI Hybrid clinical specialist/manager roles	Commitment to EBP at a national level with monitoring, reporting and benchmarking based on national quality registers, with a strong focus on medical data. Local quality improvement work based on quality improvement (QI) methods. Nurse managers have responsibility to support EBP, but limited capacity. Facilitator roles both at central and local level with responsibility to support QI and EBP.

Strategies to address the potential isolation of lone practitioners included managers undertaking 'walk-abouts' and accompanying staff on visits to patients, providing clinical staff with electronic tablets with standardized protocols and software for data capture and feedback, and holding regular safety huddles.

3.3 Challenges of Leading EBP

This third theme encompasses the challenges interviewees described in leading EBP, relating to the preparation they had received for this role and the perceived barriers they encountered. Whilst interviewees could clearly articulate their role in EBP, very few had received any educational preparation specifically targeted to implementing EBP. Some had undertaken modules in EBP as part of post-graduate study or a leadership development program, but for many the development of knowledge and skills in EBP had been an experiential process.

I suppose I've learnt as I've gone along. I mean I've done some further education but that's not learning and research, ... No-one's shown me how to do it. [A-M1-A]

Also, in the Swedish interviews a need for more knowledge was expressed:

. . . .the main challenge is knowledge and how to adopt that which actually works. I believe there is knowledge available that science has found/produced that could work well when tried in practice and be followed up. However, it feels like care and welfare should be able to find much evidence that could be introduced/adopted but time, knowledge and education is needed to be able to adopt new working practices. [S-M7-A]

Similarly, interviewees reported minimal use of implementation theories and frameworks, even in Canada where the Canadian Institutes for Health Research (CIHR) actively promoted the Knowledge-To-Action framework (Straus et al., 2009) as a planned change approach to implementing EBP. Where reference was made to frameworks, these tended to be more generic practice development, change management or quality improvement methodologies.

I guess the main thing is [you] need a method for doing it. . . . You need to commit to a method, so we've committed to the model for improvement and testing change via PDSA. You need to commit to a method and try and teach that method as deeply and as widely as you possibly can within your organisation otherwise people, in my experience, can flounder. [E-F4-A]

Connecting EBP to audit and quality improvement processes such as PDSA was one of the main enabling factors identified, alongside a supportive infrastructure (including evidence resources, technology and facilitator roles) and communication mechanisms such as safety huddles.

Barriers to EBP appeared less of a concern in the Canadian sites, which had the longest history and arguably the most extensive infrastructure (with human and non-human elements) to support EBP. In other countries, the key barriers identified from the perspective of middle level leaders related to time and workload pressures. A particular issue highlighted in the Swedish data was the dominant role of the medical profession in leading EBP, which resulted in the marginalization of nursing.

I think if staff were given more time people would gain more knowledge and gain more evidence and be more innovative with that evidence, in putting it into practice . . . . At the moment everyone's just too busy and you try and talk to people about putting stuff in place and they're like 'we're just too busy. Please don't give us anything else to do'. [A-F2-C]

It is very difficult to break through all this physician-centred- ness . . . but I believe that we are getting better and better at that too, but we have a long way to go, we need a paradigm shift to do that; and I almost feel that we are managing to move towards it, but it will probably take another 10–15 years. [S-F4-C]

In countries such as Australia where there was a strong emphasis on following policies and procedures guidance, concerns were raised that this could lead to a lack of critical thinking and reflection amongst front-line staff. This was most apparent in the acute care setting, compared to the community where the existence and influence of policies and procedures was less prominent.

I think they know that there's an expectation that they use evidence based practice but I think a lot of the time if you practically look at people it tends to be based on rote learning or based on procedures that dictate the way things are done. I don't know whether they necessarily understand the evidence process that's gone into informing those procedures. [A-EF2-A/C]

4 DISCUSSION

The findings demonstrate that a number and combination of different roles, strategies and processes are used to enact EBP. Moreover, there is an apparent relationship between different leadership roles, the context in which implementation is taking place and approaches used to embed EBP.

As previous studies have highlighted, context proved to be an important mediating factor between roles, mechanisms and the use of evidence in practice. At the macro level, differences were observed across countries, which appear to be linked to a mix of historical, policy and regulatory influences. For example, in countries such as Canada with a long history in EBP, a well-developed supporting infrastructure was apparent at both a strategic and clinical level, including individuals in dedicated facilitator roles with delegated authority to support implementation. In Australia and England, where the policy focus was on regulation and accreditation, there was a greater tendency to emphasise 'hard' systems and structures such as standards, policies and procedures to embed and monitor the implementation of evidence into clinical practice. In Sweden, national quality registers provide a substantial basis for EBP, but did not seem to have a strong impact on local quality improvement work within nursing. This highlights the need to take account of wider policy influences, beyond the immediate clinical and organisational setting, when considering barriers and enablers of EBP (McCormack et al., 2002; Harvey and Kitson, 2016). Equally, it is apparent that regardless of the policy environment, in most countries similar barriers relating to workload and time were observed, reflecting international pressures on nursing and health systems more generally.

At the front-line level of nursing leadership – for example, nurse unit managers or practice development facilitators – our findings show that contrasting mechanisms were used, which reflected contrasting leadership behaviours. Managerial leaders emphasised the management and monitoring aspects of their role, aligned to meeting the strategic objectives of the organisation, particularly around expected performance standards. In turn, this linked to an approach of 'hard-wiring' evidence into practice through policies and procedures, standards, audit and routine monitoring. By contrast, facilitative leaders emphasised processes concerned with relationships, communication and making connections, for example, by working alongside, engaging and talking with nursing staff.

Looking at the findings through a lens of organisational learning, aspects of both single and double loop learning are apparent (Argyris and Schon, 1996). The more formal, managerial mechanisms, with a focus on meeting external standards and using audit as a monitoring tool, tended to reinforce single loop learning. By comparison, facilitative approaches were more concerned with enabling and supporting others to implement, typically through local quality improvement approaches whereby front-line staff were engaged in identifying and seeking solutions to clinical problems. This aligns closely with the concept of meta-routines proposed by Berta and colleagues (Berta et al., 2015), creating a link between facilitation and higher-order (double and triple-loop) learning and "overcoming normal human tendencies to take reductionist approaches to problem-solving that afford only lower- order learning" (p.11).

Both types of activity played a part in achieving EBP. The key appeared to be achieving a balance; for example, too great a focus on managing performance against standards could promote unquestioning practice. Or, from an organisational learning perspective, too much single loop learning could be at the expense of double and triple-loop learning. This is where executive and senior nursing leaders needed to take an important strategic role, balancing external regulatory requirements with internal processes and infrastructure for creating an evidence-based culture and encouraging and supporting critical thinking at the clinical level. This reinforces findings from previous research, which highlight the need for different approaches, encompassing transactional and transformational strategies that focus on task, relational and change-oriented goals (Cummings et al., 2008; Gifford et al., 2017, 2013; Aarons, 2006). However, our study highlights that it is not about identifying particular individuals or nursing roles that have prime responsibility for leading and developing EBP. Rather, the focus should be on how best to achieve complementarity between the mechanisms required to optimise EBP and the network of roles needed to enact these mechanisms.

The study findings also highlight the potential for hybrid roles to blend managerial and facilitation mechanisms. The concept of hybridity is a subject that has previously attracted some interest in relation to implementing evidence into nursing practice. For example, an English study examined nurse consultants as a form of hybrid role, proposing that it could combine a strategic translational focus with the ability to influence both professional and managerial hierarchies (Spyridonidis and Currie, 2016). It may also be useful to consider hybridity at the organisational level. Rather than focusing on the formal merging of clinical/professional and managerial roles in one person, there could be benefit in looking strategically at the blending of skills required for implementing EBP and how this needs to be configured in relation to the prevailing context in which implementation is occurring. For example a strong external emphasis on national standards and accreditation, may create a tendency towards more formal, managerial approaches to EBP. To counter-balance this, more attention to facilitator-led, relationship-focused strategies at a local and organisational level may be warranted.

Overall, the study highlights that effective leadership for EBP is not role-specific. Rather certain mechanisms need to be enacted, mechanisms that are influenced by and need to be responsive to contextual influences at the micro, meso and macro level. This requires a strategic, yet dynamic network of roles, activities and relationships. In turn, this has implications for building capacity and capability for EBP within nursing. Previous work has highlighted the need to develop skills at different levels of complexity (for example, from learning basic skills such as audit and feedback through to more adaptive capabilities), through a combination of acquisitive and experience-based learning (Kislov et al., 2014). Yet in the sample of nursing leaders we studied, most interviewees reported that they drew on generalist knowledge

relating to leadership and change management to inform their role in EBP. The majority had not received any specific education or training on EBP; nor was the use of frameworks or theories to guide the process of implementation commonplace. As EBP has been listed as one of the key core competencies for all health professionals for the provision of safe, quality care it is notable that the nursing leaders had limited preparation in this field (Cronenwett et al., 2007). This indicates an important area for future educational development.

4.1 Study Strengths and Limitations

Our study was designed to provide more detailed insights into the nursing leadership roles and processes required to optimise the implementation of EBP. The international and cross-sectoral nature of the research enabled us to look across a breadth of different settings and roles and specifically examine the influence of macro-level contextual factors. It is important to acknowledge the limitation of having only one or two sites per country and we cannot claim that data saturation was achieved, nor that the study sites fully represented the national picture within the respective host countries. The purposive nature of sampling added a level of variability, as the study sites were not directly comparable at a cross-country level. However, the emergent pattern of a relation- ship between the policy context, organisational drivers for EBP, and related roles and implementation processes suggests trustworthiness of the study findings. The logistics of conducting a qualitative study across five different settings with multiple interviewers also posed challenges in terms of data collection, analysis and interpretation, issues that we addressed through our project management structure and face to face meetings at key points in the research process. Furthermore, we took steps to enhance the trustworthiness, confirmability and dependability of our findings by encouraging reflexivity during research team meetings. For example, organising two-day, face-to-face meetings at key stages of data analysis and interpretation meetings, enabled research team members to engage in critically constructive discussion about their own and each other's data. Additionally, the study findings were presented to local stakeholder group meetings in two of the four countries (Sweden and Australia) to sense-check interpretation of the data at a local level.

4.2 Conclusion

National policies around quality and performance shape priorities relating to EBP at an organisational level. This, in turn, influences the roles and mechanisms for implementation that are given prominence. There is a need to maintain a balance between the mechanisms of managing and monitoring performance versus facilitating critical questioning and reflection in and on practice. This requires a careful blending of managerial and facilitative leadership. The findings have implications for theory, practice, education and research relating to the implementation of EBP, both within nursing and at a wider inter-professional level. From a theoretical perspective, commonly applied EBP implementation frameworks such as the Consolidated Framework for Implementation Research (CFIR) (Damschroder et al., 2009), the Promoting Action on Research Implementation in Health Services framework (PARIHS) (Kitson et al., 1998; Harvey and Kitson, 2016) and the Knowledge to Action framework (K2A) (Straus et al., 2009) emphasise the mediating effect of context and the need for attention to the processes of implementation. Findings from this research provide a more detailed insight into the specific mechanisms that leaders need to enact and could add further detail to these type of implementation frameworks, particularly in terms of providing a more detailed explication of macro and meso-level context-mechanism relationships. In relation to practice, executive leaders need to be alert to the prevailing policy and regulatory environment in which they are operating and focus on achieving an appropriate balance between hard-wiring evidence into practice versus facilitating

implementation. Future research could involve designing and testing an implementation intervention that explicitly blends managerial and facilitative leadership strategies at an organisational and operational level. This could include further exploration of the concept of hybridity, at both an individual and collective level. Finally, more attention to educational preparation of staff to engage in and lead EBP is warranted. As a core competence for future healthcare leaders, EBP and implementation skills need to be addressed within undergraduate, postgraduate and continuing professional development educational programmes for all healthcare professionals.

REFERENCES

Schuster, M., McGlynn, E., & Brook, R. (1998). How good is the quality of health care in the United States? *Milbank Q, 76*, 517–563.

Grol, R. (2001). Successes and failures in the implementation of evidence-based guidelines for clinical practice. *Med. Care, 39*, 1146–1154.

Runciman, W. B., Coiera, E. W., Day, R. O., Hannaford, N. A., Hibbert, P. D., Hunt, T. D., et al. (2012). Towards the delivery of appropriate health care in Australia. *Med. J. Aust., 197*(2), 78–81.

Kitson, A., Brook, A., Harvey, G., Jordan, Z., Marshall, R., O'Shea, R., et al. (2017). Using complexity and network concepts to inform healthcare knowledge translation. *Int. J. Health Policy Manage., 7*(3), 231–243.

Braithwaite, J., Churruca, K., Long, J. C., Ellis, L. A., & Herkes, J. (2018). When complexity science meets implementation science: a theoretical and empirical analysis of systems change. *BMC Med, 16*(1), 63.

Sackett, D. L., Rosenberg, W. M., Gray, J. A., Haynes, R. B., & Richardson, W. S. (1996). Evidence based medicine: what it is and what it isn't. *Br. Med. J., 312*(7023), 71–72.

Greenhalgh, T., Howick, J., & Maskrey, N. (2014). Evidence based medicine: a movement in crisis? *Br. Med. J., 348*, g3725.

Bodenheimer, T., & Fernandez, A. (2005). High and rising health care costs. Part 4: can costs be controlled while preserving quality? *Ann. Intern. Med., 143*(1), 26–31.

Cosgrove, D. M., Fisher, M., Gabow, P., Gottlieb, G., Halvorson, G. C., James, B. C., et al. (2013). Ten strategies to lower costs, improve quality, and engage patients: the view from leading health system CEOs. *Health Aff, 32*(2), 321–327.

Cummings, G., Lee, H., Macgregor, T., Davey, M., Wong, C., Paul, L., et al. (2008). Factors contributing to nursing leadership: a systematic review. *J. Health Serv. Res. Policy, 13*(4), 240–248.

Rudman, A., Gustavsson, P., Ehrenberg, A., Boström, A.-M., & Wallin, L. (2012). Registered nurses' evidence-based practice: a longitudinal study of the first five years after graduation. *Int. J. Nurs. Stud., 49*(12), 1494–1504.

Aiken, L. H., Sloane, D., Griffiths, P., Rafferty, A. M., Bruyneel, L., McHugh, M., et al. (2017). Nursing skill mix in European hospitals: cross-sectional study of the association with mortality, patient ratings, and quality of care. *BMJ Qual. Saf., 26*(7), 559–568.

Kitson, A., Harvey, G., & McCormack, B. (1998). Enabling the implementation of evidence based practice: a conceptual framework. *Qual. Health Care, 7,* 149–159.

Damschroder, L., Aron, D., Keith, R., Kirsh, S., Alexander, J., & Lowery, J. (2009). Fostering implementation of health services research findings into practice: a consolidated framework for advancing implementation science. *Implement. Sci., 4,* 50.

McCormack, B., Kitson, A., Harvey, G., Rycroft-Malone, J., Titchen, A., & Seers, K. (2002). Getting evidence into practice: the meaning of' context. *J. Adv. Nurs., 38*(1), 94–104.

Gifford, W. A., Holyoke, P., Squires, J. E., Angus, D., Brosseau, L., Egan, M., et al. (2014). Managerial leadership for research use in nursing and allied health care professions: a narrative synthesis protocol. *Syst. Rev., 3,* 57.

Cummings, G. G., Tate, K., Lee, S., Wong, C. A., Paananen, T., Micaroni, S. P. M., et al. (2018). Leadership styles and outcome patterns for the nursing workforce and work environment: a systematic review. *Int. J. Nurs. Stud., 85,* 19–60.

Aarons, G., Ehrhart, M., & Farahnak, L. (2014). The implementation leadership scale (ILS): development of a brief measure of unit level implementation leadership. *Implement. Sci., 9,* 45.

Gifford, W., Graham, I. D., Ehrhart, M. G., Davies, B. L., & GA, A. (2017). Ottawa model of implementation leadership and implementation leadership scale: mapping concepts for developing and evaluating theory-based leadership interventions. *J. Healthc. Leadersh., 9,* 15–23.

Birken, S. A., S-YD, Lee, & Weiner, B. J. (2012). Uncovering middle managers' role in healthcare innovation implementation. *Implement. Sci., 7,* 28.

Gifford, W. A., Davies, B. L., Graham, I. D., Tourangeau, A., Woodend, A. K., & Lefebre, N. (2013). Developing leadership capacity for guideline use: a pilot cluster randomized control trial. *Worldviews Evid. Nurs., 10*(1), 51–65.

Tistad, M., Palmcrantz, S., Wallin, L., Ehrenberg, A., Olsson, C. B., Tomson, G., et al. (2016). Developing leadership in managers to facilitate the implementation of national guideline recommendations: a process evaluation of feasibility and usefulness. *Int. J. Health Policy Manage., 5*(8), 477–486.

Wilkinson, J. E., Nutley, S. M., & Davies, H. T. O. (2011). An exploration of the roles of nurse managers in evidence-based practice implementation. *Worldviews Evid. Nurs., 8*(4), 236–246.

Gunningberg, L., Brudin, L., & Idvall, E. (2010). Nurse Managers' prerequisite for nursing development: a survey on pressure ulcers and contextual factors in hospital organisations. *J. Nurs. Manage., 18*(6), 757–766.

Ehrenberg, A., Gustavsson, P., Wallin, L., Bostrom, A. M., & Rudman, A. (2016). New graduate nurses' developmental trajectories for capability beliefs concerning core competencies for healthcare professionals: a national cohort study on patient-centered care, teamwork, and evidence-based practice. *Worldviews Evid. Based Nurs., 13*(6), 454–462.

Harvey, G., Loftus-Hills, A., Rycroft-Malone, J., Titchen, A., Kitson, A., McCormack, B., et al. (2002). Getting evidence into practice: the role and function of facilitation. *J. Adv. Nurs., 37*(6), 577–588.

Cranley, L. A., Cummings, G. G., Profetto-McGrath, J., Toth, F., & Estabrooks, C. A. (2017). Facilitation roles and characteristics associated with research use by healthcare professionals: a scoping review. *BMJ Open, 7*(8).

Berta, W., Cranley, L., Dearing, J. W., Dogherty, E. J., Squires, J. E., & Estabrooks, C. A. (2015). Why (we think) facilitation works: insights from organisational learning theory. *Implement. Sci., 10,* 141.

Argyris, C., & Schon, D. A. (1996). Organisational Learning II: Theory, Method and Practice. Reading, Mass: Addison-Wesley.

Baskerville, N. B., Liddy, C., & Hogg, W. (2012). Systematic review and meta-analysis of practice facilitation within primary care settings. *Ann. Fam. Med., 10*(1), 63–74.

Persson, L. A., Nga, N. T., Malqvist, M., Thi Phuong Hoa, D., Eriksson, L., Wallin, L., et al. (2013). Effect of facilitation of local maternal-and-newborn stakeholder groups on neonatal mortality: cluster-randomized controlled trial. *PLoS Med, 10*(5), e1001445.

Seers, K., Rycroft-Malone, J., Cox, K., Crichton, N., Edwards, R., Eldh, A., et al. (2018). Facilitating implementation of research evidence (FIRE): a randomised controlled trial evaluating two models of facilitation informed by the promoting action on research implementation in health services (PARIHS) framework. *Implement. Sci* In review.

van der Zijpp, T. J., Niessen, T., Eldh, A. C., Hawkes, C., McMullan, C., Mockford, C., et al. (2016). A bridge over turbulent waters: illustrating the interaction between managerial leaders and facilitators when implementing research evidence. *Worldviews Evid. Nurs., 13*(1), 25–31.

Cummings, G. G., Estabrooks, C. A., Midodzi, W. K., Wallin, L., & Hayduk, L. (2007). Influence of organisational characteristics and context on research utilization. *Nurs. Res., 56*(4 Suppl), S24–S39.

Fitzgerald, L., Ferlie, E., Wood, M., & Hawkins, C. (2002). Interlocking interactions, the diffusion of innovations in health care. *Hum. Relat., 55*(12), 1429–1449.

Colorafi, K. J., & Evans, B. (2016). Qualitative descriptive methods in health science research. *HERD, 9*(4), 16–25.

Peterson, M. F. (2009). Cross-cultural comparative studies and issues in international research collaboration. In D. A. Buchanan, & A. Bryman (Eds.), The Sage Handbook of Organisational Research Methods (pp. 328–345). London: Sage Publications.

Sandelowski, M. (2000). Whatever happened to qualitative description?. *Res. Nurs. Health, 23*(4), 334–340.

Institute for Healthcare Improvement. (2003). *The Breakthrough Series: IHI's Collaborative Model for Achieving Breakthrough Improvement. (IHI Innovation Series White Paper)*. Boston: Institute for Healthcare Improvement.

Straus, S., Tetroe, J., & Graham, I. D. (2009). *Knowledge Translation in Health Care: Moving From Evidence To Practice*. West Sussex, UK: Blackwell Publishing Ltd..

Harvey, G., & Kitson, A. (2016). PARIHS revisited: from heuristic to integrated framework for the successful implementation of knowledge into practice. *Implement. Sci., 11*, 33.

Aarons, G. A. (2006). Transformational and transactional leadership: association with attitudes toward evidence-based practice. *Psychiatr. Serv., 57*(8), 1162–1169.

Spyridonidis, D., & Currie, G. (2016). The translational role of hybrid nurse middle managers in implementing clinical guidelines: effect of, and upon, professional and managerial hierarchies. *Br. J. Manage., 27*(4), 760–777.

Kislov, R., Waterman, H., Harvey, G., & Boaden, R. (2014). Rethinking capacity building for knowledge mobilisation: developing multilevel capabilities in healthcare organisations. *Implement. Sci., 9*, 166.

Cronenwett, L., Sherwood, G., Barnsteiner, J., Disch, J., Johnson, J., Mitchell, P., et al. (2007). Quality and safety education for nurses. *Nurs. Outlook, 55*, 122–131.

INTRODUCTION TO CRITIQUE 1

The preceding article (Harvey et al., 2019) is an example of a generic qualitative descriptive approach in which qualitative methods are used without alignment to a particular paradigm or philosophical approach, as described in Chapter 2. The article is critically examined here for its rigour as a qualitative descriptive study, its contribution to nursing, and its usefulness in practice. The criteria listed in Box 19.1, as well as the checklist from Figure 19.1, are used to guide the critique. Keep in mind that due to page constraints in the journal, the authors needed to make judgements about what was important to include, and it may not have been possible to address all of these criteria in a single report. There is no perfect research report, so the comments and critique are offered to help with developing your critical thinking and critical reading skills.

Authors

The authors listed all have academic affiliations at universities in nursing, health, or business. These disciplines align with, and would be relevant to, the topic of leadership in nursing practice. Although their credentials are not included, it is presumed that they have the education and experience to lead this type of research. In addition, they are from various institutes from around the world, which supports their claim in this being international research.

In the *Introduction* section it is clear the authors have studied leadership in nursing previously as they cite themselves frequently. This indicates that they may be very knowledgeable about the topic, and this is part of a program of research. It is not clear how their previous experiences might influence their perspectives or views on this topic, as they do not explicitly reflect on this in the paper. In the *Data Analysis* section, the authors describe that most of them are "working in the field of knowledge translation and implementation science, with both theoretical and practical knowledge" (Harvey et al., 2019, p. 24).

Title

The title of the article captures some components of the study. The key words of mechanisms and evidence-based practice could have been added for clarity.

Abstract

This is a structured abstract. It provides a good overview of the study, although there are a significant number of key words and concepts that are introduced, and it is not clear how they are all connected.

Background

In the introduction section, Harvey et al. (2019) review relevant bodies of literature on concepts such as: implementation of research into practice (evidence-based practice); the significance of nursing as the largest workforce in health care; and previous work on the influence of leadership in knowledge translation and implementation. They conclude from this review of the literature that leaders have a role in implementing evidence-based practice; however, there is limited understanding of macro-level roles and context in supporting these changes. The background section leads logically to the study objectives.

Purpose

The purpose of the study is clearly stated with a primary objective and three research questions. Given the background presented in the introduction, it appears to be an important topic for nursing. It is presumed by the reader, and not explicitly stated, that the question of context will be addressed by conducting the study in four different countries. Further on in the report it becomes apparent that different contexts are introduced by examining acute care and community care areas.

Method

The method used in the study is described in a section called *Methods*. As described earlier, the authors used a qualitative descriptive approach, citing an article by Colorafi and Evans (2016) to support this method. This method was chosen because "the aim was to develop a rich description of the phenomenon under study" (Harvey et al., 2019, p. 23). While qualitative research, in general, offers rich descriptions, the specific choice of this method was not stated. Grounded theory might have been selected to uncover the leadership processes involved in implementing EBP. Interpretive description might have been selected if they wanted the analysis to generate findings applicable specifically to nursing practice.

Sampling

The study was carried out in four countries: Australia, Canada, England, and Sweden. The authors contacted nursing executive leaders in their respective countries, who helped with recruitment of nurses in different sectors and roles (Harvey et al., 2019). Participants were recruited through purposive sampling. The authors present this sampling information in two tables in the research report. The inclusion criteria included managers who had a responsibility to manage nurses and nursing care and facilitators who were involved in education and practice development of nursing staff. Participants represented executive level leadership as well as clinical/frontline-level leadership. This purposive sampling allowed the researchers to examine different leadership roles and the potential impact on evidence-based practice. The recruitment reflected different clinical areas, as well as different countries, and so was suitable to their purpose. If the authors were further interested in supporting their findings through triangulation, they may consider interviewing nursing staff who are not in leadership roles, and ask them to reflect on how leaders influence their ability to engage in evidence-based practice.

Ethical Considerations

At the end of the article the authors list the ethics approval received from five different institutions. They declared they had no conflicts of interest and reported the funding sources that supported the study.

Participants were invited to participate via e-mail and given information about the study. There is no obvious coercion or deception used in the study.

Data Collection

Data was generated through semi-structured interviews with 55 participants. The authors described who conducted the interviews and where the interviews were conducted. Although they stated that three interview guides were created, these were not included for the reader. In addition, the authors reported that the interview guides were developed with input from a local stakeholder group (Harvey et al., 2019), but the composition and recruitment of this group was not described.

Data Analysis

Harvey et al. (2019) claimed to use qualitative content analysis to analyze the data using NVivo software. Keep in mind that this software helps with data management but still requires researchers to analyze the findings, creating codes, and themes. Although not explicitly stated, it is assumed that all interviews were completed prior to the beginning of analysis, so there was no concurrent data collection and data analysis.

In general, the measure of rigour in qualitative research is trustworthiness. Trustworthiness includes the concepts of credibility, auditability, and fittingness (see Chapter 15). There is sufficient description of data collection and analysis; however, there is minimal discussion of researcher reflexivity, and Harvey et al. (2019) did not include field notes. The authors do provide a credible account of the findings—for example, they explain the various roles in a manner that seems supported by the quotes they selected. However, given that the interviews were 30–60 minutes, there was no prolonged engagement with the participants, which may limit the findings. Because the interview guides were not included, it is not clear how much of this organization was according to pre-existing questions and themes, or how much further interpretation occurred (see Chapter 16).

Findings

Harvey et al. (2019) presented their findings organized into three main themes. This was an appropriate way to present the findings given their qualitative descriptive method. The participant quotes supported the authors' summaries under each theme. Two tables are presented in the findings section that describe the policy and organizational contexts in each of the four countries, and descriptions of policy and organizational contexts dominate the second theme: *Roles shaped by context: policy, organizational, and service delivery levels.* While examining policy and organizational contexts might have been useful to answer the research questions, and used to triangulate some of the data from the participants, the authors do not sufficiently explain data collection or data analysis processes related to the appearance of this data in their findings. For example, in Table 19C1.4 they state Canada has a "long history of supporting EBP" (Harvey et al., 2019, p. 27), but it is not clear how this was determined. It is not clear what constitutes a *long* history, nor how this compares to the length of time the other countries have been supporting EBP. Does a long time mean 30 years? Would 20 years not be considered a long time? Or were other countries only supportive of EBP for 3 years?

Conclusions, Implications, and Recommendations

In the discussion section, the authors describe the relationships between different leadership roles, the context of implementation, and approaches used to support EBP (Harvey et al., 2019). Unfortunately, the discussion on context (i.e., Canada having a long history of EBP and Australia and England having "hard" systems) is not reliably linked to the design or findings of the study. Further on in the discussion section, the authors do relate their findings to other research studies. For example, their participants described what seems to reflect single-loop or double-loop learning. This is an appropriate use of literature in a discussion section and helps to position new findings in an existing body of knowledge. You will also notice that the authors cited several of their own papers in the discussion section—just over one-third of the references in the paper include one of the authors. This is not necessarily a weakness of the study—often if researchers are experts in their field of study, it may be appropriate to do this. However, in a qualitative study, it may also raise concerns if authors are seeking to confirm what they already know and are not doing the challenging work of exploring other possible interpretations.

The authors provide several recommendations for practice and education, and likely future research, although this was not explicitly stated. In terms of limitations, the authors suggest that they did not reach data saturation; however, they did discover an emergent pattern (Harvey et al., 2019). In addition, they described challenges of working internationally.

In summary, there is some confusion in the research report surrounding the collection and analysis of policy and organizational data. The authors did suggest that they presented their findings to two stakeholder groups to "sense-check" the interpretation; however, nowhere in the study is the composition of this stakeholder group described, nor why there were only stakeholders from Australia and Sweden. About one-third of the references used in the article include one or more of these authors. As mentioned previously, this may reflect their programs of research and expertise in the area, but readers should be cautious that the background and discussion may be dominated by what these authors already believe to be true, rather than introduction of new ideas. In terms of strengths, the description of the analysis and presentation of findings was congruent with what would be expected of a qualitative descriptive project—there were ample quotes provided and the analysis stayed close to these original quotes. In terms of using this research in practice, nurses may find it provides some insights when developing EBP projects, particularly further understanding of leadership roles.

CRITIQUE 2

The study "Development and Implementation of the Family Caregiver Decision Guide" by Robinson et al. (2019) is critiqued here. The article is presented in its entirety and is followed by the critique on pp. 458–460.

Development and Implementation of the Family Caregiver Decision Guide

Carole A. Robinson[1,*], Joan L. Bottorff[1], Barbara Pesut[1], Janelle Zerr[1]

ABSTRACT

Care provided by family is the backbone of palliative care in Canada. The critical roles performed by caregivers can at the same time be intensely meaningful and intensely stressful. However, experiences of caregiving can be enhanced when caregivers feel they are making informed and reflective decisions about the options available to them. With this in mind, the purpose of this five-phase research project was to create a Family Caregiver Decision Guide (FCDG). The Guide entails four steps: thinking about the current caregiving situation, imagining how the caregiving situation may change, exploring available options, and considering best options if caregiving needs change. The FCDG was based on available evidence and was developed and refined using focus groups, cognitive interviewing, and a feasibility and acceptability study. Finally, an interactive version of the Guide was created for online use (https://www.caregiver-decisionguide.ca). In this article, we describe the development, evaluation, and utility of the FCDG.

KEYWORDS: psychosocial aspects; cancer; interventions; support groups; caregivers; caretaking; palliative care; decision making; life-threatening; terminal; illness and disease; qualitative; focus groups; cognitive interviewing; implementation science; British Columbia

Robinson, C. A., Bottorff, J. L., Pesut, B., & Zerr, J. (2019). Development and Implementation of the Family Caregiver Decision Guide. *Qualitative Health Research*, 30(2), 303–313. https://doi.org/10.1177/1049732319887166

[1]The University of British Columbia, Kelowna, British Columbia, Canada
*Corresponding Author: Carole A. Robinson, Professor Emeritus Nursing, Faculty of Health and Social Development, The University of British Columbia, 1147 Research Road, Kelowna, British Columbia, Canada V1V 1V7. Email: Carole.robinson@ubc.ca

INTRODUCTION

Globally, people are both aging and living longer with multiple chronic illnesses (Leeson, 2014). Indeed, the number of Canadian seniors above the age of 65 is projected to more than double between 2005 and 2036, placing increasing and unsustainable demands on the health care system (Fowler & Hammer, 2013). Despite the fact that the majority of Canadians die in hospital (Statistics Canada, 2012), most prefer to live at home for as long as possible, which, for many, means dying at home (Stajduhar & Davies, 2005; Wilson, Cohen, Deliens, Hewitt, & Houttekier, 2013). The preference to die at home has also been found in studies conducted in the United States (National Academies of Sciences, Engineering, and Medicine, 2016), England and Wales (Leeson, 2014), Europe (Higginson et al., 2014), and Japan (Fukui, Yoshiuchi, Sawai, & Watanabe, 2011). Regardless of the place of death, the demand for families to provide care at home is increasing. For example, almost three million Canadians aged 45 years and older provide 80% of care for family members with chronic and life-limiting illnesses (Statistics Canada, 2013a, 2013b). One in four Canadians are caregivers and half of them are aged between 45 and 65 years, their peak earning years (Statistics Canada, 2013a, 2013b). This means that more than six million carers are juggling their work and labor intensive caregiving responsibilities (Statistics Canada, 2013a, 2013b). Caring for an ill spouse requires about 14 hours per week, roughly equivalent to a part-time job (Funk et al., 2010). While caregiving can be rewarding, it is also stressful and can be associated with negative psychological, social, spiritual, and physical consequences (Funk et al., 2010; Topf, Robinson, & Bottorff, 2013). There are also financial implications to caregiving based on reports that caregivers have significant out-of-pocket expenditures (Keating, Fast, Lero, Lucas, & Eales, 2014; Round, Jones, & Morris, 2015; Rowland, Hanratty, Pilling, van den Berg, & Grande, 2017).

The caregiving role becomes even more critical in the advanced and end-of-life phases of illness. Estimates suggest that family caregivers are responsible for 75% to 90% of hospice palliative care provided in the home (Dunbrack, 2005). On average, Canadian family caregivers allocate approximately 54 hours per week to the care of a dying loved one at home (Canadian Hospice Palliative Care Association, 2012). The results of a recent national survey in England indicate that caregiving increases significantly in the last 3 months of life with the median hours of care reaching nearly 70 hours/week for over 50% of family caregivers (Rowland et al., 2017). Responsibilities often include shopping, housekeeping, coordinating, and accompanying their ill family member to medical appointments in addition to attending to their family member's physical, psychosocial, and spiritual care needs. These additional responsibilities can have immense impacts on family caregivers' daily lives and put them at risk of compromised quality of life and physical and mental morbidities (Grov, Dahl, Moum, & Fossa, 2005; Williams & McCorkle, 2011). Taking on the role of caregiver is often automatic and unreflected, something that Erlingsson, Magnusson, and Hanson (2012) term "sliding sideways into caregiving." Caregivers are challenged by lack of preparation, lack of information about what to expect, and inadequate support (Grande et al., 2009; Mastel-Smith & Stanley-Hermanns, 2012; Robinson, Pesut, & Bottorff,

2012). The experience of providing care to an ill family member is well understood, but how to effectively support family caregivers is not (Grande et al., 2009). There is a critical need to develop interventions that enable family caregivers to provide the kind and level of care they are committed to providing, and that the health care system depends upon.

The need to develop interventions to support the valuable work that family caregivers do led to the development of the Family Caregiver Decision Guide (FCDG), a resource designed to help family caregivers make decisions common to their caregiving role. The Guide was developed based upon several studies (Robinson et al., 2012; Topf et al., 2013) where we found family caregivers' need to provide excellent care was compromised by lack of knowledge about what they were getting into, lack of preparation for the role, lack of understanding about what to expect in terms of illness progression and at end of life, and difficulty accessing professional support as well as critical resources in a timely fashion. These findings are supported by others (Flemming, Atkin, Ward, & Watt, 2019; Oechsle, 2019; Wang, Molassiotis, Chung, & Tan, 2018). In particular, we observed that family caregivers had difficulty identifying the caregiving decisions they had made or needed to make and how to go about making those decisions. Furthermore, although decision aids have been identified as helpful resources, there was no decision aid available to assist them. Therefore, the purpose of this study was to develop and evaluate an intervention to support family caregiver decision making.

METHOD AND FINDINGS

This multiphased study began with a literature review (Phase 1) and was followed by three phases of qualitative research conducted using a sequential multiple method design (Mafuba & Gates, 2012; Morse, 2003). The iterative, user-centered design process involved intended users to create

TABLE **19C2.1**

OVERVIEW OF THE PHASES OF THE DEVELOPMENT OF THE FAMILY CAREGIVER DECISION GUIDE			
PHASE	**AIM/OBJECTIVES**	**ACTIVITIES**	**GUIDE DEVELOPMENT**
Phase 1: Literature reviews	Identify essential knowledge, skills, values, decision points, and resources that address family palliative caregiver needs	• Systematic literature reviews were conducted focused on palliative caregiving, and caregiving and gender • Gray literature was searched to identify caregiver resources	• Development of foundational assumptions and aims and objectives for the Guide • Principles to guide development and implementation • Initial version of the Guide
Phase 2: Focus group study	Engage experienced family caregivers in evaluating the comprehensiveness, understandability, applicability, and usefulness of the initial version of the Guide	• Focus groups held with family caregivers of persons who had died of cancer	• Findings guided revisions to the Guide that included adding inviting images and colors, removing tables, altering language for clarity and readability, and reformatting sections
Phase 3: Cognitive interview study	Engage current family caregivers in working through the Guide to understand rational and emotional responses and guide further refinements	• Cognitive interviews with current family caregivers (five women, three men) who worked through the Guide with the researcher	• Findings informed further refinements and implementation recommendations for the Guide
Phase 4: Implementation study	Evaluate the utility and applicability of the Guide as well as elucidate optimal implementation strategies from perspectives of family caregivers and health providers	• Current family caregivers, supported by trained hospice palliative care volunteers or palliative nurses, were invited to use the Guide. Data were collected via follow-up survey, along with semi-structured interviews with purposive sample • Providers participated in focus group discussions	• Developed guidelines for use/implementation of the Guide, along with training program for providers • Refinements to Guide based on findings
Phase 5: Dissemination	Enhance accessibility and adoption of the Guide into practice	• Developed interactive version of the Guide and website • Developed and implemented dissemination plan	• The Guide is available to print from both the website (https://www.caregiver-decisionguide.ca) and from (http://hdl.handle.net/2429/59786) and online, in an interactive format

an accessible and effective intervention to support family caregivers (see Table 19C2.1). Phases 2 to 4 received ethical approval from the university research ethics board and relevant health care agencies. All participants (caregiver and navigator) provided written consent to participate in the study. Phase 5 focused on development of strategies to support dissemination and uptake of the intervention.

Given the wide range of caregiver relationships, we defined family caregiver as whomever provided, or was providing, the majority of unpaid care at home. Family is whoever the ill person identifies as family. This included wives, husbands, partners, mothers, fathers, daughters, sons, and close friends. Support for family caregiver decision making was conceptualized as a palliative intervention. This was based on defining palliative care as focused on quality of life rather than disease that begins with the diagnosis of serious chronic or life-limiting illness and extends across the illness trajectory to end of life.

Phase 1: Development of the FCDG Based on Available Evidence

Phase 1 involved a review of literature, the subsequent identification of foundational assumptions, aims and objectives for the resource, as well as principles to guide development and, finally, initial development of the resource. The review of the evidence focused on three main bodies of literature: palliative caregiving, caregiving and gender, and caregiver resources. In each search, the overall aim was to identify literature that distinguished the essential knowledge, skills, values, decision points, and resources that address family palliative caregiver needs.

The search of empirical palliative caregiving was based on a rapid review strategy (Khangura, Konnyu, Cushman, Grimshaw, & Moher, 2012), prioritizing evidence from quality systematic reviews, and, when relevant, including high-quality primary studies and landmark and/or oft-cited studies. Our search yielded 24 articles that comprised literature reviews (12) and research studies (10 qualitative and two quantitative). Data were extracted in relation to method/sample, major findings, themes, and implications for development of the intervention. Major themes included caregiver decision making, challenges, needs, positive experiences, rural caregiving, and interventions.

Our second search of empirical literature focused on gender and caregiving for the purpose of informing a gender sensitive approach.

Twenty-six articles were reviewed and included literature reviews (four) and research studies (18 quantitative, three qualitative, and one mixed method). Data were extracted in relation to women and caregiving, men and caregiving, and implications for development of the intervention. Major findings were summarized within each of those categories (Robinson, Bottorff, Pesut, Oliffe, & Tomlinson, 2014).

Finally, we searched the gray literature for caregiver resources (11) to explore current practices in supporting family caregivers with the aim of identifying best practices, key knowledge and skills being targeted, how the support was being offered, and existing decision aids/ supports. Data were extracted in relation to aim of the resource, key components, limitations/concerns, and implications for development of the new resource.

Subsequent to our synthesis of findings, we developed the underpinnings of the FCDG, which included assumptions, aims, objectives, and principles (Table 19C2.2) as well as content for inclusion.

In addition, we took our knowledge of family caregiving acquired from previous studies as well as clinical work into account in development. Despite conceptualizing the resource as a palliative intervention, we were aware of the problematic association of the word "palliative" with death and dying, and the constraints this places on decision making. For example, palliative care is often resisted because of the belief that it is a lesser kind of care offered when there is no hope. Yet the evidence supports that early receipt of palliative care enhances quality of life and may even extend life (Temel et al., 2017; Temel et al., 2010). This led the team to purposely avoid using the word "palliative" in naming and describing the intervention. Instead the term "lifelimiting illness" was used, which we anticipated would make the intervention more acceptable, especially prior to the advanced phase of illness and caregiving.

TABLE **19C2.2**

UNDERPINNINGS OF THE FAMILY CAREGIVER DECISION GUIDE

Assumptions	Caregiving is an ongoing process involving multiple decisions over time in response to changes in the caregiving situation.
	Family caregivers need
	• To be(come) caregivers
	• To be skilled and to know more, that is, become excellent caregivers
	• To navigate competing wishes, needs, demands, and priorities
	• To have an "extra pair of hands," that is, to have help that does not take them away from providing direct care.
Aims	• Support the achievement of desired outcomes for caregivers who provide care for a family member with life-limiting illness.
	• Educate and prepare family caregivers; identify caregiving options and support decision making over time.
Objectives	• Support caregivers to clarify their values by reflecting on their own needs, preferences, and beliefs related to the caregiving process.
	• Help caregivers identify what they perceive to be the most important aspects of caregiving to assist with decision making.
	• Help caregivers determine which aspects of caregiving they may be willing to give up if caregiving becomes too burdensome or problematic.
	• Facilitate dialogue and shared decision making between caregiver and ill person.
	• Help caregivers anticipate and prepare for potential challenges and issues that may arise throughout the caregiving trajectory.
	• Support ongoing reflection about how things are going, what is needed, and how to carry on.
	• Build caregiver self-efficacy and increase problem-solving capacity.
	• Support caregiver health and well-being during and after caregiving.
	• Create space for options—If home is viewed as the best place to die, but commitment to following this path may have serious unintended negative consequences, how can we support consideration of options?
	• Facilitate therapeutic conversations between caregivers and providers.
Guiding principles for resource development	• *Flexible*—useful over time and illness progression in communities with differing availability of resources (e.g., rural vs. urban communities).
	• *Applicable* for both male and female caregivers. Men and women experience caregiving and chronic illness differently. Therefore, interventions need to be gender sensitive.
	• *Comprehensive* but not too detailed or burdensome to deter use.
	• *Understandable*—plain and acceptable language.
Guiding principles for resource implementation	• Options and supports for caregivers and their families need to align with the patient's and family's personal, cultural, and spiritual beliefs as well their readiness to deal with certain aspects of end-of-life care.
	• Caregivers' ideas of caregiving may change over time as illness progresses and caregiver burden increases. Promises to provide care may change throughout illness trajectory and should therefore be framed as provisional.
	• Caregivers need to be aware of their options throughout the different stages of caregiving. Resources for caregivers should empower caregivers to make informed decisions and promote awareness of formal and informal supports and resources.
	• Caregiving is a process; it is constructed of a series of domains and activities—not an "all or nothing" task. It involves making decisions over time. Caregivers have the right to choose which aspects of caregiving they are comfortable undertaking and which tasks they may need assistance with or choose not to do.

Continued

TABLE 19C2.2

UNDERPINNINGS OF THE FAMILY CAREGIVER DECISION GUIDE—*cont'd*

- Caregivers need to have the opportunity to fully comprehend the benefits and challenges associated with the various aspects of caregiving so that they make informed decisions. Providing care at home can result in drastic shifts in the lives of caregivers to fulfill the duties associated with caregiving; this needs to be addressed and revisited throughout the caregiving process.
- The need to create patient comfort and maximize well-being is paramount for caregivers. This means that caregivers need to feel informed, secure, and confident with the care that they are providing.
- Caregivers are more willing to accept support if it does not take away from time spent with the ill person. Therefore, resources will be more successful if they facilitate skill building and focus on caregiver strengths and resources.
- The caregiving process will have better outcomes when the needs and preferences of both the caregiver and the ill person are ascertained during decision-making processes. Strategies and resources need to facilitate dialogue between family members to promote shared decision making and mutual goal setting when possible.
- Support strategies for family caregivers are an essential component of family caregiving. Without support strategies, the needs and well-being of both the caregiver and ill person are at risk.
- Supporting family caregivers requires a proactive approach where, to a certain extent, the challenges associated with end-of-life care need to be anticipated. This will help ensure that potential issues and concerns are addressed before they develop into crisis situations.
- Caregivers must care for themselves to be able to provide care for someone else. Without recognition of their own needs, caregivers are at risk for emotional, physical, and financial hardship. Therefore, it is important to recognize, assess, and respond to caregiver needs and issues.

We also recognized the significant challenges to effectively supporting family caregivers, which became apparent in our previous research (Lockie, Bottorff, Robinson, & Pesut, 2010; Pesut, Robinson, & Bottorff, 2013; Robinson, Bottorff, McFee, Bissell, & Fyles, 2017; Robinson et al., 2012; Topf et al., 2013). Family caregivers often prioritized the needs and wishes of the ill person over all other issues, including their own health, preferences, and, at times, safety. For example, a caregiver explained that her husband only wanted to receive care from her but as he was prone to falling, she risked her own physical health in her attempts to get him off the floor. She recounted that she honored his wish until it simply became too dangerous for her to continue. The priority focus on meeting the ill person's needs, wishes, and preferences, coupled with recognition of limited paid health care provider time, often led to caregiver reluctance to engage health care professionals' focus and time for their own needs. This was viewed as diverting a precious resource away from the person who needed it most. Furthermore, caregivers reported that they withheld information from health care providers about struggling to provide care for fear of negative judgments about their abilities. They worried that care would be taken from them. Another reported challenge was the professional practice of noting concern for the caregiver but then giving them another job, to take care of their own health and well-being in addition to providing care for the ill person. Although family caregivers often recounted appreciation for expressions of concern, the recommendation of a new job was viewed as nonsupportive and evidence of lack of understanding of the demands of caregiving. The common coping strategy among caregivers of "taking one day at a time," which prevented being overwhelmed with what might be ahead, also acted to constrain necessary planning and preparing for likely changes. Finally, we were aware of the severe constraint to decision making that occurred when caregivers made an implicit or explicit promise to care at home until death because options were not considered. When a home death did not occur, these caregivers suffered greatly because of the "broken promise" (Martz & Morse, 2017; Topf et al., 2013). All of these constraints challenge our ability to effectively support family caregivers and were addressed in the development phase.

The final factor that influenced development was the unique nature of the decisions that attend family caregiving. Most decision aids are created to facilitate decisions that result in simple yes/no outcomes that are bounded by time. For example, the decision to take a particular cancer treatment at a particular time of diagnosis might be one suitable for a decision aid. However, caregiving decisions are different; the caregiving process changes over time and involves multiple decision points that coincide with changes in the caregiving situation that are ill person, caregiver, or health system related. This necessitated adaptation of the internationally recognized process for decision aid development (Coulter et al., 2013) while following accepted international standards (Elwyn et al., 2006) for decision support tools.

Taking account of these various factors, we developed the first prototype of the FCDG. The FCDG is organized around a four-step process: thinking about the current caregiving situation, thinking about how the caregiving situation may change (this section includes values clarification for both caregiver and care recipient), exploring caregiving options in the area, and best options if the needs for caregiving change. Multiple iterations of the FCDG were reviewed by team members with expertise in palliative research and palliative clinical work until we had a stable version to begin testing. Three phases of testing were conducted following approval by a university ethics committee.

Phase 2: Focus Group Study to Evaluate the First Prototype of the FCDG

In Phase 2, past family caregivers of persons who had died of cancer participated in focus groups designed to evaluate the first prototype's comprehensiveness, understandability, applicability, and usefulness. We recruited family caregivers who were well into the bereavement period (minimum 6 months postdeath) because we felt they were experienced enough to critique the FCDG and were far enough into the bereavement period that the experience would not exacerbate their grief or be overly burdensome. Eleven women and three men provided informed consent and participated in three focus groups, which were audiorecorded but not transcribed verbatim. Individual participants worked through the FCDG and then engaged in group conversation about their experience prompted by questions about what they liked, did not like, structure and flow of the FCDG, areas lacking clarity, whether their experiences as caregivers were captured, and their assessment of the potential usefulness of the FCDG. Audiotapes were reviewed and detailed handwritten notes were recorded to capture important points made about each section of the FCDG, paying close attention to diverse views, areas of consensus, and suggestions for improvement. Notes were later transcribed, reviewed by the team, and areas for refinement were specifically identified and determined by consensus (Zerr, 2015).

Participants told us that despite containing useful information, they did not think they would access the FCDG based on its appearance. There were too many tables and little aesthetic appeal. This was new learning in relation to the accepted process for decision aid development, which did not prompt us to consider aesthetics. Participants identified many language issues that were either confusing or unacceptable. Furthermore, they requested that the FCDG be more explicit about end-of-life issues including use of the word "palliative" rather than "life-limiting illness" on the cover page. This particular recommendation was not immediately taken up because we were concerned that these participants' perspective, based on having experienced the death of their ill person, might not be shared by caregivers who were earlier in the caregiving trajectory.

Participants were concerned when the focus of the FCDG was on the family caregiver, specifically their self-care, instead of the ill family member. This deemphasis of their ill family member, and subsequent emphasis on caregivers' responsibilities for their own health, disrupted what they described as their connection to the FCDG, which in turn compromised the effectiveness of the intervention. Finally, it was noted that the FCDG was useful in raising many relevant questions but held few answers and participants requested more resources to address those questions. The FCDG was redesigned to include inviting images and colors, tables were removed, language was altered for clarity and readability, sections were reformatted, and resources were added.

Phase 3: Cognitive Interview Study to Evaluate the Second Prototype of the FCDG

This phase involved testing the second prototype of the FCDG with eight current family caregivers (five women and three men) for someone with advanced cancer, using cognitive interviewing (Zerr, 2015). Following informed consent, participants worked through the FCDG alongside a researcher with a focus on understanding rational and emotional responses to the resource. The aim was to further refine the acceptability, understandability, and applicability of the FCDG. We found that the Phase 2 redesign of the FCDG was largely successful. Overall, participants found that the images created a warm, caring, and personal feel to the FCDG. Two images were described as unhelpful (e.g., one showing a man who looked sad) and were subsequently replaced. Lack of ethnic diversity in the images was noted by the caregiver participants. It became clear during our interviews that participants personally and emotionally connected to the FCDG via images that

represented them or their situation, which led the team to include more diverse pictures.

Language was viewed by the caregiver participants as understandable and applicable, except in a few instances. When the language did not fit, this caused participants to disconnect from the FCDG, with the thought that the writer of the FCDG clearly did not understand their situation. One example of this was the question of how caregivers were managing with "exercising and staying active." Similar to the findings in Phase 2 focus groups, participants found the idea of exercising (self-care) made no sense in their demanding circumstances, so this was removed. Two further significant changes involved using first person rather than second person throughout the FCDG (e.g., this Decision Guide is for *me* rather than you) and to remove the term "loved one" for the recipient of care and replace it with the more neutral term "family member." We learned in the previous research (Robinson et al., 2017) that love is only one of many motivations behind family caregiving. Furthermore, in contrast to the feedback we got from Phase 2 focus groups with family caregivers in the bereavement period, these participants were not supportive of more explicit language regarding palliation, disease progression, and death and dying because they found it to be too aggressive and upsetting. Finally, participants pointed out that the FCDG was missing a critical piece of caregiving—exhaustion, as one reason why caregiving at home might be curtailed. The FCDG was further refined based on participant feedback. Despite the identified concerns, the overall content of the FCDG was reported to be useful in that it invited reflection and supported planning as well as providing a "map" for essential conversations with the ill family member, which caregivers had not initiated. The FCDG prototype was then professionally redesigned to further enhance its aesthetic appeal and usability.

We concluded that the FCDG showed promise as an effective intervention but that it raised many questions for caregivers and offered very few answers. In addition, caregivers were not likely to seek answers because of fatigue, life demands, or unwillingness to draw attention to themselves. Therefore, we concluded that the FCDG should not be used as a stand-alone tool; instead, it was essential to accompany it with navigational support, particularly in relation to available resources.

Phase 4: Implementation Study of the Revised FCDG

Phase 4 was an implementation study designed to further evaluate the feasibility, utility, and applicability of the revised FCDG in real-world situations and in a broader illness context. In particular, we wanted to determine how navigational support might enhance the utility of the FCDG for family caregivers of someone with serious illness (not limited to cancer and including dementia), as well as identify optimal implementation strategies. The FCDG was evaluated with current family caregivers in a rural setting, who were receiving home care services (20 caregivers), using specially trained hospice palliative care volunteers as navigators and in an urban setting (12 caregivers) using palliative nurses as navigators. An implementation science approach informed by action research was used. The implementation process, including the education (~2 hours) of involved navigators that aimed to build local capacity, was developed and tailored to each setting in consultation with our community-based partners. Both the planning phase of the implementation process and the post-implementation evaluation phase included engagement with local opinion leaders.

After providing informed consent, caregiver participants were introduced to the FCDG by their navigator who then negotiated how the FCDG would be used and how support would be offered based on caregiver preferences. For example, some caregivers wished to work completely through the FCDG on their own and then discuss

their thoughts and questions with their navigator. Other caregivers preferred to work through a section at a time with their navigator alongside. All volunteer navigators made at least two in-person visits to the family caregiver and many supplemented these visits with telephone conversations. Nurse navigators made regular, scheduled home visits as part of their care of the ill person.

Data from caregiver participants were collected following completion of the FCDG. Caregivers completed a brief survey focused on the acceptability and usefulness of the FCDG as well as key implementation questions such as when the FCDG should be introduced. Individual, semi-structured interviews were also conducted with four purposively selected key family caregiver informants. Questions explored such things as whether the FCDG was useful and, if so, how; optimal timing for introducing the Guide; most effective process for using the Guide; and perceived outcomes including communication with providers, effectiveness of support, and caregiver wellbeing. The interviews were audio-recorded, transcribed verbatim, and analyzed using constant comparison.

In addition, appropriateness and utility of the FCDG as well as the implementation process were evaluated from the navigator perspective via focus groups, which were conducted at mid- and end-of-study. The mid-study focus groups were designed to facilitate implementation successes and ameliorate challenges. Topics addressed in the end-of-study focus group included implementation successes and challenges, the FCDG's usefulness in enhancing communication as well as the understanding of family caregiver values and needs, navigators' perceived ability to provide effective support, and exploration of the navigator's role. The focus group discussions were audio-recorded and analyzed thematically.

There was overwhelming consensus among the Phase 4 participants (caregivers and navigators) that the FCDG was feasible, useful, understandable, and comprehensive. Navigators commented that it helped educate and raise awareness for caregivers. They noted that caregivers were grateful for the recognition of their work, concerns, experiences, and burnout—they felt "not so alone." Some suggestions for additional content were made (e.g., related to financial planning) and the FCDG was modified as appropriate.

All participants stated that the FCDG should be used with support from a trusted, knowledgeable health care provider/navigator. Participants identified many ways that the FCDG could be approached, for example, working through it step by step with a provider, working through all steps independently and then discussing with a provider, or working through a step at a time followed by subsequent discussion with a provider. The majority of participants thought that the FCDG should be introduced as early as possible in the illness experience and used repeatedly as things change. Caregiver participants frequently commented that the FCDG came too late for optimum utility and suggested that family physicians make the initial introduction. Volunteer navigators found the experience rewarding and commented that the FCDG gave their interactions and conversations focus and direction. They got to know their caregiver partners in a deep and meaningful way.

The caregiver participants received the FCDG when they were deep into the illness trajectory, yet even then, they reported the resource to be useful. For example, they found the FCDG to be affirming because it "let's you know how much you know" and have done. As one woman said, "I know a lot more than I thought I did." Navigators commented that this gave caregivers comfort. Furthermore, the FCDG solidified previous decisions. "You can see more clearly how you made decisions, and can talk about them more clearly." Working through the FCDG validated and clarified the path caregivers were on. Even for these experienced caregivers, the FCDG was effective in raising questions such as "Do I know enough about this?"

Implementation advice was specific and helpful. For example, volunteer navigators recommended introducing the FCDG by first recognizing and acknowledging the importance of caregivers' work and stating that the goal of the FCDG is to support family caregivers in their caregiving and in living life to the fullest by helping them get what they need in their unique situation. Commendations for the caregiver, especially in front of the ill person, were viewed as extremely supportive and it was recommended that providers look for ways to specifically commend the caregiver during the implementation process of the FCDG.

Navigators offered several important tips. Volunteer navigators emphasized that follow-up with caregivers needs to be initiated by the navigator because of caregivers' reluctance to draw attention to themselves and away from their ill family member. They were particularly effective in this regard. Nurse navigators acknowledged this need but identified how difficult this was for them with their busy schedules. Sometimes family caregivers were exhausted and did not have the energy to make necessary connections or seek required supports (e.g., equipment), so providing information was not viewed as adequate or effective; volunteer navigators often offered to do the work. They noted that simply expecting caregivers to act on new or existing knowledge was unrealistic in the circumstance of exhaustion. In addition, the idea that the FCDG is meant to be revisited over time as things change was confusing to some caregivers. Navigators suggested using different colors for each time the FCDG was completed. They also suggested comparing it with a Will, which people revisit as there are new additions to the family. Most important for the navigators was knowledge about resources that caregivers could reliably access when needed and an appreciation of how the caregiver was faring emotionally.

Phase 5: Dissemination

Phase 5 focused on final refinements to the FCDG, development of an interactive version of the resource for online use, and the creation of a website to enhance accessibility and adoption of the resource into practice (https://www. caregiverdecisionguide.ca). The FCDG may now be used in two formats. Online, caregivers can work through each step in their own time and save as they go to return at a later date, or complete in one sitting. When the FCDG is completed, it can be printed and includes both questions and responses, which can then be used to focus conversations with a trusted health provider. The FCDG is also available to print from both the website and from "http://hdl.handle.net/2429/59786" for people who prefer to work offline or who may not have computer access. It is an open access resource that can be printed by health care providers for caregivers. The FCDG has been successfully implemented in 2-hour, urban and rural community workshops with groups of over 30 people including those with serious illness, current caregivers, and those anticipating becoming caregivers. One key to the success of the community-based workshops was including local health care providers knowledgeable about available resources. In addition, the print version of the FCDG has been translated into Portuguese by the Portuguese Palliative Care Association and made available throughout the country.

LIMITATIONS

During the study period, palliative nurse navigators' caseloads increased significantly, accompanied by a dramatic decrease in patient time on program (less than 6 weeks, which was the duration of study participation). This means that people were accessing palliative care closer to death than had been previously experienced and overall workload intensity increased because patients were sicker. More than half our recruited urban caregivers did not complete the study because their ill person died shortly after the FCDG was introduced. Our belief that optimal implementation of the FCDG should be early rather than late in the serious illness experience was confirmed.

The FCDG may assist in preparing caregivers for decisions at end of life, but when introduced for the first time in this phase of the trajectory it was not a useful resource because caregiving was too intense and there were such rapid changes in the ill person's condition. Furthermore, the nurse navigators had difficulty integrating follow-up with caregivers into their home visits due to the intensity of care for the ill person.

DISCUSSION

The sequential multiple methods study reported here was designed to address the pressing need for interventions to support family members caring for seriously ill people at home. Family was conceptualized as whoever the ill person accepts as family. Following international standards and user-centered, iterative approaches for the development of decision aids, the FCDG was created and subsequently refined. To our knowledge, this is the first intervention for family caregivers that focuses on supporting their decision making in planning care for their family member. The multiphased approach proved valuable in translating evidence into the development of a novel intervention through the engagement of intended users (in this case both caregivers and providers). We were particularly sensitive to the possibility of added burden for caregivers at a time when vulnerabilities may be high and multiple complex issues at play; however, the process proved feasible. The results of each phase determined the focus and methods associated with the next phase. This approach allowed us to make important iterative adjustments and refinements to the intervention as well as implementation guidelines for the FCDG to maximize acceptability and utility. Whereas initial phases focused on caregivers for someone with cancer, the implementation phase expanded to a wide variety of lifelimiting illnesses and proved applicable.

The inclusion of family caregivers and providers in the development of interventions has been recognized as important in supporting implementation into practice (Ugalde et al., 2019). Although caregiver interventions have received increasing research attention and randomized control trials report improved outcomes for family caregivers (Ferrell & Wittenberg, 2017), there has been limited focus on the potential for moving interventions into real-world settings. In a systematic review of cancer caregiver interventions conducted by Ugalde et al. (2019), fewer than half of the studies reported on the acceptability of interventions from the caregivers' perspectives, and only two studies involved caregivers in the development of interventions. The sequential multiple method approach we used in this study provides a model for including family caregivers and providers in the development and use of evidence-informed interventions to support implementation into practice. Others have also suggested that sequential multiple methods designs are more likely to produce valid and reliable knowledge than a single method (Mafuba & Gates, 2012).

Decision aids have been developed to assist people when making difficult choices that require balancing risks and benefits in the light of personal values (O'Connor et al., 1999). Providing care at home for someone with serious illness involves many value-sensitive decisions, particularly when time may be short, which have potential for negative long-term consequences (Topf et al., 2013). These decisions are complicated when caregivers are not aware of their choices or decision making (Robinson et al., 2012). Decision aids aim to address factors associated with suboptimal decision making, such as lack of knowledge, unrealistic expectations, lack of clarity about personal values, unwanted pressure, and inadequate support (Coulter et al., 2013; O'Connor et al., 1999). They are not meant to be used alone, but as part of a process that involves conversation with a knowledgeable health care provider where the discussion can be focused on what is most important to the caregiver (O'Connor et al., 1999). According

to our family caregiver participants, the FCDG effectively met the aims of decision aids. Across all the study phases, we consistently found that the FCDG was not sufficient to meet caregivers' needs on its own. Discussion with providers was required to address gaps in knowledge (e.g., about the anticipated course of illness or about resources) and support as well as unrealistic expectations regarding outcomes. The FCDG has potential to enable focused discussions between caregivers and providers so that priority needs can be identified and the response tailored to the uniqueness of each situation to be most helpful. Given the realities of our cost and time constrained health care environment, the FCDG shows promise in enabling providers to maximize the effectiveness of communication with caregivers.

Rabow, Hauser, and Adams (2004) emphasize the importance of a care partnership between physicians and caregivers that rests on excellent communication, including careful assessment of caregiver beliefs, values, and preferences as well as proactive information to support decision making. Yet caregivers often experience the opposite of partnership—being powerless, invisible, and unsupported (Erlingsson et al., 2012). The FCDG is a time-efficient tool to support the creation of a care partnership where caregivers have an active voice because they can complete it at home and at their own pace or in a group setting. Care preferences may change over time as the illness changes, which supports the idea that communication should begin early in the illness trajectory and be revisited over time. Caregivers often do not know what they don't know (Rabow et al., 2004; Robinson et al., 2012) and the FCDG was effective in raising caregivers' questions and concerns. Caregiving circumstances are diverse, which calls for diverse interventions (Chi & Demiris, 2015) to enact truly family centered care through caregiver-centered support (LaValley, 2018). Our webbased interactive version of the FCDG addresses this issue.

IMPLICATIONS FOR PRACTICE

Study findings indicate that the FCDG should be introduced to family caregivers along with assurances about their valued and essential work. These assurances are particularly important in situations where caregivers are reluctant to divert provider attention from their ill person to themselves. Caregivers can be invited to go through the FCDG at home, with a follow-up visit scheduled by the provider to review and identify needs. Once the FCDG is completed, needs, questions, and concerns can be addressed in relation to their priority to caregiving. The FCDG needs to be introduced early in the caregiving trajectory and revisited at key transitions, such as illness progression, hospitalization, and functional decline. The use of trained volunteer navigators was highly effective, with provider backup and support to address illness-related questions and problems (e.g., pain and symptom management). This makes the FCDG a potentially valuable intervention in settings where the availability of trained palliative care professionals is limited and a strong community-based volunteer system is in place (e.g., in rural settings). Furthermore, the FCDG was applicable to a variety of life-limiting illnesses.

CONCLUSION

Family caregivers are the backbone of life-limiting illness care. While there is growing recognition of the importance of their work, care for the caregiver remains sadly lacking. The FCDG is a promising intervention designed to assist caregivers to identify their needs, think ahead, and make informed decisions through focused conversations with supportive health care providers.

REFERENCES

Canadian Hospice Palliative Care Association. (2012). *Fact sheet: Hospice palliative care in Canada.* Retrieved from http://www.qelccc.ca/media/10821 /fact_sheet_hpc_in_canada_may_2012_final.pdf.

Chi, N. C., & Demiris, G. (2015). A systematic review of telehealthtools and interventions to support family caregivers. *Journal of Telemedicine and Telecare, 21,* 37–44. doi:10.1177/1357633X14562734.

Coulter, A., Stilwell, D., Kryworuchko, J., Mullen, P. D., Ng, C. J., & van der Weijden, T. (2013). A systematic development process for patient decision aids. *BMC Medical Informatics and Decision Making, 13*(Suppl. 2). doi:10.1186/1472-6947-13-S2-S2.

Dunbrack, J. (2005). *The informational needs of informal caregivers involved in providing support to a critically ill loved one.* Retrieved from http://www.hc-sc.gc.ca /hcs-sss/pubs/homedomicile/2005-info-caregiver-aidant/index-eng.php#a6.

Elwyn, G., O'Connor, A., Stacey, D., Volk, R., Edwards, A., Coulter, A., & Butow, P. (2006). Developing a quality criteria framework for patient decision aids: Online international Delphi consensus process. *British Medical Journal, 333,* Article 417. doi:10.1136/ bmj.38926.629329.AE.

Erlingsson, C. L., Magnusson, L., & Hanson, E. (2012). Family caregivers' health in connection with providing care. *Qualitative Health Research, 22,* 640–655. doi:10.1177/1049732311431247.

Ferrell, B., & Wittenberg, E. (2017). A review of family caregiving intervention trials in oncology. *CA: A Cancer Journal for Clinicians, 67,* 318–325. doi:10.3322/caac.21396.

Flemming, K., Atkin, K., Ward, C., & Watt, I. (2019). Adult family carers' perceptions of their educational needs when providing end-of-life care: A systematic review of qualitative research. *AMRC Open Research, 1.* doi:10.12688/amrcopenres. 12855.1.

Fowler, R., & Hammer, M. (2013). End-of-life care in Canada. *Clinical and Investigative Medicine, 36,* e127–e132. doi:10.25011/cim.v36i3.19723.

Fukui, S., Yoshiuchi, K., Fujita, J., Sawai, M., & Watanabe, M. (2011). Japanese people's preference for place of endof- life care and death: A population-based nationwide survey. *Journal of Pain Symptom Management, 42,* 882–892. doi:10.1016 /j.jpainsymman.2011.02.024.

Funk, L., Stajduhar, K. I., Toye, C., Aoun, S., Grande, G. E., & Todd, C. J. (2010). Part 2: Home-based family caregiving at the end of life: A comprehensive review of published qualitative research (1998-2008). *Palliative Medicine, 24,* 594–607. doi:10.1177/0269216310371411.

Grande, G., Stajduhar, K., Aoun, S., Toye, C., Funk, L., Addington-Hall, J., & Todd, C. (2009). Supporting lay carers in end of life care: Current gaps and future priorities. *Palliative Medicine, 23*, 339–344. doi:10.1177/0269216309104875.

Grov, E. K., Dahl, A. A., Moum, T., & Fossa, S. D. (2005). Anxiety, depression, and the quality of life in caregivers of patients with cancer in late palliative phase. *Annals of Oncology, 16*, 1185–1191. doi:10.1093/annonc/mdi210.

Higginson, I. J., Gomes, B., Calanzani, N., Gao, W., Bausewein, C., & Daveson, B. A. .... Project PRISMA. (2014). Priorities for treatment, care and information if faced with serious illness: A comparative population-based survey in seven European countries. *Palliative Medicine, 28*, 101–110. doi:10.1177/0269216313488989.

Keating, N. C., Fast, J. E., Lero, D. S., Lucas, S. J., & Eales, J. (2014). A taxonomy of the economic costs of family care to adults. *The Journal of the Economics of Ageing, 3*, 11–20. doi:10.1016/j.jeoa.2014.03.002.

Khangura, S., Konnyu, K., Cushman, R., Grimshaw, J., & Moher, D. (2012). Evidence summaries: The evolution of a rapid review approach. *Systematic Reviews, 1*, Article 10. doi:10.1186/2046-4053-1-10.

LaValley, S. A. (2018). End-of-life caregiver social support activation: The roles of hospice clinicians and professionals. *Qualitative Health Research, 28*, 87–97. doi:10.1177/1049732317732963.

Leeson, G. W. (2014). Increasing longevity and the new demography of death. *International Journal of Population Research*, Article 521523. doi:10.1155/2014/521523.

Lockie, S. J., Bottorff, J. L., Robinson, C. A., & Pesut, B. (2010). Experiences of rural family caregivers who assist with commuting for palliative care. *Canadian Journal of Nursing Research, 42*, 74–91.

Mafuba, K., & Gates, B. (2012). Sequential multiple methods as a contemporary method in learning disability nursing practice research. *Journal of Intellectual Disabilities, 16*, 287–296. doi:10.1177/1744629512462178.

Martz, K., & Morse, J. M. (2017). The changing nature of guilt in family caregivers: Living through care transitions of parents at the end of life. *Qualitative Health Research, 27*, 1006–1022. doi:10.1177/1049732316649352.

Mastel-Smith, B., & Stanley-Hermanns, M. (2012). It's like we're grasping at anything": Caregivers' education needs and preferred learning methods. *Qualitative Health Research, 22*, 1007–1025. doi:10.1177/1049732312443739.

Morse, J. M. (2003). Principles of mixed methods and multimethod research design. In A. Tashakkori, & C.

Teddlie (Eds.), *Handbook of mixed methods in social & behavioral research* (pp. 189–208). Thousand Oaks, CA: Sage.

National Academies of Sciences, Engineering, and Medicine. (2016). *Families caring for an aging America*. Washington, DC: The National Academies Press. doi:10.17226/23606.

O'Connor, A. M., Drake, E. R., Fiset, V., Graham, I. D., Laupacis, A., & Tugwell, P. (1999). The Ottawa patient decision aids. *Effective Clinical Practice: ECP, 2*, 163–170.

Oechsle, K. (2019). Current advances in palliative & hospice care: Problems and needs of relatives and family caregivers during palliative and hospice care—An overview of current literature. *Medical Sciences, 7*, 43. doi:10.3390/medsci7030043.

Pesut, B., Robinson, C. A., & Bottorff, J. L. (2013). Among neighbors: An ethnographic account of social responsibilities in rural palliative care. *Palliative & Supportive Care, 12*, 127–138. doi:10.1017/S1478951512001046.

Rabow, M. W., Hauser, J. M., & Adams, J. (2004). Supporting family caregivers at the end of life: They don't know what they don't know. *Journal of the American Medical Association, 291*, 483–491. doi:10.1001/jama.291.4.483.

Robinson, C. A., Bottorff, J. L., McFee, E., Bissell, L. J., & Fyles, G. (2017). Caring at home until death: Enabled determination. *Journal of Supportive Care in Cancer, 25*, 1229–1236. doi:10.1007/s00520-016-3515-5.

Robinson, C. A., Bottorff, J. L., Pesut, B., Oliffe, J. L., & Tomlinson, J. (2014). The male face of caregiving: A scoping review of men caring for a person with dementia. *American Journal of Men's Health, 8*, 409–426. doi:10.1177/1557988313519671.

Robinson, C. A., Pesut, B., & Bottorff, J. L. (2012). Supporting rural family palliative caregivers. *Journal of Family Nursing, 18*, 467–490. doi:10.1177/1074840712462065.

Robinson, C. A., Pesut, B., & Bottorff, J. L. (2015). *A family caregiver decision guide*. Kelowna, BC: University of British Columbia.

Round, J., Jones, L., & Morris, S. (2015). Estimating the cost of caring for people with cancer at the end of life:A modelling study. *Palliative Medicine, 29*, 899–907. doi:10.1177/0269216315595203.

Rowland, C., Hanratty, B., Pilling, M., van den Berg, B., & Grande, G. (2017). The contributions of family care-givers at end of life: A national post-bereavement census survey of cancer carers' hours of care and expenditures. *Palliative Medicine, 31*, 346–355. doi:10.1177/0269216317690479.

Stajduhar, K. I., & Davies, B. (2005). Variations in and factors influencing family members' decisions for palliative home care. *Palliative Medicine, 19*, 21–32. doi:10.1191/026921 6305pm963oa.

Statistics Canada. (2012). *The Canadian population in 2011: Age and sex*. Available from www.statscan .gc.ca.

Statistics Canada. (2013a). *Caregivers in Canada*. Available from https://www150.statcan.gc.ca/n1/daily-quotidien/130910/dq130910a-eng.pdf.

Statistics Canada. (2013b). *Family caregiving: What are the consequences?* Available from http://www. statcan.gc.ca/pub/75-006-x/2013001/article/11858 -eng.pdf.

Temel, J. S., Greer, J. A., El-Jawahri, A., Pirl, W. F., Park, E. R., Jackson, V. A., & Rinaldi, S. P. (2017). Effects of early integrated palliative care in patients with lung and GI cancer: A randomized clinical trial. *Journal of Clinical Oncology, 35*, 834–841. doi:10.1200/JCO.2016.70.5046.

Temel, J. S., Greer, J. A., Muzikansky, A., Gallagher, E. R., Admane, S., Jackson, V. A., & Billings, J. A. (2010). Early palliative care for patients with metastatic non– small-cell lung cancer. *New England Journal of Medicine, 363*, 733–742. doi:10.1056 /NEJMoa1000678.

Topf, L., Robinson, C. A., & Bottorff, J. L. (2013). When a desired home death does not occur: The consequences of broken promises. *Journal of Palliative Medicine, 16*(8), 1–6. doi:10.1089/jpm.2012.0541.

Ugalde, A., Gaskin, C. J., Rankin, N. M., Schofield, P., Boltong, A., Aranda, S., & Livingston, P. M. (2019). A systematic review of cancer caregiver interventions: Appraising the potential for implementation of evidence into practice. *Psycho-Oncology, 28*, 687–701. doi:10.1002/pon.5018.

Wang, T., Molassiotis, A., Chung, B. P. M., & Tan, J. Y. (2018). Unmet care needs of advanced cancer patients and their informal caregivers: A systematic review. *BMC Palliative Care, 17*, Article 96. doi:10.1186/ s12904-018-0346-9.

Williams, A. L., & McCorkle, R. (2011). Cancer family caregivers during the palliative, hospice and bereavement phases: A review of the descriptive psychosocial literature. *Palliative & Supportive Care, 9*, 315–325. doi:10.1017/S1478951511000265.

Wilson, D. M., Cohen, J., Deliens, L., Hewitt, J. A., & Houttekier, D. (2013). The preferred place of last days: Results of a representative population-based public survey. *Journal of Palliative Medicine, 16*, 502–508. doi:10.1089/jpm.2012.0262.

Zerr, J. R. (2015). *An evaluation of a family caregiver decision guide* (Master's thesis). Available from http://open.library.ubc.ca.

INTRODUCTION TO CRITIQUE 2

The preceding article by Robinson et al. (2020) is an example of a multi-phased, sequential multiple method design. The article is critically examined here for its rigour as a qualitative study, its contribution to nursing, and its usefulness in practice. The criteria listed in Box 19.1, as well as the checklist from Figure 19.1, are used to guide the critique.

Authors

The authors all have an academic affiliation with the University of British Columbia. Based on the information provided in the introduction, it appears that this project is part of a larger program of research on palliative care and family caregivers. The authors cite some of their previous work in this area, which may indicate this is part of a larger program of research and that the researchers have expertise in this area.

Title

The title of the article concisely captures the content of the article. They could have added a brief phrase about the method used.

Abstract

The abstract meets the requirements of a good abstract. It is a narrative abstract that outlines the significance of the topic to society and accurately reflects the content of the report.

Background

The authors review several pieces of relevant literature in the introduction section to provide background to the study. Robinson et al. (2020) described several trends in aging, caregiving, palliative and end-of-life care, and specifically the immense role of family caregiving at end-of-life. This helps to build the rationale for the importance of interventions for family caregivers and thus, the study. The authors provided information about what caregivers struggle with (i.e., lack of knowledge or understanding and difficulty identifying caregiving decisions); however, it was not explicitly clear in the introduction why a decision-making tool would be the most appropriate intervention.

PURPOSE

The purpose is clearly stated in this section: "The purpose of this study was to develop and evaluate an intervention to support family caregiver decision making" (Robinson et al., 2020, p. 304).

METHOD

The method used in this study is identified in the "Methods and Findings" section. Because it is a multi-phase study, the authors also detail the various phases in a table (Robinson et al., 2020, p. 305). The aims of each phase of the study are included, as well as the associated activities and how each phase contributed to the development of the family caregiver decision guide (FCDG). This multi-phased, multi-method project included development, implementation, and dissemination of this intervention. All of the phases are presented in this article, and so the paper is organized somewhat differently than most research articles. Each phase is presented in terms of the aim, activity, data collection, and findings so the reader can move chronologically through the study. For the purposes of this critique, the steps of the research process of each phase are separated and described.

SAMPLING

In phase 1 (literature review), Robinson et al. (2020) provided a detailed overview of the types of literature that they searched to support the development of the FCDG. One of these reviews included a review of existing resources for caregivers, and perhaps it was in this review that the need for a FCDG was identified. The authors included several objectives underpinning the development of this guide, including educating caregivers and facilitating therapeutic conversations, which indicates some breadth beyond a decision-aid.

Phase 2 involved focus groups with family caregivers of people who had died of cancer. The deaths had occurred at least 6 months prior to participation in the focus group. This included 11 women and 3 men. It was not stated how these participants were recruited. This information would have helped the reader to determine the type of sampling method, as well as any previously existing relationship to the researchers.

Phase 3 involved individual cognitive interviews with eight current family caregivers. Again, it was not stated how these family caregivers were recruited, or if they had a pre-existing relationship with the researchers.

Phase 4 was an implementation stage and involved 32 caregivers along with palliative care navigators. All caregivers completed a survey about the tool, and four caregivers were purposively selected for semi-structured interviews. The navigators were also included in focus groups in this phase. It was not stated how many navigators participated in the focus groups—they were composed of volunteer navigators from a rural area, as well as palliative care nurse navigators in an urban area. The criteria for selecting the four caregivers for an interview was not stated.

ETHICS

Following phase 1, ethics approval was received from a university ethics committee to continue with the remaining phases of the study (Robinson et al., 2020). It is assumed that the method of recruitment was stated in the ethics application, and this process was deemed acceptable, although further information about the recruitment process would have strengthened this report. The authors also listed their funding sources at the conclusion of the article. There does not appear to be any conflict of interest related to funding sources.

DATA GENERATION AND ANALYSIS

Phase 1 data was generated by literature reviews, focusing on quality systematic reviews and high-quality primary studies (Robinson et al., 2020).

Phases 2, 3, and 4 involved generating qualitative data from participant focus groups and individual interviews. In phase 2 the focus was evaluating the comprehensiveness, understandability, applicability, and usefulness of the tool (Robinson et al., 2020), and this information was used to make changes to the FCDG tool. Phase 3 used cognitive interviewing (see Zerr, 2015) as a technique for gathering emotional and rational responses to the tool (Robinson et al., 2020). In phase 4 data were collected from family caregivers and analyzed using constant comparison; data from navigators were analyzed using thematic analysis. The focus of this final phase was to understand feasibility, utility, and applicability of the FCDG.

Throughout the descriptions of the phases, the researchers engage in reflexivity by describing their previous thoughts and concerns and stating how these changed through the research process. For example, initially they used the term "loved one," but after collecting data in focus groups and interviews, the decision was made to use "family member." They also included reflections about the use of the term "palliative care."

FINDINGS

The findings of the various phases of the project are presented chronologically in the paper, according to the phase. Phase 1 findings from the literature review are found in a table presented in the paper (Robinson et al., 2020, p. 306). This summary of literature and resources appears comprehensive and credible. Findings in phase 2 also appeared credible and reliable. Although no direct quotes were presented in these findings, the authors presented a balanced perspective of the strengths and limitations of the tool, as reported by the participants.

In phase 3, the authors summarized findings, although no participant quotes were presented. Further changes were made to the tool based on participant feedback. In phase 4, the authors presented some participant quotes and provided summary information from the data collected. It was not always clear which data came from which source—for example, which data were gathered from the caregiver surveys versus interviews.

Phase 5 did not involve any further data collection or analysis and represents the dissemination of the project. The authors provide websites and links to the completed tool.

CONCLUSIONS, IMPLICATIONS, AND RECOMMENDATIONS

In the discussion section, Robinson et al. (2020) suggested that this tool is the first of its kind. This helps the reader to understand the significance of the tool, and the research report. In addition, they describe the inclusion of caregivers and providers in the development of the tool and how their decision aid is different from other decision aids found in the literature. They describe the implications for practice that would assist others in implementing the FCDG more successfully in their practice.

Overall, the strength of this article is its auditability. The reader can clearly follow the decision-making trail of the researchers to understand how the conclusions were reached. One aspect that would have improved this would be the inclusion of the questions used in the survey and semi-structured interviews, as well as further details on sampling. If the journal allows it, sometimes this information is included in supplementary materials available online. In this case, the FCDG is available as a supplementary file. In terms of using this in practice, this article would provide important background information if you were looking to implement a family caregiver decision support tool.

Evidence-Informed Practice Tip
Qualitative research may generate basic knowledge, hypotheses, and theories to be used in the design of other types of qualitative or quantitative studies. However, qualitative research is not necessarily a preliminary step to another type of research. It is a complete and valuable end in itself.

CRITICAL THINKING CHALLENGES

- Discuss the similarities and differences between the stylistic considerations of reporting a qualitative study versus a quantitative study in a professional journal.
- Are critiques of qualitative studies in the role of either a student or a practising nurse valid? Which type of qualitative study is the most difficult to critique? Discuss what assumptions led you to this determination.
- Discuss how nurses would go about incorporating qualitative research in evidence-informed practice. Give an example.

CRITICAL JUDGEMENT QUESTIONS

1 Why is it important for researchers to publish the development of an intervention, such as Robinson et al. (2020)?

   a Researchers are incentivized to publish as many articles as possible

   b Knowing the theoretical basis for an intervention improves implementation in other settings

   c To capture the lived experiences of the participants, especially in an area that is not well understood

   d Researchers need to account for their research grant spending in an ethical manner

2 Why is it important to examine the authors' positions and previous work?

   a It is important to only use research published by nurses

   b Researchers need to establish a program of research to improve credibility of their work c Authors should not cite their previous work in the publication because it reflects their opinions

d To be aware of possible motivations for presenting certain data and conclusions

3 What is an appropriate application of the study by Harvey et al. (2019) in nursing practice?

a Increased awareness of how leadership style and roles impact evidence-based practice

b Implementing evidence-based practice requires facilitative and managerial leadership

c Evidence-based practice is better supported with hard systems and a long history of policy

d There are insufficient data to apply these findings in practice

📶 FOR FURTHER STUDY

Go to Evolve at http://evolve.elsevier.com/Canada /LoBiondo/Research for the Audio Glossary.

REFERENCES

Barbour, R. S., & Barbour, M. (2003). Evaluating and synthesizing qualitative research: The need to develop a distinctive approach. *Journal of Evaluation in Clinical Practice, 9*, 179–186.

Critical Appraisal Skills Programme. (2020). *CASP Checklists*. https://casp-uk.net/casp-tools-checklists/.

Colorafi, K. J., & Evans, B. (2016). Qualitative descriptive methods in health science research. *HERD: Health Environments Research & Design Journal, 9*(4), 16–25. https://doi.org/10.1177 /1937586715614171.

Harvey, G., Gifford, W., Cummings, G., et al. (2019). Mobilising evidence to improve nursing practice: A qualitative study of leadership roles and processes in four countries. *International Journal of Nursing Studies, 90*, 21–30. https://doi.org/10.1016/j. ijnurstu.2018.09.017.

Ingham-Broomfield, R. (2008). A nurses' guide to the critical reading of research. *Australian Journal of Advanced Nursing, 26*(1), 102. https://search.informit. com.au/documentSummary;dn=182293025623125;res =IELHEA.

International Journal of Nursing Studies (IJNS). (2020). *Guide for Authors*. https://www.elsevier.com/journals /international-journal-of-nursing-studies/0020-7489 /guide-for-authors.

Moore, G., Audrey, S., Barker, M., Bond, L., Bonell, C., & Hardeman, W. (2015). Process evaluation of complex interventions: UK Medical Research Council (MRC) Guidance *www. ioe. ac. uk/MRC_PHSRN _Process_evaluation_guidance_final (2)*.

Robinson, C. A., Bottorff, J. L., Pesut, B., & Zerr, J. (2020). Development and Implementation of the Family Caregiver Decision Guide. *Qualitative Health Research, 30*(2), 303. https://doi.org/10.1177 /1049732319887166.

Schepner-Hughes, N. (1992). *Death without weeping: The violence of everyday life in Brazil*. Berkeley: University of California Press.

Stahlke Wall, S., & Rawson, K (2016). The nurse practitioner role in oncology: Advancing patient care. *Oncology Nursing Forum, 4*(*43*), 489–496. https://doi .org/10.1188/16.ONF.489-496.

Thorne, S. (2008). *Interpretive description*: Left Coast Press.

Thorne, S. (2020). Beyond theming: Making qualitative studies matter. *Nursing Inquiry, 27*(1), e12343. https:// doi.org/10.1111/nin.12343.

Tong, A., Sainsbury, P., & Craig, J. (2007). Consolidated criteria for reporting qualitative research (COREQ): A 32-item checklist for interviews and focus groups. *International Journal for Quality in Health Care, 19*(6), 349–357. https://doi.org/10.1093/intqhc /mzm042.

Williams, V., Boylan, A. M., & Nunan, D. (2020). Critical appraisal of qualitative research: Necessity, partialities and the issue of bias. *BMJ Evidence-Based Medicine, 25*(1), 9–11. http://dx.doi.org/10.1136 /bmjebm-2018-111132.

Zerr, J. R. (2015). *An evaluation of a family caregiver decision guide* (Master's thesis). http://open.library. ubc.ca.

CHAPTER 20

Critiquing Quantitative Research

Ramesh Venkatesa Perumal | Mina D. Singh

LEARNING OUTCOMES

After reading this chapter, you will be able to do the following:

- Identify the purpose of the critiquing process for a quantitative research report.
- Describe the criteria of each step of the critiquing process for a quantitative research report.
- Evaluate the strengths and weaknesses of a quantitative research report.
- Discuss the implications of the findings of a quantitative research report for nursing practice.
- Construct a critique of a quantitative research report.

KEY TERM

scientific merit

STUDY RESOURCES

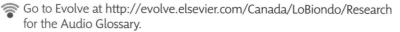 Go to Evolve at http://evolve.elsevier.com/Canada/LoBiondo/Research
for the Audio Glossary.

AS REINFORCED THROUGHOUT EACH CHAPTER of this book, it is important not only to conduct and read research but also to use research for evidence-informed practice. As nurse researchers increase the depth (quality) and breadth (quantity) of research methods from descriptive research designs to randomized clinical trials, the data to support clinical interventions and quality outcomes are becoming more readily available. Each published study, regardless of its design, reflects a *level of evidence,* but the critique of each study covers much more than the level of evidence produced by the design. When you critique a research study, examine each component to determine the merit of the report. Key to the critique is the strength of evidence that each study produces individually and collectively.

This chapter presents critiques of two studies in which research questions were tested with different quantitative designs. The critiquing criteria designed to assist research consumers in judging the relative value of a research report are found at the end of previous chapters. These critiquing criteria have been summarized to create an abbreviated set of questions that will be used as a framework for the two sample research critiques (Box 20.1). These critiques exemplify the process of evaluating reported research for potential application to practice, thus extending the research base for nursing. For clarification, refer to earlier chapters for detailed presentations of the critiquing criteria and explanations of the research process. The criteria and examples in

BOX **20.1**

MAJOR CONTENT SECTIONS OF A RESEARCH REPORT AND RELATED CRITIQUING GUIDELINES

PROBLEM STATEMENT AND PURPOSE (SEE CHAPTER 4)

1. What is the problem explored in, or the purpose of, the research study?
2. Does the statement about the problem or purpose express a relationship between two or more variables (e.g., between an independent variable and a dependent variable)? If so, what is the relationship? Is it testable?
3. Does the statement about the problem or purpose specify the nature of the population being studied? What is it?
4. What significance of the problem—if any—has the investigator identified?

REVIEW OF THE LITERATURE AND THEORETICAL FRAMEWORK (SEE CHAPTERS 2 AND 5)

1. What concepts are included in the review? Of particular importance, note which concepts are the independent and dependent variables and how they are conceptually defined.
2. Does the literature review make the relationships among the variables explicit or place the variables within a theoretical or conceptual framework? What are the relationships?
3. What gaps or conflicts in knowledge of the problem are identified? How is this study intended to fill those gaps or resolve those conflicts?
4. Are the references cited by the author mostly primary or secondary sources? Give an example of each.
5. What are the operational definitions of the independent and dependent variables? Do they reflect the conceptual definitions?

HYPOTHESES OR RESEARCH QUESTIONS (SEE CHAPTER 4)

1. What hypotheses or research questions are stated in the study? Are they appropriately stated?
2. If research questions are stated, are they used in addition to hypotheses or to guide an exploratory study?
3. What are the independent and dependent variables in the statement of each hypothesis or research question?
4. If hypotheses are stated, is the form of the statement statistical (null) or research?
5. What is the direction of the relationship in each hypothesis, if indicated?
6. Are the hypotheses testable?

SAMPLE (SEE CHAPTER 13)

1. How was the sample selected?
2. What type of sampling method is used in the study? Is it appropriate for the design?
3. Does the sample reflect the population as identified in the problem or purpose statement?
4. Is the sample size appropriate? How is it substantiated?
5. To what population may the findings be generalized? What are the limitations in generalizability?

RESEARCH DESIGN (SEE CHAPTERS 11 AND 12)

1. What type of design is used in the study?
2. What is the rationale for the design classification?
3. Does the choice of design seem logical for the proposed research problem, theoretical framework, literature review, and hypothesis?

INTERNAL VALIDITY (SEE CHAPTER 10)

1. Discuss each threat to the internal validity of the study.
2. Does the design have controls at an acceptable level for the threats to internal validity?

EXTERNAL VALIDITY (SEE CHAPTER 10)

1. What are the limits to generalizability in terms of external validity?

RESEARCH APPROACH (SEE CHAPTERS 8 AND 12)

1. Does the research approach fit with the purpose of the study?
2. Is a mixed-methods approach, if used, appropriate for the study?

METHODS (SEE CHAPTER 14)

1. What data-collection methods are used in the study?
2. Are the data-collection procedures similar for all participants?

Continued

BOX 20.1

MAJOR CONTENT SECTIONS OF A RESEARCH REPORT AND RELATED CRITIQUING GUIDELINES—cont'd

LEGAL/ETHICAL ISSUES (SEE CHAPTER 6)
1. Have the rights of participants been protected? How?
2. What indications are given that informed consent of the participants was ensured?

INSTRUMENTS (SEE CHAPTER 14)
1. Physiological measurement
   a. Is a rationale given for why a particular instrument or method was selected? If so, what is it?
   b. What provision is made for maintaining the accuracy of the instrument and its use, if any?
2. Observational methods
   a. Who did the observing?
   b. How were the observers trained to minimize bias?
   c. Did the observers have an observational guide?
   d. Were the observers required to make inferences about what they saw?
   e. Is there any reason to believe that the presence of the observers affected the behaviour of the participants?
3. Interviews
   a. Who were the interviewers? How were they trained to minimize bias?
   b. Is there evidence of any interviewer bias? If so, what is it?
4. Questionnaires
   a. What is the type or format of the questionnaires (e.g., Likert-type, open-ended)? Are they consistent with the conceptual definitions?
5. Available data and records
   a. Are the records that were used appropriate to the problem studied?
   b. Were the data used to describe the sample or for hypothesis testing?

RELIABILITY AND VALIDITY (SEE CHAPTER 15)
1. What type of reliability is reported for each instrument?
2. What level of reliability is reported? Is it acceptable?
3. What type of validity is reported for each instrument?
4. Does the validity of each instrument seem adequate? Why?

ANALYSIS OF THE DATA (SEE CHAPTER 17)
1. What level of measurement is used to measure each of the major variables?
2. What descriptive or inferential statistics are reported?
3. Were these descriptive or inferential statistics appropriate for the level of measurement for each variable?
4. Are the inferential statistics used appropriate for the intent of the hypotheses?
5. Does the author report the level of significance set for the study? If so, what is it?
6. If tables or figures are used, do they meet the following standards?
   a. They supplement and economize the text.
   b. They have precise titles and headings.
   c. They do not repeat the text.

CONCLUSIONS, IMPLICATIONS, AND RECOMMENDATIONS
1. If hypothesis testing was done, were the hypotheses supported or not supported?
2. Are the results interpreted in the context of the problem or purpose, hypothesis (see this chapter), and theoretical framework or literature reviewed?
3. What does the investigator identify as possible limitations or problems in the study in relation to the design, methods, and sample?
4. What relevance for nursing practice does the investigator identify, if any?
5. What generalizations are made?
6. Are the generalizations within the scope of the findings or beyond the scope of the findings?
7. What recommendations for future research are stated or implied?

BOX **20.1**

MAJOR CONTENT SECTIONS OF A RESEARCH REPORT AND RELATED CRITIQUING GUIDELINES—*cont'd*

APPLICATION AND UTILIZATION (SEE CHAPTER 21)
1. Does the study appear to be valid? In other words, do its strengths for nursing practice outweigh its weaknesses?
2. Do other studies have similar findings?
3. What risks or benefits are involved for patients if the research findings are used in practice?
4. Is direct application of the research findings feasible in terms of time, effort, money, and legal/ethical risks?
5. How and under what circumstances are the findings applicable to nursing practice?
6. Should these results be applied to nursing practice?
7. Would it be possible to replicate this study in another clinical practice setting?

this chapter are applicable to quantitative studies in which researchers used experimental, quasiexperimental, and nonexperimental research designs that provided levels II, III, and IV evidence.

STYLISTIC CONSIDERATIONS

As an evaluator, you should be aware of several aspects of publishing before you begin to critique research studies. First, different journals have different publication goals, and they target specific professional nursing specialties. For example, the *Canadian Journal of Nursing Research* publishes articles on the conduct or results of research in nursing. The *Canadian Oncology Nursing Journal* also publishes research articles; however, because its ephasis is broader, this journal also contains clinical and theoretical articles relating to knowledge, experience, trends, and policies in oncological nursing. Consequently, the style and content of a manuscript will vary according to the type of journal to which it is being submitted.

Second, the author of a research article prepares the manuscript by using both personal judgement and specific journal guidelines. *Personal judgement* refers to the researcher's expertise that is developed in the course of designing, executing, and analyzing the study. As a result of this expertise, the researcher is in a position to judge which content is most important to communicate to the profession. The decision is a function of the following:
- The research design: experimental or nonexperimental

- The focus of the study: basic or clinical
- The audience to whom the results will be most appropriately communicated

Each journal provides the guidelines for preparing research manuscripts for publication, and usually the following major headings are essential sections of a research manuscript or research report:
- Introduction
- Method
- Results
- Discussion

Depending on the stylistic considerations related to the author's preferences and the journal's requirements, the content included in the research report is specific to each of the sections just mentioned.

Stylistic variations (as factors influencing the presentation of the research study) are very distinct features of a research report and can deter from the focus of evaluating the reported research for **scientific merit**—that is, judging the overall quality or validity of a study. This means that sometimes, the real scientific merit of a study may be missed by digressing into commenting on stylistic variations. Constructive evaluation is based on objective appraisal of the study's strengths and limitations. This step precedes consideration of the relative worth of the findings for clinical application to nursing practice. Judgements of the scientific merit of a research study are the hallmark of promoting a sound evidence base for quality nursing practice.

CRITIQUE 1

The study "The Impact of Pain Invisibility on Patient-Centered Care and Empathetic Attitude in Chronic Pain Management" by Paul-Savoie et al. (2018) is critically appraised here. The article is presented in its entirety and is followed by the critique on pp **477–479** (From *Pain Research and Management* (2018)).

"The Impact of Pain Invisibility on Patient-Centered Care and Empathetic Attitude in Chronic Pain Management"

Paul-Savoie et al. (2018)

ABSTRACT

OBJECTIVES. The use of interdisciplinary patient-centered care (PCC) and empathetic behaviour seems to be a promising avenue to address chronic pain management, but their use in this context seems to be suboptimal. Several patient factors can influence the use of PCC and empathy, but little is known about the impact of pain visibility on these behaviours. The objective of this study was to investigate the influence of visible physical signs on caregiver's patient-centered and empathetic behaviours in chronic pain context.

METHODS. A convenience sample of 21 nurses and 21 physicians participated in a descriptive study. PCC and empathy were evaluated from self-assessment and observer's assessment using a video of real patients with chronic pain.

RESULTS. The results show that caregivers have demonstrated an intraindividual variability: PCC and empathetic behaviours of the participants were significantly higher for patients who have visible signs of pain (rheumatoid arthritis and complex regional pain syndrome) than for those who have no visible signs (Ehler–Danlos syndrome and fibromyalgia) ($p < 0.001$). Participants who show a greater difference in their patient-centered behaviour according to pain visibility have less clinical experience.

DISCUSSION. The pain visibility in chronic pain patients is an important factor contributing to an increased use of PCC and empathy by nurses and physicians, and clinical experience can influence their behaviours. Thus, pain invisibility can be a barrier to quality of care, and these findings reinforce the relevance to educating caregivers to these unconscious biases on their behaviour toward chronic pain patients.

1 INTRODUCTION

Chronic pain is a common public global health problem, associated with significant disability and many social consequences (Goldberg and McGee, 2011). Chronic pain affects people of all ages, with a particularly high prevalence in adults, ranging from 10 to 55% (Elzahaf et al., 2012). People with chronic pain are known to consult health professional frequently, leading in a heavy economic burden (Gaskin and Richard, 2012, Pizzo and Clark, 2012). To be effective, the treatment of chronic pain must consider biological, psychological, and social factors simultaneously (Jacobson and Mariano, 2001). Thus, the use of interdisciplinary patient-centered care (PCC) seems to be a promising avenue to address chronic pain management (Carter et al., 2014, Goertz et al., 2017).

There are many definitions of PCC in the context of nursing and medicine, but four dimensions are common to most cited definitions: patient-as-person, biopsychosocial perspective, sharing power and responsibility, and therapeutic alliance (Bilodeau et al., 2013, Hudon et al., 2011, McCormack and McCance, 2006). The use of this approach is related with many clinical benefits for patients with chronic pain (Goertz et al., 2017, Alamo et al., 2002, Monsivais and Engebretson, 2011, Taverner et al., 2014). More specifically, researchers have shown that PCC resulted in a decrease in the number of tender points and psychological distress in fibromyalgia patients (Alamo et al., 2002). Qualitative findings support that

PCC allows nurses to improve their assessment and to provide better anticipatory guidance and coaching (Monsivais and Engebretson, 2011).

In addition, many researchers suggest that empathy is necessary for the use of PCC (Bilodeau et al., 2013, Krasner et al., 2009, Passalacqua and Segrin, 2011). In the model of Bilodeau et al., "having an empathetic presence" is an important dimension of PCC (Bilodeau et al., 2013). In healthcare, empathy is defined as a cognitive attribute involving an understanding of the patient's experience and perspective, as a separate individual, combined with an ability to communicate that understanding to the patient (Hojat et al., 2002). Interestingly, it has been suggested that high levels of empathy were related to positive outcomes for patients (Larson and Yao, 2005, Neumann et al., 2007, Rakel et al., 2009) and especially with chronic pain patients (Canovas et al., 2017).

Although many studies support the benefits of PCC, (Haidet et al., 2002) its use in chronic pain management seems to be challenging and suboptimal (Canovas et al., 2017, Parsons et al., 2012). Patient-centered behaviour or communication does not necessarily translate into a "unique recipe," and caregivers seem to use a flexible style according to patient characteristics (Epstein et al., 2005). Over the last years, it has been suggested that several patient factors can influence the use of PCC, such as age, gender, and level of education (Bertakis and Azari, 2011, Willems et al., 2005, Zandbelt et al., 2006). For example, caregivers would tend to use more PCC behaviour with women, older, and nonsmoker patients (Bertakis and Azari, 2011, Zandbelt et al., 2006). Moreover, some authors have shown that physicians tend to use more PCC when patients reported more physical symptoms, such as nausea, dry mouth, or constipation, and when they rated patients' health condition as more severe (Zandbelt et al., 2006). However, in chronic pain context, little is known about the impact of the "visibility" of physical signs on patient-centered behaviour.

Patient factors may also influence caregivers' empathy. Indeed, both behavioral and functional neuroimaging measures have demonstrated that some stigma or prejudice could modulate empathy (Decety et al., 2009). Since many patients with chronic pain do not display any visible physical symptoms and remain stoic when they feel pain (Monsivais, 2013), it is important to assess the impact of this specific factor on patient-centered care and empathetic behaviour.

Various methods have been used for measuring the use of PCC and empathy, such as self-rating and observer rating (Hudon et al., 2011, Epstein et al., 2005, Hemmerdinger et al., 2007). Self-assessment instruments are the most common strategy used for measuring PCC and empathy, but they do not consider the influence of different patient factors such as the presence or absence of visible physical signs. The observation of PCC and empathy in real clinical encounters may raise some ethical and methodological issues, including the inability to have standardized visits, which introduces confounding variables. The use of standardized patient simulations is a very expensive strategy (Childs, 2002). Videos of real patients with chronic pain could overcome these limitations by allowing a standardized and repetitive assessment of attitudes and behaviours of caregivers (Paul-Savoie et al., 2015b).

Thus, the main objective of this study was to investigate the influence of the presence of visible physical signs on patient-centered and empathetic behaviours of nurses and physicians using videos of real patients suffering from chronic pain. In view of the limited knowledge on the topic, we also sought to identify, in an exploratory fashion, the characteristics of the caregivers who respond differently to the presence or absence of visible signs of pain.

2 MATERIALS AND METHODS

2.1 Study Design and Settings

This study is part of a larger study which investigated PCC and empathy in chronic pain management

(Paul-Savoie, n.d). A descriptive design was used, conducted from May to November 2013, in the province of Quebec, Canada. The Scientific and Human Ethics Committee of the institution where the study took place approved the research protocol. A population composed of nurses and physicians has been targeted since interdisciplinary pain management is recommended (Bilodeau et al., 2013). A convenience sampling approach was chosen, and participants were recruited through advertisements and referrals. Participants were recruited from 16 different healthcare centres, including urban, semiurban, and rural centres, in the province of Quebec, Canada.

2.2 Participants

All participants gave their written, informed consent, and a coding system was used to keep the data confidential. To take part in the study, the participants need to (i) be active members of the Quebec Board of Nurses or the Quebec College of Physicians, (ii) have chronic pain patients in their routine practice, and (iii) speak French. After signing the informed consent, a sample of 21 nurses and 21 physicians took part in the study. A minimum of 38 participants was needed to detect a moderate difference ($d = 0.5$) between visible and invisible pain conditions with a power of 85% and a type-1 error of 5%. Participants did not know the detailed purpose of the study to avoid social desirability bias, but they were informed that pain management was investigated.

2.3 Self-Assessment Measures

The practice orientation of each participant was measured with the French version of the Patient Practitioner Orientation Scale (F-PPOS) (Paul-Savoie et al., 2015a). (is self-administered questionnaire is designed for the assessment of practitioners' or future-practitioners' attitudes and orientations in their care approach. This scale contains 18 items divided into two subscales: "sharing" and "caring," and the four dimensions of PCC are represented. For each item, the caregiver is asked to indicate his or her level of agreement on a 6-point Likert scale (strongly agree to strongly disagree). A total score, ranging from patient-centered (a score of 6.00) to disease-centered (a score of 1.00), can be calculated with the addition of the two subscales. Th original version of the PPOS has good face validity and acceptable internal consistency for the total scale (an alpha of 0.89) (Krupat et al., 2000). The French version of the PPOS has good content validity and acceptable internal consistency for the total scale an (alpha of 0.60) (Krupat et al., 2000), since the minimum threshold is 0.50 (McHorney et al., 1994).

The self-rated empathy was measured with the French version of the Jefferson Scale of Physician Empathy (F-JSPE) (P. Bourgault, S. Lavoie, and M. Grégoire et al., unpublished data, June 2009). This self-administered questionnaire comprises 20 items divided into 4 dimensions: (i) adopting the patient's perspective, (ii) understanding the patient's experiences, feelings, and signals, (iii) ignoring the patient's perspective, and (iv) adopting the patient's way of thinking. The F-JSPE also includes a single item measuring the value placed on empathy. Participants respond to items on a 7- Likert scale. The total score, ranging from not empathic (a score of 20) to empathic (score of 140), can be calculated with the addition of all the items. The original version of the JSPE has good criterion-related validity with the Empathic Concern Scale of the Interpersonal Reactivity Index ($r = 0.40$), internal consistency (an alpha of 0.87 to 0.89), test-retest reliability (test-retest reliability coefficient = 0.65), and construct validity (Hojat et al., 2002, Hojat et al., 2003). The F-JSPE has good content validity and acceptable internal consistency (an alpha of 0.77) (P. Bourgault, S. Lavoie, and M. Gr´egoire et al., unpublished data, June 2009).

2.4 Observers' Assessment Measures

The PCC behaviour of each participant was measured with the Sherbrooke Observation Scale of patient-centered care (SOS-PCC) (Paul-Savoie et al., 2015b). (is instrument has been developed for the assessment of PCC behaviour of a professional caregiver by a trained observer, in the experimental clinical setting. Nine items divided into 4 dimensions (patient-as-person, biopsychosocial perspective, sharing power and responsibility, and therapeutic alliance) are measured on a 4-points Likert scale. The instrument was originally developed in French for a population of nurses and physicians. A total score, ranging from disease-centered (a score of 9) to patient-centered (a score of 36), can be calculated by the addition of all items. This instrument has good content validity, internal consistency (an alpha of 0.88), and inter-rater reliability (an intraclass coefficient (ICC) of 0.93) (Paul-Savoie et al., 2015b).

An adapted French version of Reynolds Empathy Scale (F-RES) has been used for the assessment of empathetic behaviour by a trained observer (Gosselin et al., 2015). The F-RES consists of 9 items with a categorical rating scale ("yes," "no," or "incomplete"). This instrument has good internal consistency (an alpha of 0.70) and inter-rater reliability (an ICC of 0.85) (Chan and Ahmad, 2011). In this study, we used a 7-item version with a 4-point Likert scale to make it more responsive to the context of videos. A total score, ranging from not empathetic (a score of 7) to empathetic (a score of 28), can be calculated by adding all items.

2.5 Procedure

All study participants watched four videos of real patients with chronic pain and were subsequently interviewed individually. These 4-minute videos showed female patients aged between 16 and 45 years-old, with different pathologies in which chronic pain was experienced (rheumatoid arthritis, complex regional pain syndrome (CRPS), Ehlers–Danlos syndrome, and fibromyalgia). A more detailed description of the development and content of these videos is available elsewhere (Paul-Savoie et al., 2015b). In these videos, some patients had no visible physical signs (Ehlers–Danlos syndrome and fibromyalgia) and others had obvious visible deformities in the upper limb (rheumatoid arthritis and CRPS). After viewing the videos, participants had to describe the management plan that they would provide for each patient, and these answers were video recorded. At the end of the session, each participant responded to the self-administrated questionnaires. After the data collection (n = 42 participants), three external observers watched the recorded interviews of each participant (4 interviews/participant). The group of observers consisted of a resident in psychiatry, a nurse, and a PhD student in the healthcare field. The observers were selected based on their experience in the healthcare field (more than five years) and their complementary expertise (medicine, nursing, and research). To ensure the standardization in their assessment, they had previously been trained by the research team to complete the observation scale. They evaluated the PCC and empathetic behaviour demonstrated by participants for each video using the SOS-PCC and the F-RES. Figure 20C1.1 showed the conduct of the study.

2.6 Data Analysis

Statistical analyzes were performed using the software SPSS version 18.0. To describe continuous variables, mean (standard deviation) was used, whereas frequency (percentage) was used for nominal and categorical variables. To compare patient-centered and empathetic behaviour of the participants (n = 42) according to the presence or absence of visible physical signs in the patients presented in the videos, paired T-tests were used on the mean score of the three observers. To investigate if the clinical experience can influence the modification of the behaviours according to the pain visibility, for each study participant, we calculated the difference of SOS-PCC and F-RES between the his/her behaviour for the patients with visible signs and the patients without visible signs. We divided the participants into two groups according to these differences: the participants who rated the two

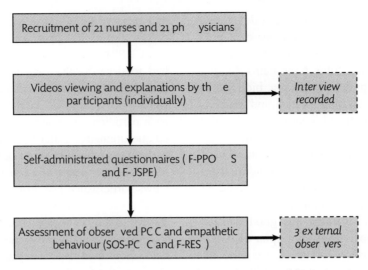

FIG. 20C1.1 Conduct of the study. F-PPOS indicates the French version of the Patient-Practitioner Orientation Scale, F-JSPE indicates the French version of the Jefferson Scale of Physician Empathy, PCC indicates patient-centered care, SOS-PCC indicates Sherbrooke Observation Scale of patient-centered care, and F-RES indicates the French version of the Reynolds Empathy Scale.

groups of patients similarly and those who rated the two groups of patients differently. To determine whether a participant showed similar or different behaviours, we have used the mean scores of SOS-PCC and F-RES for the thresholds. We used paired T-tests to compare the differences in clinical experience between the two groups study participants. The statistical level of significance was set at p < 0.05. We do not have any missing data.

3 RESULTS AND DISCUSSION

3.1 Participants' Characteristics

The sample included 42 native French-speaking caregivers ranging from 27 to 67 years (M= 46.12 years; SD = 10.84) and the majority was women (69%). Twenty-one (50%) of the participants were nurses, and 21 (50%) were physicians. Our sample was composed of nurses working in different settings, general practitioners, and medical specialists (physiatrist, rheumatologist, orthopaedist, radiologist, nephrologist, neurologist, and psychiatrist). The nurses and physicians had an average of 19.74 years of clinical experience. In this group, participants self-reported a mean overall orientation for PPC of 4.82. More specifically, the mean was 4.49 for the sharing subscale and 5.16 for the caring subscale. The participants self-reported a mean of 116.53 for empathy. These results suggest moderate levels of PCC and empathy when participants assess themselves. For the observer's assessment with observation scales, the results are presented for each video. For observed PCC, the mean for the 4 videos was 25.94, and for observed empathy, the mean was 20.70.

Table 20C1.1 shows the characteristics of these participants.

3.2 Patient-Centered and Empathetic Behaviour according to the Presence or Absence of Visible Physical Signs

In total, 168 interviews in response to the videos were videotaped successfully. We divided these interviews in two groups: (i) interviews in response to the videos presenting patients with visible physical signs (rheumatoid arthritis and

TABLE 20C1.1	
RESULTS OF SELF-ADMINISTRATED QUESTIONNAIRES.	
	PARTICIPANTS (N= 42)
Age, mean (SD)	46.12 (10.84)
Gender, n (%)	
Male	13 (31)
Female	29 (69)
Profession, n (%)	
Nurse	21 (50)
Physician	21 (50)
Clinical experience, mean (SD)	19.74 (10.34)
F-PPOS total, mean (SD)	4.82 (0.39)
Sharing, mean (SD)	4.49 (0.59)
Caring, mean (SD)	5.16 (0.37)
F-JSPE, mean (SD)	116.53 (9.80)
SOS-PCC, mean (SD)	25.94 (3.86)
Patient with rheumatoid arthritis, mean (SD)	27.12 (3.88)
Patient with CRPS, mean (SD)	27.38 (4.30)
Patient with Ehlers–Danlos syndrome, mean (SD)	26.02 (4.38)
Patient with fibromyalgia, mean (SD)	24.87 (5.11)
F-RES, mean (SD)	20.70 (3.41)
Patient with rheumatoid arthritis, mean (SD)	21.89 (3.59)
Patient with CRPS, mean (SD)	22.30 (3.25)
Patient with Ehlers–Danlos syndrome, mean (SD)	20.34 (3.81)
Patient with fibromyalgia, mean (SD)	18.94 (4.05)

SD = standard deviation; F-PPOS = French version of Patient-Practitioner Orientation Scale; F-JSPE = French version of Jefferson Scale of Physician Empathy; SOS-PCC = Sherbrooke Orientation Scale of patient-centered care; CRPS = complex regional pain syndrome; F-RES = French version of Reynolds Empathy Scale.

CRPS) and (ii) interviews in response to the videos presenting patients without visible physical signs (Ehlers–Danlos syndrome and fibromyalgia). Regarding the observed patient-centered

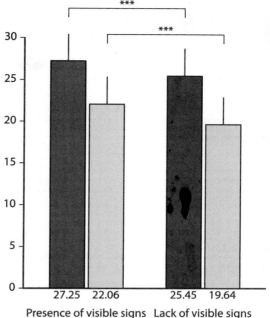

FIG. 20C1.2 Influence of pain visibility on patient-centered care and empathy. Patient-centered care and empathy behaviours were observed by external raters. SOS-PCC indicates Sherbrooke Orientation Scale of patient-centered care, and F-RES indicates French version of the Reynolds Empathy Scale.

and empathetic behaviours, the mean for SOS-PCC and F-RES was calculated for both groups. The results support that patient-centered and empathetic behaviour was significantly higher for the group of patients with visible physical signs ($p < 0.001$) (Figure 20C1.2). The group of participants who show a greater difference in their patient-centered behaviour according to pain visibility have less clinical experience than the group that had similar behaviour for both patients with and without physical visible signs ($p = 0.03$). For empathetic behaviour, the difference is not statistically significant ($p = 0.23$) (Table 20C1.2).

TABLE **20C1.2**

INFLUENCE OF CLINICAL EXPERIENCE ON CAREGIVERS' BEHAVIOURS IN THE PRESENCE OR ABSENCE OF PHYSICAL VISIBLE SIGNS.

	SIMILAR RATINGS	DIFFERENT RATINGS	P VALUE
PATIENT-CENTERED BEHAVIOUR			
n	14	28	
Clinical experience, years (SD)	24.64 (8.68)	17.29 (10.36)	0.03
EMPATHETIC BEHAVIOUR			
n	20	22	
Clinical experience, years (SD)	20.35 (9.73)	19.18 (11.05)	0.23

SD = standard deviation.

4 DISCUSSION

The results suggest that our sample of caregivers have moderate levels of self-reported PCC and empathy. In comparison with other studies, nurses and physicians who have participated in our study used more PCC than other groups of nurses and physicians with similar sociodemographic characteristics (Chan and Ahmad, 2011, Grilo et al., 2014). For self-reported empathy, our sample was comparable to other nurses and physicians (Fields et al., 2004).

The main purpose of this descriptive study was to investigate the influence of the presence or absence of visible physical signs on caregiver behaviours and attitudes in chronic pain management. PCC and empathy were assessed from two perspectives, using a combination of self-administrated questionnaires and observation scales using innovative videos of real patients with chronic pain. Our results show that nurses and physicians show intraindividual variability. Indeed, we found that PCC and empathetic behaviour of nurses and physicians vary according to the presence or absence of visible physical signs in patients with chronic pain. Interestingly, another research team have demonstrated that residents in internal medicine have displayed more patient-centered behaviour when they consider that the patient has a more severe health condition and

more visible physical symptoms (Zandbelt et al., 2006). In the same vein, another research group has demonstrated that patient-centered practice style of physicians was positively related with higher patient self-reported physical health status (Bertakis and Azari, 2011). Although the severity of the disease is not automatically associated with the presence of visible physical symptoms, the results of clinical observations have shown that patients with more severe diseases were given longer consultations and the opportunity to talk more about their medical condition (Graugaard et al., 2005). These observations have a great importance in the context of chronic pain, since these patients often have no visible physical signs, and can remain stoic when they feel pain (Monsivais, 2013) because their condition is often present for several years. For example, patients with neuropathic pain suffer from allodynia and hyperalgesia, but they often have no obvious physical signs. Moreover, some authors have suggested that professional caregivers were baffled by the lack of correlation between pain intensity verbally and nonverbally expressed by chronic pain patients and their medical condition (Allaz, 2003).

It has been shown that physicians tend to rely on their initial assessment of the pain of their patients with chronic pain even when this initial assessment underestimates the pain subsequently reported verbally by the patients (Riva et al., 2011). Thus, if chronic pain patients are not asked about their preoccupations and their medical condition's severity, stoic patients and those with less visible physical signs are more likely to receive suboptimal personalized care, with a more disease-centered orientation and less empathetic behaviour. These findings suggest that nurses and physicians adjust their practice orientation and empathy according to the clinical condition. It could explain why many patients with chronic pain are frustrated after their clinical encounters. This has a particular impact since these interactions are prominent in their experience (Riva et al., 2011).

Interestingly, we found that the clinical experience can influence the behaviours of nurses and physicians. Indeed, caregivers with more years of experience are less likely to change their behaviour were according to the presence or absence of physical visible signs. Many studies have investigated the influence of clinical experience on PCC and empathy (Neumann et al., 2011, Tsimtsiou et al., 2012), but little is known about how clinical experience could modulate these variables. A brain imaging study showed that clinical exposure could reduce empathy for pain (Cheng et al., 2007). More specifically, the authors investigated cortical activity among physicians and control subjects exposed to a series of visual stimuli with body parts in painful and painless situations. Their results indicated that the cortical structures associated with empathy for pain were significantly activated in the control subjects, but not in physicians. It is suggested that these observations are the consequence of a protective regulatory mechanism in people who work daily with pain in order to prevent their distress (Cheng et al., 2007). Thus, it is possible to believe that the behaviours of the most experienced caregivers are less influenced by the presence of visible signs of pain. However, our results show no difference in PCC and empathy levels according to the clinical experience ($p > 0.05$). It is also possible that the most experienced caregivers are more aware of the impact of pain visibility, and they consider this potential bias in their interventions. One potential limitation of our study is the lack of a real interaction between participants and patients in the videos. As a result of its methodological advantages and low cost, we used standardized videos of real chronic pain patients. However, the observation scales used for the assessment of PCC and empathetic behaviours were adapted for this kind of situation. Another potential limitation is the reactivity bias. It is possible that participants have positively modified their answers regarding the treatment plan that they would provide in reality. However, many efforts have been made to mitigate this potential bias. First, the participants did not know the variables under study at the time of data collection. Secondly, the questionnaires were distributed at the end of the experimental session in order to avoid a modification in behaviour, conscious or not, from participants.

5 CONCLUSIONS

In the last years, several studies have shown that practice orientation and empathy of professional caregivers could be influenced by many patients' factors (Riva et al., 2011, Tsimtsiou et al., 2012, Cheng et al., 2007), and our results are consistent with these previous findings. To our knowledge, this is the first study showing a direct influence of visible physical signs on PCC and empathy in the context of chronic pain management. Those observations are to be considered since chronic pain patients often do not show any apparent physical signs. (us, these patients are more likely to receive suboptimal pain management, more disease centered and devoid of empathic behaviour. (is raises the importance of educating caregivers and future caregivers to these unconscious biases and the potential impact on chronic pain patients. The impact of the presence or absence of apparent physical signs must also be considered for research in chronic pain since it is a potential confounding factor. Future studies could utilize real clinical encounters and other populations to replicate these results.

DATA AVAILABILITY

The data used to support the findings of this study are available from the corresponding author upon request.

DISCLOSURE

This work is part of a doctoral study. (is article is based on the thesis "Paul-Savoie E, Identification des caractéristiques des soignants liées à l'utilisation d'une approche centrée sur le patient dans un contexte de douleur chronique" (published doctoral thesis; https://doi.org/10.13039/100009874) (Université de Sherbrooke, Sherbrooke, Canada, https://savoirs. usherbrooke.ca/handle/11143/6974).

CONFLICTS OF INTEREST

The authors declare that there are no conflicts of interest.

ACKNOWLEDGMENTS

E. Paul-Savoie had at the time of the study a doctoral scholarship from the Canadian Institute of Health Research (CIHR) and was supported by the medicine and health science faculty of the Université de Sherbrooke. P. Bourgault was at the time of the study a Junior 1 Clinician Investigator with the Quebec Fund for Health Research FRQS) and researcher at the Centre de recherche du Centre hospitalier universitaire de Sherbrooke (CR-CHUS). S. Potvin was at the time of the study a Junior 1 Young Investigator from the FRQS and was supported by the Centre de recherche de l'Institut universitaire en santé mentale de Montréal and the Louis-H Lafontaine Hospital Foundation. E. Gosselin had doctoral scholarships from the FRQS, the Ministère de l'éducation supérieure, de la recherche et des sciences (MESRS)-Universités, and the Réseau de recherche en interventions en sciences infirmières du Québec. S. Lafrenaye was supported by the medicine and health science faculty of the Université de Sherbrooke and a researcher at the CRCHUS.

REFERENCES

Alamo, M. M., Moral, R. R., & de Torres, L. A. P. (2002). Evaluation of a patient-centred approach in generalized musculoskeletal chronic pain/fibromyalgia patients in primary care. *Patient Education and Counseling, 48*(1), 23–31.

Allaz, A. (2003). *Le Messager Boiteux: Approche Pratique des Douleurs Chroniques Rebelles, Genève: Médecine et Hygiène, in French, Lavoisier S.A.S.* Switzerland: Ch^ene-Bourg.

Bertakis, K. D., & Azari, R. (2011). Determinants and outcomes of patient-centered care. *Patient Education and Counseling, 85*(1), 46–52.

Bilodeau, K., Dubois, S., & Pepin, J. (2013). Contribution des sciences infirmières au développement des savoirs interprofessionnels. *Recherches en soins infirmiers, 113*(2), 43–50.

Canovas, L., Carrascosa, A. J., Garcia, M., et al. (2017). Impact of empathy in the patient-doctor relationship on chronic pain relief and quality of life: a prospective study in Spanish pain clinics. *Pain Medicine, 19*(7), 1304–1314.

Carter, J., Watson, A. C., & Sminkey, P. V. (2014). Pain management: screening and assessment of pain as part of a comprehensive case management process. *Professional Case Management, 19*(3), 126–134.

Chan, C. M. H., & Ahmad, W. A. W. (2011). Differences in physician attitudes towards patient-centredness: across four medical specialties. *International Journal of Clinical Practice, 66*(1), 16–20.

Cheng, Y., Lin, C. P., Li, H. L., et al. (2007). Expertise modulates the perception of pain in others. *Current Biology, 17*(19), 1708–1713.

Childs, J. (2002). Clinical resource centers in nursing programs. *Nurse Educator, 27*(5), 232–235.

Decety, J., Echols, S., & Correll, J. (2009). The blame game: the effect of responsibility and social stigma on empathy for pain. *Journal of Cognitive Neuroscience, 22*(5), 985–997.

Elzahaf, R. A., Tashani, O. A, Unsworth, B. A, et al. (2012). The prevalence of chronic an analysis of countries with a human development index less than 0.9: a systematic review without meta-analysis. *Current Medical Research and Opinion, 28*(7), 1221–1229.

Epstein, R. M., Franks, P., Fiscella, K., et al. (2005). Measuring patientcentered communication in patient-physician consultations: theoretical and practical issues. *Social Science and Medicine, 61*(7), 1516–1528.

Fields, S. K., Hojat, M., Gonnella, J. S., et al. (2004). Comparisons of nurses and physicians on an operational measure of empathy. *Evaluation and the Health Professions, 27*(1), 80–94.

Gaskin, D. J., & Richard, P. (2012). The economic costs of pain in the United States. *Journal of Pain, 13*(8), 715–724.

Goertz, C. M., Salsbury, S. A., Long, C. R., et al. (2017). Patient centered professional practice models for managing low back pain in older adults: a pilot randomized controlled trial. *BMC Geriatrics, 17*, 235–248.

Goldberg, D. S., & McGee, S. J. (2011). Pain as a global public health priority. *BMC Public Health, 11*(1), 770.

Gosselin, E., Paul-Savoie, E., Lavoie, S., et al. (2015). Reliability and validity of the French version of the Reynolds Empathy Scale in nursing. *Journal of Nursing Measurement, 23*, E16–E26.

Graugaard, P. K., Holgersen, K., Eide, H., et al. (2005). Changes in physician-patient communication from initial to return visits: a prospective study in a haematology outpatient clinic. *Patient Education and Counseling, 57*(1), 22–29.

Grilo, A. M., Santos, M. C., Rita, J. S., et al. (2014). Assessment of nursing students and nurses' orientation toward patient centeredness. *Nurse Education Today, 34*(1), 35–39.

Haidet, P., Dains, J. E., Paterniti, D. A., et al. (2002). Medical student attitudes toward the doctor-patient relationship. *Medical Education, 36*(6), 568–574.

Hemmerdinger, J. M., Stoddart, S., & Lilford, A. (2007). A systematic review of tests of empathy in medicine. *BMC Medical Education, 7*(1), 24.

Hojat, M., Gonnella, J. S., Mangione, S., et al. (2003). Physician empathy in medical education and practice: experience with the Jefferson scale of physician empathy. *Seminars in Integrative Medicine, 1*(1), 25–41.

Hojat, M., Gonnella, J. S., Nasca, T. J., et al. (2002). Physician empathy: definition, components, measurement, and relationship to gender and specialty. *American Journal of Psychiatry, 159*(9), 1563–1569.

Hudon, C., Fortin, M., Haggerty, J. L., et al. (2011). Measuring patients' perceptions of patient-centered care: a systematic review of tools for family medicine. *Annals of Family Medicine, 9*(2), 155–164.

Jacobson, L., & Mariano, A. J. (2001). General considerations of chronic pain. In J. D. Loeser, S. H. Butler, R. Chapman, & D. C. Turk (Eds.), *Bonica's Management of Pain* (pp. 241–254). Philadelphia, PA, USA: Lippincott Williams & Wilkins. Eds.

Krasner, M. S., Epstein, R. M., Beckman, H., et al. (2009). Association of an educational program in mindful communication with burnout, empathy, and attitudes among primary care physicians. *JAMA, 302*(12), 1284–1293.

Krupat, E., Rosenkranz, S. L., Yeager, C. M., et al. (2000). The practice orientations of physicians and patients: the effect of doctor patient congruence on satisfaction. *Patient Education and Counseling, 39*(1), 49–59.

Larson, E. B., & Yao, X. (2005). Clinical empathy as emotional labor in the patient-physician relationship. *JAMA, 293*(9), 1100–1106.

McCormack, B., & McCance, T. (2006). Developing a conceptual framework for person-centred nursing. *Journal of Advanced Nursing, 56*(5), 472–479.

McHorney, C. A., Ware, J. E., Lu, J. F. R., et al. (1994). The MOS 36-item short-form health survey (SF-36): III. Tests of data Pain Research and Management quality, scaling assumptions, and reliability across diverse patient groups. *Medical Care, 32*(1), 40–66.

Monsivais, D. B. (2013). Decreasing the stigma burden of chronic pain. *Journal of the American Association of Nurse Practitioners, 25*(10), 551–556.

Monsivais, D. B., & Engebretson, J. C. (2011). Cultural cues: review of qualitative evidence of patient-centered care in patients with nonmalignant chronic pain. *Rehabilitation Nursing, 36*(4), 166–171.

Neumann, M., Edelhauser, F., Tauschel, D., et al. (2011). Empathy decline and its reasons: a systematic review of studies with medical students and residents. *Academic Medicine, 86*(8), 996–1009.

Neumann, M., Wirtz, M., Bollschweiler, E., et al. (2007). Determinants and patient-reported long-term outcomes of physician empathy in oncology: a structural equation modelling approach. *Patient Education and Counseling, 69*(1–3), 63–75.

Parsons, S., Harding, G., Breen, A., et al. (2012). Will shared decision making between patient with chronic musculoskeletal pain and physiotherapists, osteopaths and chiropractors improve patient care?. *Family Practice, 29*(2), 203–212.

Passalacqua, S. A., & Segrin, C. (2011). The effect of resident physician stress, burnout, and empathy on patient-centered communication during the long-call shift. *Health Communication, 27*(5), 449–456.

Paul-Savoie, E., Bourgault, P., Gosselin, E., et al. (2015a). Assessing patient-centered care: validation of the French Version of the Patient-Practitioner

Orientation Scale (PPOS. *European Journal for Person Centered Healthcare, 3*(3), 295–302.

Paul-Savoie, E., Bourgault, P., Gosselin, E., et al. (2015b). Assessing patient-centered care for chronic pain: validation of a new research paradigm. *Pain Research and Management, 20*(4), 183–188.

Paul-Savoie, E. (2021). *Identification des caractéristiques des soignants liées à l'utilisation d'une approche centrée sur le patient dans un contexte de douleur chronique.* Canada: Sherbrooke Published doctoral thesis.

Pizzo, P. A., & Clark, N. M. (2012). Alleviating suffering 101–pain relief in the United States. *New England Journal of Medicine, 366*(3), 197–199.

Rakel, D. P., Hoeft, T. J., Barrett, B. P., et al. (2009). Practitioner empathy and the duration of the common cold. *Family Medicine, 41*(7), 494–501.

Riva, P., Rusconi, P., Montali, L., et al. (2011). The influence of anchoring on pain judgement. *Journal of Pain and Symptom Management, 42*(2), 265–277.

Taverner, T., Closs, S. J., & Briggs, M. (2014). The journey to chronic pain: a grounded theory of older adults' experience of pain associated with leg ulceration. *Pain Management Nursing, 15*, 186–198.

Tsimtsiou, Z., Benos, A., Garyfallos, A. A., et al. (2012). Predictors of physicians' attitudes toward sharing information with patients and addressing psychosocial needs: a cross-sectional study in Greece. *Health Communication, 27*(3), 257–263.

Willems, S., De Maesschalck, S., Deveugele, M., et al. (2005). Socioeconomic status of the patient and doctor-patient communication: does it make a difference?. *Patient Education and Counseling, 56*(2), 139–146.

Zandbelt, L. C., Smets, E. M., Oorf, F. J., et al. (2006). Determinants of physicians' patient-centred behaviour in the medical specialist encounter. *Social Science and Medicine, 63*(4), 899–910.

INTRODUCTION TO CRITIQUE 1

The article "The Impact of Pain Invisibility on Patient-Centered Care and Empathetic Attitude in Chronic Pain Management" by Paul-Savoie et al. (2018) is examined here in terms of its quality and the potential usefulness of the findings for application to nursing practice. The design of this study is level VI, inasmuch as it is a descriptive study.

Title

The title of the article captures the essence of the study succinctly.

Abstract

The abstract meets the requirements of a good abstract; it includes objectives, methods, results, and discussion.

Problem and Purpose

The significance of the problem was introduced clearly at the beginning of the article in the following statement: "the use of interdisciplinary patient-centered care (PCC) seems to be a promising avenue to address chronic pain management" (p. 466), but "several patient factors can influence the use of PCC and empathy, but little is known about the impact of pain visibility on these behaviours." (p. 467). In addition, the authors indicated that "caregivers seem to use a flexible style [of PCC] according to patient characteristics" (p. 467), and that "little is known about the impact of the "visibility" of physical signs on patient-care behaviour" (p. 467). This statement of the problem clearly presents a persuasive argument for the research. Paul-Savoie et al. (2018) stated that the overall purpose of the study was "to investigate the influence of the presence of visible physical signs on patient-centered and empathetic behaviours of nurses and physicians using videos of real patients suffering from chronic pain" (p. 467). This purpose statement includes the aim of the study and suggests the manner in which the research sought to study the problem, by using the word "investigate" (see Chapter 4).

Review of the Literature and Definitions

Paul-Savoie et al. (2018) used headings such as "Introduction" in which they present both the statement of the problem and the literature review. The introduction section guides the reader through the concepts of patient-centred care (PCC) and empathy.

Regarding patient-centred care, the authors reported that there are four dimensions to the concept. They are "patient-as-person, biopsychosocial perspective, sharing power and responsibility, and therapeutic alliance." The authors also have included studies that had shown clinical benefits of using the four dimensions in reducing chronic pain. The literature review also includes findings from qualitative studies that PCC allowed nurses to improve their assessment and provide better care.

The authors review the concept of empathy as it relates to PCC. After defining the concept of empathy, the authors explain the significance of empathy in reducing chronic pain and have used appropriate literature to support their claim. The authors argue that the use of PCC with chronic pain has been challenging or suboptimal. The literature review also includes different methodologies used with measuring PCC and empathy and highlighted some of the limitations of the methodologies used. In addition, Paul-Savoie et al. (2018) specified that "the observation of PCC and empathy in real clinical encounters may raise some ethical and methodological issues, including the inability to have standardized visits, which introduces confounding variables. The use of standardized patient simulations is a very expensive strategy (Childs, 2002). Videos of real patients with chronic pain could overcome these limitations by allowing a standardized and repetitive assessment of attitudes and behaviours of caregivers" (p. 467). This statement adds more credence to the rationale for the research. The authors concluded that the use of videos of real patients with chronic pain will address the limitations identified in the previous studies. All of the references were primary sources. The literature review provides a logical argument for Paul-Savoie et al's. (2018) study.

Development of a Conceptual Framework

Paul-Savoie et al. (2018) did not use any conceptual framework for the study.

Hypotheses and Research Question

There was no explicitly stated research question or hypotheses, but possible hypotheses could be "visible signs of chronic pain increase the use of PCC and empathy," and "pain invisibility is a barrier for PCC and empathy."

Sample

Paul-Savoie et al. (2018) described the sample, which consisted of 21 nurses and 21 physicians. The inclusion criteria were that the participants had to be (i) active members of the Quebec Board of Nurses or the Quebec College of Physicians, (ii) have chronic pain patients in their routine practice, and (iii) speak French. There were no exclusion criteria. The authors stated that a minimum of 38 participants was needed to detect a moderate difference (d = 0.5) between visible and invisible pain conditions with a power of 85% and a type-1 error of 5%; thus, the authors had an adequate sample size. Participants did not know the detailed purpose of the study to avoid social desirability bias, but they were informed that pain management was investigated.

Research Design

Paul-Savoie et al. (2018) stated that their design was a descriptive design that was appropriate for this study. Participants completed self-report scales on French version of the Patient Practitioner Orientation Scale (F-PPOS) and French version of the Jefferson Scale of Physician Empathy (F-JSPE).

Participants were shown videos of patients with and without physical signs of chronic pain, as it was deemed not ethical to use real clinical encounters. A trained member observed the PCC using Sherbrooke Observation Scale of patient-centred care (SOS-PCC) and empathy using French version of Reynolds Empathy Scale (F-RES). Training was done to increase reliability of the data.

Internal Validity

Although threats to internal validity are germane to research, researchers need to pay attention to factors in a nonexperimental design that may potentially compromise a study. Possible threats to internal validity include reactivity bias as participants knew that they were being observed.

External Validity

Generalizability is limited to this particular sample because the individuals were from a specific geographical area in Canada, Quebec and French-speaking participants. Thus, generalizing to other populations would be questionable. Also, the sample size limits generalizability.

Legal/Ethical Issues

Ethical approval was received from the Scientific and Human Ethics Committee of the institution where the study took place; this was necessary before the study could proceed.

Instruments

From the literature review, the authors chose the French version of the Patient Practitioner Orientation Scale (F-PPOS), French version of the Jefferson Scale of Physician Empathy (F-JSPE), Sherbrooke Observation Scale of Patient-Centered Care (SOS-PCC) for direct observation of PCC by a trained personnel, and the French version of Reynolds Empathy Scale (F-RES) for the assessment of empathetic behavior by a trained observer. The authors indicated how the items on each scale are rated.

Reliability and Validity

French version of the Patient Practitioner Orientation Scale (F-PPOS) is a valid tool with an alpha of 0.60, which is acceptable. The French version of the Jefferson Scale of Physician Empathy (F-JSPE) has a good alpha of 0.77 and Sherbrooke Observation Scale of patient-centred care (SOS-PCC) is with an alpha of 0.88, which is very good, and an interrater reliability of 0.93, which is excellent. The French version of Reynolds Empathy Scale (F-RES) has an alpha of 0.70 and an interrater reliability of 0.85.

Analysis of the Data and Findings

The demographic variables mentioned in the article are on a nominal scale of measurement. Gender, age, profession, and clinical experiences are measured on a nominal scale. There are no ordinal scale variables.

Descriptive statistics were reported as means and standard deviations in Table 20C1.1 (see p. 471). The authors report that the participants had a moderate level of PCC and empathy measured through the self-reported questionnaires.

The answer to the hypothesis lies in the following results. The results indicate that patient-centred and empathetic behaviour was significantly higher for the group of patients with visible physical signs ($p < 0.001$). The group of participants who show a greater difference in their patient-centred behaviour according to pain visibility have less clinical experience than the group that had similar behaviour for both patients with and without physical visible signs ($p = 0.03$). For empathetic behaviour, the difference is not statistically significant ($p = 0.23$). The interpretations and conclusions were based on the statistical inferences.

Discussion

The findings were explained within the context of previous research, similarities, and differences. Nurses and doctors often adjust their practice orientation and empathy according to the clinical condition. PCC and empathetic behaviours of nurses and doctors vary according to the presence or absence of visible physical signs in patients with chronic pain. The authors concluded that patients with chronic pain often did not have physical signs of chronic pain, and invisible physical signs of chronic pain is a barrier for optimal care.

Implications and Recommendations

Paul-Savoie et al. (2018) discussed the impact of chronic pain and the lack of visible signs of pain among patients experiencing chronic pain. The authors also made several recommendations to educate caregivers (present and future) to be conscious of the unconscious biases and understand the potential impact of chronic pain that will help in providing optimal care to patients experiencing chronic pain.

Study Limitation

The authors stated that the lack of interaction with the real patients is one of the limitations of the study. The authors also indicated that the tools that were used in this study were adapted for similar situation. The second limitation mentioned by the authors is the reactivity bias, and authors have taken steps like not informing the details of the study to the participants and administering the questionnaire after the observation to reduce this bias.

This study has significant contributions to the field of patient-centred care and empathetic behaviours of health care workers towards patients with obvious physical signs of pain. However, the results have to be viewed in the context of not having real patients but videotapes, and the PPC and empathy were assessed through self-reported questionnaires.

CRITIQUE 2   The study "The minimally effective dose of sucrose for procedural pain relief in neonates: a randomized controlled trial" by Stevens et al. (2018) is critiqued here. The article is presented in its entirety and is followed by the critique on pp. 491–493. (From *BMC Paediatrics*, 18(85),

The minimally effective dose of sucrose for procedural pain relief in neonates: a randomized controlled trial

Bonnie Stevens, Janet Yamada, Marsha Campbell-Yeo, Sharyn Gibbins, Denise Harrison, Kimberley Dionne, Anna Taddio, Carol McNair, Andrew Willan, Marilyn Ballantyne, Kimberley Widger, Souraya Sidani, Carole Estabrooks, Anne Synnes, Janet Squires, Charles Victor, Shirine Riahi

ABSTRACT

BACKGROUND: Orally administered sucrose is effective and safe in reducing pain intensity during single, tissue damaging procedures in neonates, and is commonly recommended in neonatal pain guidelines. However, there is wide variability in sucrose doses examined in research, and more than a 20-fold variation across neonatal care settings. The aim of this study was to determine the minimally effective dose of 24% sucrose for reducing pain in hospitalized neonates undergoing a single skin-breaking heel lance procedure.

METHODS: A total of 245 neonates from 4 Canadian tertiary neonatal intensive care units (NICUs), born between 24 and 42 weeks gestational age (GA), were prospectively randomized to receive one of three doses of 24% sucrose, plus non-nutritive sucking/pacifier, 2 min before a routine heel lance: 0.1 ml (Group 1; n = 81), 0.5 ml (Group 2; n = 81), or 1.0 ml (Group 3; n = 83). The primary outcome was pain intensity measured at 30 and 60 s following the heel lance, using the Premature Infant Pain Profile-Revised (PIPP-R). The secondary outcome was the incidence of adverse events. Analysis of covariance models, adjusting for GA and study site examined between group differences in pain intensity across intervention groups.

RESULTS: There was no difference in mean pain intensity PIPP-R scores between treatment groups at 30 s (P = .97) and 60 s (P = .93); however, pain was not fully eliminated during the heel lance procedure. There were 5 reported adverse events among 5/245 (2.0%) neonates, with no significant differences in the proportion of events by sucrose dose (P = .62). All events resolved spontaneously without medical intervention.

CONCLUSIONS: The minimally effective dose of 24% sucrose required to treat pain associated with a single heel lance in neonates was 0.1 ml. Further evaluation regarding the sustained effectiveness of this dose in reducing pain intensity in neonates for repeated painful procedures is warranted.

TRIAL REGISTRATION: ClinicalTrials.gov: NCT02134873. Date: May 5, 2014 (retrospectively registered).

KEYWORDS: Adverse event, Analgesia, Heel lance, Neonates, NICU, Pain, PIPP-R, Preterm infants, Sucrose

Paul-Savoie, E., Bourgault, P., Potvin, S., Gosselin, E., & Lafrenaye, S. (2018). The impact of pain invisibility on patient-centered care and empathetic attitude in chronic pain management. *Pain Research and Management, 2018.* https://doi.org/10.1155/2018/6375713

Stevens, B., Yamada, J., Campbell-Yeo, M., Gibbins, S., Harrison, D., Dionne, K., Taddio, A., McNair, C., Willan, A., Ballantyne, M., Widger, K., Sidani, S., Estabrooks, C., Synnes, A., Squires, J., Victor, C., & Riahi, S. (2018). The minimally effective dose of sucrose for procedural pain relief in neonates: A randomized controlled trial. *BMC Pediatrics, 18*(1), 85. https://doi.org/10.1186/s12887-018-1026-x

BACKGROUND

Multiple trials and recent systematic reviews with meta- analyses have shown that sweet solutions, including orally administered sucrose, are effective and safe in reducing pain intensity (using clinical observational or composite measures) during single, tissue-damaging procedures in neonates (Bueno et al., 2013, Stevens et al., 2016). These solutions are commonly recommended in neonatal pain guidelines (Lee et al., 2014). However, there is wide variability in sucrose doses examined in research, and more than a 20-fold variation across neonatal care settings (Taddio et al., 2009b). Despite the large number of randomized controlled trials in the 2016 Cochrane review (Stevens et al., 2016), an optimal dose of sucrose could not be determined due to the wide range of volumes and concentrations (0.05 ml of 24% to 2.0 ml of 50% solution) studied, and due to variation in study methods (e.g., administration techniques, types of painful procedures, outcome measures, and co-interventions). There are no definitive conclusions about the minimally effective dose of sucrose associated with a clinically significant reduction in pain intensity scores in neonates.

To our knowledge, there have been no direct comparisons of different volumes of sucrose at the same concentration. In this study, we evaluated the three smallest doses of sucrose most commonly reported to be effective in previous research (i.e., 0.1 ml, 0.5 ml, and 1.0 ml of 24% sucrose) (Stevens et al., 2016) to determine the minimally effective dose for neonates undergoing a skin-breaking heel lance procedure while in the neonatal intensive care unit (NICU). Doses smaller than 0.1 ml were not included in the study due to challenges posed by accurate measurement and delivery. All neonates received sucrose for procedural pain (i.e., there was no placebo or no- treatment group), which was consistent with neonatal pain guidelines and in keeping with the ethical conduct of clinical trials in newborns (Bellieni and Johnston, 2016, Campbell-Yeo, 2016, Harrison et al., 2010). We hypothesized that (a) there was no difference in pain intensity between the sucrose doses, measured at 30 and 60 s following the heel lance using the Premature Infant Pain Profile-Revised (PIPP-R), and (b) adverse events would be minimal.

METHODS

A prospective multi-centered single-blind randomized controlled trial was conducted from July 2013–April 2015 at 4 Canadian tertiary NICUs following research ethics approval. The inclusion criteria were neonates 24 to 42 weeks gestational age (GA) at birth and less than 30 days of life/or less than 44 weeks GA at the time of the intervention, scheduled to receive a heel lance, and who had not received opioids within 24 h prior to the heel lance. The exclusion criteria were neonates with a contraindication for sucrose administration (e.g., were too ill or unstable as per neonatologist's assessment, unable to swallow, pharmacologically muscle relaxed) and/or inability to assess behavioral responses to pain accurately (e.g., the neonate's face was blocked with taping). We did not use the diagnosis of neurological impairment as an exclusion criterion because the timing of diagnosis and determining the severity of impairment can be very difficult in this population. However, inability to swallow had the effect of excluding neonates with severe neurologic impairment from hypoxic-ischemic encephalopathy. Observation of the procedure was timed to ensure that no additional sucrose doses were provided within the previous 4 h. All parents or legal guardians provided informed consent.

Randomization was performed using a web-based privacy protected randomization service (Randomize.net 2015). Randomization was block stratified by GA at birth (< 29 weeks or 29– 42 weeks) to enhance balanced intervention groups. A research nurse, aware of group allocation, drew up the assigned sucrose dose into an amber colored syringe. The dose was double-checked by a second nurse, not involved with the study, and documented on the medication administration record as per unit protocol. The research nurse followed a standard dose administration time to blind the bedside nurse performing the heel lance to the sucrose volume. The syringes used to administer sucrose were also shielded from view by the re-search nurse from the bedside nurse and video recording. No other study personnel had access to the treatment allocation.

The treatment intervention was videotaped and included 4 phases. (a) Baseline observation of the neonate for 2 min prior to the heel lance. (b) Administering the total volume of 24% sucrose [0.1 ml(Group 1), 0.5 ml (Group 2), or 1.0 ml (Group 3)] drop-by-drop via syringe over the anterior surface of the tongue, allowing for individual neonate swallowing rates over a period of 1–2 min (for the largest dose). A pacifier was offered to all neonates immediately following sucrose administration to facilitate non-nutritive sucking, which has been shown to enhance sucrose efficacy in a synergistic way (Stevens et al., 1999). (c) Conducting the heel lance procedure with an automated lancet approximately 2 min after the sucrose administration, to allow for peak effects (Blass and Shide, 1994). (d) Observation of return-to-baseline pain indicator values over 30 s to several minutes. The bedside nurse conducted the heel lance according to the specific unit policy, while the research nurse experienced in NICU care ensured complete data collection.

We did not limit participating neonates from receiving other pain-relieving parent-initiated interventions (e.g., skin-to-skin/kangaroo care and breastfeeding) (Pillai Riddell et al., 2015) as per unit protocols. These were documented by the research nurse, so any group differences could be controlled for in the analysis. Pharmacological interventions shown to be ineffective in reducing heel lance pain (e.g., acetaminophen) (Ohlsson and Shah, 2015) were not administered.

OUTCOME MEASURES

The primary outcome was pain intensity measured with the PIPP-R (Gibbins et al., 2014, Stevens et al., 2014), which has demonstrated construct validity in neonates of varying GA (Gibbins et al., 2014, Stevens et al., 2014,

Lee and Stevens, 2014). The PIPP-R includes 2 physiological (heart rate, oxygen saturation), 3 behavioral (brow bulge, eye squeeze, nasolabial furrow) and 2 contextual (GA, behavioral state) variables known to modify pain responses. Throughout the treatment intervention, physiological and behavioral/facial indicators of pain intensity were collected using an infant monitoring system developed and used extensively by the research team over the past decade. The research nurse placed pulse oximetry probes on the neonate to record heart rate and oxygen saturation continuously, and positioned a digital video recorder to capture facial movements. Electronic event markers synchronized all physiological and behavioral data and demarcated the 4 phases of the treatment intervention.

Two trained coders, blinded to group allocation and study purpose, viewed the physiological and behavioral data captured by the infant monitoring system, and coded neonates' pain intensity using the PIPP-R. An inter-rater reliability > 0.9 was achieved on a random sample of 5 neonates, early in the study and with each 25% of data collected.

The secondary outcome was frequency of a priori specified adverse event/tolerance criteria (heart rate > 240 beats/min or heart rate < 80 beats/min for > 20 s; oxygen saturation < 80% for > 20 s; no spontaneous respirations for > 20 s; and choking/gagging). Adverse event data were collected by the research nurse during the intervention. The research nurse kept a record of 'rescue doses' administered (i.e., additional doses of sucrose given on direction of the nurse caring for the neonate, if the neonate became overly distressed during the procedure).

STATISTICAL ANALYSES

We estimated a sample size of 71 neonates per group (total sample size of 213). The sample size calculation accounts for multiple testing due to 3 intervention groups, and is based on a type I error probability of 5%, a power of 80%, and a smallest minimally clinic- ally significant difference of 1 on the PIPP-R with a standard deviation (SD) of 2. Consistent with previous research, this minimally clinically significant difference was justifiable given the lack of a treatment control in this study versus preceding studies (Campbell-Yeo et al., 2012). To account for potential missing data (e.g., equipment failure), we increased the sample size by 15% to 245. Analysis of covariance models adjusting for GA and study site examined between group differences in PIPP-R scores.

RESULTS
Randomization and demographic characteristics

The trial profile is presented in Fig. 20C2.1. Of the 4172 neo- nates screened for eligibility, 248 were enrolled and randomly allocated to Group 1, 2 or 3. Three neonates were excluded following randomization, as they did not undergo a heel lance, leaving 245 for the outcomes analyses. Demographic characteristics in all 3 groups were adequately matched (Table 20C2.1). These included GA at birth, days since birth, birth weight, sex, severity of illness assessed using the Score for Neonatal Acute Physiology Perinatal Extension-II (SNAPPE-II) (Harsha and Archana, 2015, Richardson et al., 2001), number of prior painful procedures, number of previous doses of sucrose, and concurrent use of non- pharmacologic pain strategies. As standard care in each unit included parent-initiated non-pharmacologic strategies (e.g., swaddling, skin-to-skin/kangaroo care, and breastfeeding) we could not ethically disallow these interventions during the painful procedure. However, there was no difference in the use of parent-initiated pain strategies across groups (Table 20C2.1). All neonates were offered a pacifier for non-nutritive sucking following sucrose administration. Overall 204/ 245 (83.2%) sucked on the pacifier, while the remainder refused or did not receive the pacifier due to medical considerations (e.g., intubated, or not tolerated well). We noted a discrepancy between the number of painful procedures documented and the number of sucrose doses documented since birth. Information on non-pharmacologic interventions was often not available in the neonates' medical records; therefore, it was difficult to discern if the discrepancy was an administration or documentation issue.

Pain intensity

The mean pain intensity [SD] PIPP-R scores at 30 s post heel lance (Group 1 6.8[3.5]; Group 2 6.8[3.2]; Group 3 6.7[3.4]) were not statistically different after adjusting for GA and research site (F[6233] = 0.01, P= .97; Table 20C2.2). Similarly, there were no significant differences in mean PIPP-R scores between groups at 60 s (F [2229] = 0.10, P = .93; Table 20C2.2). Mean pain intensity PIPP-R scores at 30 and 60 s were inversely associated with GA (P < .001) and significantly different when stratified by site (P < .001; Table 20C2.3); therefore both factors were controlled for in the analysis. Mean PIPP-R scores ranged from 6.03 (3.37) for neonates > 36 weeks GA to 9.07 (4.00) for neonates < 28 weeks GA at 30 s and 5.70 (3.31) for neonates > 36 weeks GA to 9.43 (4.04) for neonates < 28 weeks GA. No associations were found between pain intensity scores and other demographic characteristics [i.e., SNAPPE-II/ severity of illness on admission, gender, concurrent use of non-pharmacologic pain strategies (e.g. breastfeeding and skin-to-skin care), and number of painful procedures and sucrose doses since birth; Table 20C2.3]. Pain intensity scores across the 3 groups equated to mild pain for the majority of neonates (scores of < 7 on the PIPP-R; Table 20C2.4).

ADVERSE EVENTS AND RESCUE DOSES

There were 5 reported adverse events among 5/245 (2.0%) neonates as defined by the a priori criteria. These events included 3 neonates who

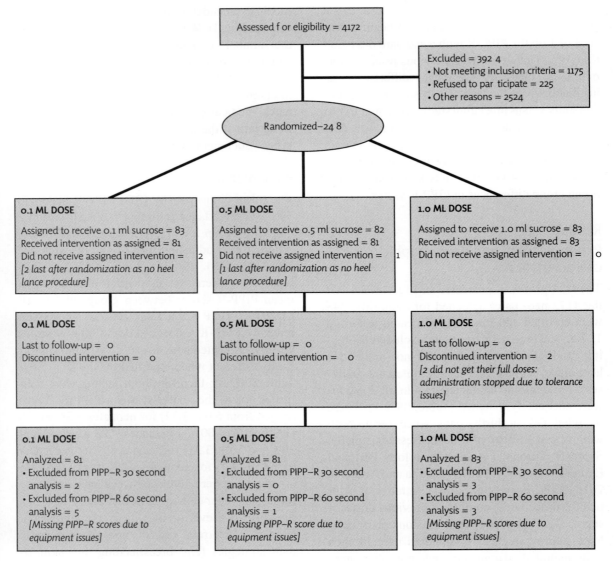

FIG. 20C2.1 Consort flow diagram of all neonates in participating NICUs screened for eligibility and randomized to sucrose intervention groups. Reasons for exclusion included not meeting inclusion criteria, refusals to participate, and other reasons [e.g., exclusion criteria, medical refusal (palliative care, social issues, and multiple research studies), isolation precautions, and researcher or parents unavailable for consent discussion].

gagged/choked, 1 with heart rate < 80 bpm and 1 with oxygen saturation < 80% following sucrose administration. All events resolved spontaneously without medical intervention. The neonate who experienced oxygen saturation < 80%, was repositioned and recovered quickly. There were no significant differences in the proportion of adverse events by sucrose group (P = .62); however, a higher proportion of younger neonates experienced an adverse event (6.7% < 29 weeks versus 1.0% 29–42 weeks; P = .044). In 13/245 (5.3%) neonates, the bedside nurse perceived that

TABLE 20C2.1

DEMOGRAPHIC CHARACTERISTICS OF THE SUCROSE INTERVENTION GROUPS

	INTERVENTION		
	0.1 ml *n* = 81	0.5 ml *n* = 81	1.0 ml *n* = 83
Sex, n (%)			
–Female	44 (54.3)	32 (39.5)	41 (49.4)
– Male	37 (45.7)	49 (60.5)	42 (50.6)
Gestational age in weeks, mean (SD)	32.6 (4.2)	32.5 (4.1)	32.7 (4.1)
Weight in grams, mean (SD)	2002.3 (859.5)	1933.0 (927.0)	2055.5 (886.0)
Day of life, median (interquartile range)	6 (4 to 9)	7 (4 to 10)	6 (4 to 9)
Birthplace, n (%) (55 missing)			
– Inborn	31 (52.5)	33 (51.6)	40 (59.7)
– Outborn	28 (47.5)	31 (48.4)	27 (40.2)
SNAPPE-II score on admission, median (interquartile range)	5.0 (0 to 19)	5.0 (0 to 18)	8.0 (0 to 18)
Number of painful procedures since birth, median (interquartile range)	22 (14 to 34)	23 (15 to 37)	23 (13 to 40)
Number of sucrose doses since birth, median (interquartile range)	5 (2 to 8)	5 (3 to 9)	6 (3 to 9)
Use of concurrent non-pharmacologic pain strategies, n (%)	27 (33.3)	31 (35.2)	30 (34.1)

SNAPPE-II scores range from 0 to 158. Higher scores indicate greater severity of illness

TABLE 20C2.2

MEAN PAIN INTENSITY SCORES AT 30S AND 60S POST HEEL LANCE

	INTERVENTION			P
	0.1 ml	0.5 ml	1.0 ml	
PIPP-R 30s	n= 79	n= 81	n= 80	
	Mean (SD): 6.8 (3.5)	Mean (SD): 6.8 (3.2)	Mean (SD): 6.7 (3.4)	0.97
	Min: 0	Min: 1.0	Min: 0	
	Max: 17.5	Max: 16.3	Max: 18.7	
PIPP-R 60s	n= 76	n= 80	n= 80	
	Mean (SD): 7.0 (3.3)	Mean (SD): 6.9 (3.6)	Mean (SD): 6.7 (3.4)	0.93
	Min: 0	Min: 0	Min: 0	
	Max: 17.0	Max: 18.0	Max: 18.7	

PIPP-R scores range from 0 to 21. Higher scores indicate greater pain intensity

the intervention was not effective in minimizing pain during the procedure, and the research nurse (at the discretion of the bedside nurse) administered a "res- cue" dose of sucrose (amount determined by the unit standard/policy). There was no significant difference in the number of rescue doses by sucrose group (P = .33), site (P = .070), or GA (P = .47).

TABLE **20C2.3**

ASSOCIATION OF MEAN PAIN INTENSITY SCORES WITH SITE AND DEMOGRAPHIC CHARACTERISTICS

	PIPP-R 30 SECONDS		PIPP-R 60 SECONDS	
	MEAN (SD)	P	MEAN (SD)	P
Site		< 0.001		< 0.001
1	5.68 (3.31)		5.66 (3.26)	
2	7.55 (3.58)		8.09 (4.16)	
3	6.13 (2.31)		6.05 (2.54)	
4	8.21 (3.87)		8.23 (3.55)	
SNAPPE-II score on admission		0.087		0.058
– Median or below (0 to 5)	6.35 (3.06)		6.38 (3.22)	
– Above Median (6+)	7.03 (3.53)		7.17 (3.70)	
Gender	0.31 (3.32)	0.44	−0.05 (3.49)	0.90
Concurrent use of non-pharmacologic pain strategies during heel lance	0.38 (3.31)	0.33	0.10 (3.49)	0.82
Gestational age	Spearman's correlation (r_s)−0.26	$P < 0.001$	Spearman's correlation (r_s)− 0.30	$P < 0.001$
Number of painful procedures	0.07	0.24	0.03	0.61
Number of sucrose doses since birth	0.004	0.95	−0.02	0.74

PIPP-R scores range from 0 to 21. Higher scores indicate greater pain intensity. SNAPPE-II scores range from 0 to 158. Higher scores indicate greater severity of illness

TABLE **20C2.4**

FREQUENCY OF PAIN INTENSITY SCORES BY SEVERITY AT 30S AND 60S POST HEEL LANCE

	INTERVENTION			P
	0.1 ml	0.5 ml	1.0 ml	
PIPP-R at 30s, n (%)	n = 79	n = 81	n = 80	0.74
– None (0)	2 (2.5)	0 (0.0)	2 (2.5)	
– Mild (1 to 6.9)	40 (50.6)	46 (56.8)	39 (48.8)	
– Moderate (7 to 11.9)	30 (38.0)	27 (33.3)	33 (41.3)	
– Severe (12+)	7 (8.9)	8 (9.9)	6 (7.5)	
PIPP-R at 60s, n (%)	n = 76	n = 80	n = 80	0.97
– None (0)	1 (1.3)	1 (1.3)	2 (2.5)	
– Mild (1 to 6.9)	38 (50.0)	44 (55.0)	41 (51.3)	
– Moderate (7 to 11.9)	29 (38.2)	26 (32.5)	30 (37.5)	
– Severe (12+)	8 (10.5)	9 (11.3)	7 (8.8)	

PIPP-R scores range from 0 to 21. Higher scores indicate greater pain intensity

DISCUSSION

Oral administration of a very small dose of sucrose (0.1 ml) appears to be equally effective at reducing pain in neonates during a single painful procedure as larger doses. Sucrose administration in the clinical setting was associated with very few adverse events. This trial was more closely aligned with a pragmatic design on the continuum between pragmatic and exploratory trials (Patsopoulos, 2011). Unlike explanatory trials that test interventions under optimal conditions, pragmatic trials are more generalizable; however, they are also more prone to co- intervention.

Although site was controlled for in the primary out- come analyses, there was a difference in PIPP-R scores across sites (Table 20C2.3) that may be partially explained by organizational contextual factors that were not con- trolled for or assessed in the analyses. For example, although we enrolled neonates in the first 30 of days of life and collected information on exposure to painful procedures and sucrose received since birth, it is possible that sucrose administration and documentation practices differed due to clinical practice guidelines or organizational contextual factors (e.g., workload/staff ratios, unit culture, and the research or clinical experience of the bedside nurses) (Estabrooks et al., 2011). We also found higher pain scores were associated with more preterm neonates (P < .001; Table 20C2.3) and they experienced a slightly greater proportion of adverse events (3 versus 2 in neonates > 29 weeks GA), although total numbers were very small. Despite higher pain scores with lower GA, there was no difference in the number of rescue doses across GA, which might be explained by site differences in sucrose administration practices.

We could think of two possible explanations for why PIPP-R scores were significantly higher in the least mature group of neonates: (a) the PIPP-R measure inherently scores younger GA higher, or b) sucrose is less effective in these babies (e.g., they are less able to mount an endogenous opioid response that is the underlying mechanism of action of sweet taste (Johnston et al., 2008)). Differences seen in mean pain intensity were not thought to be due to additional weighting in the PIPP-R measure by GA [< 28 weeks (+ 3), 28–31 weeks and 6 days (+ 2), 32 weeks to 35 weeks and 6 days (+ 1), and ≥ 36 weeks (0)], as there were no corresponding incremental differences seen by GA group. In terms of the latter explanation (b), this needs to be further researched with an adequate sample size of extremely premature neonates (< 28 weeks GA).

Our findings are consistent with past research (primarily in animals) that demonstrated that the analgesic effects of sucrose were primarily mediated by exposure and not dose (Blass and Shide, 1994, Anseloni et al., 2002). Although there was no difference in pain intensity at 30 and 60 s, pain was not fully eliminated during the heel lance procedure. Mean pain intensity scores equated to mild pain (Table 20C2.2), or approximately 3/10 if converted to the more common 10- point scale metric. As pain intensity was measured on a continuum, and treatment failure was not defined, the incidence of treatment failure was not determined. How- ever, severe pain could definitely be considered a treatment failure and this occurred in 7.5 to 11.3% of neonates (Table 20C2.4) across sucrose doses. These results are similar to systematic reviews of other behavioral interventions, including breastfeeding (Shah et al., 2012) and skin-to-skin care (Johnston et al., 2014). Given that the majority of previous studies have used a single procedure, it is uncertain if the wide variably in neonatal pain response is attributed to the intervention or other factors which remain unknown (Cignacco et al., 2009). Future work in the repeated use of interventions is warranted. In the meantime, we would recommend that if the initial dose of sucrose does not appear to be ameliorating the pain that additional rescue doses be provided during the procedure up to a specified amount. We would also recommend that multiple non-pharmacologic strategies be implemented simultaneously including swaddling, facilitated tucking, skin-to-skin/ kangaroo care, breastfeeding, and/ or pacifiers.

Knowledge is lacking on the long-term effects of sucrose with repeated administration. Of the studies that have evaluated repeated doses of sucrose (Johnsston et al., 2002, Stevens et al., 2005, Gaspardo et al., 2008, Taddio et al., 2009a, Harrison et al., 2009), none have evaluated long-term outcomes of using sucrose for all painful procedures performed throughout the neonate's stay in the NICU. Johnston (Johnsston et al., 2002, Johnston et al., 2007) reported that 107 pre-term infants < 31 weeks GA who were exposed to > 10 doses of sucrose per day in the first 7 days of life, after which time no pain relief was used, were more likely to exhibit poorer attention and motor development on the Neurobehavioral Assessment of Preterm Infants (NAPI) scale in the early months of life. Conversely, Banga (Banga et al., 2016) reported that of 93 neonates randomized to either repeated doses of sucrose or water for painful procedures for 7 consecutive days, there were no significant differences in NAPI scores or adverse events. Stevens (Stevens et al., 2005) found no statistically significant differences between sucrose plus pacifier, water plus pacifier, or the standard care group on neurobiological risk status outcomes. Future research needs to address the repeated use of minimally effective doses of sucrose on the neurodevelopment of neonates and effective- ness over time.

Approximately 2% of neonates suffered adverse events. These all resolved spontaneously without medical intervention or with minimal caregiver intervention (e.g. positioning). Most adverse events occurred at one site, where the highest proportion of the sickest neonates is cared for, although this is not represented in the study sample. This adverse event rate is consistent with the 2016 Cochrane sucrose review (Stevens et al., 2016). Although researchers are becoming more vigilant in observing and reporting adverse events, it remains unclear how adverse events are reported (i.e., chart review is considerably different from careful direct observation of every newborn infant who is receiving the intervention).

A few study limitations need mention. Pain intensity did not differ significantly between the 30 and 60-s time points. Although these time intervals have been used in multiple research studies of acute procedural pain, they are arbitrary and designed based on mean behavioral response time; observing neonates for longer periods of time may demonstrate additional responses of less typical responders or other types of responses (e.g. physiologic, cortical). Although there has been significant validation and updating of the PIPP-R measure, there remains no gold standard for measuring pain in infants that may influence the de- termination of the effectiveness (or lack thereof) of pain relieving interventions. The future, which includes novel strategies for better understanding of the developing cortical pain circuitry, will pave the way for better prevention and treatment of pain in this vulnerable population.

Finally, we were limited by the documentation in the medical records, which may not have included all pain-relieving strategies such as sucrose and non-pharmacologic interventions. Although we believe infants should receive some form of intervention for all painful procedures, it is difficult to speculate on whether the discrepancy between number of documented painful procedures and pain-relieving interventions an administration or documentation issue is. As the number of painful procedures included since birth was extensive (e.g., tape removals, bloodwork, injections, vascular access attempts/insertions, NG/ OG tube insertions and suctioning, chest tube attempts/insertions, lumbar punctures, eye exams, and urinary catheterizations), it is possible oral sucrose is not routinely administered for each of these types of procedures, depending on unit standards/practices.

CONCLUSIONS

No difference in pain intensity was shown among 3 doses of sucrose during an acute tissue-damaging procedure in hospitalized neonates. The 0.1 ml of 24% sucrose dose was the minimally effective dose that can be recommended for use out of the 3 doses most commonly reported to be effective in previous research. Subsequent study is required to determine the sustained effectiveness of this dose in reducing pain intensity during painful procedures neonates experience in the NICU over time and across GA, and the long-term effects of cumulative sucrose use.

ABBREVIATIONS

GA: Gestational age; NAPI: Neurobehavioral assessment of preterm infants; NICU: Neonatal intensive care unit; PIPP-R: Premature infant pain profile- revised; SD: Standard deviation; SNAPPE-II: Score for neonatal acute physiology perinatal extension- II

REFERENCES

Anseloni, VC, Weng, HR, Terayama, R, Letizia, D, Davis, BJ, Ren, K, et al. (2002). Age- dependency of analgesia elicited by intraoral sucrose in acute and persistent pain models. *Pain, 97*(1–2), 93–103.

Banga, S, Datta, V, Rehan, HS, & Bhakhri, BK. (2016). Effect of sucrose analgesia, for repeated painful procedures, on short-term neurobehavioral outcome of preterm neonates: a randomized controlled trial. *J Trop Pediat, 62*(2), 101–106.

Bellieni, CV, & Johnston, CC. (2016). Analgesia, nil or placebo to babies, in trials that test new analgesic treatments for procedural pain. *Acta Paediatr, 105*(2), 129–136.

Blass, EM, & Shide, DJ. (1994). Some comparisons among the calming and pain- relieving effects of sucrose, glucose, fructose and lactose in infant rats. *Chem Senses, 19*(3), 239–249.

Bueno, M, Yamada, J, Harrison, D, Khan, S, Ohlsson, A, Adams-Webber, T, et al. (2013). A systematic review and meta-analyses of nonsucrose sweet solutions for pain relief in neonates. *Pain Res Manage, 18*(3), 153–161.

Campbell-Yeo, M. (2016). First, do no harm'–the use of analgesia or placebo as control for babies in painful clinical trials. *Acta Paediatr, 105*(2), 119–120.

Campbell-Yeo, ML, Johnston, CC, Joseph, KS, Feeley, N, Chambers, CT, & Barrington, KJ. (2012). Cobedding and recovery time after heel lance in preterm twins: results of a randomized trial. *Pediatrics, 130*(3), 500–506.

Cignacco, E, Denhaerynck, K, Nelle, M, Buhrer, C, & Engberg, S. (2009). Variability in pain response to a non-pharmacological intervention across repeated routine pain exposure in preterm infants: a feasibility study. *Acta Paediatr, 98*(5), 842–846.

Estabrooks, CA, Squires, JE, Hutchinson, AM, Scott, S, Cummings, GG, Kang, SH, et al. (2011). Assessment of variation in the Alberta context tool: the contribution of unit level contextual factors and specialty in Canadian pediatric acute care settings. *BMC Health Ser Res, 11*(1), 1.

Gaspardo, CM, Miyase, CI, Chimello, JT, & Martinez, FE (2008). Martins Linhares MB. Is pain relief equally efficacious and free of side effects with repeated doses of oral sucrose in preterm neonates?. *Pain, 137*(1), 16–25.

Gibbins, S, Stevens, BJ, Yamada, J, Dionne, K, Campbell-Yeo, M, Lee, G, et al. (2014). Validation of the premature infant pain profile-revised (PIPP-R). *Early Hum Dev, 90*(4), 189–193.

Harrison, D, Bueno, M, Yamada, J, Adams-Webber, T, & Stevens, B. (2010). Analgesic effects of sweet-tasting solutions for infants: current state of equipoise. *Pediatrics, 126*(5), 894–902.

Harrison, D, Loughnan, P, Manias, E, Gordon, I, & Johnston, L. (2009). Repeated doses of sucrose in infants continue to reduce procedural pain during prolonged hospitalizations. *Nurs Res, 58*(6), 427–434.

Harsha, SS, & Archana, BR. (2015). SNAPPE-II (score for neonatal acute physiology with Perinatal extension-II) in predicting mortality and morbidity in NICU. *J Clin Diagn Res, 9*(10) Sc10–2.

Johnston, C, Campbell-Yeo, M, Fernandes, A, Inglis, D, Streiner, D, & Zee, R. (2014). Skin- to-skin care for procedural pain in neonates. *Cochrane Database Syst Rev*(1), Article Cd008435.

Johnston, CC, Fillion, F, Campbell-Yeo, M, Goulet, C, Bell, L, McNaughton, K, Byron, J, Aita, M, Finley, GA, & Walker, CD. (2008). Kangaroo mothercare diminishes pain from heel lance in very preterm neonates: a crossover trial. *BMC Pediatr, 8*(1), 13.

Johnston, CC, Filion, F, Snider, L, Limperopoulos, C, Majnemer, A, Pelausa, E, et al. (2007). How much sucrose is too much sucrose?. *Pediatrics, 119*(1), 226.

Johnsston, CC, Filion, F, Snider, L, Majnemer, A, Limperopoulos, C, Walker, CD, et al. (2002). Routine sucrose analgesia during the first week of life in neonates younger than 31 weeks' postconceptional age. *Pediatrics, 110*(3), 523–528.

Lee, GY, & Stevens, BJ. (2014). Neonatal and infant pain assessment. In PJ McGrath, BJ Stevens, SM Walker, & WT Zempsky (Eds.), *Oxford textbook of paediatric pain* (1st ed) (pp. 353–369). Oxford: Oxford University Press.

Lee, GY, Yamada, J, Kyololo, O, Shorkey, A, & Stevens, B. (2014). Pediatric clinical practice guidelines for acute procedural pain: a systematic review. *Pediatrics, 133*(3), 500–515.

Ohlsson, A, & Shah, PS. (2015). Paracetamol (acetaminophen) for prevention or treatment of pain in newborns. *Cochrane Database Syst Rev*(6), Article Cd011219.

Patsopoulos, NA. (2011). A pragmatic view on pragmatic trials. *Dialogues Clin Neurosci, 13*(2), 217–224.

Pillai Riddell, RR, Racine, NM, Gennis, HG, Turcotte, K, Uman, LS, Horton, RE, et al. (2015). Non-pharmacological management of infant and young child procedural pain. *Cochrane Database Syst Rev*(12), Article Cd006275.

Randomize.net. A comprehensive internet-based randomization service for clinical trials. http://www.randomize.net (2015). Accessed 11 Apr 2017.

Richardson, DK, Corcoran, JD, Escobar, GJ, & Lee, SK. (2001). SNAP-II and SNAPPE-II: simplified newborn illness severity and mortality risk scores. *J Pediat, 138*(1), 92–100.

Shah, PS, Herbozo, C, Aliwalas, LL, & Shah, VS. (2012). Breastfeeding or breast milk for procedural pain in neonates. *Cochrane Database Syst Rev, 12,* Article Cd004950.

Stevens, B, Johnston, C, Franck, L, Petryshen, P, Jack, A, & Foster, G. (1999). The efficacy of developmentally sensitive interventions and sucrose for relieving procedural pain in very low birth weight neonates. *Nurs Res, 48*(1), 35–43.

Stevens, B, Yamada, J, Beyene, J, Gibbins, S, Petryshen, P, Stinson, J, et al. (2005). Consistent management of repeated procedural pain with sucrose in preterm neonates: is it effective and safe for repeated use over time?. *Clin J Pain, 21*(6), 543–548.

Stevens, B, Yamada, J, Ohlsson, A, Haliburton, S, & Shorkey, A. (2016). Sucrose for analgesia in newborn infants undergoing painful procedures. *Cochrane Database Syst Rev, 7*(7), Article CD001069.

Stevens, BJRNP, Gibbins, SRNP, Yamada, JRNP, Dionne, KRNMN, Lee, GRNM, Johnston, CRNDF, et al. (2014). The premature infant pain profile-revised (PIPP-R): initial validation and feasibility. *Clin J Pain, 30*(3), 238–243.

Taddio, A, Shah, V, Atenafu, E, & Katz, J. (2009a). Influence of repeated painful procedures and sucrose analgesia on the development of hyperalgesia in newborn infants. *Pain, 144*(1–2), 43–48.

Taddio, A, Yiu, A, Smith, RW, Katz, J, McNair, C, & Shah, V. (2009b). Variability in clinical practice guidelines for sweetening agents in newborn infants undergoing painful procedures. *Clin J Pain, 25*(2), 153–155.

INTRODUCTION TO CRITIQUE 2

The article "The minimally effective dose of sucrose for procedural pain relief in neonates: A randomized controlled trial" (Stevens et al., 2018) is examined in terms of its quality and the potential usefulness of the findings for application to nursing practice. The design of this study was level II, inasmuch as it was a randomized controlled trial.

Title

The title reflects the captures the essence of the study succinctly.

Abstract

The abstract meets the requirements of thoroughness. It contains the background, methods, the research design, the findings, the results, and conclusion.

Problem and Purpose

The identification of the research problem is very well organized with an easy flow of the linkages between its elements. Stevens et al. (2018) outlined the significance of the study by stating that sweet solutions like sucrose are effective and safe in reducing pain intensity among neonates. "However, there is more than 20-fold variations in sucrose doses examined in research. Despite the large number of randomized controlled trials in the 2016 Cochrane review, an optimal dose of sucrose could not be determined due to the wide range of volumes and concentrations (0.05 ml of 24% to 2.0 ml of 50% solution) studied, and due to variation in study methods (e.g., administration techniques, types of painful procedures, outcome measures, and co-interventions)," and they continued on with "there have been no direct comparisons of different volumes of sucrose at the same concentration" (p. 481).

The authors continue to describe that there is no conclusive evidence on the optimal dose of sucrose with previous experimental studies. The authors also stated that there is no research done

yet comparing three different volumes of sucrose with same concentration. This statement adds strength to the rationale for conducting the study.

Stevens et al. (2018) stated that the purpose of the study was to determine the minimally effective dose of 24% sucrose for reducing pain in hospitalized neonates undergoing a single skin-breaking heel lance procedure. This is a good purpose statement as it includes what the researchers hope to achieve with the research.

Review of the Literature and Definitions

The authors combined a brief literature review with the study background. The literature reviewed and documented seems adequate to give a rationale for the study.

Theoretical Framework

There is no theoretical framework, but variables and outcome measures are clearly articulated. Conceptual definitions of the variables would assist the reader in replicating the study.

Hypotheses and Research Question

Stevens et al. (2018) stated the research hypotheses as follows: "(a) there was no difference in pain intensity between the sucrose doses, measured at 30 and 60 s following the heel lance using the Premature Infant Pain Profile-Revised (PIPP-R), and (b) adverse events would be minimal" (p. 481).

The primary outcome was the pain intensity measured with PIPP-R. The secondary outcome was frequency of a priori specified adverse event/tolerance criteria (heart rate > 240 beats/min or heart rate < 80 beats/min for > 20 s; oxygen saturation < 80% for > 20 s; no spontaneous respirations for > 20 s; and choking/gagging).

No research question was stated but such a statement could be articulated from the hypothesis as follows: What is the minimally effective dose of 24% sucrose for reducing pain in hospitalized neonates undergoing a single skin-breaking heel lance procedure?

Sample

Samples were chosen based on specific inclusion and exclusion criteria. Randomization was done using a web-based randomization service. Randomization was block stratified by gestational age at birth (< 29 weeks or 29–42 weeks). Neonates 24 to 42 weeks gestational age (GA) at birth and less than 30 days of life/or less than 44 weeks GA at the time of the intervention, scheduled to receive a heel lance, and who had not received opioids within 24 h prior to the heel lance were included in the study. The authors excluded neonates with a contraindication for sucrose administration (e.g., were too ill or unstable as per neonatologist's assessment, unable to swallow, pharmacologically muscle relaxed) and/or inability to assess behavioral responses to pain accurately (e.g., the neonate's face was blocked with taping).

The sample size calculation accounted for multiple testing due to three intervention groups and is based on a type I error probability of 5%, a power of 80%, and a smallest minimally clinically significant difference of 1 on the PIPP-R with a standard deviation (SD) of 2. To account for potential missing data (e.g., equipment failure), the sample size was increased by 15% to 245.

Research Design

Stevens et al. (2018) stated that this was a prospective, multi-centred, single-blind, randomized controlled trial. There were three arms to the study. Neonates were randomly assigned to one of the three intervention groups (0.1 ML dose, 0.5 ML dose, and 1.0 ML dose). This design is consistent with the purpose of the research. The intervention was different doses of sucrose solution, and the dependent variable was the pain intensity measured through PIPP-R, which included two physiological, three behavioral, and two contextual variables. The pain intensity was measured at 30 s and 60 s.

All three groups had matching demographic variables such as gestational age at birth, birthweight, sex, and severity of illness assessed using the Score for Neonatal Acute Physiology Perinatal Extension-II (SNAPPE-II). The research design chosen fits well with the question at hand. The data collection has been done according to the protocol.

Internal Validity

Stevens et al. (2018) have designed the study in a way that had addressed the potential threats to internal validity. First, there was strict randomization and the researchers/data collectors were blinded to the study groups. Second, the interrater reliability of the researchers who coded the pain intensity using the tool was more than 0.9. Third, the construct validity of the tool that was used to measure the pain intensity (PIPP-R) had been demonstrated through research. The alpha value of 0.9 indicates that this instrument is highly reliable.

External Validity

The study has a wide generalizability based on the strength of the randomized design.

Legal/Ethical Issues

The authors have obtained approval from the research and ethics boards at all the hospitals where the study was conducted. The authors also have obtained informed consent from a parent prior to enrolling the neonate into the study.

Instruments

Stevens et al. (2018) used PIPP-R tool to collect data on the pain intensity of neonates at 30-s and 60-s intervals. This instrument has demonstrated construct validity in neonates of varying gestational age, thus it was appropriate to use. The tool includes two physiological (heart rate, oxygen saturation), three behavioural (brow bulge, eye squeeze, nasolabial furrow), and two contextual variables (gestational age, behavioural state).

Reliability and Validity

Stevens et al. (2018) has described the construct validity and interrater reliability of the tool PIPP-R. Two trained coders, blinded to group allocation and study purpose, were used to view the physiological and behavioural data captured by the infant monitoring system, and coded neonates' pain intensity using the PIPP-R. An interrater reliability > 0.9, indicating consistency of observations between two or more observers, was achieved on a random sample of five neonates, early in the study and with each 25% of data collected.

Results

Stevens et al. (2018) used descriptive statistics to present the demographic characteristics of the three intervention groups; these data are presented in Table 20 C2.1, with their mean and standard deviations. The mean pain scores at 30 s and 60 s are presented in Table 20 C2.2.

A description of the participants' results was also presented in the text (Stevens et al., 2018, p. 483). Evidence to support the hypothesis was detailed in text as follows: "Pain intensity scores across the three groups equated to mild pain for the majority of neonates (scores of < 7 on the PIPP-R)."

Regarding the secondary outcomes, the authors have reported that there were 2% of the adverse events reported that resolved spontaneously.

Discussion

Stevens et al. (2018) stated that their finding related to the dose of sucrose was consistent with previous research findings. The authors have done an extensive literature search and have compared the results of the findings with the previous studies. The authors have also explained some of the potential weaknesses in the present design stating that the contextual factors of the various organizations could not be well controlled. The authors also stated that there was no difference in the pain intensity among the neonates in different intervention groups; however, the pain was not eliminated completely. So, the authors recommend using additional doses of sucrose and non-pharmacological measures to reduce pain.

The authors also have stated that future research should focus on the long-term effects of sucrose and neurodevelopment of neonates. The authors have substantiated this argument with the literature available.

Limitations and Conclusion

Stevens et al. (2018) mentioned that the decision to measure pain intensity at 30 s and 60 s was arbitrary and would be considered a limitation. The authors also have stated that the study is limited by the data collected from medical records that may not have included documentation of all the pain-relieving strategies.

The authors have concluded that there was no difference between the doses of 0.1 ML, 0.5 ML, and 1.0 ML and suggest that 0.1 ML is enough to reduce the pain intensity. However, the authors also suggest future studies to assess the sustained effectiveness of sucrose.

The findings of the study are relevant in the area of pain control among neonates undergoing painful procedures. However, the results have to be viewed with caution, as they are not generalizable across the population due to the identified limitations.

CRITICAL THINKING CHALLENGES

- Discuss the ways in which the stylistic considerations of a journal affect the researcher's ability to present the research findings of a quantitative study.

- Are critiques of quantitative studies valid when a student or a practising nurse writes them? What level of quantitative study is best for you as a consumer of research to critique? What assumptions did you use to make this determination?

- What is essential for you as a consumer of research to use when you critique a quantitative research study? Discuss the ways you might use Internet resources now or in the future when you critique studies.

CRITICAL JUDGEMENT QUESTIONS

1 The purpose of critiquing an article is to
   a Identify the mistakes in a study
   b Appraise the level of evidence
   c Provide feedback to the researcher
   d Support the researcher

2 Stylistic variations of a research report might influence:
   a The reader's ability to identify mistakes
   b Ability to judge the overall quality or validity of the study
   c The presentation of results in an organized manner
   d The repeatability of the study

3 Which of the following is the most relevant question to critique the research design of a quantitative study?
   a What type of research design is used in this study?
   b Does the choice of design seem logical for the proposed problem?
   c Is the design based on a philosophical foundation?
   d Has the researcher mentioned about a pilot study and its findings?

 FOR FURTHER STUDY

Go to Evolve at http://evolve.elsevier.com/Canada/LoBiondo/Research for the Audio Glossary.

REFERENCES

Paul-Savoie, E., Bourgault, P., Potvin, S., Gosselin, E., & Lafrenaye, S. (2018). The impact of pain invisibility on patient-centered care and empathetic attitude in chronic pain management. *Pain Research and Management, 2018*, Article 6375713. https://doi.org/10.1155/2018/6375713.

Stevens, B., Yamada, J., Campbell-Yeo, M., Gibbins, S., Harrison, D., Dionne, K., Taddio, A., McNair, C., Willan, A., Ballantyne, M., Widger, K., Sidani, S., Estabrooks, C., Synnes, A., Squires, J., Victor, C., & Riahi, S. (2018). The minimally effective dose of sucrose for procedural pain relief in neonates: A randomized controlled trial. *BMC Pediatrics, 18*(1), 85. https://doi.org/10.1186/s12887-018-1026-x.

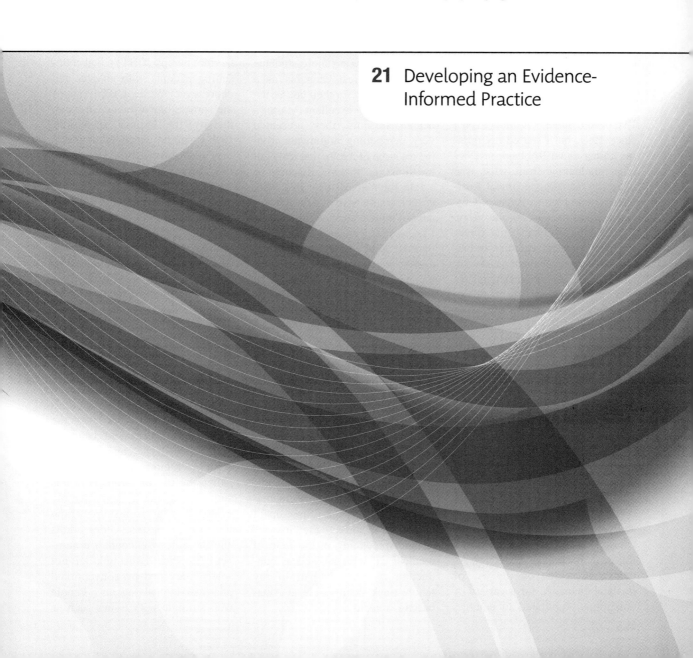

PART SEVEN

Application of Research: Evidence-Informed Practice

RESEARCH **VIGNETTE**

The Influence of NP Program Students in My Current Research Portfolio: Exploring Medical Cannabis and Applying It to Clinical Practice

Luisa Barton, NP-PHC, BScN, MN, DNP
Assistant Professor
Athabasca University
Alberta

I've been a nurse practitioner (NP) since 1997, but I started my nursing career as an RN back in 1989 after graduating from what was once Ryerson Polytechnical Institute (now known as Ryerson University). For the past 30-plus years, I can honestly say that my career has been colourful, exciting, and lucrative. It gives me great pleasure to share my research journey thus far.

I've been very fortunate to work in a variety of specialties and environments in my seasoned career path. I've worked in the academic setting, teaching in various NP programs at universities for over 20 years. Through my role as a professor, I became interested in medical cannabis. About 5 years ago, I had several NP program students in the classroom setting who shared their clinical experiences about preceptors who were providing their patients with medical cannabis options. These students were inspired by the clinical successes they were witnessing in their clinical practicum. As evidence/research on the use of medical cannabis, for a variety of conditions, continued to emerge,

I was encountering more students choosing medical cannabis as a topic of interest for their course assignments. As excellent Master's degree students, they presented very compelling arguments from the research literature that truly got me thinking, "there really could be a role for medical cannabis." So, as luck would have it, a former student of mine contacted me to see if I knew of any recent NP graduates that would be interested in joining a new start-up medical cannabis company. I quickly responded that I was very interested in practicing in the field. I have now been working as an NP with the company since December 2018. As an NP at Northstar Wellness, I practice mostly via telemedicine, but we also offer in-person appointments at our clinics throughout Ontario. My major responsibilities include: performing medical assessments (to determine patients' suitability for medical cannabis), health teaching about medical cannabis, completing medical documentation/prescribing, and follow-ups. I am fortunate to have the "luxury" of both practicing in the field of medical cannabis as well as conducting research as part of my tenure-track faculty role at Athabasca University.

As an NP in active practice, I am encountering more people struggling with anxiety and depression than ever before in my career history. According to large population-based surveys, up to 33.7% of the population are affected by an anxiety disorder during their lifetime (Carpenter et al., 2018). As a consultant in a downtown Toronto clinic, I have been able to apply my training of cognitive behavior t herapy (CBT) when counselling patients with anxiety and depression. While CBT remains the cornerstone of evidence-based therapy for various conditions such as anxiety, medical cannabis may also have a role as adjunctive therapy in mental health as well as other health conditions in adults and older adults (Blessing et al., 2015). For example, in Canada, cannabis consumption among those >65 years old has been accelerating at a much faster pace than it has among other age groups (Statistics Canada, 2019). There are several hundred natural compounds, including over 120 cannabinoids, that have been isolated from cannabis species. Both THC (delta-9-tetrahydrocannabinol) and CBD (cannabidiol) are most relevant in medical cannabis (Hatcher et al., 2018). CBD is the second most prevalent cannabinoid found in the cannabis plant. As more regions in the world legalize the use of cannabis, it has surged in popularity and scientific evidence as a promising therapy for many illnesses. Older adults and the elderly encounter a number of medical issues that are not solely alleviated by conventional pharmacological agents. People who struggle with issues such as poor sleep, pain, as well as anxiety and delusions from diagnoses such as dementia and PTSD too often don't have their symptoms fully resolved with pharmacological agents, which way too often can lead to polypharmacy. Medical cannabis has had a significant positive impact on their health outcomes and improved quality of life (Abuhasira, Schleidger, Machoulam, & Novack, 2018; Katz, Katz, Shoenfeld, & Porat-Katz, 2017; Minerbi, Häuser, & Fitzcharles, 2019). Although research continues to be limited, recent studies are showing promising results from the use of cannabis therapy.

Fortunately, as an NP practicing in Ontario, I am in a unique position to offer patients a variety of options, particularly both CBT and CBD/medical cannabis, along with other conventional therapies that are mutually agreed upon. While my practice in this area is very rewarding, as an NP and researcher, it behooves me to study the health impact of medical cannabis as a form of therapy in adults and older adults with mental and physical health conditions. In fact, mental and physical are not two separate entities; to address both is truly considered a holistic approach. To be clear, my research endeavour is ***not*** to do randomized control studies (RCTs) per se (many patients are already using medical cannabis for their illnesses). Rather, it is to review studies and anecdotal evidence in practice in order to offer practice tools and pearls of wisdom to health care providers in primary health care. In this way, my research is framed within knowledge translation. According to CIHR (2016), "Knowledge Translation is defined as a dynamic and iterative process that includes synthesis, dissemination, exchange and ethically-sound application of knowledge to improve the health of Canadians, provide more effective health services and products and strengthen the health care system."

It is my hope that my research portfolio will provide health care practitioners with the evidence and tools they need to be in a better position and to have more confidence in offering medical cannabis as an option to their patients. ■

REFERENCES

Abuhasira, R., Schleidger, L. B., Machoulam, R., & Novack, V. (2018). Epidemiological characteristics, safety and efficiency of medical cannabis in the elderly. *European Journal of Internal Medicine, 49,* 44–50.

Blessing, E. M., Steenkamp, M. M., Manzanares, J., & Marmar, C. R. (2015). Cannabidiol as a potential treatment for anxiety disorders. *Neurotherapeutics: The Journal of the American Society for Experimental NeuroTherapeutics, 12*(4), 825–836.

Canadian Institutes of Health Research (2016). Knowledge Translation: About Us. https://cihr-irsc.gc.ca/e/29418.html.

Carpenter, J. K., Andrews, L. A., Witcraft, S. M., Powers, M. B., Smits, J. A. J., & Hofmann, S. G. (2018). Cognitive behavioral therapy for anxiety and related disorders: A meta-analysis of randomized placebo-controlled trials. *Depression and Anxiety, 35*(6), 502–514. https://doi.org/10.1002/da.22728.

Hatcher, L., MacCallum, C., & Schecter, D. (2018). Insights into cannabis-based medicines, *Medical Cannabis 2018 Conference. Proceedings presented at 2018 Medical Cannabis Conference.*

Katz, I., Katz, D., Shoenfeld, Y., & Porat-Katz, B. S. (2017). Clinical evidence for cannabinoids in the elderly. *The Israel Medical Association Journal: IMAJ, 19*(2), 71.

Minerbi, A., Häuser, W., & Fitzcharles, M. (2019). Medical cannabis for older patients. *Drugs & Aging, 36*(1), 39–51.

Statistics Canada. (2019). *National Cannabis Survey, third quarter 2019.* Retrieved from https://www150.statcan.gc.ca/n1/daily-quotidien/191030/dq191030a-eng.htm.

CHAPTER 21

Developing an Evidence-Informed Practice

Lorraine Thirsk

LEARNING OUTCOMES

After reading this chapter, you will be able to do the following:

- Differentiate among conduct of nursing research, research utilization, and evidence-informed practice.
- Describe the steps of evidence-informed practice.
- Identify three barriers to evidence-informed practice and strategies to address each.
- List three sources for finding evidence.
- Describe strategies for implementing evidence-informed practice changes.
- Identify steps for evaluating an evidence-informed change in practice.
- Use research findings and other forms of evidence to improve the quality of care.

KEY TERMS

clinical practice guidelines
conduct of research
dissemination
evaluation
evidence-based practice

evidence-informed decision-
 making
evidence-informed practice
knowledge-focused triggers
knowledge translation

opinion leaders
problem-focused triggers
research utilization
translation science

STUDY RESOURCES

 Go to Evolve at http://evolve.elsevier.com/Canada/LoBiondo/Research
for the Audio Glossary.

THERE ARE SEVERAL TERMS THAT YOU MAY ENCOUNTER regarding use of evidence in nursing practice. The Canadian Nurses Association (CNA, 2010) defines **evidence-informed decision-making** as "a continuous interactive process involving the explicit, conscientious and judicious consideration of the best available evidence to provide care" (p. 1). Evidence is further defined as information acquired through research and scientific practices (CNA, 2010). As described in Chapter 1, the evidence-based medicine movement began over two decades ago (Sackett et al., 1996). Other, similar terms that you may come across include evidence-informed practice and evidence-based practice (CNA, 2020). Melnyk and Fineout-Overholt (2019) offer that evidence-based practice is "a problem-solving approach to clinical practice" (p. 8) that involves integrating high-quality research, clinical expertise, and patient/family values (Figure 21.1). The overarching theme amongst all these definitions, and a major tenet of the evidence movement, is that using high-quality research in nursing practice will improve patient outcomes when combined with individual patient values and clinical expertise from nurses. Although the CNA (2020) has decided on the term evidence-informed decision-making and nursing practice, you will notice most definitions of evidence-based practice also include components of clinical expertise and patient/family values (see, for example, Melnyk & Fineout-Overholt, 2019).

Availability of high-quality research does not ensure that the findings will be used to affect patient outcomes. Evidence-based practice, unfortunately, remains a low priority (Melnyk et al., 2016) even though it is necessary to achieve high-quality health care, improve patient outcomes, reduce costs, and empower clinicians (Melnyk & Fineout-Overholt, 2019). The use of evidence-informed practices is now an expected standard in many institutions. However, implementing such evidence-informed safety practices is a challenge and requires use of strategies that address the complexity and systems of care, individual practitioners, senior leadership, and, ultimately, changing health care cultures to be evidence-informed practice environments (Melnyk & Fineout-Overholt, 2011a; Melnyk, 2016b).

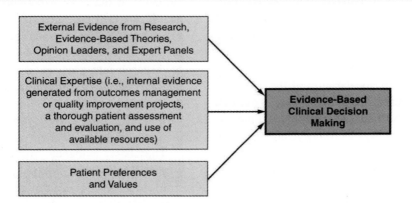

FIG. 21.1   Components of Evidence-Based Practice.
Melnyk, B.M., & Fineout-Overholt, E. (2011b). *Evidence-based practice in nursing & healthcare. A guide to best practice.* Berlin: Wolters Kluwer.

Conducting research is only the first step in improving practice. Because of the gap between discovery and use of knowledge in practice (Melnyk et al., 2014; Squires et al., 2015; Titler, 2008), efforts must be concentrated on developing methods to speed translation of research findings into practice. There is an overwhelming amount of information available to clinicians and pre-appraisal and synthesis is needed to support the use of evidence in practice (Alper & Haynes, 2016; Djulbegovic & Guyatt, 2017). Development and dissemination of evidence-informed practice guidelines, or clinical practice guidelines, are essential steps, but each alone does little to promote knowledge uptake by direct care providers. Melnyk et al. (2014) identified multiple barriers to implementing evidence into practice, including the following:

- The perception that it takes too much time
- A lack of evidence-informed practice knowledge and skills among clinicians
- A focus in health professional education on the research process rather than evidence-informed practice
- Lack of support in organizations
- Lack of evidence-informed practice mentors and appropriate resources
- Resistance from colleagues, managers, leaders, and physicians

Overcoming these barriers is an active process that is facilitated partly by modelling and imitation of other health care providers who have successfully adopted an innovation, by an organizational culture that values and supports use of evidence, and by localization of the evidence for use in a specific health care setting (Melnyk & Fineout-Overholt, 2011a; Melnyk & Fineout-Overholt, 2019; Rogers, 2003). Understanding and mitigating the barriers will promote the widespread adoption of evidence-informed practice. This chapter presents an overview of evidence-informed practice, the process of implementing evidence in practice to improve patient outcomes, and a description of translation science.

OVERVIEW OF EVIDENCE-INFORMED PRACTICE

The purpose of this book thus far has been to familiarize yourself with the process of **conducting research**. Traditionally, conducting research has included **dissemination** of findings through research reports in journals and at scientific conferences. Dissemination is the communication of research findings; dissemination activities take many forms, including publications, conferences, consultations, and training programs (Adams & Titler, 2010), but promoting knowledge uptake and changing practitioner behavior requires active interchange with those in direct care (Scott, Plotnikoff, Karunamuni, et al., 2008; Titler, Herr, Brooks, et al., 2009).

The terms *research utilization* and *evidence-informed practice* are sometimes used interchangeably. However, although these two terms are related, they are not one and the same. Research utilization is the process of using research findings to improve patient care, often based on a single study (Melnyk & Fineout-Overholt, 2019). *Evidence-informed practice* is a broader term that encompasses not only research utilization but also the use of case reports and expert opinion in deciding the practices to be used in health care. If evidence-informed practice is defined as the conscious and judicious use of the current "best" evidence in the care of patients and delivery of health care services, then research utilization is a subset of evidence-informed practice that focuses on the application of research findings. Translation of research into practice is a multifaceted, systemic process of promoting adoption of evidence-informed practices in delivery of health care services that goes beyond dissemination of evidence (Rogers, 2003).

The best evidence for practice includes empirical evidence from systematic reviews, from randomized controlled trials, and from other scientific methods such as descriptive and qualitative research. When enough research evidence is available, practice should be guided by this evidence, in conjunction with clinical expertise and patients' values. In some cases, however, a sufficient research base may not be available, and health care decision-making is derived principally from non-research evidence sources such as expert opinion, scientific principles (Titler et al., 2001), evidence-based theories, and local/internally generated practice projects (Melnyk & Fineout-Overholt, 2019). When more research is completed in a specific area, the research evidence must be incorporated into evidence-informed practice.

Use of Evidence in Practice

Nursing has a rich history of using research in practice, pioneered by Florence Nightingale, who used data to change practices that contributed to high mortality rates in hospitals and communities (Nightingale, 1858, 1859, 1863a, 1863b). Although during the early and mid-1900s few nurses built on the solid foundation of research utilization exemplified by Nightingale (Titler, 1994), the nursing profession has provided major leadership for improving care through application of research findings in practice. While the scientific body of nursing knowledge is growing (Estabrooks, Derksen, Winther, et al., 2008; Titler, 2008; Titler et al., 2009), the majority of research on nursing practice is from single descriptive and qualitative studies (Melnyk, 2016a; Richards, et al., 2018). While nurses rely on many forms of knowledge, such as the personal and ethical, in their nursing practice, they need to be clear about what constitutes evidence (Thorne & Sawatzky, 2014; Thorne, 2018).

Cronenwett (1995) and others have described two forms of using research evidence in practice: conceptual and decision driven (Estabrooks, 2004). Conceptual forms influence the thinking of the health care provider but not necessarily the action. Exposure to new scientific knowledge occurs, but the new knowledge may not be used to change or guide practice. An integrative review of the literature, formulation of a new theory, or generating of new hypotheses may be the result. Use of knowledge in this way is referred to as *knowledge creep* or *cognitive application*. It is often used by individuals who read and incorporate research into their critical thinking (Weiss, 1980). Decision-driven forms of using evidence in practice encompass application of scientific knowledge as part of a new practice, policy, procedure, or intervention. In this type of application of research findings, a critical decision is reached to endorse current practice or to change it on the basis of review and critique of studies applicable to that practice. Examples of decision-driven models of using research in practice are the Iowa Model Revised: Evidence-Based Practice to Promote Excellence in Health Care (Iowa Model Collaborative, 2017), the Ottawa Model of Research Use (OMRU; Logan & Graham, 1998), the Promoting Action on Research Implementation in Health Services (i-PARIHS) model (Kitson & Harvey, 2016), and the Conduct and Utilization of Research in Nursing (CURN) model (Haller, Reynolds, & Horseley, 1979; Horsley, Crane, Crabtree, et al., 1983).

Multifaceted active dissemination strategies are needed to promote use of research evidence in clinical and administrative health care decision making, and they must address both the individual practitioner's and the organization's perspectives (Titler, 2008). When nurses decide individually what evidence to use in practice, considerable variability in practice patterns results, which can potentially lead to adverse patient outcomes. For example, a solely "individual" perspective of evidence-informed practice would leave the decision about use of pressure injury prevention practices to each nurse. Some nurses may be familiar with the research findings for pressure injury prevention, whereas others may not be. As a result, different nurses may use conflicting practices, especially since shifts change every 8 to 12 hours. From an organizational perspective, policies and procedures are based on research, and then adoption of these practices by nurses is systematically promoted in the organization (Squires, Moralejo, & LeFort, 2007). A culture that is supportive of EIP is a necessity (Melnyk, 2016b).

Models of Evidence-Informed Practice

Multiple models have been developed to guide the implementation and sustainment of evidence-informed practice (Dang et al., 2019). Common elements of these models are syntheses of evidence, implementation, evaluation of the effect on patient care, and consideration of the context/ setting in which the evidence is implemented. Grol, Bosch, Hulscher, and associates (2007) have provided a summary of models. Included in their summary relevant to quality improvement and implementation of change in health care are cognitive, educational, motivational, social interactive, social learning, social network, and social influence theories, as well as models related to team effectiveness, professional development, and leadership. Additional work by the Improved Clinical Effectiveness through Behavioural Research Group (ICEBeRG) has resulted in the development of a database consisting of planned action models, frameworks, and theories that explicitly describe both the concepts and action steps to be considered or taken. This database was developed from a search of social science, education, and health literature that focused on practitioner or organizational change.

Implementing evidence in practice must be guided by a conceptual model to organize the strategies being used and to clarify extraneous variables (e.g., behaviours and facilitators) that may influence adoption of evidence-informed practices (e.g., organizational size, characteristics of users; ICEBeRG, 2006). Although a thorough review of these models is beyond the scope of this chapter, three models are explored here: the Iowa Model of Evidence-Based Practice to Promote Quality Care, the Ottawa Model of Research Use, and the i-PARIHS model.

The Iowa Model of Evidence-Based Practice to Promote Quality Care

An overview of the Iowa Model Revised: Evidence-Based Practice to Promote Excellence in Health Care (Iowa Model Collaborative, 2017), as an example of a practice model, is illustrated in Figure 21.2. This model has been widely disseminated and adopted in academic and clinical settings since the original publication (see Titler, et al., 1994). It is an organizational, collaborative model that incorporates conduct of research, use of research evidence, and other types of evidence (Titler et al., 2001). Titler and colleagues adopted the definition of *evidence-based practice* as the conscientious and judicious use of current best evidence to guide health care decisions. Levels of evidence range from randomized controlled trials to case reports and expert opinion.

In this model, knowledge- and problem-focused "triggers" lead staff members to question current nursing practice and whether patient care can be improved through the use of research findings. If, through the process of literature review and critique of studies, staff members find that the number of scientifically sound studies is not sufficient for use as a base for practice, they consider conducting a study. Nurses in practice collaborate with scientists in nursing and other disciplines to conduct clinical research that addresses practice problems encountered in the care of patients. Findings from such studies are then combined with findings from existing scientific knowledge to develop and implement these practices. If research is insufficient for guiding practice, and if conducting a study is not feasible, other types of evidence (e.g., case reports, expert opinion, scientific principles, theory) are used or combined with available research evidence to guide practice. Priority is given to projects in which a high proportion of practice is guided by research evidence. Practice guidelines usually reflect research and non-research evidence and therefore are called *evidence-informed practice guidelines*.

An evidence-informed practice guideline is developed from the available evidence. The recommended practices, based on the relevant evidence, are compared with current practice, and a decision is made about the necessity for a practice change. If a practice change is warranted, changes are implemented through a process of planned change. The practice is first implemented with a small group of patients, and it is evaluated. The evidence-informed practice is then refined on the basis of evaluation data, and the change is implemented with additional patient populations for which it is appropriate. Patient/family, staff, and fiscal outcomes are monitored. Organizational support and administrative support are important factors for success in the use of evidence in care delivery.

The Ottawa Model of Research Use

Logan and Graham (1998) developed the OMRU, a model for interdisciplinary health care research use. The framework was created to "be used by policymakers seeking to increase the use of health research by practitioners, as well as by researchers interested in studying the process by which research becomes integrated into practice" (p. 228). They identified the following six components of research utilization: (1) the practice environment, (2) potential adopters, (3) the evidence-informed innovation, (4) transfer strategies, (5) adoption, and (6) health-related and other outcomes. Constant assessment, monitoring, and evaluation parallel the progression through the components. As barriers are identified, strategies are developed to surmount them and to enhance supports.

Promoting Action on Research Implementation in Health Services (i-PARIHS)

The i-PARIHS model is widely used to introduce knowledge into practice. Kitson and Harvey (2016) spent several years refining the original model, known as PARIHS, into the updated version (i-PARIHS). The aim of this model is to help nurses determine the most appropriate facilitation methods to change practice. The model considers three key elements:

Evidence—the quality and type of evidence
Context—the characteristics of the setting in which the change would occur
Facilitation—the support needed to implement the change into practice

In the newest model, iPARIHS, the *i* stands for *innovation* and includes a practical set of instructions on how to use the model. Harvey and Kitson (2015) have also developed a clinical resource to facilitate implementation of the PARIHS model.

STEPS OF EVIDENCE-INFORMED PRACTICE

The Iowa Model Revised: Evidence-Based Practice to Promote Excellence in Health Care (Iowa Model Collaborative, 2017; see Figure 21.2), in conjunction with Rogers' (1995, 2003) diffusion of innovations model, provides guiding steps in actualizing evidence-informed practice. A team approach is most helpful in fostering a specific evidence-informed practice, with one person in the group providing leadership for the project. Melnyk and Fineout-Overholt (2019) stress that the first step for successful EIP is creating a spirit of inquiry. This means organizations support a culture and environment where nurses are "comfortable and excited about asking questions…as well as challenging current institutional or unit-based practices" (Melnyk & Fineout-Overholt, 2019, p. 16).

Selection of a Topic

Step one of an evidence-informed practice project is to select a topic. Ideas for evidence-informed practice come from several sources categorized as problem- and knowledge-focused triggers. Problem-focused triggers are research ideas identified by staff through quality improvement, risk surveillance, benchmarking data, financial data, or recurrent clinical problems. For example, the increased incidence of *Clostridium difficile*

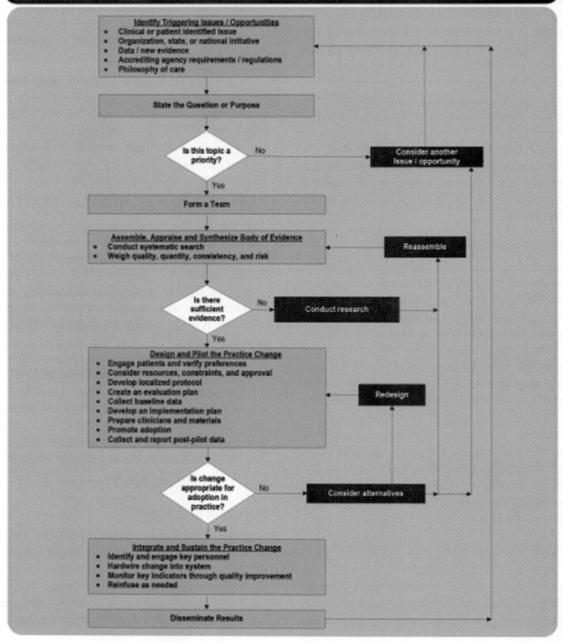

FIG. 21.2   The Iowa Model Revised: Evidence-Based Practice to Promote Excellence in Health Care. (Iowa Model Collaborative, 2017).

on a long-term care unit, resulting in increased morbidity, is a problem-focused trigger because it raises concern among hospital staff.

Knowledge-focused triggers are research ideas generated when staff members read research, listen to scientific papers at research conferences, or encounter evidence-informed practice guidelines published by federal agencies or specialty organizations. Examples of such triggers include ideas about pain management, assessing placement of nasogastric and nasointestinal tubes, and use of saline to maintain patency of arterial lines. Sometimes topics arise from a combination of problem- and knowledge-focused triggers, such as the length of bed rest time after femoral artery catheterization. In selecting a topic, nurses must consider how the topic fits with organization, department, and unit priorities in order to garner support from leaders within the organization and the necessary resources to successfully complete the project.

Individuals should work collectively to achieve consensus in topic selection. Working in groups to review performance improvement data, brainstorm about ideas, and achieve consensus about the final selection is helpful. For example, a unit staff meeting may be used to discuss ideas for evidence-informed practice; quality improvement committees may identify several practice areas in need of attention (e.g., urinary tract infections in older patients, reducing the incidence of pressure injuries); an evidence-informed practice task force may be appointed to select and address a clinical practice issue (e.g., pain management); or surveying a panel of experts may be used to prioritize areas for evidence-informed practice. Criteria to consider when a topic is selected are outlined in Box 21.1.

Research Hint

Regardless of which method is used to select an evidence-informed practice topic, it is critical that the staff members who will implement the potential practice changes are involved in selecting the topic and view it as contributing significantly to the quality of care.

BOX 21.1

SELECTION CRITERIA FOR AN EVIDENCE-INFORMED PRACTICE PROJECT

1. The priority of this topic for nursing and for the organization
2. The magnitude of the problem (small, medium, large)
3. Applicability to several or few clinical areas
4. Likelihood of the change to improve quality of care, decrease length of stay, contain costs, or improve patient satisfaction
5. Potential problems associated with the topic and capability to diffuse them
6. Availability of baseline quality improvement or risk data that will be helpful during evaluation
7. Multidisciplinary nature of the topic and ability to create collaborative relationships to effect the needed changes
8. Interest and commitment of staff to the potential topic
9. Availability of a sound body of evidence, preferably research evidence

Forming a Team

A team is responsible for development, implementation, and evaluation of the evidence-informed practice. The team or group may be an existing committee, such as the quality improvement committee, the practice council, or the research committee. A task force approach also may be used, in which a group is appointed to address a specific practice issue and use research findings or other evidence to improve practice. The composition of the team is directed by the topic selected and should include interested stakeholders in the delivery of care. For example, a team working on evidence-informed pain management should be interdisciplinary and include pharmacists, nurses, physicians, and psychologists. In contrast, a team working on the evidence-informed practice of bathing might include a nurse expert in skin care, assistive nursing personnel, and staff nurses.

In addition to forming a team, key stakeholders who can facilitate the evidence-informed practice project or put up barriers against successful implementation should be identified. A *stakeholder* is a key individual or group of individuals who are directly or indirectly affected by the implementation of the evidence-informed practice. Examples of key stakeholders are nurse managers, nurse educators, researchers, nursing supervisors, chairs of committees or councils that must approve system changes (e.g., policy/procedure revisions; changes in documentation forms), and patients/families. Questions to consider in identification of key stakeholders include the following:

- How are decisions made in the practice areas in which the evidence-informed practice will be implemented?
- What types of system changes will be needed?
- Who is involved in decision-making?
- Who is likely to lead and champion implementation of the evidence-informed practice?
- Who can influence the decision to proceed with implementation of an evidence-informed practice?
- What type of cooperation is needed from which stakeholders to be successful?

Use Figure 21.3 to think about the status of key stakeholders and to strategize about interventions to engage various types of stakeholders for your evidence-informed practice project.

An important early task for the evidence-informed practice team is to formulate the evidence-informed practice question. This helps set boundaries around the project and assists in retrieval of the evidence. A clearly defined question should specify the types of people/patients, interventions or exposures, outcomes, and relevant study designs (Higgins & Green, 2011). For types of people, the team should specify the diseases or conditions of interest, the patient population (e.g., age, gender, educational status), and the setting. For example, if the topic for the evidence-informed practice project is pain, the team needs to specify the type of pain (e.g., acute, persistent, cancer), the age of the population (e.g., children, neonates, adults, older adults), and the setting (e.g., inpatient, outpatient, ambulatory care, home care, primary care). For intervention, the types of interventions of interest to the project and the comparison interventions

(e.g., standard care, alternative treatments) need to be specified. In the example of pain, the interventions of interest might include pharmacological treatment, analgesic administration methods (e.g., patient-controlled analgesia, epidural, intravenous), pain assessment, nonpharmacological treatment, and patient/family education regarding self-care pain management. For outcomes, the team should select outcomes of primary importance and consider the type of outcome data that will be needed for decision-making (e.g., benefits, harm, cost). Outcomes that may be interesting but of little importance to the project should be excluded.

Finally, it is important to consider the types of study designs that are likely to provide reliable data to answer the question, and the team must search for the highest level of evidence available. A similar type of approach to formulating the practice question is PICOT: patient, population, or problem; intervention/treatment; comparison intervention/treatment; outcomes; and time frame (Melnyk & Fineout-Overholt, 2011b; see Chapter 4).

Evidence Retrieval

Once a topic is selected, relevant research and related literature must be retrieved and should include clinical studies, meta-analyses, integrative literature reviews, and existing evidence-informed practice guidelines. As more evidence is available to guide practice, professional organizations and federal agencies are developing and making available evidence-informed practice guidelines, often called clinical practice guidelines. It is important that these guidelines are accessed as part of the literature retrieval process. Table 21.1 includes a list of resources for practice guidelines and current best evidence from specific studies of clinical problems.

In 1999, the Registered Nurses' Association of Ontario (RNAO) initiated the Nursing Best Practice Guidelines Project to develop practice guidelines for nurses providing patient care. The

STAKEHOLDER INFLUENCE

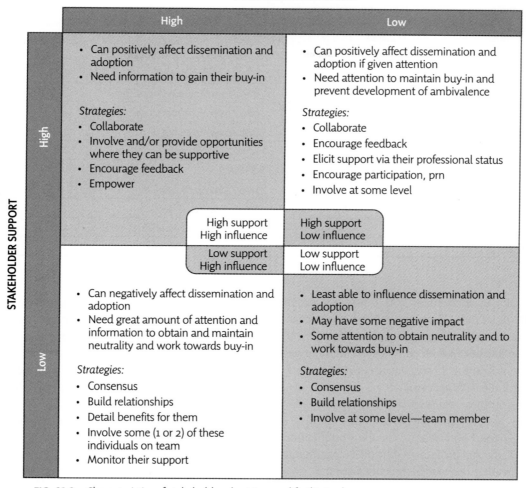

	High	Low
High	• Can positively affect dissemination and adoption • Need information to gain their buy-in *Strategies:* • Collaborate • Involve and/or provide opportunities where they can be supportive • Encourage feedback • Empower	• Can positively affect dissemination and adoption if given attention • Need attention to maintain buy-in and prevent development of ambivalence *Strategies:* • Collaborate • Encourage feedback • Elicit support via their professional status • Encourage participation, prn • Involve at some level
	High support High influence	High support Low influence
	Low support High influence	Low support Low influence
Low	• Can negatively affect dissemination and adoption • Need great amount of attention and information to obtain and maintain neutrality and work towards buy-in *Strategies:* • Consensus • Build relationships • Detail benefits for them • Involve some (1 or 2) of these individuals on team • Monitor their support	• Least able to influence dissemination and adoption • May have some negative impact • Some attention to obtain neutrality and to work towards buy-in *Strategies:* • Consensus • Build relationships • Involve at some level—team member

(STAKEHOLDER SUPPORT)

FIG. 21.3 Characteristics of stakeholders (resistors and facilitators). (Used/reprinted with permission from the University of Iowa Hospitals and Clinics, Copyright 2002. For permission to use or reproduce these figures, please contact the University of Iowa Hospitals and Clinics at 319-384-9098 or uihcnursingresearchandebp@uiowa.edu.)

project has produced 50 completed guidelines, with additional guidelines under development. These guidelines cover a broad range of topics relevant to nursing practice including social issues, chronic disease, nursing education and leadership, workplace health, and health promotion. The RNAO best practice guidelines are readily available to nurses through an application for personal electronic devices (e.g., iPhone and Android). Details are provided at the website: http://rnao.ca/bpg/app.

Another electronic database, Evidence-Based Medicine Reviews (EBMR) from Ovid Technologies (http://www.ovid.com/site/catalog/databases/904.jsp), combines several electronic databases, including the Cochrane Database of Systematic Reviews, Cochrane Database of Methodology Reviews (CDMR), and MEDLINE,

TABLE 21.1	
SOURCES FOR EVIDENCE-INFORMED PRACTICE GUIDELINES AND STUDIES OF CLINICAL PROBLEMS	
ORGANIZATION	**WEBSITE**
PROFESSIONAL ORGANIZATIONS THAT PUBLISH EVIDENCE-INFORMED PRACTICE GUIDELINES	
American Association of Critical-Care Nurses	http://www.aacn.org
American Pain Society	http://americanpainsociety.org/
Canadian Heart and Stroke Foundation	http://www.strokebestpractices.ca
National Institute for Health and Care Excellence	http://www.nice.org.uk
Registered Nurses' Association of Ontario (RNAO)	http://www.rnao.ca
SOURCES FOR BEST EVIDENCE FROM STUDIES OF CLINICAL PROBLEMS	
American College of Physicians	http://www.acponline.org
Centre for Health Evidence	http://www.cche.net
Cochrane Library	http://www.cochranelibrary.com
Joanna Briggs Institute	http://joannabriggs.org

plus links to more than 200 full-text journals. EBMR links these databases to one another; if a study on a topic of interest is found on MEDLINE and also has been included in a systematic review in the Cochrane Library, the review also can be readily and easily accessed.

In using these sources, it is important to identify key search terms and to use the expertise of health science librarians in locating publications relevant to the project. Additional information about locating the evidence is in Chapter 5.

Once the literature is located, it is helpful to classify the articles as clinical (non-research), integrative research reviews, theory articles, research articles, synthesis reports, meta-analyses, and evidence-informed practice guidelines. Table 21.2 defines the different types of reviews that you may encounter in the literature. Before you read and critique the research, it is useful to read theoretical and clinical articles to have a broad view of the nature of the topic and related concepts and to then review existing evidence-informed practice guidelines. It is helpful to read articles in the following order:

1. Clinical articles, to understand the state of the practice

2. Theory articles, to understand the various theoretical perspectives and concepts that may be encountered when you critique studies
3. Systematic review articles and synthesis reports, to understand the state of the science
4. Evidence-informed practice guidelines and evidence reports
5. Research articles, including meta-analyses

 Research Hint _____

Remember that even though an article is published in a peer-reviewed journal, it still needs to be appraised to determine the quality.

The volume of information available makes it important to access pre-appraised evidence, such as systematic reviews or clinical practice guidelines, when available (Alper & Haynes, 2016; Djulbegovic & Guyatt, 2017). These also need to be appraised for their quality. It may be helpful to review the 6S pyramid, presented in Chapter 5, to help in understanding levels of pre-appraised evidence.

Schemas for Grading the Evidence

There is no consensus among professional organizations or across health care disciplines

TABLE **21.2**

EXAMPLES OF EVIDENCE-INFORMED PRACTICE RATING SYSTEMS

GRADE WORKING GROUP (2004)	REGISTERED NURSES' ASSOCIATION OF ONTARIO (2012)	U.S. PREVENTIVE SERVICES TASK FORCE (2008; HARRIS ET AL., 2001)
STRENGTH OF EVIDENCE/QUALITY OF EVIDENCE	**LEVELS OF EVIDENCE**	**LEVELS OF CERTAINTY REGARDING NET BENEFIT**

High: Further research is very unlikely to change our confidence in the estimate of effect. Scientific evidence provided by well-designed, well-conducted, controlled trials (randomized and non-randomized) with statistically significant results that consistently support the guideline recommendation.

Moderate: Further research is likely to have an important impact on our confidence in the estimate of effect and may change the estimate.

Low: Further research is very likely to have an important impact on our confidence in the estimate of effect and is likely to change the estimate.

Very Low: Any estimate of effect is very uncertain.

Note: The type of evidence is first ranked as follows:

Randomized trial = high.
Observational study = low.
Any other evidence = very low.
Limitations in study quality, important inconsistency of results, uncertainty about the directness of the evidence, imprecise or sparse data, and high probability of reporting bias can lower the grade of evidence. Expert opinion supports the guideline recommendation because the available scientific evidence did not present consistent results or because controlled trials were lacking. Grade of evidence can be increased if there is (1) strong evidence of association—significant relative risk of >2 (<0.5) based on consistent evidence from two or more observational studies, with no plausible confounders (1); (2) very strong evidence of association—significant relative risk of >5 (<0.2) based on direct evidence with no major threats to validity (2); (3) evidence of a dose response gradient (1); and (4) all plausible confounders would have reduced the effect (1).

Ia: Evidence obtained from meta-analysis or systematic review of randomized controlled trials
Ib: Evidence obtained from at least one randomized controlled trial
IIa: Evidence obtained from at least one well-designed controlled study without randomization
IIb: Evidence obtained from at least one other type of well-designed quasiexperimental study
III: Evidence obtained from well-designed nonexperimental descriptive studies, such as comparative studies, correlation studies, and case studies
IV: Evidence obtained from expert committee reports or opinions and/or clinical experiences of respected authorities

High: The available evidence usually includes consistent results from well-designed, well-conducted studies in representative primary care populations. These studies assess the effects of the preventive service on health outcomes. This conclusion is therefore unlikely to be strongly affected by the results of future studies.

Moderate: The available evidence is sufficient to determine the effects of the preventive service on health outcomes, but confidence in the estimate is constrained by such factors as the following:

- The number, size, or quality of individual studies
- Inconsistency of findings across individual studies
- Limited generalizability of findings to routine primary care practice
- Lack of coherence in the chain of evidence

As more information becomes available, the magnitude or direction of the observed effect could change, and this change may be large enough to alter the conclusion.

Low: The available evidence is insufficient to assess effects on health outcomes. Evidence is insufficient because of one or more of the following:

- The limited number or size of studies
- Important flaws in study design or methods
- Inconsistency of findings across individual studies
- Gaps in the chain of evidence
- Findings not generalizable to routine primary care practice
- Lack of information on important health outcomes.

More information may allow estimation of effects on health outcomes.

Continued

TABLE **21.2**

EXAMPLES OF EVIDENCE-INFORMED PRACTICE RATING SYSTEMS—cont'd

STRENGTH OF RECOMMENDATIONS	GRADES OF RECOMMENDATION	GRADES OF RECOMMENDATION
Strong: Confident that the desirable effects of adherence to a recommendation outweigh the undesirable effects. **Weak:** The desirable effects of adherence to a recommendation probably outweigh the undesirable effects, but the developers are less confident. ***Note:*** Strength of recommendation is determined by the balance between desirable and undesirable consequences of alternative management strategies, quality of evidence, variability in values and preferences, and resource use.	A: There is good evidence to recommend the clinical preventive action. B: There is fair evidence to recommend the clinical preventive action. C: The existing evidence is conflicting and does not allow making a recommendation for or against use of the clinical preventive action; however, other factors may influence decision making. D: There is fair evidence to recommend against the clinical preventive action. E: There is good evidence to recommend against the clinical preventive action. I: There is insufficient evidence (in quantity and/or quality) to make recommendations; however, other factors may influence decision making.	A: The USPSTF recommends the service. There is high certainty that the net benefit is substantial. Practice: Offer or provide this service. B: The USPSTF recommends the service. There is high certainty that the net benefit is moderate or there is moderate certainty that the net benefit is moderate to substantial. Practice: Offer or provide this service. C: The USPSTF recommends against routinely providing the service. There may be considerations that support providing the service in an individual patient. There is at least moderate certainty that the net benefit is small. Practice: Offer or provide this service only if other considerations support the offering or providing the service in an individual patient. D: The USPSTF recommends against the service. There is moderate or high certainty that the service has no net benefit or that the harms outweigh the benefits. Practice: Discourage the use of this service. I: The USPSTF concludes that the current evidence is insufficient to assess the balance of benefits and harms of the service. Evidence is lacking, of poor quality, or conflicting, and the balance of benefits and harms cannot be determined. Practice: Read the clinical considerations section of USPSTF Recommendation Statement. If the service is offered, patients should understand the uncertainty about the balance of benefits and harms.

USPSTF, U.S. Preventive Services Task Force.
From Registered Nurses' Association of Ontario (RNAO). (2011). Rating system described by Canadian Task Force on Preventive Health Care. (CTFPHC). (1997). Quick tables by strength of evidence. Available at http://www.canadiantaskforce.ca and http://rnao.ca/sites/rnao-ca/files/storage/related/618_BPG_Falls_summary_rev05.pdf.

regarding the best system to use for denoting the type and quality of evidence or for grading schemas to denote the strength of the body of evidence (Djulbegoivc & Guyatt, 2017). For example, the Scottish Intercollegiate Guidelines Network has an extensive method detailed on their website for appraising research and setting forth guideline recommendations (http://www.sign.ac.uk/methodology.html).

The Grading of Recommendations Assessment, Development, and Evaluation (GRADE) Working Group, initiated in 2000, is an informal collaboration of individuals interested in addressing grading schema in health care (http://www.gradeworkinggroup.org). In setting forth practice recommendations, the GRADE system first rates the quality of the evidence as high, moderate, low, or very low and then grades the strength of the evidence as strong or weak (GRADE Working Group, 2004; Guyatt, Oxman, Kunz, et al., 2008a, 2008b; Table 21.2). Their methods are available on their website, with grading software (GRADEpro) available.

The National Guidelines Clearinghouse classifies submitted guidelines according to methods used by developers to accomplish two goals: (1) to assess the quality and strength of the evidence through expert consensus (committee or expert panel method), through subjective review, through weighting according to a rating scheme provided by the developers, or through weighting according to a rating scheme not provided by the developers; and (2) to formulate recommendations through various types of expert consensus (e.g., expert manual method, nominal group technique, consensus development conference) and balance sheets.

The RNAO (2012) guidelines for best practices are based on scientific evidence after a thorough review of the literature. Each of the studies is rated to determine whether it should be included in the guideline. The rating system used for the level of evidence and the grades of recommendation are illustrated in Table 21.2.

Before critiquing research articles, reading relevant literature, and reviewing evidence-informed practice guidelines, an organization or group responsible for the review must agree on methods for noting the type of research, rating the quality of individual articles, and grading the strength of the body of evidence. Users must evaluate which systems are most appropriate for the task being undertaken, the length of time to complete each instrument, and its ease of use. It is also important to decide how the strength of the evidence will be reflected in the guideline.

Critique of Evidence-Informed Practice Guidelines

As the number of evidence-informed practice guidelines proliferate, it becomes increasingly important that nurses critique these guidelines with regard to the methods used for formulating them and consider how they might be used in their practice. Critical areas that should be assessed when evidence-informed practice guidelines are critiqued include the following:

1. Date of publication or release
2. Authors of the guideline
3. Endorsement of the guideline
4. A clear purpose of what the guideline covers and patient groups for which it was designed
5. Types of evidence (research, non-research) used in formulating the guideline
6. Types of research included in formulating the guideline (e.g., "We considered only randomized and other prospective controlled trials in determining efficacy of therapeutic interventions.")
7. A description of the methods used in grading the evidence
8. Search terms and retrieval methods used to acquire research and non-research evidence used in the guideline
9. Well-referenced statements regarding practice
10. Comprehensive reference list
11. Review of the guideline by experts
12. Whether the guideline has been used or tested in practice and, if so, with what types of patients and in what types of settings

Evidence-informed practice guidelines, formulated through the use of rigorous methods, provide a useful starting point for nurses to understand the evidence base of certain practices. However, more research may have become available since the publication of the guideline, and refinements may be needed. Although information in well-developed, national, evidence-informed practice guidelines is a helpful reference, it is usually necessary to localize the guideline through the use of institution-specific, evidence-informed policies, procedures, or standards before the guideline is applied within a specific setting. A useful tool for critiquing clinical practice guidelines is the AGREE II tool (available at http://www.agreetrust.org/).

As evidence-informed practice guidelines are used more extensively in practice, research is becoming available on whether the utilization of the guidelines results in better patient outcomes. For example, MacDougall et al. (2019) tested the implementation of pediatric pain guidelines for vaccinations, which validated the pain management guidelines.

Critique of Evidence

Critique of each resource found should involve the same methodology, and the critique process should be a shared responsibility. Review Chapter 3, as well as the critiquing criteria throughout this book. Keep in mind the Levels of Evidence and 6S Pyramid (Chapter 5). It is important for evidence-informed practice that you are using the best evidence, determining what is unreliable, and making practice changes that are based on high-quality studies (Fineout-Overholt & Stevens, 2019). Other tips for critiquing include:

- Using a journal club to discuss critiques performed by each member of the group
- Pairing a novice and expert to do critiques
- Eliciting assistance from students who may be interested in the topic and want experience performing critiques
- Making a class project of critique and synthesis of research for a given topic

Several resources are available to assist with the critique process, including *Evidence-Based Practice in Nursing and Healthcare (*Melnyk & Fineout-Overholt, 2019*)* and *Evidence-Based Nursing: A Guide to Clinical Practice* (DiCenso, Guyatt, & Ciliska, 2005). If you wish to start your own journal club, refer to Silversides (2011) for practical advice and further references.

Research Hint_____
Keep critique processes simple and encourage participation by nurses who are providing direct patient care.

Synthesis of the Research

Once studies are critiqued, a decision is made regarding use of each study in the synthesis of the evidence for application in clinical practice. Factors that should be considered for inclusion of studies in the synthesis of findings are overall scientific merit of the study; type (e.g., age, gender, pathological condition) of participants enrolled in the study and their similarity to the patient population to which the findings will be applied; and relevance of the study to the topic of question. For example, if the practice area is prevention of deep venous thrombosis in patients after surgery, a descriptive study with a heterogeneous population of medical patients is not appropriate for inclusion in the synthesis of findings. To synthesize the findings from research critiques, it is helpful to use a summary table in which critical information from studies can be documented (see Chapter 5).

Setting Forth Evidence-Informed Practice Recommendations

On the basis of the critique of evidence-informed practice guidelines and synthesis of research, recommendations for practice are set forth. The type and strength of evidence used to support the practice need to be clearly delineated. Box 21.2 is a useful tool to assist with this activity.

The following are examples of practice recommendation statements, with evidence ratings:
- "Implement individualized breastfeeding self-efficacy interventions throughout the perinatal period to enhance breastfeeding confidence including:
  - One-on-one counseling prior to discharge from the childbirth setting and
  - follow-up post-discharge."

BOX 21.2

CONSISTENCY OF EVIDENCE FROM CRITIQUED RESEARCH AND APPRAISALS OF EVIDENCE-INFORMED PRACTICE GUIDELINES

1. Are studies replicated with consistent results?
2. Are the studies well designed?
3. Are recommendations consistent among systematic reviews, evidence-informed practice guidelines, and critiqued research?
4. Are risks to the patient identified from evidence-informed practice recommendations?
5. Are benefits to the patient identified?
6. Have cost analysis studies been conducted with regard to the recommended action, intervention, or treatment?
7. Are summary recommendations about assessments, actions, and interventions or treatments available from the research, systematic reviews, and evidence-informed guidelines with an assigned evidence grade?
8. Is one of the following examples of grading the evidence used?
   a. Evidence from well-designed meta-analysis or other systematic reviews
   b. Evidence from well-designed controlled trials, both randomized and nonrandomized, with results that consistently support a specific action (e.g., assessment), intervention, or treatment
   c. Evidence from observational studies (e.g., correlational descriptive studies) or controlled trials with inconsistent results
   d. Evidence from expert opinion or multiple cases

(Used/reprinted with permission from the University of Iowa Hospitals and Clinics, Copyright 2002. For permission to use or reproduce these figures, please contact the University of Iowa Hospitals and Clinics at 319-384-9098 or uihcnursingresearchandebp@uiowa.edu.)

(Strength of recommendation = Ia, Ib) (RNAO, 2018, p. 19)
- "Nurses understand the common signs and symptoms present during the last days and hours of life" (Strength of recommendation = IIb-IV) (RNAO, 2011, p. 5).
- "We recommend asking children and youth (age 5–18 yr) or their parents about tobacco use by the child or youth and offering brief* information and advice, as appropriate, during primary care visits† to prevent tobacco smoking among children and youth" (weak recommendation, low-quality evidence) (Canadian Task Force on Preventive Health Care, 2017).

Research Hint

Use of a summary form helps identify commonalities across several studies with regard to study findings and the types of patients to which study findings can be applied. It also helps in synthesizing the overall strengths and weakness of the studies as a group.

Decision to Change Practice

After studies are critiqued and synthesized and evidence-informed practices are set forth, the next step is to decide whether findings are appropriate for use in practice. The following criteria should be considered in making these decisions:
- Relevance of evidence for practice
- Consistency in findings across studies, guidelines, or both
- A significant number of studies, evidence-informed practice guidelines, or both in which sample characteristics are similar to those to which the findings will be applied
- Consistency among evidence from research and other non-research evidence
- Feasibility for use in practice
- The risk–benefit ratio (risk of harm; potential benefit for the patient)

Evidence-Informed Practice Tip

A good rule of thumb to use when considering a practice change is as follows:

Level of evidence + quality of evidence = strength of evidence and confidence to act and change practice (Melnyk & Fineout-Overholt, 2019).

Synthesis of study findings and other evidence may result in supporting current practice, making minor practice modifications, undertaking major practice changes, or developing a new area of practice.

An example of evidence-informed practice change was reported by Thier (2019) regarding a project to improve pain during IV initiation in an outpatient clinic. After reviewing the recent research literature on use of intradermal lidocaine prior to IV insertion, the team at this clinic decided that use of intradermal lidocaine was warranted and proceeded with the practice change. They monitored the patient outcomes and saw an improvement in patient satisfaction/patient experience scores.

Development of Evidence-Informed Practice

The next step is to put in writing the evidence base of the practice (Haber, Feldman, Penney, et al., 1994) the grading schema that has been agreed upon should be used. When results of the critique and synthesis of evidence support current practice or suggest a change in practice, a written evidence-informed practice standard (e.g., policy, procedure, guideline) is warranted. This is necessary so that professionals in the organization (1) know that the practices are based on evidence and (2) know which type of evidence (e.g., randomized controlled trial, expert opinion) was used in developing the evidence-informed standard. Several different formats can be used to document evidence-informed practice changes. The format chosen is influenced by what the document is and how it will be used. Written evidence-informed practices should be part of the organizational policy and procedure manual and should include linkages to the references for the parts of the policy and procedure that are based on research and other types of evidence.

Clinicians (e.g., nurses, physicians, pharmacists) who adopt evidence-informed practices are influenced by the perceived participation they have had in developing and reviewing the protocol (Titler, 2008). It is imperative that once the evidence-informed practice standard is written, key stakeholders have an opportunity to review it and provide feedback to the person or persons responsible for writing it. Focus groups can provide discussion about the evidence-informed standard and identify key areas that may be potentially troublesome during the implementation phase. It may be necessary to design and implement a pilot practice change initially, and consideration should be given to also involving patients in the proposed practice change (Dang et al., 2019).

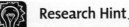

Research Hint

Use a consistent approach to writing evidence-informed practice standards and referencing the research and related literature.

Implementing the Practice Change

If a practice change is warranted, the next steps are to make the evidence-informed changes in practice. This step goes beyond writing a policy or procedure that is evidence informed; it requires interaction among direct care providers to champion and foster evidence adoption, leadership support, and system changes. Rogers's (2003) seminal work on diffusion of innovations is extremely useful for selecting strategies for promoting adoption of evidence-informed practices. Other investigators describing barriers to and strategies for adoption of evidence-informed practices have used Rogers's (2003) model (Gravel et al., 2006; Scott et al., 2008; Thompson et al., 2007).

According to this model, adoption of innovations, such as evidence-informed practices, is influenced by the nature of the innovation (e.g., the type and strength of evidence; the clinical topic) and the manner in which it is communicated (disseminated) to members (nurses) of a social system (organization, nursing profession; Rogers, 2003). Strategies for promoting adoption of evidence-informed practices must address these areas within a context of participative, planned change. The RNAO (2012) published *Toolkit: Implementation of Best Practice Guidelines* to assist staff in health care settings to successfully integrate the guidelines into clinical practice. The toolkit outlines seven essential components of knowledge translation:

1. Identify the problem: identify, review, select knowledge tools/resources
2. Adapt knowledge tools/resources to local context

3. Assess barriers and facilitators to knowledge use
4. Select, tailor, and implement interventions
5. Monitor knowledge use
6. Evaluate outcomes
7. Sustain knowledge use

Nature of the Innovation/Evidence-Informed Practice

Characteristics of an innovation or evidence-informed practice topic that affect adoption include the relative advantage of the evidence-informed practice (e.g., effectiveness, relevance to the task, social prestige); the compatibility with values, norms, work, and perceived needs of users; and complexity of the evidence-informed practice topic (Rogers, 2003). For example, evidence-informed practice topics that are perceived by users as relatively simple (e.g., influenza vaccines for older adults) are more easily adopted in less time than those that are more complex (e.g., acute pain management for hospitalized older adults).

Strategies to promote adoption of evidence-informed practices related to characteristics of the topic include practitioner review and "reinvention" of the evidence-informed practice guideline to fit the local context, use of quick reference guides and decision aids, and use of clinical reminders (Doebbeling et al., 2006).

An important principle to remember for planning implementation of an evidence-informed practice project is that the attributes of the evidence-informed practice topic as perceived by users and stakeholders (e.g., ease of use, valued part of practice) are neither stable features nor sure determinants of their adoption. Rather, it is the interaction among the characteristics of the evidence-informed practice topic, the intended users, and a particular context of practice that determines the rate and extent of adoption (Rogers, 2003).

Studies suggest that clinical systems, computerized decision support, and prompts/quick reference guides that support practice (e.g., decision-making algorithms) have a positive effect on aligning practices with the evidence base (Doebbeling et al.,

2006; Titler et al., 2006). Computerized knowledge management has consistently demonstrated significant improvements in provider performance and patient outcomes (Wensing et al., 2006). These systems are designed to present pre-appraised evidence to clinicians and are an important part of the evidence-based movement in providing timely updates and dissemination of knowledge (Djulbegovic & Guyatt, 2017).

One example of this computerized decision-support system (CDSS) was reported by Johansson-Pajala et al. (2018). They studied the use of a CDSS during medication reviews in a long-term care setting. The CDSS was helpful in identifying more potential adverse drug reactions than standard care (i.e., nurse review only), while nursing knowledge of individual residents identified issues such as lack of adherence.

Methods of Communication

Interpersonal communication methods and influence among social networks of users affect adoption of evidence-informed practices (Rogers, 2003). Use of opinion leaders, change champions, consultation with experts in the field, and education are strategies tested to promote adoption of evidence-informed practices. Education is necessary, and research has demonstrated that attending conferences and in-service programs is effective (Squires et al., 2011). Education should not only focus on overcoming knowledge gaps (i.e., what needs to change) but also *why* a change will be beneficial, and the evidence to support the change (Rodgers et al., 2019).

It is important that staff know the scientific basis and improvements in quality of care anticipated by the changes. Disseminating information to staff needs to be done creatively. A staff in-service may not be the most effective method, and it may not reach the majority of the staff. Although it is unrealistic for all staff to have participated in the critique process or to have read all studies used, it is important that they know the myths and realities of the practice. Staff education must also include ensuring competence in the skills necessary to carry out the new practice.

Use of stories and telling experiences of the practice change can raise emotions and engage stakeholders, motivating them towards change (Rodgers et al., 2019). Visibly identifying those who have learned the information and are using the evidence-informed practice (e.g., through wearing buttons, ribbons, pins) stimulates interest in others who may not have internalized the change. As a result, the "new" learner may begin asking questions about the practice and be more open to learning. Other educational strategies such as train-the-trainer programs, webinars, and competency testing are helpful in education of staff.

Several studies have demonstrated that opinion leaders are effective in changing behaviours of health care practitioners (Dopson et al., 2010; Doumit et al., 2007), especially in combination with educational outreach or performance feedback. Opinion leaders are from the local peer group, viewed as a respected source of influence, considered by associates as technically competent, and trusted to judge the fit between the innovation and the local situation (Dobbins et al. 2009; Doumit et al., 2007). The key characteristic of an opinion leader is that he or she is trusted to evaluate new information in the context of group norms. To do this, an opinion leader must be considered by associates as technically competent and a full and dedicated member of the local group (Rogers, 2003).

Social interactions such as "hallway chats," one-on-one discussions, and addressing questions are important yet often overlooked components of translation (Jordan et al., 2009). If the evidence-informed practice that is being implemented is interdisciplinary, discipline-specific opinion leaders should be used to promote the change in practice. Role expectations of an opinion leader are in Box 21.3.

Because nurses prefer interpersonal contact and communication with colleagues rather than Internet or traditional sources of practice knowledge (Estabrooks et al., 2005), it is imperative that one or two "change champions" be identified for each patient care unit or clinic where the

---

BOX 21.3

ROLE EXPECTATIONS OF AN OPINION LEADER

1. Be or become an expert in the evidence-informed practice.
2. Provide organizational or unit leadership for adopting the evidence-informed practice.
3. Implement various strategies to educate peers about the evidence-informed practice.
4. Work with peers, other disciplines, and leadership staff to incorporate key information about the evidence-informed practice into organizational/unit standards, policies, procedures, and documentation systems.
5. Promote initial and ongoing use of the evidence-informed practice by peers.

Modified from Titler, M. G., Herr, K., Everett, L. Q., et al. (2006). *Book to bedside: Promoting and sustaining EBPs in elders* (Final Progress Report to AHRQ, Grant No. 2R01 HS010482-04). Iowa City: University of Iowa College of Nursing.

---

change is being made so that evidence-informed practices can be enacted by direct care providers (Titler et al., 2006). Staff nurses are some of the best change agents for evidence-informed practice. The change champion believes in an idea; will not take "no" for an answer; is undaunted by insults and rebuffs; and, above all, persists. Conferencing with opinion leaders and change champions periodically during implementation is helpful in addressing questions and providing guidance as needed (Titler et al., 2006).

Additionally, clinical nurse educators can provide one-on-one consultation to staff regarding use of the evidence-informed practice with specific patients, assist staff in troubleshooting issues in application of the practice, and provide feedback on provider performance regarding use of the evidence-informed practice. It is important to build excitement for the practice change, create discomfort with the status quo, and develop shared ownership for the success of the project (Rodgers et al., 2019).

Users of the Evidence-Informed Practice

Members of a social system (e.g., nurses, physicians, clerical staff) influence how quickly and widely evidence-informed practices are adopted (Rogers, 2003). Audit and feedback, performance gap assessment (PGA), and trying the evidence-informed practice are strategies that have been tested (Hysong et al., 2006; Ivers et al., 2012; Jamtvedt et al., 2010; Titler et al., 2006). PGA (baseline practice performance) informs members at the beginning of change about a practice performance and opportunities for improvement. Specific practice indicators selected for PGA are related to the practices that are the focus of the practice change, such as every-4-hour pain assessment for acute pain management (Titler et al., 2006).

The practice of audit and feedback involves ongoing auditing of performance indicators, aggregating data into reports, and discussing the findings with practitioners during the practice change (Ivers et al., 2012; Jamtvedt et al., 2010; Titler et al., 2006). This strategy helps staff know and see how their efforts to improve care and patient outcomes are progressing throughout the implementation process.

Social System

Clearly, the social system or context of care delivery matters when implementing evidence-informed practices (Kochevar & Yano, 2006; Rogers, 2003). As part of the work of implementing evidence-informed practices, it is important that the social system (e.g., unit, service line, clinic) ensure that policies, procedures, standards, clinical pathways, and documentation systems support the use of the evidence-informed practices (Titler, 2004). Documentation forms or clinical information systems may need revision to support practice changes; documentation systems that fail to readily support the new practice thwart change. For example, if staff members are expected to reassess and document pain intensity within 30 minutes after administration of an analgesic agent, documentation forms must reflect this practice standard. It is the role of leadership to ensure that organizational documents and systems are flexible and supportive of the evidence-informed practices.

A learning organizational culture and proactive leadership that promotes knowledge sharing are important components for building an evidence-informed practice (Gallagher-Ford et al., 2019). Additional components of a receptive context for evidence-informed practice include the following:

- Strong leadership
- Clear strategic vision
- Good managerial relations
- Visionary staff in key positions
- A climate conducive to experimentation and risk taking
- Effective data-capture systems

Leadership support is critical for promoting use of evidence-informed practices and is expressed verbally and by providing necessary resources, materials, and time to fulfill responsibilities (Stetler, et al., 2006). Senior leadership needs to create an organizational mission, vision, and strategic plan that incorporates evidence-informed practice, implements performance expectations for staff that include evidence-informed practice work, integrates the work of evidence-informed practice into the governance structure of the health care system, demonstrates the value of evidence-informed practices through administrative behaviours, and establishes explicit expectations that nurse leaders will create microsystems that value and support clinical inquiry (Titler, 2002).

In summary, making an evidence-informed change in practice involves a series of action steps in a complex, nonlinear process. The time needed to implement the change depends on the nature of the practice change. Merely increasing staff knowledge about an evidence-informed practice and passive dissemination strategies are not likely to work, particularly in complex health care settings. Strategies that seem to have a positive effect on promoting use of evidence-informed practices include audit and feedback, use of clinical reminders and practice prompts, involvement of opinion leaders and change champions, interactive education, mass media, educational outreach/academic detailing, and the context of care delivery (e.g., leadership, learning, questioning). It is important that senior leadership and those leading evidence-informed practice improvements are aware of change as a process and continue to encourage and teach peers about the change in practice. The new practice must be continually reinforced and sustained or the practice change will be intermittent and soon fade, allowing more traditional methods of care to return.

Evaluation

Evaluation provides an opportunity to collect and analyze data with regard to use of a new evidence-informed practice and then to modify the practice as necessary. It is important that the evidence-informed change is evaluated, both at the pilot testing phase and when the practice is changed in additional patient care areas. The importance of the evaluation cannot be overemphasized; it provides information for performance gap assessment, audit, and feedback, and it provides information necessary to determine whether the evidence-informed practice should be retained, modified, or eliminated. Steps of the evaluation process are summarized in Box 21.4.

Evaluation should include both process and outcome measures. The process component focuses on how the practice change is being implemented. It is important to know if staff are using the practice and implementing the practice as noted in the evidence-informed practice guideline. Evaluation of the process also should note (1) barriers that staff encounter in carrying out the practice (e.g., lack of information, skills, or necessary equipment); (2) differences in opinions among health care providers; and (3) difficulty in carrying out the steps of the practice as originally designed (e.g., shutting off tube feedings 1 hour before aspirating contents for checking placement of nasointestinal tubes). Process data can be collected from staff and/or patient self-reports, medical record audits, or observation of clinical practice. Examples of process and outcome questions are shown in Table 21.3.

Outcome data are an equally important part of evaluation. The purpose of outcome evaluation is

---

BOX 21.4

STEPS OF EVALUATION FOR EVIDENCE-INFORMED PRACTICE

1. Identify process and outcome variables of interest.
   Examples:
   Process variable: For patients older than 65 years, a Braden scale will be completed on admission.
   Outcome variable: Presence/absence of nosocomial pressure injury; if present, determine stage as I, II, III, or IV.
2. Determine methods and frequency of data collection.
   Example:
   Process variable: Chart audit of all patients older than 65 years, 1 day a month
   Outcome variable: Assessment of all patients older than 65 years, 1 day a month
3. Determine baseline and follow-up sample sizes.
4. Design data-collection forms.
   Example:
   Process variable: chart audit abstraction form
   Outcome variable: pressure injury assessment form
5. Establish content validity of data-collection forms.
6. Train data collectors.
7. Assess interrater reliability of data collectors.
8. Collect data at specified intervals.
9. Provide "on-site" feedback to staff regarding the progress in achieving the practice change.
10. Provide feedback of analyzed data to staff.
11. Use data to assist staff in modifying or integrating the evidence-informed practice change.

---

to assess whether the patient, staff, and/or fiscal outcomes expected are achieved. Therefore, it is important that baseline data be used for a preintervention/postintervention comparison (Titler et al., 2001). The outcome variables measured should be those that are projected to change as a result of changing practice. For example, research demonstrates that less restricted family visiting practices in critical care units result in improved satisfaction with care. Thus, patient and family member satisfaction should be an outcome measure that is evaluated as part of changing visiting practices in adult critical care units. Outcome measures should be measured before the change in practice is implemented, after implementation, and every 6 to 12 months thereafter. Findings must be provided to clinicians to reinforce the impact of the change and to ensure that they are incorporated into quality improvement programs. When

			NEITHER AGREE NOR		STRONGLY

TABLE 21.3

EXAMPLES OF EVALUATION MEASURES

EXAMPLE OF PROCESS QUESTIONS	STRONGLY DISAGREE	DISAGREE	NEITHER AGREE NOR DISAGREE	AGREE	STRONGLY AGREE
1. I feel well prepared to use the Braden Scale with older patients.	1	2	3	4	5
2. Malnutrition increases patient risk for pressure injury development.	1	2	3	4	5

EXAMPLE OF OUTCOME QUESTION

Patient: On a scale of 0 (no pain) to 10 (worst possible pain), how much pain have you experienced over the past 24 hours? _____ (Pain intensity)

(Used/reprinted with permission from the University of Iowa Hospitals and Clinics, Copyright 2002. For permission to use or reproduce these figures, please contact the University of Iowa Hospitals and Clinics at 319-384-9098 or uihcnursingresearchandebp@uiowa.edu.)

collecting process and outcome data for evaluation of a practice change, it is important that the data collection tools are user-friendly, short, concise, and easy to complete and have content validity. Focus must be on collecting the most essential data. Those responsible for collecting evaluative data must be trained on data-collection methods and be assessed for interrater reliability. Those individuals who have participated in implementing the protocol can be very helpful in evaluation by collecting data, providing timely feedback to staff, and assisting staff to overcome barriers encountered when implementing the changes in practice.

One question that often arises is how much data are needed to evaluate this change. The preferred number of patients (N) is somewhat dependent on the size of the patient population affected by the practice change. For example, if the practice change is for families of critically ill adult patients and the organization has 1000 adult critical care patients annually, 50 to 100 satisfaction responses preimplementation and 25 to 50 responses postimplementation, at 3 and 6 months, should be adequate to look for trends in satisfaction and possible areas that need to be addressed in continuing this practice (e.g., more bedside chairs in patient rooms). The rule of thumb is to keep the evaluation simple, because data often are collected by busy clinicians who may lose interest if

the data collection, analysis, and feedback periods are too long and tedious. The evaluation process includes planned feedback to staff who are making the change. The feedback includes verbal and/or written appreciation for the work and visual demonstration of progress in implementation and improvement in patient outcomes. The key to effective evaluation is to ensure that the evidence-informed change in practice is warranted (e.g., will improve quality of care) and that the intervention does not bring harm to patients.

TRANSLATION SCIENCE

Translation science, mentioned previously in this chapter, is "rigorous research that studies how evidence-based interventions are translated to real-world clinical settings" (Melnyk & Fineout-Overholt, 2019, p. 9). It includes research to (1) understand context variables that influence adoption of evidence-informed practices and (2) test the effectiveness of interventions to promote and sustain use of evidence-informed health care practices. Translation science denotes both the systematic investigation of methods, interventions, and variables that influence adoption of evidence-informed health care practices, as well as the organized body of knowledge gained through such research (Eccles & Mittman, 2006; Rubenstein & Pugh, 2006; Sussman et al., 2006; Titler et al., 2007). Researchers in Canada may use the terms *research utilization, knowledge-to-action, knowledge transfer,* or *knowledge translation* interchangeably, whereas researchers in the United States, the United Kingdom, and Europe may be more likely to use the term *implementation* or *research translation* to express similar concepts (Graham et al., 2006). Kitson and Harvey (2016) state that knowledge translation "describes the process by which knowledge moves from where it was first created and refined to where it has to get to in order to make an impact on clinical practice and patient care" (p. 294).

The goals of the Canadian Institutes of Health Research (CIHR) are to not only support the development of new knowledge through research but also ensure that the knowledge is translated into practice. The CHIR define knowledge translation "as a dynamic and iterative process that includes synthesis, dissemination, exchange and ethically sound application of knowledge to improve the health of Canadians, provide more effective health services and products and strengthen the health care system" (CIHR, 2016). The CIHR lists the steps of knowledge to action as follows:

A. Creating Knowledge
   1. Deriving knowledge from primary studies, such as randomized controlled trials (knowledge inquiry)
   2. Synthesizing primary studies to form secondary knowledge, such as systematic reviews or meta-analyses
   3. Generating knowledge tools or products (third-generation knowledge) such as practice guidelines, decision aids, or care pathways based on best available evidence distilled from synthesized knowledge

B. Applying Knowledge
   4. Identifying the problem and identifying, reviewing, and selecting knowledge
   5. Adapting knowledge to local context
   6. Assessing barriers and facilitators to knowledge use

   7. Selecting, tailoring, and implementing intervention to address barriers to knowledge use
   8. Monitoring knowledge use
   9. Evaluating outcome of knowledge use
   10. Developing mechanisms to sustain knowledge use

The CIHR website is an excellent reference for further study on knowledge translation (http://www.cihr-irsc.gc.ca/e/39128.html).

FUTURE DIRECTIONS

Use of research across health care systems for improving the quality of care is essential. As professionals continue to understand the science of nursing and synthesize this science for application in practice, it will become increasingly necessary to test and understand how to best promote the use of this science in daily practice. There are many roles for nurses in the future of evidence-informed practice. Nurses in roles of providing direct patient care can identify areas where practice needs to be improved and be involved and supportive of improvements to practice. Nurses with graduate education, and particularly PhDs, are needed to conduct primary research studies, such as nursing intervention studies. In education and administrative roles nurses can champion evidence-informed practices to create a culture for improving patient care. In advanced practice roles—such as clinical nurse specialists and nurse practitioners—nurses can develop and engage in research in clinical areas where there is insufficient research. Although less common in Canada than other jurisdictions, the Doctor of Nursing Practice degree has a focus of developing experts to lead evidence-informed practice throughout organizations and institutions (Melnyk, 2016).

Education of nurses must include knowledge and skills in the use of research evidence in practice. Nurses are increasingly being held accountable for practices informed by scientific evidence. Thus, nurses must integrate into their profession the expectation that all nurses have a professional responsibility to read and use research in their practice and to communicate with nurse scientists the many and varied clinical problems for which a scientific basis for practice does not yet exist.

CRITICAL THINKING CHALLENGES

- Discuss the differences among nursing research, research utilization, and evidence-informed practice. Support your discussion with examples.

- Why would it be important to use an evidence-informed practice model, such as the Ottawa Model of Health Care Research, to guide a practice project focused on justifying and implementing a change in clinical practice?

- You are a staff nurse working on a cardiac step-down unit. Many of your colleagues do not understand evidence-informed practice. How would you help them to understand how evidence-informed practice is relevant to providing optimal care to this patient population?

- What barriers do you see to applying evidence-informed practice in your clinical setting? Discuss strategies to use in overcoming these barriers.

CRITICAL JUDGEMENT QUESTIONS

1. Identifying a practice issue for an evidence-informed practice project is the responsibility of:
   a. All registered nurses
   b. Clinical nurse educators
   c. Doctors of nursing practice
   d. Healthcare managers

2. How do you know if you should make a practice change?
   a. Levels of evidence reflect mostly RCTs
   b. There is a need to improve patient care
   c. High levels and high quality of evidence
   d. Computerized decision-support systems

3. What is the foundation of evidence-informed practice change?
   a. Identifying the problem using a PICOT format
   b. Creating a spirit of inquiry
   c. Selection of a topic
   d. Dissemination and implementation

KEY POINTS

- According to the Iowa Model Revised: Evidence-Based Practice to Promote Excellence in Health Care (Iowa Model Collaborative, 2017), the steps of evidence-informed practice are as follows: selecting a topic, forming a team, retrieving the evidence, grading the evidence, developing an evidence-informed practice standard, implementing the evidence-informed practice, and evaluating the effect on staff, patient, and fiscal outcomes.

- Adoption of evidence-informed practice standards requires education and dissemination to staff and use of change strategies, such as communication with opinion leaders, change champions, a core group, and consultants.

- It is important to evaluate the change. Evaluation provides data for performance gap assessment, audit, and feedback and provides information necessary to determine whether the practice should be retained.

- Evaluation includes both process and outcome measures.

- It is important for organizations to create a culture of evidence-informed practice. Creating this culture requires an interactive process. To create this culture, organizations need to provide access to information, access to individuals who have skills necessary for evidence-informed practice, and a written and verbal commitment to evidence-informed practice in the organization's operations.

- The terms *research utilization* and *evidence-informed practice* are sometimes used interchangeably. These terms, although related, are not one and the same. Research utilization is the process of using research findings to improve practice. Evidence-informed practice is a broad term that encompasses the use of not only research findings but also other types of evidence, such as case reports and expert opinion, in deciding the evidence base that informs practice.

- There are two forms of evidence use: conceptual and decision driven.
- There are several models of evidence-informed practice. A key feature of all models is the judicious review and synthesis of research and other types of evidence to develop an evidence-informed practice standard.

🛜 FOR FURTHER STUDY

Go to Evolve at http://evolve.elsevier.com/Canada/LoBiondo/Research for the Audio Glossary.

REFERENCES

Adams, S. L., & Titler, M. G. (2010). Building a learning collaborative. *Worldviews on Evidence-Based Nursing, 7*(3), 165–173.

Alper, B. S., & Haynes, R. B. (2016). EBHC pyramid 5.0 for accessing preappraised evidence and guidance. *BMJ Evidence-Based Medicine, 21*(4), 123–125. http://dx.doi.org/10.1136/ebmed-2016-110447.

Canadian Nurses Association (CNA). (2010). *Position statement: Evidence-informed decision-making and nursing practice.* https://www.cna-aiic.ca/-/media/nurseone/page-content/pdf-en/evidence-informed-decision-making-and-nursing-practice.pdfCanadian.

Canadian Nurses Association. (2020). *Evidence-based practice: Definitions galore.* https://www.cna-aiic.ca/en/nursing-practice/evidence-based-practice/definitions-galore.

Canadian Institutes of Health Research (CIHR). (2016). *Knowledge translation.* Retrieved from http://www.cihr-irsc.gc.ca/e/29418.html.

Canadian Task Force on Preventive Health Care. (2017). Recommendations on behavioral interventions for the prevention and treatment of cigarette smoking among school-aged children and youth. *CMAJ, 189,* E310–E316. https://doi.org/10.1503/cmaj.161242.

Cronenwett, L. R. (1995). Effective methods for disseminating research findings to nurses in practice. *Nursing Clinics of North America, 30,* 429–438.

Dang, D., Melnyk, B. M., Fineout-Overholt, E., Yost, J., Cullen, L., Cvach, M., Larabee, J. H., Rycroft-Malone, J., Schultz, A. A., Stetler, C. B., & Stevens, K. R (2019). In B. M. Melnyk, & E. Fineout-Overholt (Eds.), *Evidence-based practice in nursing and healthcare: A guide to best practice* (4th ed., pp. 378–427): Wolters Kluwer.

DiCenso, A., Guyatt, G., & Ciliska, D. (2005). *Evidence-based nursing: A guide to clinical practice.* St. Louis: Elsevier.

Djulbegovic, B., & Guyatt, G. H. (2017). Progress in evidence-based medicine: a quarter century on. *The Lancet, 390*(10092), 415–423. https://doi.org/10.1016/S0140-6736(16)31592-6.

Dobbins, M., Robeson, P., Ciliska, D., Hanna, S., Cameron, R., O'Mara, L., DeCorby, K., & Mercer, S. (2009). A description of a knowledge broker role implemented as part of a randomized controlled trial evaluating three knowledge translation strategies. *Implementation Science, 4*(23), 1–9. https://doi.org/10.1186/1748-5908-4-23.

Doebbeling, B. N., Chou, A. F., & Tierney, W. M. (2006). Priorities and strategies for the implementation of integrated informatics and communications technology to improve evidence-based practice. *Journal of General Internal Medicine, 21*(S2), S50–S57.

Dopson, S., FitzGerald, L., Ferlie, E., et al. (2010). No magic targets! Changing clinical practice to become more evidence based. *Health Care Management Review, 27*(3), 35–47.

Doumit, G., Gattellari, M., Grimshaw, J., et al. (2007). Local opinion leaders: Effects on professional practice and health care outcomes. *Cochrane Database of Systematic Reviews*(1), CD000125.

Eccles, M. P., & Mittman, B. S. (2006). Welcome to implementation science. *Implementation Science, 1,* 1.

Estabrooks, C. A. (2004). Thoughts on evidence-based nursing and its science: A Canadian perspective. *Worldviews on Evidence-Based Nursing, 1*(2), 88–91.

Estabrooks, C. A., Chong, H., Brigidear, K., et al. (2005). Profiling Canadian nurses' preferred knowledge sources for clinical practice. *Canadian Journal of Nursing Research, 37*(2), 119–140.

Estabrooks, C. A., Derksen, L., Winther, C., et al. (2008). The intellectual structure and substance of the knowledge utilization field: A longitudinal author co-citation analysis, 1945–2004. *Implementation Science, 3,* 49.

Fineout-Overholt, E., & Stevens, K. R (2019). Critically appraising knowledge for clinical decision making. In B. M. Melnyk, & E. Fineout-Overholt (Eds.), *Evidence-based practice in nursing and healthcare: A guide to best practice* (4th ed., pp. 109–123): Wolters Kluwer.

Gallagher-Ford, L., Buck, J. S., & Melnyk, B. M (2019). Leadership strategies for creating and sustaining evidence-based practice organizations. In B. M. Melnyk, & E. Fineout-Overholt (Eds.), *Evidence-based practice in nursing and healthcare: A guide to best practice* (4th ed., pp. 328–343): Wolters Kluwer.

GRADE Working Group. (2004). Grading quality of evidence and strength of recommendations. *British Medical Journal, 328,* 1490–1494.

Graham, I. D., Logan, J., Harrison, M. B., et al. (2006). Lost in knowledge translation: Time for a map?. *Journal of Continuing Education in the Health Professions, 26*(1), 13–24.

Gravel, K., Légaré, F., & Graham, I. D. (2006). Barriers and facilitators to implementing shared decision-making in clinical practice: A systematic review of health professionals' perceptions. *Implementation Science, 1,* 16.

Grol, R. P., Bosch, M. C., Hulscher, M. E., et al. (2007). Planning and studying improvement in patient care: The use of theoretical perspectives. *The Milbank Quarterly, 85*(1), 93–138.

Guyatt, G. H., Oxman, A. D., Kunz, R., et al. (2008a). Rating quality of evidence and strength of recommendations: What is "quality of evidence" and why is it important to clinicians?. *British Medical Journal, 336*(7651), 995–998.

Guyatt, G. H., Oxman, A. D., Kunz, R., et al. (2008b). Rating quality of evidence and strength of recommendations: Incorporating considerations of resources use into grading recommendations. *British Medical Journal, 336*(7654), 1170–1173.

Haber, J., Feldman, H. R., Penney, N., Carter, E., Bidwell-Cerone, S., & Hott, J. R. (1994). Shaping nursing practice through research-based protocols. *The Journal of the New York State Nurses' Association, 25*(3), 4–12.

Haller, K. B., Reynolds, M. A., & Horsley, J. O. (1979). Developing research-based innovation protocols: Process, criteria, and issues. *Research in Nursing & Health, 2*(2), 45–51.

Harris, R. P., Helfand, M., Woolf, S. H., Lohr, K. N., Mulrow, C. D., Teutsch, S. M., & Atkins, D. Methods Work Group Third U.S. Preventive Services Task Force. (2001). Current methods of the US Preventive Services Task Force: a review of the process. *American Journal of Preventive Medicine, 20*(3), 21–35. https://doi.org/10.1016/S0749-3797(01)00261-6.

Harvey, G., & Kitson, A. (2015). *Implementing evidence-based practice in healthcare. A facilitation guide.* New York: Routledge.

Higgins, J. P. T., & Green, S. (Eds.). (2011). *Cochrane handbook for systematic reviews of interventions 5.1.* Retrieved from http://handbook.cochrane.org/.

Horsley, J. A., Crane, J., Crabtree, M. K., et al. (1983). *Using research to improve nursing practice: A guide.* New York: Grune & Stratton.

Hysong, S. J., Best, R. G., & Pugh, J. A. (2006). Audit and feedback and clinical practice guideline adherence: Making feedback actionable. *Implementation Science, 1,* 9.

ICEBeRG. (2006). Designing theoretically informed implementation interventions: The improved clinical effectiveness through behavioural research group. *Implementation Science, 1,* 4.

Iowa Model Collaborative. (2017). Iowa model of evidence-based practice: Revisions and validation. *Worldviews on Evidence-Based Nursing, 14*(3), 175–182. doi:10.1111/wvn.12223.

Ivers, N., Jamtvedt, G., Flottorp, S., et al. (2012). Audit and feedback: Effects on professional practice and healthcare outcomes. *Cochrane Database of Systematic Reviews*, (6), Article CD000259.

Jamtvedt, G., Young, J. M., Kristoffersen, D. T., et al. (2010). Audit and feedback: Effects on professional practice and health care outcomes (Review). *Cochrane Database of Systematic Reviews*, (7), Article CD000259.

Johansson-Pajala, R. M., Martin, L., & Blomgren, K. J. (2018). Registered nurses' use of computerised decision support in medication reviews: Implications in Swedish nursing homes. *International Journal of Health Care Quality Assurance, 31*(6), 531–544. https://0-doi-org.aupac.lib.athabascau.ca/10.1108/IJHCQA-01-2017-000.

Jordan, M. E., Lanham, H. J., Crabtree, B. F., et al. (2009). The role of conversation in health care interventions: Enabling sensemaking and learning. *Implementation Science, 4,* 15.

Kitson, A. L., & Harvey, H. (2016). Methods to succeed in effective knowledge translation in clinical practice. *Journal of Nursing Scholarship, 48*(3), 294–302.

Kochevar, L. K., & Yano, E. M. (2006). Understanding health care organization needs and context: Beyond performance gaps. *Journal of General Internal Medicine, 21,* S25–S29.

Logan, J., & Graham, I. (1998). Toward a comprehensive interdisciplinary model of health care research use. *Science Communication, 20*(2), 229.

MacDougall, T., Cunningham, S., Whitney, L., & Sawhney, M. (2019). Improving pediatric experience of pain during vaccinations: A quality improvement project. *International Journal Of Health Care Quality Assurance, 32*(6), 1034–1040. https://doi.org/10.1108/IJHCQA-07-2018-0185.

Melnyk, B. M. (2016a). Level of evidence plus critical appraisal of its quality yields confidence to implement evidence-based practice changes. *Worldviews on Evidence-Based Nursing, 13*(5), 337–339. https://doi.org/10.1111/wvn.12181.

Melnyk, B. M. (2016b). Culture eats strategy every time: What works in building and sustaining an evidence-based practice culture in healthcare systems.

Worldviews on Evidence-Based Nursing, 13(2), 99–101.

Melnyk, B. M., & Fineout-Overholt, E. (2011a). *Implementing evidence-based practice for nurses: Real-life success stories*. Indianapolis, IN: Sigma Theta Tau.

Melnyk, B. M., & Fineout-Overholt, E. (2011b). *Evidence-based practice in nursing & healthcare. A guide to best practice*. Berlin: Wolters Kluwer.

Melnyk, B. M., & Fineout-Overholt, E. (2019). Making the case for evidence-based practice and cultivating a spirit of inquiry. In B. M. Melnyk, & E. Fineout-Overholt (Eds.), *Evidence-based practice in nursing and healthcare: A guide to best practice* (4th ed., pp. 7–32): Wolters Kluwer.

Melnyk, B. M., Gallagher-Ford, L., Long, L. E., et al. (2014). The establishment of evidence-based practice competences for practicing registered nurses and advanced practice nurses in real-world clinical settings: Proficiencies to improve healthcare quality, reliability, patient outcomes, and costs. *Worldviews on Evidence-Based Nursing, 11*(1), 5–15.

Melnyk, B. M., Gallagher-Ford, L., Thomas, B. K., Troseth, M., Wyngarden, K., & Szalacha, L. (2016). A study of chief nurse executives indicates low prioritization of evidence-based practice and shortcomings in hospital performance metrics across the United States. *Worldviews on Evidence-Based Nursing, 13*(1), 6–14. https://doi.org/10.1111/wvn.12133.

Nightingale, F. (1858). *Notes on matters affecting the health, efficiency, and hospital administration of the British Army*. London: Harrison and Sons.

Nightingale, F. (1859). *A contribution to the sanitary history of the British Army during the late war with Russia*. London: John W. Parker and Sons.

Nightingale, F. (1863). *Notes on hospitals*. London: Longman, Green, Roberts, and Green.

Nightingale, F. (1863). *Observation on the evidence contained in the statistical reports submitted by her to the Royal Commission on the Sanitary State of the Army in India*. London: Edward Stanford.

Registered Nurses Association of Ontario (RNAO). (2011). *End-of-life care during the last days and hours*.https://rnao.ca/sites/rnao-ca/files/End-of-Life_Care_During_the_Last_Days_and_Hours_0.pdf.

Registered Nurses' Association of Ontario. (2012). *Toolkit: Implementation of best practice guidelines* (2nd ed.). Toronto, ON: Author.

Registered Nurses Association of Ontario. (2018). *Breastfeeding - promoting and supporting the initiation, exclusivity, and continuation of breastfeeding for newborns, infants, and young children* (3rd ed.). https://rnao.ca/sites/rnao-ca/files/bpg/breast_feeding_BPG_WEB_updated_Oct_2_1.pdf.

Richards, D. A., Hanssen, T. A., & Borglin, G. (2018). The second triennial systematic literature review of European nursing research: Impact on patient outcomes and implications for evidence-based practice. *Worldviews on Evidence-Based Nursing, 15*(5), 333–343. https://doi.10.1111/wvn.12320.

Rodgers, C. C., Brown, T. L., & Hockenberry, M. J. (2019). Implementing evidence in clinical settings. In B. M. Melnyk, & E. Fineout-Overholt (Eds.), *Evidence-based practice in nursing and healthcare: A guide to best practice* (4th ed., pp. 269–292). Berlin: Wolters Kluwer.

Rogers, E. (1995). *Diffusion of innovations*. New York: Free Press.

Rogers, E. M. (2003). *Diffusion of innovations* (5th ed.). New York: Free Press.

Rubenstein, L. V., & Pugh, J. A. (2006). Strategies for promoting organizational and practice change by advancing implementation research. *Journal of General Internal Medicine, 21*, S58–S64.

Sackett, D. L., Rosenberg, W. M., Gray, J. M., Haynes, R. B., & Richardson, W. S. (1996). Evidence based medicine: What it is and what it isn't. *British Medical Journal, 71*(7023), 312. https://doi.org/10.1136/bmj.312.7023.71.

Scott, S. D., Plotnikoff, R. C., Karunamuni, N., et al. (2008). Factors influencing the adoption of an innovation: An examination of the uptake of the Canadian Heart Health Kit (HHK). *Implementation Science, 3*, 41.

Silversides, A. (2011). Journal clubs: A forum for discussion and professional development. *Canadian Nurse, 107*(2), 18–23. http://doi:10.1186/1748-5908-3-59.

Squires, J. E., Estabrooks, C. A., Gustavsson, P., et al. (2011). Individual determinants of research utilization by nurses: A systematic review update. *Implementation Science, 6*(1), 1–20.

Squires, J. E., Graham, I. D., Hutchinson, A. M., et al. (2015). Identifying the domains of context important to implementation science: A study protocol. *Implementation Science, 10*(135), 1–9.

Squires, J. E., Moralejo, D., & LeFort, S. M. (2007). Exploring the role of organizational policies and procedures in promoting research utilization in registered nurses. *Implementation Science, 2*, 17.

Stetler, C. B., Legro, M. W., Wallace, C. M., et al. (2006). The role of formative evaluation in implementation research and the QUERI experience. *Journal of General Internal Medicine, 21*, S1–S8.

Sussman, S., Valente, T. W., Rohrbach, L. A., et al. (2006). Translation in the health professions: Converting science into action. *Evaluation and the Health Professions, 29*(1), 7–32.

Thier, A. (2019). Intradermal lidocaine intervention on the ambulatory unit: An evidence-based implementation project. In B. M. Melnyk & E. Fineout-Overholt (Eds.), *Evidence-based practice in nursing and healthcare: A guide to best practice* (4th ed., pp. 257–264). Berlin: Wolters Kluwer.

Thompson, D. S., Estabrooks, C. A., Scott-Findlay, S., et al. (2007). Interventions aimed at increasing research use in nursing: A systematic review. *Implementation Science, 2*, 15.

Thorne, S. (2018). What can qualitative studies offer in a world where evidence drives decisions? *Asia-Pacific Journal of Oncology Nursing, 5*(1), 43. https://doi.org/10.4103/apjon.apjon_51_17.

Thorne, S., & Sawatzky, R. (2014). Particularizing the general: Sustaining theoretical integrity in the context of an evidence-based practice agenda. *Advances in Nursing Science, 37*(1), 5–18. https://doi.org/10.1097/ANS.0000000000000011.

Titler, M. G. (1994). Critical analysis of research utilization (RU): An historical perspective. *American Journal of Critical Care, 2*(3), 264.

Titler, M. G. (2002). *Toolkit for promoting evidence-based practice.* Iowa City: University of Iowa Hospitals and Clinics, Department of Nursing Services and Patient Care.

Titler, M. G. (2004). Methods in translation science. *Worldviews on Evidence-Based Nursing, 1*, 38–48.

Titler, M. G. (2008). The evidence for evidence-based practice implementation. In R. Hughes (Ed.), *Patient safety and quality—An evidence-based handbook for nurses.* Rockville, MD: Agency for Healthcare Research and Quality.

Titler, M. G., Everett, L. Q., & Adams, S. (2007). Implications for implementation science. *Nursing Research, 56*(Suppl. 4), S53–S59.

Titler, M. G., Herr, K., Brooks, J. M., et al. (2009). A translating research into practice intervention improves management of acute pain in older hip fracture patients. *Health Services Research, 44*(1), 264–287.

Titler, M. G., Herr, K., Everett, L. Q., et al. (2006). *Book to bedside: Promoting & sustaining EBPs in elders (Final Progress Report to AHRQ, Grant No. 2R01 HS010482-04).* Iowa City: University of Iowa College of Nursing.

Titler, M. G., Kleiber, C., Steelman, V. J., et al. (1994). Infusing research into practice to promote quality care. *Nursing Research, 43*(5), 307–313.

Titler, M. G., Kleiber, C., Steelman, V. J., et al., (2001). *The Iowa model of evidence-based practice to promote quality care.* Critical care nursing clinics of North America, *13*(4), 497–509. https://doi.org/10.1016/S0899-5885(18)30017-0.

U.S. Preventive Services Task Force (2008). *U.S. Preventive Services Task Force grade definitions.* http://www.uspreventiveservicestaskforce.org/supstf/grades.htm.

Weiss, C. H. (1980). Knowledge creep and decision accretion. *Science Communication, 1*(3), 381–404.

Wensing, M., Wollersheim, H., & Grol, R. (2006). Organizational interventions to implement improvements in patient care: A structured review of review. *Implementation Science, 1*(2), https://doi.org/10.1186/1748-5908-1-2.

RESEARCH **VIGNETTE**

Cancer Survivorship Program: Cancer, Work, Fear of Cancer Recurrence

Christine Maheu, RN, PhD
Associate Professor
Ingram School of Nursing
McGill University
Montreal, Quebec

INTRODUCTION

Despite decades of improved outcomes associated with cancer treatment, an unprecedented number of cancer survivors experience consequences from their cancer and its treatment that negatively affect their physical, emotional, social, informational, spiritual, and practical well-being (Canadian Cancer Statistics, 2019; McCorkle et al., 2011). To capitalize on the rapid uptake of the Internet as an information source for cancer survivors (Castleton et al., 2011; Whitten et al., 2005) and optimize accessibility to services for cancer survivors on a wide scale, **my program of research is organized around the following objective**: to develop, implement, and evaluate SMS interventions and resources using e-health technologies to enable cancer survivors to manage their most frequent unmet needs in the emotional (fear of cancer recurrence, cancer-related distress) and practical (return to work following cancer) domains.

BACKGROUND

My program of research is built on the theoretical tenets of the supportive cancer care framework (Fitch, 2008), whereby my team works collaboratively with clinicians and cancer survivors and engages them early in the research design phase. This process allows us to determine the most pressing needs for knowledge generation and knowledge transfer and to design research that really speaks to the needs of cancer survivors and which considers the current gaps and unmet needs. As such, I had the opportunity to partner with a survey company Ipsos Reid and the Canadian Partnership Against Cancer (CPAC) to develop and implement a 2017 pan-Canadian survey conducted with 13,000 cancer survivors aged 18–65 who responded on what were their top specific unmet needs and concerns. The results showed that cancer survivors still suffer and need support for their distress from cancer-related problems, fatigue, fear of cancer recurrence (FCR), financial difficulties, and difficulty returning to work (RTW) (Canadian Partnership Against Cancer, 2018). More than 35% of survivors reported that they are not getting the help they need to address these concerns, and only half of the survivors surveyed received information that is useful in addressing them (Canadian Partnership Against Cancer, 2018). Among these post-treatment concerns, systematic reviews on FCR indicate that this concern remains the most commonly reported problem and one of the most prevalent unmet needs for cancer survivors (Simard & Savard, 2009; Ozga et al., 2015) for which they require help from professionals to cope (Hodgkinson et al., 2007; Shim et al., 2010). Fear of cancer recurrence —defined as "fear, worry, or concern relating to the possibility that cancer will come back or progress" (Lebel et al., 2016)—is characterized by high levels of worry and intrusive thoughts, maladaptive coping, excessive distress, difficulties in making future plans, and functional impairments Lebel et al., 2016). Up to 70% of survivors will experience a heightened level of FCR (Simard & Savard, 2015) that warrants professional attention (Thewes et al., 2012; Costa et al., 2016).

According to the supportive cancer care framework mapping the cancer care experience of 100% of patients entering the cancer system (Fitch, 2008), we can anticipate that 20% of patients will require basic support services; 30% will need additional information, education, and peer support; 35% to 40% will require specialized or professional intervention; whereas only 10% to 15% require complex interventions. The majority of cancer survivors who continue to struggle to manage the consequences of their cancer and treatment in the context of cancer as a complex chronic illness are facing serious demands, along with their families, that will require new skills to assume greater responsibility for their health care. The increased reliance on outpatient treatments and the responsibility for the day-to-day management of complex cancer challenges fall heavily on patients and their families (Kuijpers et al., 2013).

Self-management support (SMS) interventions offer one option to improve health and well-being while at the same time containing the cost of care for cancer survivors (Howell, 2018). Self-management refers to the "ability of the individual to manage the symptoms, treatment, physical and psychosocial consequences, and lifestyle changes inherent in living with a chronic condition and disability, to promote survival and recover health and well-being in cancer (p. 1324)" (Kuijpers et al., 2013). These interventions offer individuals and families a way to assume greater responsibility in managing their health care (McCorkle et al., 2011; Kuijpers et al., 2013; Howell, 2018). The focus of the interventions is on enhancing ability, building confidence to manage conditions effectively, as well as training and support to develop the knowledge, skills, and resources-seeking abilities (Kuijpers et al., 2013; Committee on Improving the Quality of Cancer Care, 2013) necessary to positively influence the cognitive, behavioural, and emotional responses associated with health-related quality of life (Kuijpers et al., 2013). The format of SMS interventions can be lay or professionally led, group or individual, generic or disease-specific (Kuijpers et al., 2013; Lorig & Holman, 2003). As such, SMS interventions are important,

as they can increase the patient's knowledge of issues likely to arise post-treatment, such as lingering symptoms of distress, FCR, and challenges in RTW (Howell et al., 2017).

However, **current gaps** in health care and support show that while interventions and resources have been created to meet the supportive care needs and the myriad of biopsychosocial effects of cancer, these interventions and resources are often not accessible or known to the population or are fragmented, and their evidence base is only preliminary (Howell, 2018). Further research is still needed to understand the efficacy of SMS on health outcomes across cancer supportive care needs and from the perspective of cancer survivors and their families and from the use of different formats of care delivery (Howell, 2018). My **program of research** is focused on developing, implementing, and evaluating SMS interventions and resources using among available options, e-health technologies to meet the most frequent unmet supportive care needs of cancer survivors in the emotional (FCR, cancer-distress) and practical (RTW following cancer) domains.

Four studies highlighted are:

1) Assessed and identified the transition support and services needs of cancer survivors from post-cancer treatment to primary care (**Study 1;** Outcome: identify areas of needs and unmet needs from the transition process, provide guidance for cancer survivorship program development);

2) Provided preliminary evidence on the use of SMS interventions

that can improve psychosocial functioning for individuals in the pre-cancer diagnostic phase (**Study 2**; Outcomes: cancer-distress and uncertainty) and for cancer survivors in the post-treatment phase (**Study 3**; Outcomes: FCR);

3) Developed a knowledge translation e-health resource to support RTW following cancer, in addition to the creation of e-interactive online tools for cancer patients and survivors, health care providers, and employers (**Study 4;** Outcomes: Creation of a bilingual website platform *Cancer and Work/Cancer et Travail)*.

Study 1: Cancer Survivors' Transition Survey Study.

The aim of this quality improvement study was to determine the predictors associated with cancer survivors' satisfaction with their overall care and identify the aspects of follow-up cancer care that can be modified to improve cancer survivors' overall quality of care. This national survey was a collaboration between the Canadian Partnership Against Cancer and Ipsos Reid. Thirteen thousand (13,000) cancer survivors took part in the survey (Canadian Partnership Against Cancer, 2018). I led the survey development through to focus group consultations with cancer survivors, health care providers, and policymakers and then led data interpretation. Its results have now been published by CPAC (http://www.systemperformance.ca/report/living-with-cancer-patient-experience/). **Future:** As per the survey recommendations, our program will propose a unique blend

527

of using face-to-face and e-health Internet SMS interventions with public-private-volunteer partnership designed to increase access to cancer-related follow-up services, enhance the cancer survivorship experience, and reduce health care costs.

Study 2: Feasibility Testing of a SMS Uncertainty Telephone Intervention for Breast Cancer Rapid Diagnostic Clinic (RDC).

To date, research data on the effects of psychosocial interventions to improve the psychological impact of rapid diagnostic clinics (RDC) are limited, restricted to descriptive data, and suggest the need for more effective anxiety management interventions for pa-

tients in the RDC pathway. This study tested the feasibility (recruitment, retention, and acceptability) of a nursing-led telephone intervention on levels of uncertainty, psychological distress, and coping skills in women with a suspicious breast abnormality awaiting further testing through a RDC. Recruitment at the Gattuso Rapid Diagnostic Clinic at Princess Margaret Cancer Centre in Toronto was completed in June 2018. Descriptive studies on this topic and a systematic review have been published by our team (Zanchetta Santos et al., 2015; Maheu et al., 2015; Maheu et al., 2014; Singh et al., 2017); an invited webinar on the topic of supportive care RDC was conducted for the Ca-

nadian Association of Nurses in Oncology (2014). The final study paper is currently under review.

Study 3: Efficacy of a Cognitive Existential Group Intervention to Address FCR in Women With Cancer–Ongoing, Randomized Controlled Trial.

This multisite clinical trial— the FORT study—is assessing the efficacy of a SMS cognitive-existential group intervention for the management of FCR using face-to-face. It is the only Canadian trial of its kind, following in parallel from two other produced FCR international trials for FCR management (Humphris & Ozakinci, 2008). I published our study protocol, and our final

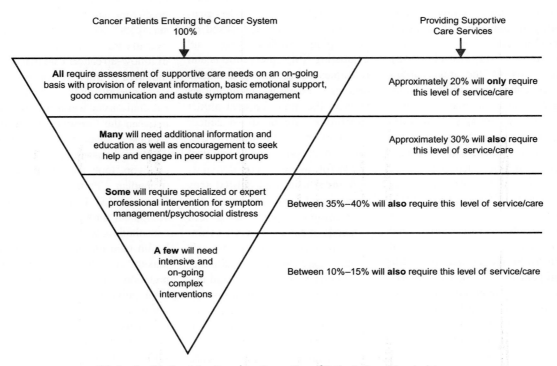

FIG. 1 Service Provision Based on Proportion of Patients Requiring Assistance

results paper will be available in 2021 (Maheu et al., 2016). This research platform supported eight parallel studies by graduate students. The results showed that the intervention was effective at reducing FCR and for over 6 months following the end of the intervention in comparison to an active control group. The intervention is currently being tested in different format, individual, telehealth, and chat, and with different cancer populations.

Study 4: Cancer and Work Website. *Co-PI: 2015–2017. Status: Complete. Funding ($290,000) Canadian Partnership Against Cancer*

With my co-lead, Ms. Parkinson, a vocational rehabilitation counselor from BC Cancer, we developed and implemented the Cancer and Work website (www.cancerandwork.ca) (Maheu & Parkinson, 2016; Parkinson & Maheu, 2019). Approximately ~450 pages of content were gathered or originally written covering 26 topic areas, producing eight online cancer and work-related tools and nine webcasts. The website is divided in three parallel and complementary sections providing written material and resources to cancer survivors, health care providers, and employers. Original written work was created in collaboration between our team and 45 invited experts in the field. To date, Cancer and Work is the only such knowledge translation resource in Canada, pulling together extensive resources in self-management support (SMS) on a single website on return to work (RTW) topics to benefit cancer patients and survivors, health care providers, and employers. **Website traffic.** Between its launch in October 2016 to August 30th, 2019, the site has received over 60,500 sessions and over 39,780 users with 26.6% of them returning, averaging ~800 visits per week. Seventy-five percent (75%) of viewers were from Canada, 10% from the US, and the rest international. Regarding page views, 21% went to the survivors' section, 28% to the health care providers' section, 32% to the section for employers, and 19% went to online tools. Cancer and Work is hosted on the McGill University server. **Award:** In July 2018, the website was recognized as a *Leading Practice* by Health Standards Organization and gets to have this recognition for 2 years.

We currently have **three ongoing studies** with our Cancer and Work website.

(1) The first study's overall objective is to generate and implement the *adoption* and *uptake* of the two selected online tools for usability testing; the job analysis and the return to work planner online tools, from the Cancer and Work website (Maheu & Parkinson, 2019).

(2) Our second study is to evaluate the satisfaction and acceptability and effectiveness of the Cancer and Work website as an e-resource intervention for supporting cancer survivors in the phases of RTW (preparing to RTW, Returned to Work after completion of treatment, sporadic RTW, and continuous work during treatment). The purpose of this study is two-fold: 1) to determine the longitudinal impact of the Cancer and Work website as an e-resource intervention as a SMS on the following primary study variables: self-efficacy, mastery, depression, uncertainty, anxiety, increased knowledge in the RTW process, and 2) to conduct an evaluation of the website using the RE-AIM framework (Glasgow et al., 2019). The secondary outcomes will be if participants stay at work or return to work earlier than planned (self-reported). This study uses a mixed-methods approach with a within-subjects repeated measures to assess for the satisfaction, acceptability, and to evaluate the effectiveness of Cancer and Work as an e-resource intervention to support cancer patients and survivors in the RTW process or staying at work.

(3) In our third study, the overarching objective of our mixed-methods study design is to investigate the usability, feasibility, acceptability, and preliminary efficacy of iCanWork, a multimodal 11-Step RTW and rehabilitation based intervention, which will provide formalized support to cancer survivors to remain in or return to work after cancer, to improve work productivity and RTW outcomes among cancer survivors. Our approach is consistent with the Medical Research Council for preclinical trial feasibility studies. We hypothesize that iCanWork will be feasible and acceptable to cancer survivors and rehabilitation

professionals. Deliverables: Completion of our study aims will provide feasibility, acceptability, and preliminary efficacy data regarding iCanWork's ability to support cancer survivors RTW in the form of a detailed feasibility report. These data will also identify the refinements that need to be made to iCanWork in preparation for a future RCT. Lastly, these data will also determine the best primary endpoint to use in future RCT by identifying which RTW measures produced the highest variance.

Contributions. The few studies to date on cancer and work have been conducted in breast cancer survivors and did not have within their primary aim to support and assist cancer survivors to return to work or stay at work but rather, to improve quality of life. Additionally, even less studies considered the concept of sustained employability during or after cancer. The findings from this study will fill a huge gap in the literature by providing knowledge on the use of an e-resource, Cancer and Work for the support of cancer survivors for preparing to RTW, RTW after completion of treatment, sporadic RTW, and continuous work during treatment. Our study is an incremental innovation carried out in participatory partnership with researchers and knowledge users to the implementation assessment of a tailored e-health intervention to provide for a valuable support and resource for returning or staying at work following cancer. ■

REFERENCES

Canadian Cancer Statistics. (2019). Canadian Cancer Statistics. Canadian Cancer Statistics - Canada.ca 2019 [Internet]. Available from: https://www.canada.ca/en/public-health/services/chronic-diseases/cancer/canadian-cancer-statistics.html.

Canadian Partnership Against Cancer. (2018). Living with Cancer: A Report on the Patient Experience. Canadian Partnership Against Cancer, editor (pp. 50). Toronto (ON): Canada: Canadian Partnership Against Cancer (pp. 50).

Castleton, K., Fong, T., Wang-Gillam, A., et al. (2011). A survey of Internet utilization among patients with cancer. *Supportive Care in Cancer, 19*(8), 1183–1190.

Committee on Improving the Quality of Cancer Care (2013). Addressing the Challenges of an Aging Population; Board on Health Care Services; Institute of Medicine. In L Levit, E Balogh, S Nass, & PA Ganz (Eds.), Delivering high-quality cancer care: Charting a new course for a system in crisis. Washington (DC): National Academies Press (US).

Costa, D. S. J., Dieng, M., Cust, A. E., Butow, P. N., & Kasparian, N. A. (2016). Psychometric properties of the Fear of Cancer Recurrence Inventory: an item response theory approach. *Psychooncology, 25*(7), 832–838.

Fitch, M. I. (2008). Supportive care framework. *Canadian Oncology Nursing Journal, 18*(1), 6–24.

Glasgow, R. E., Vogt, T. M., & Boles, S. M. (1999). Evaluating the public health impact of health promotion interventions: the RE-AIM framework. *American Journal of Public Health, 89*(9), 1322–1327.

Hodgkinson, K., Butow, P., Hunt, G. E., Pendlebury, S., Hobbs, K. M., & Wain, G. (2007). Breast cancer survivors' supportive care needs 2-10 years after diagnosis. *Supportive Care in Cancer, 15*(5), 515–523.

Howell, D. D. (2018). Supported self-management for cancer survivors to address long-term biopsychosocial consequences of cancer and treatment to optimize living well. *Current Opinion in Supportive and Palliative Care, 12*(1), 92–99.

Howell, D., Harth, T., Brown, J., Bennett, C., & Boyko, S. (2017). Self-management education interventions for patients with cancer: a systematic review. *Supportive Care in Cancer, 25*(4), 1323–1355.

Humphris, G., & Ozakinci, G. (2008). The AFTER intervention: a structured psychological approach to reduce fears of recurrence in patients with head and neck cancer. *British Journal of Health Psychology, 13*(Pt 2), 223–230.

Kuijpers, W., Groen, W. G., Aaronson, N. K., & van Harten, W. H. (2013). A systematic review of web-based interventions for patient empowerment and physical activity in chronic diseases: relevance for cancer survivors. *Journal of Medical Internet Research, 15*(2), e37.

Lebel, S., Ozakinci, G., Humphris, G., et al. (2016). From normal response to clinical problem: definition and clinical features of fear of cancer recurrence. *Supportive Care in Cancer, 24*(8), 3265–3268.

Lorig, K. R., & Holman, H. (2003). Self-management education: history, definition, outcomes, and mechanisms. *Annals of Behavioral Medicine, 26*(1), 1–7.

Maheu, C., & Parkinson M., on behalf of the Cancer and Work website core team members. (2016). Cancer and Work. https://www.cancerandwork.ca/.

Maheu, C., & Parkinson, M. (2019). Evaluation of the Cancer and Work Return to Work Tool. Oral abstract presented at the International Psycho-Oncology Society, Banff, Canada. Published abstract #135 from the 2019 October International Psycho-Oncology Society (IPOS) in the Journal of Psychosocial Oncology Research & Practice. *Journal of Psychosocial Oncology Research and Practice, 1*(1S), E9.

Maheu, C., Singh, M., McCready, D., Fawcett, S., Sarvanantham, S., Stuart-McEwen, T., Sidani, S., Lambert, S., Dubois, S., Zanchetta, M., & Howell, D. (2015–2016). Development and pilot testing of an uncertainty management telephone intervention for women attending a rapid diagnostic clinic for suspicious breast abnormality. Funded by Réseau de recherche en interventions en sciences infirmières du Québec (RRISIQ).

Maheu, C., Wang, C., McCready, D., Lord, B., & Howell, D. (2015). Rapid diagnostic assessment for a suspicious breast abnormality: Examining the impact on anxiety and uncertainty. *Canadian Oncology Nursing Journal, 25*, 361–362.

Maheu, C., Lebel, S., Courbasson, C., et al. (2016). Protocol of a randomized controlled trial of the fear of recurrence therapy (FORT) intervention for women with breast or gynecological cancer. *BMC Cancer, 16*, 291.

McCorkle, R., Ercolano, E., Lazenby, M., et al. (2011). Self-management: Enabling and empowering patients living with cancer as a chronic illness. *CA: A Cancer Journal for Clinicians, 61*(1), 50–62.

Ozga, M., Aghajanian, C., Myers-Virtue, S., et al. (2015). A systematic review of ovarian cancer and fear of recurrence. *Palliative & Supportive Care, 13*(6), 1771–1780.

Parkinson, M., & Maheu, C. (2019). Cancer and work. *Canadian Oncology Nursing Journal, 29*(4), 258–266.

Shim, E.-J., Shin, Y.-W., Oh, D.-Y., & Hahm, B.-J. (2010). Increased fear of progression in cancer patients with recurrence. *General Hospital Psychiatry, 32*(2), 169–175.

Simard, S., & Savard, J. (2009). Fear of Cancer Recurrence Inventory: development and initial validation of a multidimensional measure of fear of cancer recurrence. *Supportive Care in Cancer, 17*(3), 241–251.

Simard, S., & Savard, J. (2015). Screening and comorbidity of clinical levels of fear of cancer recurrence. *Journal of Cancer Survivorship, 9*(3), 481–491.

Singh, M., Maheu, C., Brady, T., & Farah, R. (2017). The psychological impact of the rapid diagnostic centres in cancer screening: A systematic review. *Canadian Oncology Nursing Journal, 27*(4), 348–355.

Thewes, B., Butow, P., Bell, M. L., et al. (2012). Fear of cancer recurrence in young women with a history of early-stage breast cancer: a cross-sectional study of prevalence and association with health behaviours. *Supportive Care in Cancer, 20*(11), 2651–2659.

Whitten, P., Kreps, G. L., & Eastin, M. S. (2005). Creating a framework for online cancer services research to facilitate timely and interdisciplinary applications. *Journal of Medical Internet Research, 7*(3), e34.

Zanchetta, Santos, Maheu, M., Baku, C., Nembhard, L., S., P. J., & Lemonde, M (2015). Prospective roles for Canadian Oncology nurses in breast cancer rapid diagnostic clinics. *Canadian Oncology Nursing Journal, 25*, 144–149. (English); 150–156 (French).

The Rocks and Hard Places of MAiD: A Qualitative Study of Nursing Practice in the Context of Legislated Assisted Death

Barbara Pesut[1],* | Sally Thorne[2] | Catharine J. Schiller[3] | Madeleine Greig[1] | Josette Roussel[4]

ABSTRACT

BACKGROUND: Medical Assistance in Dying (MAiD) was legalized in Canada in June 2016. The Canadian government's decision to legislate assisted dying, an approach that requires a high degree of obligation, precision, and delegation, has resulted in unique challenges for health care and for nursing practice. The purpose of this study was to better understand the implications of a legislated approach to assisted death for nurses' experiences and nursing practice.

METHODS: The study used a qualitative approach guided by Interpretive Description. Semi-structured interviews were conducted with 59 registered nurses and nurse prac-

titioners. Interviews were audio-recorded, transcribed, and managed using qualitative analysis software. Analysis followed a procedure of data immersion, open coding, constant comparative analysis, and the construction of a thematic and interpretive account.

RESULTS: Nurses in this study described great variability in how MAiD had been enacted in their work context and the practice supports available to guide their practice. The development of systems to support MAiD, or lack thereof, was largely driven by persons in influential leadership positions. Workplaces that supported a range of nurses' moral responses to MAiD were most effective in supporting nurses' well-being during this impactful change in practice. Participants cited the importance of teamwork in providing high-quality MAiD-related care, although many worked without the benefit of a team. Nursing work related to MAiD was highly complex, largely because of the need for patient-centered care in systems that were not always organized to support such care. In the absence of adequate practice supports, some nurses were choosing to limit their involvement in MAiD.

CONCLUSIONS: Data obtained in this study suggested that some workplace contexts still lack the necessary supports for nurses to confidently meet the precision required of a legislated approach to MAiD. Without accessible palliative care, sufficient providers, a supportive team, practice supports, and a context that allowed nurses to have

[1]Canada Research Chair in Health, Ethics, and Diversity, University of British Columbia Okanagan, 1147 Research Road, Okanagan, Kelowna, BC V1V 1V7, Canada.

[2]University of British Columbia, T201-2211 Wesbrook Mall, Vancouver, BC V6T 2B5, Canada.

[3]University of Northern British Columbia, Prince George, BC V2N 4Z9, Canada.

[4]Policy, Advocacy and Strategy, Canadian Nurses Association, 50 Driveway, Ottawa, Ontario K2P 1E2, Canada.

*Correspondence: Barbara Pesut, Canada Research Chair in Health, Ethics, and Diversity, University of British Columbia Okanagan, 1147 Research Road, Okanagan, Kelowna, BC V1V 1V7, Canada (Barb.pesut@ubc.ca)

a range of responses to MAiD, nurses felt they were legally and morally at risk. Nurses seeking to provide the compassionate care consistent with such a momentous moment in patients' lives, without suitable supports, find themselves caught between the proverbial rock and hard place.

KEY WORDS: assisted death, assisted suicide, euthanasia, legislation, medical assistance in dying, Nursing practice, palliative care

BACKGROUND

All forms of assisted suicide were illegal in Canada until February 2015 when the Supreme Court of Canada (SSC) released its landmark decision *Carter v Canada (Attorney General) ("Carter")* (Carter. v. Canada (Attorney General), 2015). In its ruling, the SCC struck down the *Criminal Code's* prohibition on assisted suicide for competent adults in certain clinical circumstances, on the basis that such a prohibition unjustifiably violated the *Canadian Charter of Rights and Freedoms ("Charter")*.

The SCC's ruling gave the federal government time to craft a legislative framework to regulate assisted dying. In June 2016, medical assistance in dying (MAiD) was legalized in *An Act to amend the Criminal Code and to make related amendments to other Acts (medical assistance in dying)*, a statute still colloquially known as *Bill C-14* (Bill C-14, 2016). The government had crafted a new concept, MAiD, within this legislation rather than continue to use an existing term, such as *"physician-assisted suicide"* or *"physician-assisted dying."* This new terminology represented a recognition that a team of healthcare providers, not only physicians, is typically required to implement such a complex procedure (Schiller, 2017). In *Bill C-14*, MAiD is defined as: (a) the administration by a medical practitioner or nurse practitioner of a substance to a person, at their request, that causes their death; or (b) the prescribing or providing by a medical practitioner or nurse practitioner of a substance to a person, at their request, so that they may self-administer the

substance and in doing so cause their own death. Only 6 of the 6749 medically assisted deaths recorded in Canada between December 10, 2015 and October 31, 2018 were self-administered (Health Canada, 2019).

According to *Bill C-14*, to be eligible for MAiD, an individual must meet all of the following criteria: (a) they are eligible for health services funded by a government in Canada; (b) they are at least 18 years of age and capable of making decisions with respect to their health; (c) they are suffering from a grievous and irremediable medical condition; d) they have made a voluntary request for medical assistance in dying that was not made as a result of external pressure; and (e) they give informed consent to receive medical assistance in dying after having been informed of the means that are available to relieve their suffering, including palliative care (Bill C-14, 2016). Once *Bill C-14* was passed, provincial and territorial governments, as well as provincial and territorial regulatory bodies for the health professions, became responsible for enacting policies, procedures, and processes to guide MAiD-related healthcare practice in Canada.

Implications of a Legislated Approach to MAiD

The Canadian government chose to enact legislation that would regulate assisted suicide, but there were other options available to them. Luzon modeled five approaches to assisted death based upon obligations, precision, and delegation:

> Obligation means that people are legally bound by a rule, so that their behavior is subject to examination under the general rules, procedures, and discourse of the law. Precision means that rules unequivocally define the conduct they require, authorize, permit, or prohibit. Delegation refers to the body that has been granted authority (by the public) to determine, implement, interpret, and apply the rules. All three dimensions can vary in degree. Based on these characteristics, legalization may be hard (where all three properties are maximized), soft (where some properties are maximized and others minimized), and null (where all three properties are minimized).[5] [emphasis added; p. 7]

The five possible legal framework responses to assisted death are as follows. The first would involve maintaining the *status quo*, such that assisted death would continue to be treated as a crime; this would have been an obviously problematic approach given the existence of the *Carter* decision. The second is *defense,* in which it would be recognized that there may, at times, be situations in which a valid defense to assisted death can be made. The third involves *de-prioritization*; this response would allow laws against assisted suicide to remain in place but it would not be viewed as a priority of the justice system to prosecute those who are involved in assisted dying or to impose criminal sanctions upon them. The fourth is *de-criminalization* in which no precise laws are provided; this was the approach used by the Canadian government after the *Criminal Code* prohibition on abortion was struck down by the SCC in the 1988 R v Morgentaler case. The fifth is *legislation* in which "*there is a specific binding law (high in obligation), a precise, specific, clear rule for every practice (high in precision), and the designated third party to which the state delegates authority is the legislature (high in delegation)*" (Luzon, 2018) (p. 14).

Canada chose the fifth approach to assisted death, which, according to Luzon, entails a **hard** approach characterized by a high degree of obligation, precision, and delegation (Luzon, 2018). To that end, *Bill C-14* incorporated numerous safeguards and requirements into the MAiD process. For example, eligibility for MAiD must be determined by two practitioners, either physicians or nurse practitioners, who are independent of one another (the second practitioner must also be independent of the patient). Once the patient has been determined to be eligible, he or she must then submit a written request for MAiD in the presence of two independent witnesses. In addition, there is a mandatory reflection period of at least 10 days between the signing of that written request by the patient and the day that MAiD is

actually provided, although this can be shortened in certain clinical circumstances (Bill C-14, 2016). These, and other, safeguards were written into the legislation by the government to decrease the possibility that the MAiD procedure could be used inappropriately.

The Nursing Role in MAiD

Not only has Canada taken the "hardest" approach to assisted death, but it is also the first country to allow nurse practitioners to act as MAiD assessors and providers. Although it is important to note that this role for nurse practitioners is further regulated at the provincial level and so not all nurse practitioners are allowed by the provincial health regions to act as MAiD assessors or providers. In Canada, registered nurses who do not hold a nurse practitioner credential also play important roles in MAiD. The important role of the registered nurse is also evident in studies from other countries where assisted death is legal (Denier et al., 2009, 2010a; 2010b; Dierckx de Casterle et al., 2010; van de Scheur & van der Arend, 1998; Suva et al., 2019). For example, our synthesis of qualitative studies from Belgium, the Netherlands, and Canada of registered nurses' experiences with assisted death suggested that nurses perform a central role in negotiating initial inquiries about assisted death, that nurses provide important "wrap-around" care for patients and family, and that participating in an assisted death was impactful for nurses and required significant moral work (Pesut et al., 2019a).

In consideration of the importance of the registered nursing role, and the new role for nurse practitioners in Canada, we conducted a study in which we explored the policy, practice, and ethical implications of MAiD for nursing. This was a two-phased study in which we first conducted systematic reviews of the literature (Pesut et al., 2019a, 2019b, 2019c). and then a qualitative study of Canadian nurses' experiences with MAiD. As part of the literature synthesis we gathered and analyzed nursing regulatory documents that were created to guide nursing practice in MAiD from the 10 provinces and 3 territories in Canada (Pesut et al., 2019b). We discovered substantial variability in the degree to which these regulatory bodies chose to provide additional guidelines for nurses beyond what was provided in the MAiD legislation. As such, we were interested in better understanding how nurses were experiencing the enactment of the legislation in their practice related to MAiD, and thus explored this qualitatively. In this paper, we report on findings from the qualitative phase of the study that revealed the impact of Canada's legislated approach to assisted death on nurses' experiences, and on nursing practice, in Canada.

METHODS

This qualitative study was guided by Interpretive Description, a pragmatic approach to developing knowledge for a practice discipline (Thorne, 2016).

Participants

Data were collected through 60 interviews with 59 participants (see Table A.1 for demographic data). Recruitment of this sample occurred via bulletins that were distributed to key stakeholders and prospective participants using convenience, purposive, and snowball sampling techniques. For example, we advertised through the Canadian Nurses' Association, through health regions, and through the Canadian Association of MAiD Assessors and Providers. We asked interview participants to pass the study information on to others. We sought to gain participation from all English-speaking provinces. We did not specifically target the Canadian territories as the interim reports on MAiD produced by Health Canada suggested that few cases were occurring in those areas (Health Canada, 2019). Eligibility criteria required that participants were registered nurses or nurse practitioners who

TABLE **A.1**

DEMOGRAPHICS OF STUDY PARTICIPANTS

CHARACTERISTIC	NUMBER OF PARTICIPANTS $n = 59$
Province	British Columbia: $n = 28$ (48%)
	Ontario: $n = 16$ (27%)
	Manitoba: $n = 7$ (12%)
	Alberta: $n = 5$ (9%)
	Newfoundland and Labrador: $n = 2$ (3%)
	Saskatchewan: $n = 1$ (2%)
Age	25–44: $n = 27$ (46%)
	45–64: $n = 29$ (49%)
	> 65: $n = 3$ (5%)
Gender	Female: $n = 56$ (95%)
	Male: $n = 3$ (5%)
Ethnicity	Caucasian: $n = 57$ (97%)
	Other: $n = 2$ (3%)
Designation	Registered Nurse: $n = 43$ (73%)
	Nurse Practitioner: $n = 13$ (22%)
	Clinical Nurse Specialist: $n = 3$ (5%)
Years Worked	2–4 years: $n = 4$ (7%)
	5–9 years: $n = 10$ (17%)
	10–14 years: $n = 13$ (22%)
	15–19 years: $n = 4$ (7%)
	20–24 years: $n = 6$ (10%)
	> 25 years: $n = 22$ (38%)
Work Context	Home & Community: $n = 32$ (54%)
	Acute Care: $n = 10$ (17%)
	LTC: $n = 5$ (9%)
	Hospice: $n = 4$ (7%)
	Clinic: $n = 3$ (5%)
	Other: $n = 5$ (9%)
Conscientious Objection	No/Unsure: $n = 50$ (85%)
	Yes: $n = 9$ (15%)
Spiritual or Religious Affiliation	Religious or Spiritual: $n = 33$ (56%)
	Neither: $n = 15$ (25%)
	Spiritual but not Religious: $n = 11$ (19%)

had previously cared for patients requesting or receiving MAiD, or those registered nurses or nurse practitioners who had decided, for whatever reason, not to participate in the MAiD process. No participants dropped out of the study or requested that their data be removed from the study. These 59 participants had significant experience with MAiD. For example, 24 of the 59 participants had conducted more than 25 conversations with patients about MAiD, and 11 of the 59 participants had been involved with more than 25 patients who went on to receive MAiD.

Data Collection and Analysis

Data were collected in the fall of 2018 and the spring of 2019, approximately 2 years after the MAiD legislation was enacted. Semi-structured interviews, conducted by telephone, were used to garner an in-depth understanding of nurses' experiences with MAiD. Telephone interviews were necessary to reach nurses from across Canada. Interviews were conducted by the principal investigator and research coordinator. Participants were provided with a detailed consent form at least 24 h prior to the interview to ensure that they understood the focus and objectives of the study. Interviews were conducted only after the signed consent was received. Interviewers reiterated the rationale for conducting the study prior to the interview, and participants were provided with an opportunity to ask questions. A semi-structured interview guide was developed for this study, piloted, and refined prior to data collection (Additional file 1). Examples of interview questions included: (i) Can you tell us how the process of MAiD occurs in your practice context? (ii) What resources and practice supports are available to assist you in caring for MAiD patients? (iii) Tell us about your experiences with MAiD. The average length of interviews was 55 min. In totality, 2992 min of interview data were collected and subsequently analyzed.

Interview data were audio-recorded, transcribed verbatim, de-identified, checked for accuracy, and uploaded into NVivo[12TSN] for data analysis and management. Transcripts included emotions evident during the interview (e.g., crying). All audio recordings were reviewed by the principal investigator and detailed field notes were written and referred back to during the analytic process. Data were analyzed following the logic of Interpretive Description (Thorne, 2016). Open codes were developed and negotiated by two investigators (BP & MG) after an immersion process of reading and re-reading multiple transcripts. These codes were further refined with input from two additional investigators (ST & JR). These open codes were then used to code the remaining data. Codes were further refined in an iterative process of data collection and analysis by using constant comparative data analysis techniques, a technique developed initially within Grounded Theory (Glaser & Strauss, 1967). Once all of the transcripts had been coded, data contained within these codes were summarized to construct a thematic and interpretive account of Canadian nurses' experiences with MAiD. In this paper we discuss the experiences related to Canada's legislated approach to MAiD.

RESULTS

Nurses interviewed for this study described great variability in how MAiD had been enacted within their geographic and work context and how that variability had influenced their experiences with MAiD. This variability was largely influenced by three themes: (1) the leadership taken by influential persons within systems, (2) the presence and nature of a multi-disciplinary team, and (3) the systems' complexity and capacity to support MAiD.

Systems: Influential Leaders Setting the Tone

Nurses described work contexts that ranged from a virtual absence of any MAiD-related guidelines to highly structured systems in which a comprehensive set of supports existed to guide nursing practice. In some contexts, policies and procedures were established fairly quickly. For example, one participant described how, after the legislation was passed, key leaders in the health region immediately established a working group to work intensively over a weekend to construct the policies and procedures that would guide immediate practice. However, in other contexts those first MAiD cases were done with little direction, *"We really had no idea what we were doing because we hadn't actually made any policy or guidelines yet"* (p. 42). Even many months after the legislation, some nurses were still working within a healthcare policy and procedure void. These findings were similar for both registered nurses and nurse practitioners, although nurse practitioners had the structure provided for them within *Bill C-14*. Nurses, however, sometimes found themselves trying to assist in a MAiD procedure with no practice guidelines in their places of work. This created uncertainty in their practice, particularly when nurses remained the primary caregivers of patients contemplating or undergoing MAiD, which also involved high levels of interaction with their families. *"So, my big concern is if someone does approach me with a written request, what do I do from there? And I know the health region has developed no policies pertaining to what the process is"* (p. 26).

Much of this variability in the degree of practice support was a result of the decisions (or lack of decisions) made by persons in influential leadership positions either immediately preceding or following the legalization of MAiD. For example, one participant mentioned that a change in government soon after the *Carter* decision had slowed down the development of MAiD guidelines in their province, which in turn heighted the perception of risk. *"With the change in government, things were a little bit stalled and questions weren't necessarily being answered. I think there were a lot of physicians and NPs maybe a little bit nervous about how things were working"* (p. 1). Some health authorities assigned key individuals to lead the development of practice supports. A number of innovations were developed, including regional interdisciplinary MAiD teams, designated persons to work alongside and support individuals considering whether to undergo MAiD, and therapeutic interventions designed to address the underlying suffering that had contributed to a MAiD request. However,

leaders also developed organically as they championed the MAiD process. For example, this nurse participated in a provision while her clinical leader was away. *"Because she was away, I informally became the leader of MAiD on our unit"* (p. 50).

Leaders responsible for palliative care were particularly influential in the development of structures and processes to support MAiD. The beliefs of these leaders about the acceptability of MAiD, its fit with palliative care, and perhaps most importantly, their recognition that MAiD would generate a range of moral responses in their colleagues, determined the direction and outcomes of these practice supports. For example, in one jurisdiction, MAiD assessment responsibilities were assigned to nurse practitioners who were engaged in palliative care. This decision meant that palliative care and MAiD were both integrated within nursing responsibilities. As logical as this decision seemed from a workflow perspective, it resulted in unique tensions, particularly for those palliative nurses who objected to MAiD due to either their moral values or their beliefs about its fit with a palliative care philosophy.

Another example of influence was how leaders constructed workplace policies to support a range of moral responses to MAiD. We specifically use the term *"range of moral responses,"* rather than conscientious objection, to reflect the uncertainty about MAiD that was characteristic of nurses in this study. Few openly declared themselves as conscientious objectors; instead, more were uncertain about how they felt about MAiD. Nurses described workplace policies that varied dramatically in how they accommodated their nurses' willingness or not to participate in MAiD and the uncertainty that caused. At one end of the spectrum, nurses were allowed to take a day off without pay if they were uncomfortable with MAiD and it was occurring on their unit. At the other end of the spectrum, nurses were expected to provide all non-MAiD-related care, no matter how they felt about MAiD. These policies reflected very different approaches to nurses' moral well-being. As employees of healthcare, nurses felt they had little control over the ways in which their workplaces were structured to accommodate their comfort level with MAiD. For example, one nurse stated, *"we need some sort of support groups or guidelines for conscientious objectors. I have heard that other countries have more lenient processes for conscientious objectors so that they don't feel stigmatized"* (p. 54).

Nurses perceived physicians, and in particular palliative physicians, to be important influencers in how MAiD processes developed. For example, one participant described how the medical director influenced the implementation of MAiD on her palliative unit. *"Our medical director at the time wasn't on board and that trickled down to all of us"* (p. 57). Unlike nurses who were employees of healthcare, physicians were perceived as having more latitude to choose whether, how, and to what extent they would support the MAiD process. In some cases, nurses described how physicians worked with them to seamlessly integrate MAiD with palliative care. In other cases, nurses described physicians who erected barriers to patient involvement with MAiD. These barriers could include telling patients that they were not quite ready for MAiD, or suggesting that it could not be done in the community where patients were living, or simply ignoring patient requests. The strongest type of physician resistance described by participants was the withdrawal of palliative care services once a patient had chosen MAiD. This withdrawal of services made it difficult for nurses to support good pain and symptom management while the patient was awaiting MAiD. Nurses responded strongly to this withdrawal of palliative services: *"So we have a serious practice issue here. I'm mad as hell"* (p. 24).

However, participants also suggested that relationships between those who provided palliative care and those who provided MAiD were becoming more congenial over time. *"We have come a long way because people are not so angry or defensive"* (p. 31). In some cases, this was because MAiD teams had been formed outside of palliative care teams and they had learned to work together. In other cases, palliative clinicians were becoming more comfortable with MAiD as an option, either within or outside of palliative care. Despite this apparent easing of relationships between MAiD and palliative providers, there remained significant concerns related to the inadequacy of palliative care systems in Canada and the impact that MAiD could have in the face of this inadequacy. For example, one participant suggested that the workload generated by MAiD could be a significant barrier for palliative care clinicians who were already working to maximum capacity. Another participant suggested that palliative care, which already carried a fair bit of stigma because of its relationship to death, would become further stigmatized with the introduction of MAiD. Ultimately, this perception would lead to even less acceptability and uptake of palliative care by patients. But what created wider concern for nurses was the inadequate accessibility to palliative care services for some patients in Canada. Under *Bill C-14*, clinicians are required to offer palliative care to clients who are considering a MAiD death. Participants reflected on the irony of how much attention had gone into supporting accessibility to MAiD without corresponding attention paid to overall accessibility to palliative care. *"We use this rhetoric that it's somebody's right to die and I don't want to debate that part but I think it's also their right to have access to care done by clinicians who are knowledgeable about palliative care"* (p. 23). This participant was reflecting on the paucity of specialized palliative care but also on the lack of palliative care knowledge within primary care where most palliative care happens. This same participant went on to describe how providers' lack of palliative care knowledge unwittingly contributed to patient suffering. This tension between a system that caused undue suffering because of ignorance of good palliative care, and a system designed to relieve that suffering through MAiD, put this nurse in an intense state of tension:

> This is the crazy thing for me to consider ... it's a shame and it's something that I grieve to think that our system, as it is, can contribute so much to the suffering of somebody on so many different levels. ... on top of whatever illness process that is causing suffering. But that our health care system contributes to suffering and is doing nothing about our own contribution to that suffering but then uses that very suffering to activate access to MAiD. It's absolutely ridiculous to me. (p. 23)

In light of the tensions between palliative care and MAiD, participants had thoughtfully considered what they thought might be the ideal relationship between the two systems. One participant described it as *"parallel lines with crossover points"* (p. 24). MAiD providers would work along one continuum while palliative care providers would work along the other continuum. But, if and when a client should choose to cross over from palliative care to MAiD, then palliative care would continue as an unbroken commitment to patients.

In summary, nurses in this study were working within systems that differed greatly in their response to MAiD. Some were highly organized whereas others were devoid of policies, procedures, and formal direction. Much of this variability was attributed to the way in which influential leaders, particularly those with responsibilities for palliative care, had chosen to approach MAiD. Further, perspectives of these influential palliative leaders had in turn been influenced by the broader challenges of palliative care accessibility in the Canadian context.

Teamwork: Two's a Team

Nurses in this study participated in MAiD teams to varying degrees. At one end of the spectrum, nurses worked in isolation, being lone assessors and/or providers who worked only peripherally with other assessors and providers. At the other end of the spectrum were nurses who were integrated into well-connected teams dedicated to providing MAiD. In the middle were nurses who worked organically and closely with a few physicians but who were outside of a formal team structure. Even as they found themselves with varying degrees of team support, participants described teamwork as essential to a successful MAiD process. MAiD was a new procedure, and participants described the time it took for physicians and nurses to create a MAiD process that worked well and to feel comfortable with that process. Nurses suggested that, at minimum, two people should be present at every provision of MAiD, one to do the provision and one to look after family and friends and to troubleshoot situations that arose during the process. Having a second person was particularly important in light of the impactful nature of the experience and the need to ensure a seamless, trouble-free provision. For example, this nurse talked about a difficult provision and the importance of a supportive physician. *"It was just me, the doctor and the patient and it was a bad feeling dark, no windows. Afterward I had to wait for the funeral home and I said to the physician, 'you can go.' He said, 'I'm not leaving you.' So, it was just so nice to have that support from the physician"* (p. 37). As physicians were often *"piloted in"* to perform the procedure, it was the nurses who ultimately learned what worked well and who were often in a position to provide support and mentorship to those physicians who performed the procedure less frequently. For example, one nurse remembered supporting a physician through his first provision:

> What struck me about that day was my physician colleague, how his hands were shaking. And I remember putting my hand on his shoulder and just kind of nodding because we were there together and he had never done this before but we had spent a lot of time together previously. (p. 1)

In the latter part of this quote, the nurse acknowledges that it was her previous relationship with the physician that allowed her to support him better. These supportive relationships within the MAiD team were acknowledged as an integral part of the process of a successful MAiD provision. Relationships facilitated the ability to know how each person would respond to such an impactful event, the ability for the nurse to step in and troubleshoot without offending the physician, and the ability to effectively debrief after the process. For example, this nurse described an experience of working with a physician who was unwittingly excluding the family's access to the patient at the last moment, but she did not feel that she and the physician had enough of an established relationship for her to correct him:

> She [the client] was turned towards him [the physician] and her family was at her back and I thought what a shame that we couldn't take a moment and turn her to her family. But that was the first time I'd worked with that clinician. I didn't have any relationship with him at all. (p. 2)

Another participant spoke of supporting a physician new to the MAiD process who was concerned that the patient had not died after administering the medication. Even though the nurse was certain that the patient had died, she took the stethoscope and listened for the heartbeat for a prolonged period of time so that the physician would be reassured. Such examples told a compelling story of the need for mutual support throughout the process of MAiD provision.

Participants also reflected on who might be excluded from the team, but who would nevertheless be deeply impacted by a MAiD death. For example, intravenous (IV) team members play an important role in the establishment and maintenance of the IVs upon which the success of MAiD administration rests. IV team members often establish the IV many hours before the provision to ensure that it is ready. During this insertion they often visit with patients and hear their story. As one nurse described it, you don't put in the IV before you establish the relationship. But, even though these IV team members had established a relationship with the client, they did not have the team support when the client went on to receive MAiD. This nurse described encountering

one such IV nurse. *"I remember an IV nurse starting an IV and for some reason she was waiting outside the door, the door was closed. I can't remember exactly why but she was crying and I comforted her but, you know, she does not get the support we get on the unit"* (p. 6).

Privacy issues attaching to disclosure of a MAiD death also influenced who received support as part of the team. Home care nurses, acute care nurses, and residential care aides and nurses were frequently left out of the process for privacy reasons. Home care nurses described caring for long-term clients who were not imminently dying and then being notified that they had suddenly passed away. The nurse would then follow up with the family and would be told that the client had received MAiD. It was not uncommon for these nurses to wonder why patients and families had not discussed this option with them, particularly in light of their long-term relationships. Nurses in general experienced this as being left out of the loop and, in some cases, it changed their practice in relation to MAiD:

> We had no idea they [clients and family] were thinking about it or mentioning it and no one had a clue and we'd just get notified that they'd passed away, which was really bizarre in the beginning. So, I think that was a turning point for me to make sure they knew all of their options and that they felt safe discussing all of their health with me. And no matter what they chose, they had those options on the table and that they could feel supported through the whole process if that's what they chose. (p. 12)

Stories from residential care were particularly challenging because of the close and enduring relationships that exist between clients and care aides. Clients might choose to keep their decision to access MAiD private, in part because they did not want to spend their last day saying goodbye or justifying their decisions. However, care aides were then taken by surprise by the death:

> Her request was not to tell any of the staff members until afterwards. Her care aides took that very poorly because they didn't know. They were with her right to the last minute and it was a normal day. They took her

to dinner, they took her out for a smoke, they took her back to her room. But then, they were told that she had died. (p. 28)

So, while teamwork was considered the ideal of care, many were left out of the team for various reasons, and as a result did not receive the supports that those who were directly involved in the MAiD team experienced. Further, because MAiD was an impactful experience, those who had learned to work well together formed strong teams that were difficult for others to break into. For example, much of the MAiD referral process across Canada involves a centralized coordinator, often a nurse, who then assigns the patient to willing assessors and providers. These willing individuals are often the "go to" people who work well together. As a result, others who would like to develop experience with the MAiD process may be inadvertently excluded, as was the case of the following participant:

So, you have these pairs of teams and I think it speaks to the powerfulness of the experience. You need to work with a team that you're trusting in. Right? But there's an interesting sort of dynamic with that because, if you're a primary provider and you have a secondary person you use all the time, then you're just going to ask your secondary person. (p. 2)

In summary, participants cited the importance of teamwork both to support a seamless MAiD process and to support those involved in this impactful experience. However, the ability to work within a team where relationships were well-established had benefits beyond mutual support. It also facilitated the seamless organization of what was potentially a highly complex process.

Processes: Patient-Centered Aspirations in a Complex System

Participants in this study described the complexity of facilitating a MAiD-related death. This complexity developed, in part, from the desire for a patient-oriented process. Participants recognized that MAiD would be the final act of healthcare they would perform for a client and that it would occur in a client's last moment of life. This led to an intense desire to get the MAiD process "right" and to provide the most person-centered care in the limited time that clients had left. For example, one nurse contrasted her previous practice in hospital to her current practice in MAiD using the analogy of a wheel and spokes. In her hospital practice she was the wheel and her patients were the spokes; in her MAiD practice that was reversed. However, this was a difficult aspiration to accomplish within a system that was generally not oriented toward providing patient-centered care. The achievement of such a patient-oriented perspective was plagued by difficulties.

This patient-centered perspective meant that nurses prioritized a MAiD-related request and/or provision over other duties. *"I will be dropping everything else that I'm doing when we have a MAiD case. It doesn't matter what other priorities we have on the go, and I have lots of priorities because I'm the practice lead for a few areas"* (p. 2). Priority tasks in a MAiD situation included assessing clients in a timely manner, coaching and educating clients and their families through the decision-making process, and most importantly, organizing a time and space for death in accordance with patient wishes. In some cases, this prioritization was driven by health policies that stipulated that patient requests had to be addressed within a specified time frame (typically a short one). In other cases, it was driven by the urgency of the request because clients were at risk of becoming incapacitated and then would not be able to provide the requisite final consent.

Once a request for MAiD had been initiated, nurses had to perform these priority tasks within systems that were organized to accommodate MAiD to varying degrees. This rural nurse spoke of the disruptions of continuity of care caused by the MAiD care system. *"The client goes to their doctor, he refers to the MAiD steering committee, and I don't know who those people are, they refer to my supervisor and it comes back to me. This is probably a patient that I already know"* (p. 39). In contrast, a seamless system included the presence of an organized referral system, willing MAiD assessors and providers, continuity of care with the existing system, ready access to MAiD-related paperwork and patient records, and a physical space within which to provide MAiD. However, even with all of these factors in place, the system could quickly become overwhelmed when a number of patients were requesting MAiD at the same time. For example, many patients and physicians preferred to schedule the death in the evenings or on weekends. This could prove challenging for MAiD providers, particularly for those who were engaged in MAiD as part of their regular Monday to Friday workload. One nurse described how she eventually had to set boundaries around her time. Even though she was supportive of MAiD, and was committed to its accessibility, she admitted that she did not want to spend all of her weekends providing MAiD.

Nurses also became overwhelmed when they were the only providers willing to engage in MAiD. One nurse practitioner shared that she had become the "go to" person because the physicians in her community were not willing to perform MAiD. She was not sure whether this was because of moral reasons or a lack of adequate financial remuneration. But, she was quickly coming to the end of her emotional resources as a sole provider with limited support.

Participants also described having difficulty accessing patient records for their assessment process. This was particularly challenging when requests were urgent or when assessments were conducted over holidays. Further, there was little agreement about the amount of background information that should be provided to, or shared between, independent assessors. Physical space in which to provide MAiD could also be challenging, particularly for those patients who chose not to have MAiD performed in their home. In some cases, institutions where MAiD could occur (e.g., hospital, residence, or hospice) had policies that prohibited patient admissions that were solely for

MAiD; however, nurses suggested that this accessibility was improving.

The ability to negotiate responsibilities was also an important part of system capacity. This was particularly relevant when there were dedicated MAiD teams. For example, one participant described how challenging it could be to decide whether a client should be referred to social work or to the MAiD team if a client expressed a wish for a hastened death. This was particularly the case if nurses did not have the time for the in-depth conversation that would enable them to better understand the intent of the request. Without this understanding, it was risky to do an immediate referral if the client was seeking support and it was risky to not do an immediate referral if it could be interpreted as limiting accessibility. Once a MAiD referral was made, it could be difficult to distinguish between the care responsibilities of regular providers and MAiD providers:

> So, it's been a bit of a challenge to delineate what we're doing in relationship to the request for assisted dying and what normal care still continues to be. So, that's just a lot of conversations and we go and we meet with teams to say this is our bucket and this is your bucket and we're all playing in the same sandbox to support the patient, but we all need to help each other. (p. 3)

Once a MAiD request had been confirmed, and a time set for provision, nurses were also responsible to organize the support individuals, such as the IV team or pharmacists. In some cases, the IV team required 24 h advance notice to accommodate workload and conscientious objectors. Throughout this process, participants were confronted with complex organizational tasks, within systems that supported those tasks to varying degrees, and with the expectation that they would do their very best for this patient's final hours.

Specific legislative requirements added a further layer of complexity to the system. For example, the legislation requires that one of the two MAiD assessors must also be the MAiD provider. However, in a person-centered approach, patients can indefinitely prolong the time between assessment and provision. This delay can have a number of implications. It might mean that the client presentation changes since the initial assessment, as described by this participant:

> About a month after I saw her for a secondary assessment I realized I've now become her primary provider. But because it's been so long I don't know whether to sign the Form C (clinician assessment form) or not because she actually doesn't have intolerable suffering at this point in time. She goes out for lunch every day with her friends like she's always done. But what happens if next week things turn upside down for her? Somebody else is going to have to come in and do the whole secondary assessment again. You know, without a system in place, it just makes things like that complicated that don't need to be complicated. (p. 30)

The participant in the quote above found herself becoming the provider rather than the secondary assessor, but at least she was involved in both. In other situations, nurse practitioners were expected to be providers when they had not completed either of the original two required assessments. This usually occurred when there was a long delay between assessment and provision and the original assessors were no longer available. This placed these nurses in a difficult position, particularly if their assessment differed from the original assessment.

An additional legislative complexity involved the paperwork associated with a MAiD death as well as the coroner interview required post-MAiD in some jurisdictions. This paperwork became more complex with the new reporting requirements introduced by Health Canada in 2018. Nurses described having to endure these reporting requirements right after an impactful and exhausting MAiD administration. The most troubling aspect of these new reporting requirements was the need to defend one's actions, similar to what one might do in a court of law. The legality of their participation was in question as described by this participant:

> The sense is that we have to prove that what we did was okay and that it was right. Our fear is that they're going to challenge us or ask a question that we won't have an answer to. That will put us in a position of

feeling like, "Uh oh. What did I do now?" The new legislation [reporting requirements], make it worse. (p. 30)

This same participant went on to describe the ironic nature of the self-reporting process that entailed grading one's diligence in following the legislation:

> It is a three-page table that documents in a grid format how we're going to get into trouble if we do things wrong. I mean, that blows my mind, to be honest. I'm thinking, "Is this really necessary? I'm not planning on doing anything wrong (laughs). Why do you have to grade it?" It is a bit bizarre, you know. Not having done due diligence for foreseeable death is a score of 4 which means you get reported to your college. There are some 5s that mean you get reported to the police. But you think, "Hmm, okay. So, if I have provided this service to someone who shouldn't have qualified under the law and who wasn't actually dying then I essentially killed them. That's reported to my college? That should be murder, right? (p. 30)

In this anecdote, the participant shows her struggle with the rules of a complex legislated and reporting process that determines the line between assisted death and murder and takes little account of her moral commitment to doing the right thing.

For nurses, the end result of trying to accomplish impactful patient-centered care within a complex system was excessive workload and emotional burden. This resulted in some nurses setting boundaries around their MAiD practice:

> I don't find the provisions so emotionally draining, but it's more the logistics and it's a lot of work. The logistics of filling in 16 pieces of paper and making sure they're all correct so you don't get into trouble because the consequences are pretty significant. Then there's organizing the pharmacy, going to pick up the medication, and organizing with the family, organizing with the nurse. Like, there is so much that goes into it. And that part can be so draining. And making it all happens as it should, you know, so that everything lines up. So, I think it's important not to do too many cases. And that's what I've been focusing on, making sure I'm not taking too much on. (p. 25)

This nurse was choosing to set limits on her MAiD-related practice. But for other participants, the cost of working within a system that did not adequately support them was simply too much. The risks of not providing good care or of running afoul of the legal system were just too great.

> Working in this haphazard framework you worry that patients are going to fall through the cracks because, you know, we all have busy worlds. Half of the practitioners I work with on an every-other-day basis say they're not going to do this anymore. (p. 30)

DISCUSSION

Findings from this study describe the impact of a legislated approach to assisted death on Canadian nursing practice and nurses' experience. Such findings illustrate the proverbial rock and hard place in which nurses have obligations in relation to the MAiD legislation but find themselves in the complex situation of trying to negotiate best practices with variable support. Nurses in this study described a high degree of variability in policies and procedures, system processes, and team support across Canadian jurisdictions. They further described the importance of teamwork in facilitating such an impactful event. Finally, they described the complexity of facilitating a patient-centered death within a system that was not always well structured to support their efforts. These factors influenced their experiences with assisted death, and their willingness to take part, beyond any considerations of conscientious objection.

In discussing these findings, it is important to remember the limitations of this study. This was a qualitative study that explored the experiences of 59 registered nurses and nurse practitioners. This data was gathered just 2 years post legislation. As such, it represents nurses' early experiences with MAiD and complements other early studies of nurses' experiences in the Canadian context (Beuthin, 2018; Beuthin et al., 2018). Further, these interviews were conducted by telephone rather than in person. However, in reflecting on the richness, depth, and variability of participant responses, conducting these interviews by

telephone may have provided a layer of necessary anonymity for such a controversial topic.

As discussed in the introduction to this paper, the legislated approach to MAiD requires *delegation, precision, and obligation* (Luzon, 2018). In this discussion, we will first explore some of the reasons for the variability of practice supports described in this study and relate those to the way that healthcare responsibilities are delegated in Canada. We will then discuss how adequate practice supports are essential to nurses' abilities to meet the requirements of precision under the MAiD legislation. Finally, we will highlight the tensions that arise in nursing practice as a result of particular obligations inherent in the legislation.

Delegation: Supports As a Reflection of Sociocultural Context

In a country that has chosen a "hard" (Luzon, 2018). approach to MAiD, it is intriguing that the development of nursing practice supports have been so variable across the country. In Canada, responsibility for healthcare rests with the provinces and territories. Provincial and territorial governments in turn delegate this responsibility to health authorities through policy direction and financing. Provinces and territories have structured their health authorities differently; some have one health authority for the entire province (e.g., Alberta and Manitoba), and others have multiple authorities within a province (e.g., British Columbia and Newfoundland). Health authorities are designed, in part, to be responsive to the needs of their particular population (Hurley, 2004). Having multiple health authorities across the country can be inefficient when a task as complex as generating MAiD policies and supports is required. However, the variability in available practice supports that was described in these findings may also be an artifact of the interaction between the sociocultural context of each region and the nature of MAiD.

A number of factors make MAiD a contentious healthcare policy issue. First, MAiD is unique in its healthcare outcome. The intent of MAiD, unlike any other procedure done in healthcare, is always to definitively produce death (Gamble, 2018). Second, MAiD is a morally contentious act. Canadians have a range of responses to MAiD, from believing it to be a morally repugnant act to believing it to be a deeply compassionate act to relieve suffering (Wasylenko, 2017). Third, MAiD is new to Canada. Even though healthcare providers have always received requests to hasten death, only now do they have the legal authority to do so (Rodriguez-Prat & van Leeuwen, 2018; Wright et al., 2017). Further, the experience of the death itself is vastly different from a normal death (Denier et al., 2010b). Such a different, morally complex, and new procedure is likely to be negotiated in profoundly different ways depending upon the sociocultural context. Provinces and territories are known to each be unique sociocultural contexts that are ultimately reflected in their healthcare policy and practice. Provinces in which the majority of citizens would reject MAiD as an option may also be less likely to prioritize the implementation of MAiD-related structures. As important as it is to reflect the unique values and beliefs of the individuals of a particular region, nurses and other healthcare providers can also be placed in a challenging position. Canadians in certain clinical circumstances can claim a legal right to assisted death, but nurses residing within some jurisdictions may not have adequate systems in place to support their practice in fulfilling that right.

Precision: Practice Supports in a Legislated Context

A legislated approach requires a high degree of precision, or a "*precise, specific, clear rule for every practice*" (Luzon, 2018) (p. 14). Our review of Canadian nursing regulatory documents indicated that these rules are found in legislation; regulatory guidelines; professional liability guidelines; and employer standards, guidelines, and policies (Pesut et al., 2019b). Findings from

this current study indicated that the necessary rules were present in some contexts but notably absent in others. In addition to these rules, participants spoke of a need for practice supports that would enable them to fulfill the requirements and obligations associated with a MAiD death. They understood that specific rules can only be enacted properly within a context of adequate support and, more importantly, when there was a mismatch between the required precision and contextual supports, nurses recognized that their practice was at risk. For example, the reporting guidelines required by Health Canada (Government of Canada, 2018) were precise and specific in how they evaluated whether a MAiD procedure complied with the law. But, nurses at times perceived that they did not have adequate resources to meet those requirements. This was evident when nurses indicated they did not have access to required palliative care, to a supportive team, to policies, procedures, and systems that would guide their practice, or to a sufficient number of assessors and providers to support the number of patients seeking MAiD. A perceived lack of a supportive system put some nurses in an untenable position. They were engaging in a high-risk practice that contained precise criteria to differentiate between "*MAiD and murder.*" But they were doing so within what one nurse described as "*haphazard*" systems that do not support the necessary degree of precision. Further, it is important to note that while there are reporting systems in place in Canada, there is no specific oversight and review of MAiD practices. This makes it difficult for practitioners to benchmark good practice other than through their own self-report. Also, there are little data upon which to further develop national policies and best practices. The result was that some practitioners were choosing to limit their involvement in MAiD or refuse to engage in it altogether. However, it is important to remember that, when these practice supports were in place, nurses who participated in this study felt confident in their ability to meet precision requirements.

Not all of the uncertainty in this study was related to a lack of precision at the healthcare policy level. Some related this lack of precision to ambiguity in the legislative language itself. Of particular concern is the definition given in *Bill C-14* to "grievous and irremediable medical condition," one of the eligibility requirements for MAiD. A "grievous and irremediable medical condition" is defined within *Bill C-14* as requiring four criteria to be met, two of which are that death has become *"reasonably foreseeable"* and that the *"illness, disease or disability or state of decline is causing enduring and intolerable physical or psychological suffering."* The concepts of "reasonably foreseeable" death and *"intolerable suffering"* in particular have been the subject of significant and ongoing controversy in healthcare, legal and patient advocacy communities (Reel, 2018; Downie & Scallion, 2018; Downie & Chandler, 2018). Indeed, since, Bill C-14, the Quebec Superior Court has struck down the requirement that death be *"reasonably foreseeable"* (Thanh Ha & Grant, 2019). Such controversy was reflected within this study as well. Nurses reported that a reasonably foreseeable death was being interpreted differently by different clinicians. Documents that have attempted to clarify this language from a legal perspective (e.g., 26) may not necessarily be congruent with clinicians' clinical and moral judgement. This may explain some of the findings in which nurses felt that physicians were placing access barriers in front of patients seeking MAiD. What nurses interpreted as physicians limiting accessibility by telling patients they were not ready for MAiD yet, may actually have been a physician interpretation that the patient's death was not yet *foreseeable.* If the death was not foreseeable, then provision of MAiD would violate the legislation and render the assisted death a criminal act. Such lack of precision in terminology led to divergent opinions and practice, and ultimately tensions, among clinicians.

In terms of the language of "irremediable suffering," nurses in this study believed that such

suffering could only be defined by the patient. However, this created doubt in their abilities to adhere to the legislation. This was evident in the difficulty experienced by a participant in checking the box on the reporting guidelines to confirm that the client was enduring irremediable suffering while knowing that the client was still participating in daily enjoyable activities. Such leeway in interpretation made it difficult for nurses in this study to feel as though they were fulfilling their obligation to practice within clear and specific rules. This uncertainty was compounded when nurses could not draw upon the collective wisdom of a supportive team.

Obligation: Accessibility and Participation

A legislative approach to assisted death also implies a high degree of obligation. Normally, this implies an obligation to fulfill rules in a precise manner (Luzon, 2018). But the ideal of obligation has taken on a new dimension within Canada because the MAiD legislation was developed because of an appeal to *Charter of Rights and Freedoms* guarantees. As such, MAiD in Canada has been framed as a right, and as a right, it brings issues of accessibility to the fore. If Canadians have a legal right to MAiD, then the healthcare system has a responsibility to make MAiD accessible (particularly given the *Canada Health Act*, which confirms accessibility as one of the five essential conditions of the Canadian health system). This idea has generated much debate in Canada. Some MAiD proponents have argued that accessibility means that MAiD should be discussed alongside other end-of-life options, even if the patient has not specifically requested information about MAiD.(Daws et al., 2019). Accessibility to MAiD may also be challenging in rural and remote areas where there may be few providers willing to provide MAiD, and where taking on MAiD-related responsibilities can have significant implications for those rural practitioners who also provide palliative care (Schiller, 2017; Collins & Leier,

2017). This is particularly difficult when many parts of rural and remote Canada still do not have access to good palliative care (Canadian Institute for Health Information, 2018). Gaps in accessibility to palliative care explain, in part, data in this study about how palliative care providers have resisted the development of MAiD. Some practitioners have expressed their concern that the philosophies of assisted dying and palliative care are incompatible with one another while others have argued that the two philosophies may not actually be contradictory (Radbruch et al., 2016; Dierickx et al., 2018). However, if the political will to provide accessibility to palliative care is not as strong as the political will to provide accessibility to MAiD, then inevitably it will be easier for patients to access MAiD than to access palliative care. This is of even greater concern when one considers the potential end-of-life healthcare cost savings generated by MAiD-related deaths in Canada (Trachtenberg, 2017).

The obligation to make MAiD accessible influenced nurses' experiences both positively and negatively. Some nurses worked within well-resourced teams dedicated to patient-centered access, thus fulfilling their ideal of MAiD access for patients who wanted it. However, facilitating accessibility could be more problematic outside of such a team structure. Those nurses who felt that they were obligated to provide MAiD because others in their community refused to do so found themselves in a difficult position. This was evident in the data when nurses had to erect boundaries around their involvement, either because they were trying to organize this precise act within a poorly designed system or because they were experiencing ill effects of trying to do this emotionally laborious task alone. But, in a climate that focuses on an obligation to access, it is difficult for nurses to decline to participate, particularly as employees of healthcare. For example, in this study, once a decision-maker had chosen to embed a MAiD role within a particular nursing role to improve access, it then became

difficult for nurses to decline to participate in MAiD and still fulfill their employment obligations. A number of nurses in this study reflected on how they had never imagined that they would be asked to participate in such an act within their nursing career. Notably, in this study, nurses' decision to not participate was not always because of a conscientious objection. Rather, that decision could often be attributed to a lack of resources and support, to a difference in philosophies (e.g., palliative care and MAiD), or to a belief that MAiD was inappropriately overshadowing other important healthcare priorities. These reasons for non-participation have been discussed in the literature related to institutional participation in MAiD (Shadd & Shadd, 2019). In these situations, and in situations where nurses were conscientious objectors, nurses' experiences were influenced by how responsive and respectful leaders were in accommodating their decision of whether or not to participate in MAiD.

Clinical Implications

MAiD legislation in Canada has led to a dramatically new form of practice. There is an opportunity to unpack multiple layers of nursing practice experience to better understand both the implications of the structural context of practice and the moral impact of various care settings and teamwork arrangements. Findings of this study demonstrate the powerful impact of organizational leadership on the workplace policies and culture that significantly determine how nurses experience this new care option. We can also see how the potentially conflicting worldviews of different practice sectors, in this case the specialist palliative care sector and the sector involved in MAiD provision, shape not only the care options accessible to patients but also the nuances of nursing engagement with patients who are considering or completing MAiD. These data demonstrate a full range of care cultures, from those that place all concerned in states of extreme tension to those that create space for the ambiguity and complexity characteristic of MAiD at this time in Canadian history. As more and more nurses across the international context encounter patients for whom MAiD is a possibility, it will be increasingly important that procedures and supports be put in place to support nursing practice. This is particularly essential where a legislated, or hard, approach to assisted death requires precision, obligation, and delegation. Further, robust policies, and perhaps more importantly, supportive procedures, are required to ensure that nurses can choose to participate or not in this radical new end of life care option. Those who choose to participate require supported practice; those who choose not to participate need the freedom to do so without fear that it will negatively influence their colleagues or their employment options. This will be particularly relevant in international contexts where assisted death becomes embedded within health systems, similar to how it has been enacted in Canada.

The nature of the Canadian legislation has spawned new and intimate practice teams that support practitioners to provide patient-centered, high-quality care, and mutual support during such a momentous time. However, these data also reveal the potential disruption of currently existing teams and a lack of recognition of the supportive work done by those who may not be directly involved in MAiD assessment and provision. It further reveals the difficulties encountered by those who act as MAiD assessors and providers without the presence of a supportive team. So, although the MAiD legislation provides specificity as to the roles and obligations of assessors and providers, such work cannot be solely delegated to these individuals. Comprehensive care must consider the many collateral persons who provide support throughout the care trajectory, from the time patients first consider MAiD through to the stage of bereavement. All members of the care team clearly feel the need for guidance and insight as to how to manage the moral tensions associated with providing the best care possible through to the end. Further, members of these teams require expertise in how to assess and negotiate the complex patient request for death that may or may not reflect and request for MAiD. Belgian law stipulates that the nursing team should be consulted regarding patient euthanasia requests, although no such requirement exists in the Netherlands (Pesut et al., 2019a). Evidence derived from nurses in Belgium has attested to the complexity of these conversations (Denier et al., 2010a; Denier et al., 2010b). Countries considering the legalization of assisted death should carefully consider the impact of teamwork on best practices, including those having to do with communicating with patients and families.

CONCLUSION

These findings have permitted a glimpse into the morally difficult and organizationally complex work that a legislated approach to MAiD places upon nurses who are already often coping with highly challenging work environments. Variable practice supports, leadership philosophies, team structures, and system and legislative supports greatly influenced whether nurses were able to confidently meet the hard requirements of a legislated approach. Clearly, in light of a legislated approach to MAiD that requires high degrees of delegation, precision, and obligation we have much work to do in supporting nursing through basic and continuing educational programming, care pathways and best practice guidelines, and workplace teams and environments. Further, we must continue to try to understand the important lessons that the experience of nurses of being caught "between a rock and a hard place" can offer with respect to what this radical new care options mean for all concerned.

REFERENCES

Beuthin, R. (2018). Cultivating compassion: the practice experience of a medical assistance in dying coordinator in Canada. *Qualitative Health Research, 28*(11), 1679–1691.

Beuthin, R., Bruce, A., & Scaia, M. (2018). Medical assistance in dying (MAiD): Canadian nurses' experiences. *Nursing Forum, 53,* 511–520.

Bill C-14. (2016). *An Act to amend the Criminal Code and to make related amendments to other Acts (medical assistance in dying):* Statutes of Canada. chapter 3. http://www.parl.ca/DocumentViewer /en/42-1/bill/C-14/royal-assent.

Canadian Institute for Health Information. (2018). *Access to palliative care in Canada.* https://www.cihi .ca/sites/default/files/document/access-palliative-care -2018-en-web.pdf. Accessed 15 Nov 2019.

Carter. v. Canada (Attorney General). (2015). 1SCR331. https://scc-csc.lexum.com/scc-csc/scc-csc/en/item /14637/index.do.

Collins, A., & Leier, B. (2017). Can medical assistance in dying harm rural and remote palliative care in Canada? *Canadian Family Physician, 63*(3), 186–190.

Daws, T., Landry, J. T., Viens, P., et al. (2019). *Bringing up medical assistance in dying (MAiD) as a clinical care option:* Canadian Association of MAiD Assessors and Providers. https://camapcanada.ca /wp-content/uploads/2020/01/Bringing-up-Medical -Assistance-In-Dying.pdf.

Denier, Y., Dierckx de Casterle, B., De Bal, N., & Gastmans, C. (2009). Involvement of nurses in the euthanasia care process in Flanders (Belgium): an exploration of two perspectives. *Journal of Palliative Care, 25*(4), 264–274.

Denier, Y., Gastmans, C., De Bal, N., & Dierckx de Casterle, B. (2010a). Communication in nursing care for patients requesting euthanasia: a qualitative study. *Journal of Clinical Nursing, 19*(23–24), 3372–3380.

Denier, Y., Dierckx de Casterle, B., De Bal, N., & Gastmans, C. (2010b). "It's intense, you know." Nurses' experiences in caring for patients requesting euthanasia. *Medicine, Health Care and Philosophy, 13*(1), 41–48.

Dierckx de Casterle, B., Denier, Y., De Bal, N., & Gastmans, C. (2010). Nursing care for patients requesting euthanasia in general hospitals in Flanders, Belgium. *Journal of Advanced Nursing, 66*(11), 2410–2420.

Dierickx, S., Deliens, L., Cohen, J., & Chambaere, K. (2018). Involvement of palliative care in euthanasia practice in a context of legalized euthanasia: a population-based mortality follow-back study. *Palliative Medicine, 32*(1), 114–122.

Downie, J., & Chandler, J. A. (2018). *Interpreting Canada's medical assistance in dying legislation.* Montreal, Quebec: Institute for Research on Public Policy. http://irpp.org/wp-content/uploads/2018/03/ Interpreting-Canadas-Medical-Assistance-in-Dying- Legislation-MAiD.pdf.

Downie, J., & Scallion, K. (2018). Foreseeably unclear: the meaning of the "reasonably foreseeable" criterion for access to medical assistance in dying in Canada. *Dalhousie Law Journal.* https://doi.org/10.2139 /ssrn.3126871.

Gamble, N. (2018). Can euthanasia be classified as a medically beneficial treatment? *Ethics Med, 34*(2), 103–111.

Glaser, B. G., & Strauss, A. L. (1967). *The discovery of grounded theory: strategies for qualitative research.* Chicago: Aldine Publishing Company.

Government of Canada. (2018). *Guidance for reporting on medical assistance in dying.* https://www. canada.ca/en/health-canada/services/medical -assistance-dying/guidance-reporting-summary.html.

Health Canada. (2019). Fourth Interim Report on Medical Assistance in Dying. https://www.canada .ca/en/health-canada/services/publications/health -system-services/medical-assistance-dying-interim -report-april-2019.html2019.

Hurley, J. (2004). Regionalization and the allocation of healthcare resources to meet population needs. *Healthcare Papers, 5*(1), 34–39.

Luzon, G. (2018). The practice of euthanasia and assisted suicide meets the concept of legalization. *Criminal Law and Philosophy, 13,* 329–345. https://doi. org/10.1007/s11572-018-9474-9.

Pesut, B., Thorne, S., Greig, M., Fulton, A., Janke, R., & Vis-Dunbar, M. (2019a). Ethical, policy, and practice implications of nurses' experiences with assisted death: a synthesis. *Advances in Nursing Science, 42*(3), 216–230.

Pesut, B., Thorne, S., Stager, M. L., Schiller, C., Penney, C., Hoffman, C., Greig, M., & Roussel, J. (2019b). Medical assistance in dying: a narrative review of Canadian nursing regulatory documents. *Policy, Politics, & Nursing Practice, 20*(3), 113–130.

Pesut, B., Greig, M., Thorne, S., Storch, J., Burgess, M., Tishelman, C., Chambaere, K., & Janke, R. (2019c). Nursing and euthanasia: A narrative review of the nursing ethics literature. *Nursing Ethics, 2019,* 1–16.

Radbruch, L., Leget, C., Bahr, P., et al. (2016). Euthanasia and physician-assisted suicide: a white paper from the European association for palliative care. *Palliative Medicine, 30*(2), 104–116.

Reel, K. (2018). Denying assisted dying where death is not 'reasonably foreseeable': intolerable overgeneralizations in Canadian end-of-life law. *Canadian Journal of Bioethics, 1*(3), 71–81.

Rodriguez-Prat, A., & van Leeuwen, E. (2018). Assumptions and moral understandings of the wish to hasten death: a philosophical review of qualitative studies. *Medicine, Health Care and Philosophy, 21*(1), 63–75.

Schiller, C. J. (2017). Medical assistance in dying in Canada: focus on rural communities. *Journal for Nurse Practitioners, 13*(9), 628–634.

Shadd, P., & Shadd, J. (2019). Insitutional non-participation in assisted dying: changing the conversation. *Bioethics, 33*(1), 207–214.

Suva, G., Penney, T., & McPherson, C. (2019). Medical assistance in dying: a scoping review to inform nurses' practice. *Journal of Hospice & Palliative Nursing, 21*(1), 46–53.

Thanh Ha, T., & Grant, K (2019). Quebec court strikes down restriction to medically assisted dying law, calls it unconstitutional. *Globe and Mail.*

Thorne, S. (2016). *Interpretive description: qualitative research for applied practice* (2nd ed.). New York: Routledge.

Trachtenberg, A. J. (2017). Cost analysis of medical assistance in dying in Canada. *CMAJ, 189*(3), E101–E105.

van de Scheur, A., & van der Arend, A. (1998). The role of nurses in euthanasia: a Dutch study. *Nursing Ethics, 5*(6), 497–508.

Wasylenko, E. (2017). Becoming dead: two solitudes? *Healthcare Management Forum, 30*(5), 262–265.

Wright, D. K., Chirchikova, M., Daniel, V., Bitzas, V., Elmore, J., & Fortin, M.-L. (2017). Engaging with patients who desire death: interpretation, presence, and constraint. *Canadian Oncology Nursing Journal, 27*(1), 56–64.

Lanolin for the Treatment of Nipple Pain in Breastfeeding Women: A Randomized Controlled Trial

Kimberley T. Jackson[1,2,*] | Cindy-Lee Dennis[2]

ABSTRACT

Nipple pain and damage are commonly experienced by breastfeeding women and are associated with negative breastfeeding outcomes. Health care providers often recommend the application of lanolin to treat painful/damaged nipples, yet no randomized controlled trial has evaluated the effectiveness of lanolin on nipple pain and breastfeeding outcomes. The purpose of this study was to evaluate the effect of lanolin on nipple pain among breastfeeding women with damaged nipples. A randomized, single-blind, controlled trial was conducted at a tertiary care hospital in Hamilton, Ontario, Canada. Breastfeeding women ($N = 186$) identified as having nipple pain/damage were randomized to apply lanolin (intervention group; $n = 93$) or to receive usual postpartum care (control group; $n = 93$). The primary outcome was nipple pain at 4 days post-randomization measured by the Numeric Rating Scale. Additional outcomes included nipple pain measured by the Short-Form McGill Pain Questionnaire, breastfeeding duration/exclusivity, breastfeeding self-efficacy, and maternal satisfaction with lanolin treatment versus usual care. The results revealed no significant group differences in mean pain scores at 4 days post-randomization. Women in both groups experienced clinically relevant decreases in nipple pain by 7 days post-randomization. Significantly, more women in the lanolin group reported that they were satisfied with treatment compared with those receiving usual care. No significant group differences were found for other secondary outcomes. While more women were satisfied using lanolin, its application to sore/damaged nipples was ineffective for reducing nipple pain or improving breastfeeding outcomes.

KEY MESSAGES

- Nipple pain and damage is common among breastfeeding women and is often implicated in breastfeeding cessation.
- This trial suggests that regardless of the use of lanolin or usual postpartum care, it is expected that nipple pain intensity will decrease by approximately seven to ten days postpartum.
- The findings of this study suggest that the application of lanolin to painful/damaged nipples in the immediate postpartum period does not significantly decrease nipple pain or improve breastfeeding outcomes when compared with usual care.

INTRODUCTION

Although there are many factors that contribute to a woman's decision to initiate and continue breastfeeding, evidence suggests that most women discontinue breastfeeding prematurely

[1]University of Western Ontario, London, Ontario, Canada, and

[2]Lawrence S. Bloomberg Faculty of Nursing, University of Toronto, Canada and Women's Health Research Chair, St. Michael's Hospital, Toronto, Canada

*Correspondence: Kimberley T. Jackson, Arthur Labatt Family School of Nursing, Room 134, Health Sciences Addition, London, Ontario, Canada, N6A 5C1, 519-661-2111 x 86936. Email: kim.jackson@uwo.ca

because of perceived difficulties rather than maternal choice (Dennis, 2002). Nipple pain and damage is a common occurrence for breastfeeding women in the early postpartum period (Heads & Higgins, 1995; Hewat & Ellis, 1987; Ziemer et al., 1990, Buck, Amir, Cullinane & Donath, 2014) and is often implicated in breastfeeding cessation (Fetherston, 1995; Yeoung et al., 1986). The incidence of nipple pain is high, with reports of 95% of Canadian women (Hewat & Ellis, 1987), 77–79% of Australian women (Heads & Higgins, 1995; Buck, Amir, Cullinane & Donath, 2014), 62% of women from France (Darmangeat, 2011), and 90–96% of U.S. women (Ziemer & Pigeon, 1993; Ziemer, Paone, Schupay & Cole, 1990) experiencing nipple pain in the early stages of breastfeeding.

Various interventions have been evaluated in the treatment of painful, damaged nipples including breastfeeding education (Clark, 1985; Livingstone & Stringer, 1999; Darmangeat, 2011; Cadwell, Turner-Maffei, Blair, Brimdyr & McInerney, 2004), breast shells (Gosha & Tichy, 1988), compresses (Lavergne, 1997), ointments (including lanolin) (Clark, 1985; Livingstone & Stringer, 1999; Kuscu et al., 2001; Riordan, 1985; Abou-Dakn et al., 2011; Dennis et al., 2012), LED phototherapy (Chavez et al., 2012) and tea bags (Lavergne, 1997; Riordan, 1995). Among all of the published intervention studies, no single treatment for nipple pain/damage has been demonstrated to be effective. Results from a recent Cochrane systematic review suggest that there is no evidence that any one intervention is superior to the others in the treatment of nipple pain or trauma (Dennis et al., 2014).

Health care providers often recommend the application of lanolin to treat painful and/or damaged nipples. Aside from expressed breastmilk, lanolin is the only intervention that has received continued endorsement by the La Leche League International, the most predominant global, community-based breastfeeding support network for women. Lanolin is also recommended by the International Board Certified Lactation Consultants (IBCLC) and is included in their core curriculum for lactation consultant practice (Mannel et al., 2008). Lanolin is considered a pure and safe intervention (containing no preservatives, additives, water, chemicals, or perfume), aimed at creating a moist healing environment for nipple trauma and providing a semi-occlusive barrier that promotes retention of internal moisture and prevents dryness (Martin, 2000). Lanolin may provide a moist dermal environment to prevent eschar formation, promote epithelial regrowth, and decrease nipple pain (Cable et al., 1997; Pugh et al., 1996). However, there has been no randomized controlled trial specifically evaluating the effect of lanolin. The purpose of this trial was to evaluate the effect of lanolin on nipple pain among breastfeeding women with damaged nipples.

Participants

Women were recruited from a large tertiary care hospital in Hamilton, Ontario, Canada from May 2011 to March 2012. Eligible participants were breastfeeding women who: (1) had nipple pain and visible nipple damage; (2) delivered a full-term (greater than 37 weeks gestation), singleton infant within the previous 72 h; and (3) were able to speak English. The exclusion criteria included: (1) infants not expected to be discharged home with their mother; (2) infants with a congenital abnormality that would impair breastfeeding, or ankyloglossia (tongue-tie); (3) maternal allergy to lanolin; (4) maternal health condition(s) that might interfere with breastfeeding; and (5) maternal aversion to, or, strong desire to use lanolin.

Sample Size

The sample size was estimated based upon the goal to detect a minimum 20% reduction in mean NRS pain scores for women receiving lanolin within the first 36 h postpartum. In a 2012 randomized controlled trial (Dennis et al., 2012) comparing lanolin to an all-purpose nipple ointment, mean NRS pain scores decreased by 23% from baseline to 1-week post-randomization for women using lanolin for their nipple pain. Thus, with 90% power, a 30% loss to follow-up rate and a two-tailed α error of 0.05, a sample size of 186 (93 per group) was required.

Methods

Following approval by the Hamilton Integrated Research Ethics Board and the University of Toronto Health Sciences Research Ethics Board, a randomized, single-blind, controlled trial was conducted (Fig. B.1). This trial was registered as an international randomized controlled trial with ClinicalTrials.gov, trial number NCT01420419. To recruit participants, the trial was briefly introduced to women who were identified by hospital nurses as having nipple pain and damage. Verbal consent was then obtained to have the Principal Investigator provide a detailed study explanation. Following informed consent procedures, baseline data were collected and the participants were randomized to either a control group or an intervention group. Randomization was achieved by using sealed, opaque, sequentially numbered envelopes containing randomly generated numbers. This procedure was constructed by a research assistant external to the trial. Women allocated to the control group ($n = 93$) received usual postpartum in-hospital and community care, whereas those allocated to the intervention group ($n = 93$) received usual postpartum in-hospital care, in addition to the lanolin intervention. Usual postpartum in-hospital care may have included breastfeeding education/assistance by an RN/RPN or lactation consultant. Acceptable strategies for pain relief may have included: application of warm/cool compresses to the affected nipple, analgesia (e.g., acetaminophen or ibuprofen), air drying the nipples, or the use of breast shields. Once discharged from hospital, standard community resources were available to all mothers including: public

health breastfeeding programmes, outpatient hospital breastfeeding clinics, LaLeche League, community-based breastfeeding support groups, and hospital telephone assistance. All mothers could proactively seek support from any or all of these resources. To control for contamination, women in the control group were asked not to apply lanolin to their nipples for the trial period. Nurses on the postpartum unit and in the outpatient breastfeeding clinic were also instructed not to offer or recommend lanolin to women in the control group.

A research assistant blinded to participant group allocation telephoned all women at 4 and 7 days post-randomization and at 4 and 12 weeks postpartum to determine nipple pain, breastfeeding duration and exclusivity, breastfeeding self-efficacy, and maternal satisfaction with treatment received. In addition, participants in the control group were asked at each follow-up if they used lanolin to treat their nipple pain.

Intervention

The intervention in this trial was a 40-g tube of Lansinoh® HPA® Lanolin (VA, USA) accompanied by an instruction pamphlet. Participants were instructed to wash their hands and to gently apply a pea-sized amount of lanolin to the nipple and the areola immediately surrounding the erectile portion of the nipple following every feed until resolution of symptoms or the end of the 7-day trial period. Women were free to continue using lanolin and/or other standard care resources if their symptoms had not resolved within the 7-day study period.

Outcome Measures
Nipple Pain

The primary outcome was nipple pain as measured using the Numeric Rating Scale (NRS) (McCaffery & Beebe, 1989), where participants rated their pain on a scale ranging from 0 = *no pain* to 10 = *pain as bad as it could be*. The

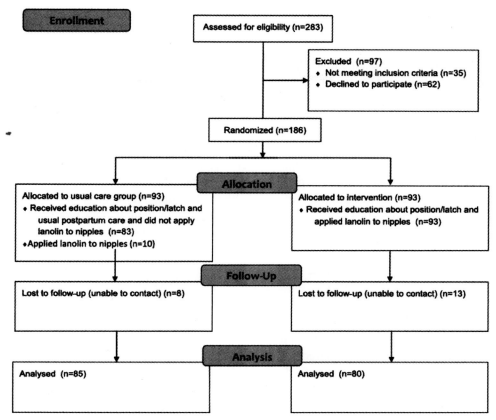

FIG. B.1   Trial schema.

NRS is commonly used to assess pain intensity among a variety of adult populations and its reliability and validity have been well established (McDowell, 2006; Jensen & Karoly, 2001). The NRS was administered at baseline and at 4 days post-randomization. For many mothers, nipple pain appears to have the greatest intensity between the third and seventh day postpartum, with a peak in severity on the third day postpartum (Hewat & Ellis, 1987; Ziemer et al., 1990). Given that participants were 1–3 days postpartum when they enrolled in the study, the follow-up at 4 days post-randomization was chosen to capture the period where pain severity tends to be the greatest, and to allow time for the intervention to take effect; that is, between 5 and 8 days postpartum.

Although the reliability and validity of the NRS have been well established among a variety of adult populations in both clinical and research settings (Jensen & Karoly, 2001), there are no studies that specifically address the validity of the NRS among breastfeeding women. As such, the Short Form McGill Pain Questionnaire (SF-MPQ) (Melzack, 1987) was also utilized to measure nipple pain intensity and quality and to provide a further description of pain at baseline and at 4 and 7 days post-randomization, as it provides other potentially valuable information beyond the sensory aspects of pain. The SF-MPQ is comprised of a Pain Rating Index (PRI) and a Present Pain Intensity (PPI) scale. The PRI is a 15-item questionnaire, which uses descriptors to evaluate sensory and affective dimensions of pain.

Participants select adjectives that best describe their pain and rank the severity on a 4-point scale from 0 = *none* to 3 = *severe*. Scores are summed to produce a total score ranging from 0 to 45. The PPI is a 6-point scale to rate intensity ranging from 0 = *mild* to 5 = *excruciating*. The SF-MPQ also includes a visual analogue scale, which was not used in this trial as follow-up data were collected via telephone. The SF-MPQ has been widely used to assess the pain experience in a variety of adult patient populations (Wilkie et al., 1990). The psychometric properties of the SF-MPQ have been well documented (Wright et al., 2001).

Breastfeeding Duration and Exclusivity

Breastfeeding duration was assessed at 4 and 12 weeks postpartum and measured by asking women if they had breastfed within the past 24 h or not. Breastfeeding exclusivity was assessed at baseline, 4 and 7 days post-randomization, and at 4 and 12 weeks postpartum and measured using Labbok & Krasovec's levels of breastfeeding (Labbok & Krasovek, 1990). Responses included: (1) exclusive breastfeeding (breastmilk only); (2) almost exclusive breastfeeding (less than one bottle per week of non-human milk or other fluid); (3) high breastfeeding (less than one bottle per day of non-human milk, other fluid or food); (4) partial breastfeeding (1 bottle per day of non-human milk); (5) token breastfeeding (breast given to comfort baby, with minimal nutritional contribution); and (6) bottlefeeding (no human milk given).

Breastfeeding Self-efficacy

This outcome was assessed at baseline and at 4 days post-randomization using the Breastfeeding Self-Efficacy Scale - Short Form (BSES-SF) (Dennis, 2003). The BSES-SF is a 14-item self-report instrument developed to measure breastfeeding confidence. All items are preceded by the phrase "I can always" and anchored with a 5-point Likert scale where 1 = *not at all confident*

and 5 = *always confident*. Scores are summed to produce a total score ranging from 14 to 70, with higher scores indicating higher levels of breastfeeding self-efficacy. The BSES-SF has been psychometrically tested and has demonstrated that it is a valid and reliable measure of breastfeeding self-efficacy (Gregory et al., 2008).

Maternal Satisfaction

This outcome was measured at 12 weeks postpartum and included questions related to satisfaction with the treatment, how likely they would use the treatment again, and if they would recommend the treatment to others. All items were rated on a 5-point scale where 1 = *very satisfied* and 5 = *very dissatisfied*. Additional questions with diverse formats were related to maternal report of side effects and adherence to the treatment protocol. Table B.1 summarizes the instruments and measurements utilized and their corresponding time points.

Data Analysis

Data were analyzed using SPSS Version 20 and an intention-to-treat approach. For continuous data, means and standard deviations were calculated and differences between groups were examined using independent samples t-tests. For categorical data, frequencies and percentages were calculated and differences between groups were examined using chi-squared tests. A two-sided significance level of 0.05 was utilized for all study outcomes.

RESULTS

Sample Characteristics

In total, 186 women were recruited into the study. Characteristics of participants are shown in Table B.2. There were no clinically important differences in baseline characteristics between the two groups. Of the women that were randomized, 21 (lanolin group, $n = 13$; control group, $n = 8$) could not be contacted by telephone, resulting in a 14% loss to follow-up (LTF) rate for the lanolin

TABLE **B.1**

SUMMARY OF INSTRUMENTS AND MEASUREMENT TIMES

STUDY VARIABLE	MEASURE	TIMING
Baseline maternal information	Baseline questionnaire	Prior to randomization
Primary outcome		Baseline and at 4 days post-randomization
1. Pain intensity	11-point NRS	
Secondary outcomes		
1. Breastfeeding duration	Breastfeeding or not	4 and 7 days post-randomization and at 4 and 12 weeks postpartum
2. Breastfeeding exclusivity	[a]Labbok & Krasovec's levels of breastfeeding	Baseline, 4 and 7 days post-randomization, and at 4 and 12 weeks postpartum
Other outcomes		
1. Pain intensity	11-point NRS	7 days post-randomization
2. Pain quality	SF-MPQ	4 days post-randomization
3. Breastfeeding self-efficacy	BSES-SF	4 days post-randomization
4. Maternal satisfaction with intervention	Maternal satisfaction questionnaire	12 weeks postpartum

[a](Labbok & Krasovec, 1990). NRS, Numeric Rating Scale; SF-MPQ, Short-Form McGill Pain Questionnaire; BSES-SF, Breastfeeding Self-Efficacy Scale Short-Form.

group, and a 8.6% LTF rate for the control group for the primary outcome (Fig. B.1). The overall LTF rate was 11.3%. For the secondary outcomes, participants who were still breastfeeding at 4 weeks postpartum ($n = 155$) were telephoned again at 12 weeks postpartum. Among the 155 participants, 22 (lanolin group, $n = 13$; control group, $n = 9$) did not complete the outcome assessment, resulting in a 16% LTF rate for the lanolin group and a 12.2% LTF rate for could not be contacted by telephone despite three telephone calls followed by an emailed request for continued participation.

Participants were considered compliant if they described using lanolin after 75% or more of the feeds for the 7-day study period: 63 (78.8%) of women in the lanolin group described using the lanolin as recommended. Almost half ($n = 39$, 49%) of the women used lanolin after every feed, 24 (30%) women used lanolin after 75% of feeds, and 17 (21%) women used lanolin after 50% of feeds or less. Among the 85 women in the control group who completed the 4 days

post-randomization outcome assessment, 10 (12%) reported using lanolin to treat their nipple pain. Among the 83 women in the control group who completed the 12-week follow-up, 13 (16%) reported that they had used lanolin at some point during the study period. Among these women, 9 (11%) reported using lanolin after every feed and 4 (5%) reported using lanolin after 75% of feeds.

Clinical Outcomes

Nipple Pain

Both groups reported less nipple pain on all pain outcome measures from baseline to 4 days post-randomization. No significant group differences were found in pain scores for the NRS or the SF-MPQ sub-scales (Table B.3). While there were clinically meaningful reductions in nipple pain on all pain outcome measures from baseline to 7 days post-randomization for both groups, no significant differences in pain scores were found between groups.

TABLE **B.2**

BASELINE CHARACTERISTICS

BASELINE CHARACTERISTIC (0–3 DAYS POSTPARTUM)	USUAL CARE n = 93	TREATMENT n = 93
Age, *mean* (SD)	29.0 (4.9) n (%)	29.5 (5.3) n (%)
Marital status		
Married/Common-law	88 (94.6)	86 (92.5)
Single	5 (5.4)	7 (7.5)
Ethnicity		
Caucasian	81 (87.1)	81 (87.1)
Non-Caucasian	12 (12.9)	12
Education		
Elementary	0	4 (4.3)
High school	24 (25.8)	14 (15.1)
College	30 (32.3)	33 (35.5)
University	39 (41.9)	42 (45.2)
Annual household income[a]		
<$39 999	19 (22.3)	14 (15.9)
$40 000–99 999	29 (34.1)	38 (43.1)
>$100 000	37 (43.5)	36 (40.9)
Breastfeeding level		
Exclusive	69 (74.2)	67 (72.0)
Almost exclusive	11 (11.8)	18 (19.4)
High	9 (9.7)	6 (6.5)
Partial	4 (4.3)	2 (2.2)
NRS, *mean* (SD)	6.5 (2.3)	6.2 (2.2)
SF-MPQ Total, *mean* (SD)	17.7 (8.4)	16.9 (7.9)
BSES-SF, *mean* (SD)	55.5 (9.2)	55.6 (8.9)

[a]Participants did not wish to disclose their annual household income (usual care group, n = 8; treatment group, n = 5). NRS, Numeric Rating Scale; SF-MPQ, Short-Form McGill Pain Questionnaire; BSES-SF, Breastfeeding Self-Efficacy Scale – Short Form.

Breastfeeding Duration and Exclusivity

At 4 weeks postpartum, 20 (24%) women in the control group had discontinued breastfeeding compared with 12 (15%) in the lanolin group. At 12 weeks postpartum, 31 (37%) women in the control group had discontinued breastfeeding compared with 22 (28%) in the lanolin group. However, these differences between groups were not statistically significant (Table B.4). Breastfeeding exclusivity levels were also similar among groups at both 4 and 12 weeks postpartum with no statistically significant differences between the groups (Table B.4).

Breastfeeding Self-efficacy

Women in both groups reported high levels of breastfeeding self-efficacy at baseline and at 4 days post-randomization (Table B.2). No significant difference was found among the groups for changes in breastfeeding self-efficacy scores at 4 days post-randomization with the control group having a mean score of 55.4 (SD = 10.4) compared with 56.3 (SD = 11.8) for the treatment group.

Maternal Satisfaction

Overall, the majority (n = 42, 53%) of women in the lanolin group were "very satisfied" with the effects of lanolin in treating their nipple pain. Conversely, only 18 (22%) women in the control group were "very satisfied" with the care they received to manage their nipple pain. This difference in maternal satisfaction between the groups was statistically significant, χ^2 (2, n = 160) = 20.8, p ≤.001). Only 1 (1%) woman in the lanolin group was "very dissatisfied" with the treatment they received compared with 11 (14%) women in the control group. No side effects were reported by those in the lanolin group.

DISCUSSION

This is the first randomized controlled trial to rigorously evaluate the effect of lanolin on nipple pain among breastfeeding women with damaged nipples. Overall, lanolin was ineffective in reducing nipple pain or improving breastfeeding duration and exclusivity rates. No significant difference was found among the groups for mean changes in nipple pain intensity scores, nor for SF-MPQ

TABLE **B.3**

NIPPLE PAIN MEASURES BETWEEN GROUPS

VARIABLE	USUAL CARE	TREATMENT	MEAN DIFFERENCE BETWEEN GROUPS (T- UC)	t(df)	P
	Δ(T2 – T1) M(SD)	Δ(T2 – T1) M(SD)	TΔ - UCΔ M(SD)		
NRS 4 Days P.R.	– 0.5(3.0)	– 0.7(3.1)	– 0.3(0.5)	– 0.5(163)	0.6
NRS 7 Days P.R.	– 2.5(3.0)	– 2.4(3.2)	– 0.0(0.5)	– 0.0(158)	0.9
SF-MPQ 4 Days P.R.	2.5(10.6)	1.3(11.4)	– 1.2(1.7)	– 0.7(163)	0.5
SF-MPQ 7 Days P.R.	– 5.3(8.6)	– 4.3(11.0)	1.0(1.6)	0.6(158)	0.5

Δ denotes change in scores over time (NRS, Numeric Rating Scale; P.R., post-randomization; SF-MPQ, Short-Form McGill Pain Questionnaire; T, treatment; UC, usual care).

TABLE **B.4**

BREASTFEEDING EXCLUSIVITY

TIME	INFANT FEEDING CATEGORY	USUAL CARE	TREATMENT	$\chi^2(df)$	P
		(n = 84)	(n = 78)		
		n (%)	n (%)		
4 weeks postpartum	Exclusive or almost exclusive	52 (61.9)	51 (63.0)	3.2(2)	0.2
	High or partial	12 (14.3)	18 (22.2)		
	Token or bottle-feeding	20 (23.8)	12 (14.8)		
		Usual care	Treatment		
		n (%)	[a]n (%)		
12 weeks postpartum	Exclusive or almost exclusive	42 (50.0)	43 (55.1)	1.5(2)	0.5
	High or partial	11 (13.1)	13 (16.7)		
	Token or bottle-feeding	31 (36.9)	22 (28.2)		

[a]n = 81.

scores at 4 or 7 days post randomization. Both groups had moderate pain (Serlin et al., 1995) at baseline (mean NRS rating between 5 and 6) and continued to have moderate pain 4 days later. At 7 days post randomization NRS scores were in the mild range (1–4) for both groups, and these findings were similar to an RCT using lanolin as a control group (Dennis et al., 2012). Based on the data from this trial and those from another study (Abou-Dakn et al., 2011), it is suggested that regardless

of the use of lanolin or usual care, it is expected that nipple pain intensity scores will decrease by approximately seven to ten days postpartum. Our baseline results did not differ from previous nipple pain studies where moderate pain levels were also found (Abou-Dakn et al., 2011; Dennis et al., 2012).

Although compliance for this trial was high, it is plausible that amount of lanolin and/or the frequency of application to the nipple were insufficient to achieve a therapeutic effect. Prior literature reporting on the use of lanolin for nipple pain has been inconsistent with respect to what is considered a therapeutic dose, and how compliance is defined and measured. The overall goal of moist wound healing is to keep wounds *continuously* moist throughout the stages of re-epithelialization. In this trial, women would not have continuous moist wound healing. Furthermore, it would be unfeasible to expect under realistic conditions that women would be able to keep their nipples covered with lanolin 100% of the time. Clothing and movement results in lanolin wearing off over time, leading to periods where the nipple tissue would become dry. As such, in this trial the reasonable and expected use of lanolin did not have an effect on the severity of nipple pain when compared with usual care.

The secondary research question addressing the effect of lanolin on breastfeeding duration and exclusivity did not find any statistical differences between the groups. In one previous trial that evaluated the effect of an all-purpose nipple ointment vs. lanolin as a control group, lanolin had no effect on breastfeeding duration and/or exclusivity at 12 weeks postpartum (Dennis et al., 2012). In this trial, no differences were found among women using lanolin vs. an all-purpose nipple ointment, and similar breastfeeding duration and exclusivity rates were found at 12 weeks postpartum.

This is the first trial to examine the effect of lanolin for the treatment of nipple pain on breastfeeding self-efficacy. Mean BSES-SF scores between study groups at baseline and 4 days postrandomization were similar with no significant differences found. Baseline scores were also high, in contrast to scores reported in an exploratory study of breastfeeding self-efficacy (Kingston et al., 2007). This study found that mothers experiencing moderate to severe nipple pain during the first 48 h postpartum had significantly lower BSES-SF scores than those experiencing no nipple pain (Kingston et al., 2007). This is in contrast

to this trial, where BSES-SF scores were high despite all women experiencing some degree of nipple pain. It is plausible that the BSES-SF scores were high for this trial as a result of the recruitment site having Baby Friendly Hospital Initiative (BFHI) (World Health Organization, 2009) status. Hospitals with BFHI assess, monitor, and educate staff on how to foster the establishment and maintenance of breastfeeding among women. As such, women who deliver their infants at BFHI accredited hospitals are more likely to receive various efficacy-enhancing experiences from staff such as the provision of assistance and guidance with breastfeeding and encouragement and verbal persuasion.

Significantly more women who received lanolin were very satisfied with the treatment they received compared with those who received usual care to manage their nipple pain. It is plausible that participants using lanolin may have felt a greater sense of control over their nipple pain by doing "something" rather than "nothing," in turn leading to a greater sense of satisfaction. This increased satisfaction is similar to results found in a trial evaluating an all-purpose nipple ointment where participants in the lanolin group had significantly higher levels of satisfaction with breastfeeding vs. those in the all-purpose nipple ointment group ($p < .01$) (Dennis et al., 2012).

Although this trial has numerous methodological strengths including random generation of group assignment, strong participant adherence to trial protocols, and several mechanisms to prevent contamination and crossover, it is not without limitations. Potential limitations of this study may include the usage of a single recruitment site and that nipple infection was neither assessed nor treated. Another limitation may be the recruitment hospital's BFHI status. It is well established that hospitals accredited with BFHI have superior breastfeeding initiation, duration, and exclusivity rates vs. non-BFHI accredited hospitals (Kramer et al., 2001). Finally, although only 12% of the control group admitted to using lanolin, there is the potential of social desirability response bias. As such, the use of lanolin by the control group may have been higher than reported.

One of the most important findings in this trial was that almost all women independent of study group allocation experienced less nipple pain after approximately 7–10 days postpartum. Numerous studies support the role of anticipatory guidance as an effective intervention to help mothers cope during the postpartum period (Meleis, 1975; Meleis & Swendsen, 1978; Swendsen et al., 1978). Noting that nipple pain peaks at around 3 days postpartum and decreases thereafter, the provision of health teaching that pain will likely subside in about a week may help sustain breastfeeding during the most painful period and beyond.

Finally, because there are no known interventions to effectively treat nipple pain (Dennis et al., 2014), the importance of preventing nipple damage and pain in the early hours and days postpartum cannot be overlooked. Nipple damage often results from improper latch or positioning at the breast (Woolridge, 1986; Tait, 2000). To prevent nipple damage and pain it is imperative to provide newly breastfeeding women with education regarding proper positioning and latch, but to also frequently observe breastfeeding in the early postpartum period and to provide hands-on assistance if needed.

CONCLUSION

The application of lanolin to painful nipples in the immediate postpartum period did not significantly decrease nipple pain, nor did it improve breastfeeding duration and exclusivity; it also did not have an effect on breastfeeding self-efficacy, a known modifiable variable predictive of breastfeeding outcomes. As such, the provision of lanolin in-hospital and/or the recommendation of lanolin by health professionals to treat breastfeeding-related nipple pain is questionable and warrants further investigation to ensure the provision of evidence-based care.

REFERENCES

Abou-Dakn, M., Fluhr, J. W., Gensch, M., & Wockel, A. (2011). Positive effect of HPA lanolin versus expressed breast milk on painful and damaged nipples during lactation. *Skin Pharmacology and Physiology, 24,* 27–35.

Buck, M. L., Amir, L. H., Cullinane, M., & Donath, S. M. (2014). Nipple pain, damage, and vasospasm in the first 8 weeks postpartum. *Breastfeeding Medicine, 9,* 56–62.

Cable, B., Stewart, M., & Davis, J. (1997). Nipple wound care: a new approach to an old problem. *Journal of Human Lactation, 13,* 313–317.

Cadwell, K., Turner-Maffei, C., Blair, A., Brimdyr, K., & McInerney, Z. M. (2004). Pain reduction and treatment of sore nipples in nursing mothers. *The Journal of Perinatal Education, 13,* 29–35.

Chavez, M. E., Araujo, A. R., Santos, S. F., Pinotti, M., & Oliveira, L. S. (2012). LED phototherapy improves healing of nipple trauma: a pilot study. *Photomedicine and Laser Surgery, 30,* 172–178.

Clark, M. (1985). A study of four methods of nipple care offered to postpartum mothers. *The New Zealand Nursing Journal, 78,* 16–18.

Darmangeat, V. (2011). The frequency and resolution of nipple pain when latch is improved in private practice. *Clinical Lactation, 2–3,* 22–24.

Dennis, C. L. (2002). Breastfeeding initiation and duration: 1990–2000 literature review. *Journal of Obstetric, Gynecologic, and Neonatal Nursing, 31,* 12–32.

Dennis, C. L. (2003). The Breastfeeding Self-Efficacy Scale: psychometric assessment of the short form. *Journal of Obstetric, Gynecologic, and Neonatal Nursing, 32,* 734–744.

Dennis, C. L., Jackson, K., & Watson, J. (2014). Interventions for treating painful nipples among breastfeeding women. *Cochrane Database of Systematic Reviews, 12,* CD007366.

Dennis, C. L., Schottle, N., Hodnett, E., & McQueen, K. (2012). An all-purpose nipple ointment versus lanolin in treating painful damaged nipples in breastfeeding women: a randomized controlled trial. *Breastfeeding Medicine, 7,* 473–479.

Fetherston, C. (1995). Factors influencing breast feeding initiation and duration in a private Western Australian maternity hospital. *Breastfeeding Review Journal, 3,* 9–11.

Gosha, J. L., & Tichy, A. M. (1988). Effect of a breast shell on postpartum nipple pain: an exploratory study. *Journal of Nurse-Midwifery, 33,* 74–77.

Gregory, A., Penrose, K., Morrison, C., Dennis, C. L., & MacArthur, C. (2008). Psychometric assessment of the Breastfeeding Self-Efficacy Scale among British women. *Public Health Nursing, 25*, 278–284.

Heads, J., & Higgins, L. C. (1995). Perceptions and correlates of nipple pain. *Breastfeeding Review Journal, 3*, 59–64.

Hewat, R. J., & Ellis, D. J. (1987). A comparison of the effectiveness of two methods of nipple care. *Birth, 14*, 15–41.

Jensen, M. P., & Karoly, P. K. (2001). Self-report scales and procedures for assessing pain in adults. In D. C. Turk, & R. Melzack (Eds.): *Handbook of Pain Assessment* (2nd edn.). New York: The Guilford Press.

Kingston, D., Dennis, C. L., & Sword, W. (2007). Exploring breastfeeding self-efficacy. *Journal of Perinatal and Neonatal Nursing, 21*, 207–215.

Kramer, M. S., Chalmers, B., Hodnett, E. D., et al. (2001). Promotion of breastfeeding intervention trial (PROBIT): a randomized trial in the Republic of Belarus. *Journal of the American Medical Association, 285*, 120–413.

Kuscu, N. K., Koyuncu, F., & Lacin, S. (2001). Collegenase treatment of sore nipples. *International Journal of Gynecology & Obstetrics, 76*, 81–82.

Labbok, M., & Krasovec, K. (1990). Toward consistency in breastfeeding definitions. *Studies in Family Planning, 21*, 226–230.

Lavergne, N. A. (1997). Does application of tea bags to sore nipples while breastfeeding provide effective relief? *Journal of Obstetric, Gynecologic, and Neonatal Nursing, 26*, 53–58.

Livingstone, V., & Stringer, L. J. (1999). The treatment of Staphylococcus aureus infected sore nipples: a randomized comparative study. *Journal of Human Lactation, 15*, 241–246.

Mannel, R., Martens, P. J., & Walker, M. (2008). *Core Curriculum for Lactation Consultant Practice* (2nd edn.). Boston: Jones and Bartlett Publishers.

Martin, J. (2000). Nipple pain: causes, treatments and remedies. *Leaven, 36*, 10–11.

McCaffery, M., & Beebe, A. (1989). *Pain: Clinical Manual for Nursing Practice*. Mosby: St. Louis, MO.

McDowell, I. (2006). *Measuring Health: A Guide to Rating Scales and Questionnaires*. Oxford University Press: New York.

Meleis, A. I. (1975). Role/insufficiency and role supplementation: a conceptual framework. *Nursing Research, 24*, 264–271.

Meleis, A. I., & Swendsen, L. (1978). Role supplementation: an empirical test of a nursing intervention. *Nursing Research, 27*, 11–18.

Melzack, R. (1987). The short-form McGill Pain Questionnaire. *Pain. 30*(2), 191–197.

Pugh, L. D., Buchko, B. L., Bishop, G. A., Cochran, J. F., Smith, L. R., & Lerew, D. J. (1996). A comparison of topical agents to relieve nipple pain and enhance breastfeeding. *Birth, 23*, 88–93.

Riordan, J. (1985). The effectiveness of topical agents in reducing nipple soreness of breastfeeding mothers. *Journal of Human Lactation, 1*, 36–41.

Serlin, R. C., Mendoza, T. R., Nakamura, Y., Edwards, K. R., & Cleeland, C. S. (1995). When is cancer pain mild, moderate or severe? Grading pain severity by its interference with function. *Pain. 61*, 277–284.

Swendsen, L. A., Meleis, A. I., & Jones, D. (1978). Role supplementation for new parents: a role mastery plan. *American Journal of Maternal/Child Nursing, 3*, 84–91.

Tait, P. (2000). Nipple pain in breastfeeding women: causes, treatment and prevention strategies. *Journal of Midwifery and Women's Health, 45*, 197–201.

Wilkie, D. J., Savedra, M. C., Holzemer, W. L., Tesler, M. D., & Paul, S. M. (1990). Use of the McGill Pain Questionnaire to measure pain: a metaanalysis. *Nursing Research, 39*, 36–41.

Woolridge, M. (1986). Aetiology of sore nipples. *Midwifery, 2*, 172–176.

World Health Organization. (2009). Baby-friendly hospital initiative. Revised, Updated and Expanded for Integrated Care. Available at: http://www.who.int/nutrition/publications/infantfeeding/bfhi_trainingcourse/en/. (Accessed 10 March 2016).

Wright, K. D., Asmundson, G. J., & McCreary, D. R. (2001). Factorial validity of the Short-Form McGill Pain Questionnaire (SF-MPQ). *European Journal of Pain, 5*, 279–284.

Yeoung, D., Pennell, M., Leung, M., & Hall, J. (1986). Breastfeeding prevalence and influencing factors. *Canadian Journal of Public Health, 72*, 323–330.

Ziemer, M. M., Paone, J. P., Schupay, J., & Cole, E. (1990). Methods to prevent and manage nipple pain in breastfeeding women. *Western Journal of Nursing Research, 12*, 732–744.

Mâmawoh Kamâtowin, "Coming together to help each other in wellness": Honouring Indigenous Nursing Knowledge

R. Lisa Bourque Bearskin | Brenda L. Cameron | Malcolm King |
Cora Weber-Pillwax | Madeleine Dion Stout | Evelyn Voyageur | Alice Reid |
Lea Bill | Rose Martial[a]

ABSTRACT

This paper is the result of coming to know and better understand Indigenous nursing experience in First Nations, Inuit, and Métis communities. Using an Indigenous research approach, I (first author) drew from the collective experience of four Indigenous nurse scholars and attended to the question of how Indigenous knowledge manifests itself in the practices of Indigenous nurses and how it can better serve individuals, families, and communities. This research framework centered on Indigenous principles, processes, and practical values as expressed in Indigenous nursing practice. The results were woven from key understandings and meanings of Indigeneity as a way of being. Central to this study was that Indigenous knowledge has always been fundamental to the ways that these Indigenous nurses have undertaken nursing practice, regardless of the systemic and historical barriers they faced in providing healthcare for Indigenous people. The results of this research demonstrated how Indigenous nurses consistently drew on their inherited Indigenous knowledge to deliver nursing care to Indigenous people. Their identity as Indigenous persons was integral to their identities as Indigenous nurses. Of significance is the personal and particular description of how these Indigenous nurse scholars developed their nursing approaches in relevance to how health and healthcare delivery must be integrated into healthcare systems as a pathway to reducing health disparities.

KEY WORDS: Indigenous nurses, Indigenous nursing knowledge, Indigenous research methodologies, Indigenous wellness, nursing practice

GLOSSARY

Indigenous Peoples: used in this article to mean First Nations, Inuit, and Métis peoples in Canada and used synonymously with the term Aboriginal Peoples enshrined in Section 35A in the Constitution Act of 1982. The Royal Commission on Aboriginal Peoples (1996) states that in over 605 different First Nations communities, some people prefer to identify themselves as part of their linguistic group, such as Cree, and/or Métis, or both.

mâmawoh kamâtowin: Cree term used to describe the meaning of Indigenous community development.

[a]Mâmawoh Kamâtowin, "Coming together to help each other in wellness": Honouring Indigenous Nursing Knowledge

***nohkum*:**   Cree for "my grandmother."
***nikawy*:**   Cree for "my mother."

AUTHORS

R. Lisa Bourque Bearskin, RN, PhD, associate professor, Thompson Rivers University. Dr. Bourque Bearskin is Cree/Métis from Beaver Lake Cree Nation, AB, specializing in Indigenous nursing knowledge research. Primary author of paper and corresponding author: 900 McGill Rd, Kamloops, BC V2C 0C8; lbourquebearskin@tru.ca, (250) 828-5056.

Brenda L. Cameron, RN, PhD, professor emerita, Faculty of Nursing, University of Alberta, Edmonton, AB. Primary PhD supervisor and expert nursing content advisor and editor.

Malcolm King, PhD, professor, Faculty of Health Sciences, Simon Fraser University, Burnaby, BC, and scientific director, CIHR Institute for Aboriginal Peoples' Health. Co-supervisor and expert researcher who guided the development of the study.

Cora Weber-Pillwax, PhD, associate professor, Education Policy Studies, Faculty of Education, University of Alberta, Edmonton, AB. She is Métis from Calling Lake, AB. Co-supervisor and expert knowledge holder of Indigenous research methodologies and community-based research; contributed to all levels of writing and editing.

Madeleine Kētēskwew Dion Stout, PhD, Kehewin First Nation, retired nurse, co-searcher, active educator, researcher, and author. Helped shape the study through her insights on Indigenous health and wellness; insistence on home-grown and complementary interventions and services; and insertion of Cree concepts to change the way this research project offers content.

Evelyn Voyageur, PhD, from the Dzawada'enuxw First Nation, is a retired RN and an Elder-in-residence at North Island College in Comox Valley, BC. Shared expert Indigenous nursing knowledge as a co-searcher, supported data analysis, and provided expert insight throughout the research process.

Alice Reid, retired RN, NP, worked extensively in northern Alberta. She is Métis from Sandy Lake, AB. Played a key role as a co-searcher, supported data analysis, and provided guidance throughout the research process.

Lea Bill, RN, BScN, from Pelican First Nation in Saskatchewan, is a project manager for Alberta First Nations Cancer Pathways project, president of Spirit Feather Consulting, and a traditional practitioner. Provided spiritual guidance in addition to her role as a co-researcher, supported data analysis, and acted as language interpreter throughout the research process.

Elder Rose Martial, Denesuline from Cold Lake First Nations, AB, is a retired community health representative who guided this work from its inception. She continues to work as a community researcher and as an Elder advisor to the Access Research Project at the University of Alberta with Dr. B. Cameron.

INTRODUCTION

The aim of this research was to draw on Cree/Métis understanding through Indigenous research methodologies (IRM), in order to explore how Indigenous knowledge systems and identity are embedded in the nursing practices of four Indigenous nurse scholars. Attention is given to Cree ways of being, knowing, and acting when situated at the intersection of nursing and the hierarchy of Western nursing knowledge. As Weber-Pillwax (1999) explained, the central tenet of IRM is that the one who searches becomes the "active center" to also reveal and present his or her own story along with the emerging stories of those who are researching from within their own worldviews. Therefore, my[1] own life experience as an Indigenous nurse was as central to the study as were the life experiences of the other four Indigenous

---

[1]This paper is written from the first-person perspective of the first author.

nurses, and all experiences were interwoven into one collective story of being Indigenous nurses in Canada. The substance of this study was grounded in the primary concern of nursing, that is the health of people, but specifically, it examined the context of delivering culturally appropriate and safe care.

Relationality

To strengthen my research approach, I drew on courses grounded in traditions of Aboriginal or Cree/Métis Peoples, offered by the University of Alberta through the Indigenous Peoples Education graduate program. For example, the Cree language graduate course[2] that I took with Elder John Crier and Cora Weber-Pillwax supported my own Indigenous knowledge system. In this relationship I was able to draw on traditional knowledge embedded within key words, and I began to accurately and critically examine the significance of Cree/Métis teachings in my inquiry on Indigenous nursing practice. Being attentive to the variances in meaning between languages was important, as not all of the four Indigenous nurses were Cree/Métis; one of the nurses was from the Dzawada' enuxw First Nation on the West Coast.

An important feature of this work is captured from a Northern Plains Cree/Métis perspective. *Mâmawoh kamâtowin* is a Cree term that I understand to mean "to help each other in a collective sense." The goal of this original research was not to separate my life from my work, but rather to support and enable me to situate myself within the work as a specific and whole

context where, as described by IRM, the "self" is a central aspect of the study and its incumbent relationships.

Locating Myself in the Context of the Research Inquiry

As a Cree/Métis woman who has survived life experiences rooted in violence, residential school, and the child welfare system, and who lives with the effects of intergenerational trauma,[3] I continue to witness many forms of violence that First Nations, Inuit, and Métis Peoples experience. As a nurse, I have come face to face with this in my everyday life. Some of those moments are imprinted in my memory forever and have shaped my thinking on many levels. What I have come to know intimately is that nurses struggle with their personal moral convictions when they are confronted with Indigenous clients. Nurses in these situations are faced with what Cameron (2006) has referred to as the *unpresentable*: cases such as the murdered and missing Aboriginal women in Canada, and the cultural genocide that stems from effects of residential schools (Truth and Reconciliation Commission of Canada, 2015). Yet, even though this history of trauma is recognized as factual and historical in Canada, Allan and Smylie (2015) found that healthcare professionals respond to Aboriginal people by offering racialized care that renders us uncivilized, without human dignity and human rights. In some cases, even human touch is denied, as was seen in the case of Brian Sinclair, an Indigenous man who waited over 34 hours in a hospital emergency department to be assessed for a simple blocked catheter and died unattended while waiting for care (as detailed in the inquest report; Preston,

---

[2]University of Alberta course EDPS 501: Meaning and Structure of Cree Language. Objective: With course instructor, a Cree language and traditional knowledge teacher and the students will examine the roots and structures of Cree words that carry significant and ancient values and root meanings related to Cree knowledge systems and ways of being.

---

[3]According to Bombay, Matheson, and Anisman (2009), *intergenerational trauma* is a term used to describe years of trauma (personal/collective) that is transmitted across generations.

2014). Dion Stout (2012) reported that nurses are not well informed about Indigenous people's histories, or their suffering as individuals, families, and communities living under poverties and policies that render them invisible and unpresentable.

Research Framework

As described by Ermine (1995, 2007), Kirkness (2013), Kovach (2009, 2013), Weber-Pillwax (1999, 2001, 2003, 2004, 2008), and Wilson (2008), the IRM framework draws on critical, self-reflexive, hermeneutic analysis, a process that helped me engage in a deeper self-understanding and unearthing of experiences used in the context of this study. Meyer (2008) and Ranco (2006) describe hermeneutic analysis as a way to understand the "other" and use it to enhance our own Indigenous ways of knowing. IRM is an approach that centers Indigenous identity (Weber Pillwax, 1999) and provides a research process (Kovach, 2009) and practical values (respect, responsibility, reciprocity, and relevance; Kirkness & Barnhardt, 2001). From these theoretical underpinnings, the research design captures four key components of the research process based on Cree understanding: creating respectful research activities; enacting ethical relationships; being responsible for the gathering, documenting, and analysis of data; and ensuring that mutual reciprocity is honored for the purposes of understanding the spectrum of Indigenous nursing knowledge as informed by the four Indigenous nurses, and more powerfully, by *nohkum, nikawy*, and myself. One of the objectives of this study was to learn and to understand what Indigenous nursing knowledge consists of and how this knowledge is infused into the practices of nursing as a means to facilitate and create healing and wellness. This objective aligns with the original research question addressing lived experiences of Indigenous nurses as practitioners and scholars.

Data Gathering

In maintaining respectful, relational, responsible, and reciprocal features of this study, the four Indigenous nurse scholars became co-researchers in the process of seeking a collective understanding of Indigenous ways of knowing and being (Meyer, 2003, 2008; Ranco, 2006; Struthers, 2001, 2003). A combination of protocols, data collection methods, and analysis techniques were used, including participant observation, self-reflexive writing, one-on-one conversations, and research circles of understanding. These activities facilitated sharing of our experiences and deepened the critical and analytical nature of our discussions, which facilitated a deepened integration of methodological features of the research phases. The Indigenous nurses became actively involved through various circles of conversation in generating, positing, sorting, questioning, understanding, and recontextualizing the data in ways that supported my constant assessment of the relationship and connections between emerging knowledge. I received their feedback and used it to extend and foster our own understanding as an effective means to "address social issues in the wider framework of self-determination, decolonization, and social justice" (Smith, 2012, p. 4).

Data Analysis

This reiterative inductive process of analysis involved a constant movement back and forth from the written text to the shared thoughts and words of the Indigenous nurse scholars. The goal of the data analysis process was to obtain a rich description that accurately depicted the statements, thoughts, and experiences of the Indigenous nurse scholars, and that was aligned with the relational commitments of our nursing work. The first analysis phase involved a line-by-line review of transcribed textual data by the researcher; the review was then mapped out and returned to the Indigenous nurse scholars. This second analysis phase involved a deep layer of thinking in which the nature of the text, both spoken and written, guided the analysis as various and distinct aspects of Cree ways of knowing and being revealed themselves to the Indigenous nurses. This allowed for the development of a collective analysis where main ideas of content themes were generated from the renewed and/or deeper collective meaning and where the collective nature of both process and outcome simultaneously enhanced reliability and rigor of the research process. Member checking and peer debriefing were embedded naturally into the IRM processes and also provided validation of our collective interpretations and ascribed meanings to the data. Research ethics were based on IRM principles, thus going beyond the minimum standards outlined by OCAP[4] and the Tri-Council (CIHR, NSERC, and SSHRC, 2014) for working "with, for, and by" Indigenous Peoples.

RESULTS

The results of this original research study were interpreted and reported as deriving from two sources of knowledge: ontological beginnings and epistemological openings. Specific to each section were particular threads of understanding that resonated across the women's lives. These threads, woven from the narratives of Indigenous nurse scholars, showed the meanings and implications of Indigenous nursing with families, communities, and Nations. Including threads of my own narrative in the results was vital to maintaining the holistic nature of this discussion of Indigenous nurses' knowledge. There were many significant results in the original study, but for the purposes of this manuscript, I drew on a few of those threads that referred to ontological beginnings and epistemological openings as the roots of the nurses' wellness statements.

---

[4]OCAP®: Ownership, Control, Access, and Possession is a registered trademark of the First Nations Information Governance Centre (FNIGC; www.fnigc.ca).

Ontological Beginnings and Epistemological Openings

The contributions of the Indigenous nurse scholars showed that they lived according to the roots of their being and that these roots were central to their identity. They constantly reminded me that "knowing who you are and where you come from" is foundational to our existence. Alice Reid affirmed the notion of identity in all of her discussions: "We are all creatures of creation, and from that sense we are all one with unique experiences." She spoke to these early roots of the nature of being, knowing, and doing; in other words, of the ontological and epistemological markers of her Cree/Métis worldview:

> It is always with us. It is a given, and it is up to us to accept it or not. It is not something we claim; it is just being who we are and what we believe and how we behave.

This state of being is the personal agency within every individual. It is always in relation to our families, deeply rooted in the underground of our history and the land of our origin.

Likewise, Evelyn Voyageur spoke about her early roots of existence and the importance of her Elders' teachings. She also talked extensively about how the notion of self is rooted in community. Evelyn shared a story that captures the philosophy of community wellness as a ceremony:

> The Spirit dance is bound in the teaching of protection, and it used to be done in the early morning. And it only belongs to the Willie family, my dad's side, and my great niece holds the dance. It happens at four o'clock in the morning, and we would go to the big house. She carries a big basket to collect all the bad energy, and then she throws it in the fire. And that was how our day often began. She was also known as a healer.

This story shows the spirit of her people, their relationship to knowledge, and their understanding of how to act in accordance with traditions in the collective to preserve health and wellness. Lea Bill also described her roots as deeply embedded in her ancestors' identity and language:

> It has always been there because right from the time I was very young my grandmother taught me. She was

a midwife and a medicine woman, if you might call her that; she was *onanatawihowew*, which translates to 'the one who helps with healing.' It has to do with *nantawih*, meaning 'to support,' or 'to bring up the body,' *natawihiehiwewin*. Or 'building up the body', *wiyaw*. So it has to do with supporting the body. So right from the time I was young, I was witness to and participated in our traditional ceremonies, and I became a helper early in my life.

When she was a young girl, Lea's connection to her grandmother set a path that she would follow for the duration of her life. Her grandmother was a midwife and traditional healer who heavily influenced Lea's commitment to healing and encouraged her to pursue nursing in the "Western way." Lea grew up immersed in the helping relationship through which she learned the principles of natural law.[5] Over the years she became skilled in ways to ground her nursing care in her own traditional healing knowledge systems.

Early roots of Indigenous knowledge. From an Indigenous perspective, our traditional Cree names represent a kindred spirit and a deeper meaning. As Madeleine Dion Stout noted, our coming to know is often grounded in the names we hold that are interconnected, interdependent on nature and natural law. Having this understanding brings us closer to our own knowing and being:

> I was always called kētēskwew at home. It was not just a ceremonial name. It is life lived as ceremony. And when you are given that kind of name, you always remember that you are, as in my case, an ancient woman or child with an ancient spirit.

It is clear from the Indigenous nursing scholars that the roots of our upbringing (being and knowing) run deeply into the familial landscape, and thus deeply into the creation of our world. Our inherited traditional knowledge comes from the roots of our ancestries (McCallum, 2014).

---

[5]Natural law is a philosophy of life that underpins Indigenous understanding of being human; it states that everything is connected and related, from the smallest particle in the cosmos to all living and non-living forms.

Their families nurtured their spirits so that their backbones became strong. They learned to share their gifts so that the far-reaching branches of knowledge could take root in the minds and hearts of others. From the blood in their veins to the inscriptions on their minds, their spiritual and traditional experiences became embedded in their being. As Couture (1991) explains, primal experience of being is the "accumulation of knowledge rooted in experience that is carried forward by oral traditions" (p. 59). He discussed this as a foundation of Indigenous existence where the inner and outer worlds meet and spiritual and physical worlds are equally real and functional. Yet it is this knowledge, that the deeper layer of consciousness is integral to wellness, that non-Indigenous people often find difficult to comprehend. Further to this, Battiste (2013) suggests that non-Indigenous people attribute this spiritual understanding to the lack of civilization amongst Indigenous Peoples. As I interpreted what the Indigenous nurse scholars said, I thought about the pedagogy of spiritual knowledge in relation to epistemological openings. *Openings* meaning those opportunities where Indigenous nurses can walk in their own way of knowing. In her research with Cree and Ojibwa healers, Struthers (2001 & 2003) recognizes that Indigenous people do not learn Indigenous knowledge from books, but from other people, and through dreams, visions, and genetic memory. The memory of the ancestors is in our blood, within our genetic makeup. This visceral level of knowledge expressed in blood memory plays a significant role in cellular development, and that cellular memory can change one's emotional state (Pert, 1997). According to Elder Lionel Kinunwa (as cited in Steinhauer, 2002):

> We have ancestral memories in our blood; they are in our muscles, they are in our bones, they are in our hair. ... These memories come out of the molecular structure of our being. ... When you hear someone speaking your language, your molecular structure picks up those vibrations, because each language has its own peculiar patterns. (p. 76)

Hampton (1995) also talked about the significance of memory coming before knowledge; it is here that I see the implications of memory and knowledge of our routes and roots in life. As Battiste (2013) suggests, "Maybe this wisdom is taking its rightful place" (p. 17). When I think about memory, I think about the circularity of knowledge because if knowledge comes from the wisdom and experiences of the people, then memory takes us back to the beginning of knowledge development. Memory is central to who we are and to our outwardly lived practices; Indigenous nurse scholars pull their ancestral knowledge into their everyday lives. Their truths, origins, and memories are central to what they share and receive. The nurse scholars told me that we have no choice in the memories that we are given, but we do have a choice in the memories we accept because they deeply shape who we are today and who we are becoming.

Integrating roots of knowledge into nursing practices. What follows is a very brief but personal and particular description of how these Indigenous nurse scholars developed some of their nursing approaches based on Indigenous teachings with which they had grown up. These Indigenous nursing scholars made visible to me the roots of their individual identities, and I saw how the nurses each manifested themselves in their own distinct approaches to holistic nursing practices. Each demonstrated their personal, intellectual, spirited, and heartfelt perspectives on their own historical relationships as Indigenous people. Each created a unique learning experience in the context of this study and I came to realize that each played a significant role in translation of Indigenous knowledge.

My experiences with Alice Reid focused on the family unit with a specific emphasis on Indigenous women and girls. Evelyn Voyageur's invitation to the village helped me to center my thinking on nursing education and the role of the community in education. The time that I spent with Madeleine Dion Stout helped me to intellectualize and concentrate on the philosophical and political aspects of Indigenous knowledge systems and maternal childcare. My final experience, with Lea Bill, led to a deeper personal understanding of Indigenous healing and self-care and its effectiveness in addressing historical trauma. Each of the Indigenous nurse scholars integrates their own knowing into nursing by relying on her understanding of Cree knowledge systems.

Alice's life and beginnings were grounded in northern Alberta. As a nurse practitioner licensed in the United States, and as licensure was not fully recognized in Canada, she worked as a registered nurse with an expanded scope of practice. She often worked in isolation in rural and remote communities. Her responsibilities included everything from nursing administration to medical treatment, to assisting in births, wakes, and environmental emergency response situations. With very few resources, limited equipment, and reduced access to clean running water or heated buildings, she pragmatically solved issues and worked with what she had.

Witnessing the impact of Christianization and colonization on families was significant to her practice. She asserts that it is as real today as it was yesterday: "We have become unknown citizens in our own lands, and we have to just keep walking." Alice's statement captures the issue of ongoing colonial experience that continues to impact individual wellness and nursing practice. Alice's Indigenous knowledge as well as her advanced nursing knowledge helped her to survive the harsh northern situation of remoteness and limited access to healthcare services. She is clear that she needed both of these knowledge bases to counteract the terror of lived residential school experience that affected the people she nursed. When she spoke about the meaning of family as if we "are one," all related by one bond, one tribe, one Nation, one Mother Earth, this notion of oneness helped me situate the importance of human-centered practice. As Alice noted, First Nations, Inuit, and Métis women are "the invisible sinews" that bind the spirit of northern Indigenous women together as a way to strengthen community healing.

For Evelyn Voyageur the heart of community was always central to her worldview. I watched her deliver a unique educational experience to nursing and allied students where the community was the teacher. It was a profound and clear example of how a community-based Indigenous knowledge teaching and learning approach had mutual benefits to cultural continuity and community development in nursing education. Discourses in cultural continuity and community development often focus on an analysis of deficit, which inadvertently perpetuates social disparities, stigmas, and mythical dogma of Indigenous people's life histories and biographical accounts in Canadian literature (Valaskakis, Dion Stout, & Guimond, 2009). What Evelyn showed me was how nursing's traditional teaching and learning approaches harmed some Indigenous nurse trainees, because traditional nursing education has not been grounded in the historical context in which Indigenous people live. In Evelyn's work the entire community educates nurses, so education comes from a lived experience perspective. This provides a more realistic picture for nurses and student nurses about resiliency and strength among community members, often providing many examples of how power dynamics in relational nursing practice can be neutralized so that clients are driving their own healing and healthcare services delivery.

During the time I spent with Madeleine Dion Stout, it was evident that her contribution to nursing was well situated at the political level. Her knowledge extended beyond the realm of practice, drawing attention to the interlocking policies of practice and revealing how detrimental Western ways of knowing and being had been inscribed into the flesh of people she worked with. Against this political backdrop Madeleine worked tirelessly to challenge the oppression and ideological constructs that she had long ago learned to survive.

Through her Cree theoretical lens, Madeleine addressed the sociocultural, historical, and contextual determinants of health. For example, in her keynote presentation *Original Instructions and the Politics of the Powerless: Nursing in First Nations* at the Philosophy in the Nurses' World: Politics of Nursing Practice conference, sponsored by University of Alberta, she explained:

> Nurses need to meet First Nations at their point of resistance and respect the fact that knowledge sharing is less a matter of seizing knowledge and cataloguing it and more about paying respect to the known, learning from the knowers, and fully participating in the knowing. The knowing of the prevailing context and conditions that shape the culture and structures we nurse in is a must.

At this point of resistance, Madeleine suggested that Indigenous nurse scholars hold their ground against these continuing forces as a way to create and preserve wellness. "We were never conquered peoples. We never gave up our identities or responsibilities to the government." In this light, her reinforcement about understanding ethics and Indigenous human rights advanced my thinking from concealment of Indigenous nursing knowledge to resurfacing it, so that our focus remains on the social constructs and cultural structures in Indigenous nursing knowledge and practice. In this context, social constructs such as race, gender, and religion have been used to advance various forms of knowledge, which undermines cultural structures such as protocols and processes for learning traditional knowledge.

The unique experience of working with Lea Bill took me to the most private and sacred parts of the mountains in the Kananaskis country of Alberta. There we spent time translating the wisdom we hold, which tells us that there is a greater life force that draws us to another's experiences. It was about a nurse's healing journey—being able to let go of pain and hardship, recognize one's own personal power, and incorporate spiritual energy into our nursing being. The acts of self-healing are often taken for granted in our nursing profession. Understanding natural law and relational nursing practice requires attributes that stem from resiliency and strength. It is our duty as Indigenous nurses to be of service and to be responsive to the suffering. Lea stated that we cannot forget those who come behind us:

> So many of our people have bought into the idea of the script that we are incapable, and we see the evidence of this when we look at the statistics of health. But this is a multigenerational message that has been imprinted in the people, and it's not just our people; it is continuing worldwide.

Madeleine further explains, "We've tried so hard to spray our Indianness away just to get by and fit in." The idea of trying to fit and be respected as human beings during a time when families were significantly marginalized was problematic.

From my nursing education, I learned to think from binary positions—Western and Indigenous, objective and subjective, mind versus spirit, and individual over community. What I wish I had learned was to value the knowledge found in the faces, spaces, and places of Indigeneity. One knowledge system must not be valued over another. We are all part of the human race, and each of us has a unique perspective and context in which we can flourish and contribute to world health. It is this Indigenous mindfulness that brings me closer to home—to my own Cree/Métis way of learning, seeing, and knowing. Eminent scholars and traditional knowledge holders have reminded me that the ways of knowing unfolding before us are considered science (Little Bear, 2000, 2009). The traditional knowledge from these teachings is a good example of this. These teachings are sacred ways of knowing and can take a lifetime to learn. In contrast, in nursing, I was trained to think from one worldview, which left my Indigeneity in nursing unexplored and yet to be unmasked.

DISCUSSION

A major aim of this original work has been to articulate a better understanding of how Indigenous knowledge is taken up in nursing. There are many questions left to answer, but for the purpose of this article the aim was to describe how Indigenous nursing knowledge could be of benefit and value to the discipline of nursing. The theme of wellness was central throughout the study and showed that Indigenous knowledge is inherent in Indigenous ways of being, knowing, and doing; that it can be understood as the anchor that supports the capacity of First Nations, Inuit, and Métis Peoples to lift up the work of our Indigenous nursing leaders and sustain health and wellness of Indigenous communities. In essence this inquiry is similar to the work of Gehl (2012), who wrote about the Anishinaabe concept "Debwewin Journey"—a model of knowing that links Western ideologies of knowing from the head to learning from the heart, the holistic nature of nursing.

This study revealed many complex issues and concepts associated with Indigenous wellness in relation to the nursing profession. This area of inquiry is extremely challenging and requires meaningful and consistent engagement, participation, and leadership of Indigenous people. Indigenous people hold the experiential understandings of their knowledge systems and their ontological and epistemological roots, which guide how they interact with and within the world. Just as important, I have come to the understanding that, regardless of our individual experiences, we as Indigenous nurses inherently bring our knowledge as Indigenous persons to our nursing practice; we know that knowledge originates within our families, communities, ancestors, and the Creator—a system that has endured for thousands of years.

The Indigenous nurse scholars talked about nursing as a "pedagogy of service" in which practice is not grounded in engagement with the other. They spoke about the need to "shift the soil" and "re-turn" to the roots of nursing, which are found within the contexts of their own Indigenous community. In recognizing the attributes and efficiency of "old" knowledge, the Indigenous nurse scholars support the creation of "new" knowledge as a means of improving the understanding of nursing services in Indigenous communities in the face of ever-growing health disparities (Fridkin, 2012). The concept of Indigenous wellness is integral to the delivery of health services, as it can offer concrete approaches and benefits that far outweigh the lack of culturally responsive nursing practice that underscores racism in nursing (McGibbon & Etowa, 2009; Vukic, Jesty, Mathews, & Etowa, 2012). The Indigenous nurse scholars support the idea of "working together" in ways that address the Truth and Reconciliation Commission of Canada's (2015) 94 Calls to Action. In accommodating this vision as a moral imperative, we need to make space for the unique contributions of Indigenous knowledge. We must recognize that "poverty of all kinds have stolen productive capacity and independence from many Indigenous people, leaving them confused, traumatized and in poor health" (Dion Stout, 2012, p. 12). We cannot sacrifice the old for the new or the new for the old; we have to bring them into balance in the center of the collective whole, for Indigenous wellness to flourish.

Limitations

The main limitation of this study is that we cannot ever fully understand or replicate someone else's story because the context is almost impossible to duplicate. Yet Archibald (2008), King (2003), and McLeod (2007) explain that while stories are not complete, and are limited in presenting a full understanding, they show us a path from which we can all learn. Although it is not necessarily a limitation of Indigenous research, the Indigenous nurse scholars were not all of Cree/Métis background. This is an extremely important consideration with IRM as it is important always to remember that Indigenous knowledge from one group cannot be generalized to that of all Aboriginal Peoples.

CONCLUSION

In conclusion, the question remains: How do we bring Indigenous knowledge into our nursing environments? This early work provides a glimpse into how these Indigenous nursing scholars integrated the roots of their being into their nursing practices to achieve wellness through their respect for, as well as engagement and relationships with the people. Here, at the intersection of ontology and epistemology, they established a foundation upon which to foster individual, family, and community wellness. A common thread in our reflexive discussions was the belief that we do not need to give up who we are in order to be able to carry out successful nursing practices and meaningful research with our communities. Rather, we must travel to the inner spaces of our deepest thoughts to engage with ancient knowledge as a way of knowing, where we can begin a new chapter, a way of being where Indigenous nurses can flourish in Indigenous nursing practice. While the research showed many features important to the delivery of nursing services to Indigenous communities, most significant was the assertion that local Indigenous people and their community knowledge systems are needed at the core of nursing. From this work our nursing team will continue to develop further research exploring Indigenous-nurse-led practice.

REFERENCES

Allan, B., & Smylie, J. (2015). *First Peoples, second class treatment: The role of racism in the health and well-being of Indigenous Peoples in Canada*. Toronto, ON: Wellesley Institute.

Archibald, J. (2008). *Indigenous storywork: Educating the heart, mind, body and spirit*. Vancouver, BC: University of British Columbia Press.

Battiste, M. (2013). *Decolonizing education: Nourishing the learning spirit*. Saskatoon, SK: Purich.

Bombay, A., Matheson, K., & Anisman, H. (2009). Intergenerational trauma: Convergence of multiple processes among First Nations people in Canada. *Journal of Aboriginal Health, 5*(3), 6–47.

Cameron, B. L. (2006). Towards understanding the unpresentable in nursing: Some nursing philosophical considerations. *Nursing Philosophy, 7*(1), 23–35. https://doi.org/10.1111/j.1466-769X.2006.00246.x.

CIHR, NSERC, & SSHRC. (2014). *Tri-council policy statement (TCPS2): Ethical conduct for research involving humans.* Canadian Institutes of Health Research, Natural Sciences and Engineering Research Council of Canada, and Social Sciences and Humanities Research Council of Canada. Retrieved from Panel on Research Ethics website: Government of Canada. http://www.pre.ethics.gc.ca/pdf/eng/tcps2 -2014/TCPS_2_FINAL_Web.pdf.

Couture, J. E. (1991). Explorations in native knowing. In W. J. Friesen (Ed.), *The cultural maze: Complex questions on Native destiny in western Canada* (pp. 53–73). Calgary, AB: Detselig Enterprises.

Dion Stout, M (2012). Ascribed health and wellness, "Atikowisi miýwâyâwin," to achieved health and wellness, "Kaskitamasowin miýw-âyâwin": Shifting the paradigm. *Canadian Journal of Nursing Research, 44*(2), 11–14.

Ermine, W. (1995). Aboriginal epistemology. In M. Battiste, & J. Barman (Eds.), *First Nations education in Canada: The circle unfolds* (pp. 101–112). Vancouver, BC: University of British Columbia Press.

Ermine, W. (2007). Ethical space of engagement. *Indigenous Law Journal, 6*(1), 193–203.

Fridkin, A. (2012). Addressing health inequities through Indigenous involvement in health policy discourses. *Canadian Journal of Nursing Research, 44*(2), 108–122.

Gehl, L. (2012). Debwewin journey: A methodology and model of knowing. *AlterNative: An International Journal of Indigenous Peoples, 8*(1), 53–65.

Hampton, E. (1995). Memory comes before knowledge: Research may improve if researchers remember their motives. *Canadian Journal of Native Education, 21*(Suppl), 46–54.

King, T. (2003). *The truth about stories.* Minneapolis, MN: University of Minnesota Press.

Kirkness, V. J. (2013). *Creating space: My life and work in Indigenous education.* Winnipeg, MB: University of Manitoba Press.

Kirkness, V. J., & Barnhardt, R. (2001). First Nations and higher education: The four R's—Respect, relevance, reciprocity, responsibility. In R. Hayoe & J. Pan (Eds.), *Knowledge across cultures: A contribution to dialogue among civilizations* (pp. 1–18). Retrieved from Assembly of First Nations website: http://www .afn.ca/uploads/files/education2/the4rs.pdf.

Kovach, M. (2009). *Indigenous methodologies: Characteristics, conversations, and context.* Toronto, ON: University of Toronto Press.

Kovach, M. (2013). Treaties, truths, and transgressive pedagogies: Re-imagining indigenous presence in the classroom. *Socialist Studies, 9*(1), 109–126.

Little Bear, L (2000). Foreword. In G. Cajete (Ed.), *Native science: Natural laws of interdependence* (pp. x–xiii). Santa Fe, NM: Clear Light.

Little Bear, L (2009). Jagged worldviews colliding. In M. Battiste (Ed.), *Reclaiming Indigenous voice and vision* (pp. 7–85). Vancouver, BC: University of British Columbia Press.

McCallum, L. M. (2014). *Indigenous women, work, and history.* Winnipeg, MB: University of Manitoba Press.

McGibbon, E. A., & Etowa, J. B. (2009). *Anti-racist health care practice.* Toronto, ON: Canadian Scholars' Press.

McLeod, N. (2007). *Cree narrative memory: From treaties to contemporary times.* Saskatoon, SK: Purich.

Meyer, M. (2003). Hawaiian hermeneutics and the triangulation of meaning: Gross, subtle, causal. *Canadian Journal of Native Education, 27*(2), 249–255.

Meyer, M. A. (2008). Indigenous and authentic: Native Hawaiian epistemology and the triangulation of meaning. In N. K Denzin, Y. S Lincoln, & L. T Smith (Eds.), *Handbook of critical and Indigenous methodologies*, 217–232. https://doi .org/10.4135/9781483385686.n11.

Pert, C. B. (1997). *Molecules of emotion: Why you feel the way you feel.* New York, NY: Scribner.

Preston, T. J. (2014). *In the Provincial Court of Manitoba: In the matter of the Fatality Inquiries Act and in the matter of Brian Lloyd Sinclair, deceased.* Winnipeg, MB: Provincial Court of Manitoba. Retrieved from http://www.manitobacourts.mb.ca /site/assets/files/1051/brian_sinclair_inquest _-_dec_14.pdf.

Ranco, D. J. (2006). Toward a Native anthropology: Hermeneutics, hunting stories, and theorizing from within. *Wicazo Sa Review, 21*(2), 61–78. https://doi .org/10.1353/wic.2006.0022.

Royal Commission on Aboriginal Peoples. (1996). *Report of the Royal Commission on Aboriginal Peoples.* Retrieved from Indigenous and Northern Affairs Canada website: http://www.aadnc-aandc. gc.ca/eng/1307458586498/1307458751962.

Smith, L. T. (2012). *Decolonizing methodologies: Research and Indigenous Peoples* (2nd ed.). London, UK: University of Otago Press.

Steinhauer, E. (2002). Thoughts on an Indigenous research methodology. *Canadian Journal of Native Education, 26*(2), 69–81.

Struthers, R. (2001). Conducting sacred research: An Indigenous experience. *Wicazo Sa Review, 16*(1), 125–133. https://doi.org/10.1353/wic.2001.0014.

Struthers, R. (2003). The artistry and ability of traditional women healers. *Health Care for Women International, 24*(4), 340–354. https://doi.org/10.1080/07399330390191706.

Truth and Reconciliation Commission of Canada. (2015). *Honouring the truth, reconciling for the future: Summary of the final report of the Truth and Reconciliation Commission of Canada.* Retrieved from http://www.trc.ca/websites/trcinstitution/File/2015/Findings/Exec_Summary_2015_05_31_web_o.pdf.

Valaskakis, G. G., Dion Stout, M., & Guimond, E (2009). *Restoring the balance: First Nations women, community and culture.* Winnipeg, MB: University of Manitoba Press.

Vukic, A., Jesty, C., Mathews, Sr. V., & Etowa, J. (2012). Understanding race and racism in nursing: Insights from Aboriginal nurses. *International Scholarly Research Notices Nursing,* 2012, 1–9. doi:10.5402/2012/196437.

Weber-Pillwax, C. (1999). Indigenous research methodology: Exploratory discussion of an elusive subject. *Journal of Educational Thought, 33*(1), 31–45.

Weber-Pillwax, C. (2001). Coming to an understanding: A panel presentation: What is Indigenous research?. *Canadian Journal of Native Education, 25*(2), 166–174.

Weber-Pillwax, C. (2003). *Identity formation and consciousness with reference to Northern Alberta Cree and Métis Indigenous Peoples* (Unpublished doctoral dissertation). Edmonton: University of Alberta.

Weber-Pillwax, C. (2004). Indigenous researchers and Indigenous research methods: Cultural influences or cultural determinants of research methods. *Pimatisiwin: A Journal of Aboriginal and Indigenous Community Health, 2*(1), 77–90.

Weber-Pillwax, C. (2008). Citizenship and its exclusions. In A. A. Abdi, & L. Shultz (Eds.), *Educating for human rights and global citizenship* (pp. 193–204). Albany, NY: State University of New York Press.

Wilson, S. (2008). *Research is ceremony: Indigenous research methods* Winnipeg, MB: Fernwood.

How Does Simulation Impact Building Competency and Confidence in Recognition and Response to the Adult and Pediatric Deteriorating Patient Among Undergraduate Nursing Students?

Sandra Goldsworthy, PhD, RN, CNCC(C), CMSN(C)[1] | J. David Patterson, RN, MN | Martie Dobbs, RN, MSc | Arfan Afzal, PhD | Shelley Deboer, RN, BN

ABSTRACT

BACKGROUND: The ability to recognize and respond to a deteriorating adult or pediatric patient is critical to prevention of poor patient outcomes. Simulation is one teaching/ learning strategy that can prepare nursing students as they plan to transition to practice. Recognition and response to hemodynamic instability, respiratory distress, cardiac arrest, a massive hemorrhage, or a pediatric seizure has the potential to save patient lives.

METHOD: In this quasi-experimental pre/post study, participants were randomly assigned to a treatment or a control group (N = 59). The treatment group received a 16-hour simulation intervention held over two days that were two weeks apart. In addition, the treatment group completed two virtual simulations (one adult and one pediatric case).

RESULTS: A new measure, Clinical Self-efficacy, was piloted in this study and showed a high internal consistency (0.91).

Significant improvement in all items on the Clinical Self-efficacy tool was seen in the treatment group after the intervention. On the contrary, there was no significant improvement in any of the Clinical Self-efficacy items in the control group.

CONCLUSION(S): The hybrid simulation intervention proved effective in improving confidence and competence in the recognition and response to deteriorating patients. Further multisite research is needed to further explore the significance of the simulation intervention.

KEY WORDS: competence, deteriorating patient, nursing, self-efficacy, simulation, undergraduate, virtual simulation

[1]Faculty of Nursing, University of Calgary, 2500 University Drive NW, Calgary AB T2N 1N4, Canada

KEY POINTS

- A new Clinical Self-efficacy measure was developed and tested in this study and showed high internal consistency (0.91).
- The treatment group showed significant increase in competence in all areas after intervention.

As simulation continues to gain traction in the preparation of undergraduate nursing students, specific strategies are being developed to enhance performance in the practice area. One such strategy includes a comprehensive high-fidelity simulation intervention that was aimed at improving recognition and response to the rapidly deteriorating patient. The intervention includes pediatric and adult-based acute care scenarios. Students are exposed to a hybrid approach to simulation with opportunities to complete both high-fidelity and virtual simulation cases. The simulation cases were developed and tested using best practices in simulation that included the following: The International Nursing Association for Clinical Simulation and Learning simulation standard IX: simulation design (Lioce et al., 2015), content expert panels, the utilization of peer-reviewed simulation case templates (Goldsworthy & Graham, 2013), and a "dry run" with subsequent refinement of all cases. Prebriefing of students was completed through required pre-readings, an overview of the learning objectives, and an orientation to the simulation learning space. In addition to the preparation of the students, the instructor team was prebriefed by reviewing and running all the cases and the evaluation tools and participating in a dry run and setup of the learning stations.

LITERATURE REVIEW

Newly graduated nurses face significant challenges when exposed to the real-life clinical situation of a rapidly deteriorating patient. The graduate nurses' challenges may be associated with limited exposure to clinical situations requiring the students to identify and manage the deteriorating patient (Bogossian et al., 2014). Limited assessment skills acquired during training decreases students' ability to recognize the key signs of acute illness and deterioration. To optimize students' skills for assessing and managing acutely ill and deteriorating patients, the National Institute for Health and Care Excellence (2007) and the UK Resuscitation Council (2010) recommend the teaching of critical assessment skills in undergraduate nursing programs. Some authors argue that didactic methods of teaching and assessing critical assessment skills do not adequately prepare students for clinical practice (Buykx et al., 2011). The authors believe that simulation represents the ideal strategy for nursing students to develop, refine, and rehearse clinical skills in recognizing and responding to patient deterioration in a safe environment. In the following section, knowledge and skills performance, self-efficacy, self-confidence, and situation awareness are explored.

Knowledge and Skills Performance

Simulation provides an opportunity for students to connect theory to practice. Competency checklists allow assessment of nursing student performance in the simulation laboratory by totalling the number of correct actions taken (Cooper et al., 2010). Skills performance can be measured using an objective structured clinical examination (Merriman, Stayt, & Ricketts, 2014) instrument, and knowledge can be assessed with the use of knowledge questionnaire (Cooper, Bogossian, Porter, & Cant 2014; Cooper et al., 2010, 2016). Objective structured clinical examinations are typically assessing singular skills (i.e., medication administration) contrasted with simulation cases that provide a comprehensive opportunity to care for a "patient" in the simulation laboratory and involve multiple skills, prioritization, and communication behaviours.

In multiple studies, investigators examined, in simulated environments, the ability of undergraduate nursing students to assess, identify, and respond to patients deteriorating or at risk of deterioration (Buckley & Gordon, 2011; Kelly, Forber, Conlon, Roche, & Stasa, 2014). The investigators found significant increases in student nurses' knowledge, skills performance, confidence, and perception of team work following simulation experiences (Buckley & Gordon, 2011; Cooper et al., 2015a, b; Davies, Nathan, &

Clarke, 2012; Kelly et al., 2014; Liaw, Zhou, Lau, Siau, & Chan, 2014).

In an exploratory study of theoretical and applied learning in response to a virtual simulation program, FIRST2ACT WEB™, investigators found enhanced knowledge and skills, improved virtual clinical performance, and increased confidence and competence in final year nursing students (Bogossian et al., 2015; Cant, Young, Cooper, & Porter, 2015; Cooper et al., 2015a, b). The benefits of face-to-face approach during these simulation events were the ability to work as a team, receive face-to-face briefings, and offer in-depth feedback (Cooper et al., 2015a, b, 2016). Combining structured education curriculum with simulation training also improves nursing students' performance in recognizing and responding to clinical deterioration (Hart et al., 2014a, b).

Theoretical Framework

This study was underpinned by Bandura's (1986) social cognitive theory, in which an individual's reactions and actions are based on what the individual has observed in others. The concept of self-efficacy arises from social cognitive theory and is broadly defined as: "… people's judgements about their capabilities to organize and execute courses of action required to attain designated types of performance; it is concerned not with the skills one has but with judgements of what one can do with whatever skills one possesses" (Bandura, 1986, p. 391).

An individual's self-efficacy can influence how they approach tasks and new challenges, such as learning situations such as a competency development in recognizing a patient that is deteriorating. Self-efficacy is conceptualized as being general or domain specific. General self-efficacy is a trait-like generality dimension defined as: "… an individual's perception of their ability to perform across a variety of situations" (Judge, Erez, & Bono, 1998, p. 170). Domain-specific self-efficacy refers to how an individual feels capable of approaching and performing specific tasks, such as competencies in

approaching and caring for a deteriorating patient (Bandura, 1986). Domain-specific self-efficacy is typically developed through mastery experiences and through vicarious learning and modelling by observing others perform the task (Bandura, 1986). Mastery experiences are largely gained through hands-on experience, as through practice in the clinical setting with patients or through practice in the simulation laboratory with simulated patients. Bandura (1986) also argued that self-efficacy develops with opportunity to repeat tasks. Individuals that have increased levels of self-efficacy feel they can have an impact on their environment, whereas individuals with low levels of self-efficacy view problems as unmanageable and insurmountable. Individuals with low self-efficacy may avoid a situation, instead of facing a task, if they may not be able to do it. Research on self-efficacy in relation to training interventions is important in the understanding of effective training. An individual with higher self-efficacy is more likely to make an effort and persist longer at a task, compared to those with lower self-efficacy.

Studies in the nursing population have explored the influence of self-efficacy and performance for specific tasks. In one study exploring self-efficacy in the nursing population, a simulation intervention was delivered to 112 undergraduate nursing students (Bambini, Washburn, & Perkins, 2009). In the intervention, the training included maternal/child scenarios that mimicked the real practice settings, which were delivered via high-fidelity patient simulators. The results showed a significant increase in the levels of self-efficacy when pretests were compared to the posttest measures (Bambini et al., 2009).

Similar results were found in a US study (N = 49 registered nurses) where high-fidelity simulation training was conducted for preeclampsia and eclampsia management. Nurse levels of self-efficacy were significantly increased when the pretest and posttest were compared (Christian & Krumwiede, 2013). In addition, the levels of self-efficacy were found to be sustained over time when the posttests were readministered at eight weeks after intervention. In this single group design, the nurses also reported being highly satisfied with simulation as an effective teaching strategy.

Sample

After ethics approval was received from the university ethics board, nursing students in their third year were recruited through common classes into the study. The participants in this research included 63 undergraduate nursing students in their final year of their Bachelor of Nursing (BN) degree. The participants were randomly assigned to either the treatment group (n = 24) or the comparison group (n = 39).

METHOD

This study used a quasi-experimental design to test the effects of a 16-hour simulation intervention on third-year undergraduate nursing students' confidence and competence in the recognition and response to the rapidly deteriorating adult and pediatric patient. Students in the comparison group completed the baseline survey and a second survey aligned with the completion of the simulation intervention in the treatment group. Students in the treatment group completed pretests before each scenario and posttests at the completion of each scenario. Students in the treatment group attended two eight-hour simulation days in which they participated in a total of six scenarios on the first day and two weeks later attended a second eight-hour simulation day where all scenarios were repeated. In addition, students in the treatment group completed two virtual simulation case studies (adult cardiac arrest scenario and a pediatric asthma scenario—see Figure D.1) in the time frame between the two high-fidelity case scenario days.

Deteriorating Patient: High-Fidelity Scenario Approach

Each high-fidelity scenario was run over one hour (Figure D.2). The prebriefing period was 15 minutes in duration and included an orientation to the simulation space, simulator, role assignment, handover report, and pretest questions that were completed individually.

Each student was assigned a role and worked on the case in teams of four. Roles included primary nurse, secondary nurse, laboratory/diagnostics, and a pharmacology role. Students switched roles after each scenario to ensure they had participated in all roles. The intent was that the primary and secondary nurse completed the initial assessment at the head of the bed and the laboratory/diagnostics and pharmacology students worked

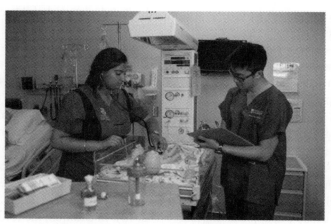

FIG. D.1 Student pediatric simulation team.

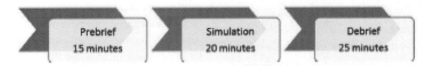

FIG. D.2 Timing of high-fidelity simulation delivery.

at the foot of the bed reviewing laboratory and diagnostic results and doctor's orders and communicating this information to the students completing the assessments. Each case was repeated on the second day of the high-fidelity simulation to allow for increased mastery of the acute care medical surgical (adult and pediatric) competencies. High-fidelity cases included the following: angina/cardiac arrest, COPD/respiratory failure, post-op hemorrhage, pediatric sepsis, pediatric asthma, neonatal seizures (Figures D.1, D.3).

All instructors were provided with a debriefing guide and debriefing questions. Because instructor experience varied in simulation debriefing and delivery of simulation, it was decided to use a plus/delta methodology for debriefing. Debriefing was completed directly at the bedside immediately after each simulation and was approximately 25 minutes in duration. In addition to debriefing, a posttest multiple choice/short answer quiz was delivered to assess knowledge after each simulation case.

Deteriorating Patient: Virtual Case Scenario Approach

In the virtual cases (VSim, Wolters Kluwer), students could repeat the cases as many times as they wanted to achieve mastery with the case. The virtual cases included an electronic preparation guide to orientate students to the program and technology before beginning the case. Each case also had suggested readings and pretest questions and answers to further prepare the student before entering each of the virtual cases. The virtual simulation program utilized allowed students to "drive" the scenario and end the scenario when they felt they had completed the needed assessments and interventions. At the conclusion of the case, the student was provided with a posttest, guided reflection questions, and a debriefing log outlining how they performed in the case. The debriefing log also included comprehensive rationales for incorrect interventions and choices.

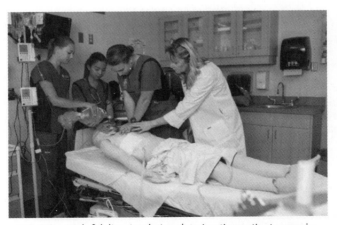

FIG. D.3 High-fidelity simulation deteriorating patient scenario.

Measures

Two primary measures were used in this study. First, a new clinical self-efficacy measure (CSE) was developed to explore confidence in ten different areas related to recognizing and responding to the deteriorating patient. The CSE tool was developed through using Bandura's (2006) guide for developing domain-specific self-efficacy tools and demonstrated a high internal consistency of 0.91 in this study. The second measure was a multiple choice knowledge assessment related to each of the six deteriorating patient simulation cases in the intervention.

Data Analysis

Descriptive statistics provided a profile of the characteristics of the students in the treatment and comparison groups. We used paired and independent t-tests to determine whether there was a statistically significant mean improvement in the CSE after the intervention, within and between the treatment and comparison groups. Furthermore, within the treatment group, we tested for significant knowledge improvement at postintervention using Wilcoxon signed-rank test.

The assumptions of the paired and independent t-tests were tested. Normality was tested using Shapiro-Wilk test as the sample sizes were less than 50. Homogeneity of variances was tested using Levene's test. If the assumption of normality did not hold, we conducted a nonparametric test using Wilcoxon signed-rank test or Mann-Whitney test, as appropriate. A p-value of less than .05 indicated statistical significance throughout all inferential analyses. For multiple comparisons, p-values were adjusted using Holm-Bonferroni method. All analyses were conducted using IBM SPSS Statistics 24.

RESULTS

Table D.1 represents the baseline characteristics of students. About 62% of the students were initially assigned to the comparison group to allow

TABLE **D.1**

BASELINE CHARACTERISTICS OF STUDENTS ACCORDING TO THE TREATMENT GROUP

VARIABLE	TREATMENT	CONTROL
n (%)	24 (38.1)	39 (61.9)
Age, Mean (SD)	26.0 (6.9)	25.2 (6.0)
Gender, n (%)		
Female	19 (79.2)	37 (94.9)
Male	5 (20.8)	2 (5.1)
English as a First Language, n (%)		
No	8 (33.3)	4 (10.3)
Yes	16 (66.7)	35 (89.7)
Highest Level of Completed Education, n (%)		
Diploma	9 (37.5)	14 (36.8)
Undergraduate	14 (58.3)	19 (50.0)
Others	1 (4.2)	5 (13.2)

Note. N = sample size; SD = standard deviation.

for attrition. The average age of the students in the treatment and comparison group were similar, being 26 years and 25 years, respectively. Other sociodemographic characteristics were also very comparable between these two groups including that the majority of the students were female, speak English as their first language, and completed undergraduation as the highest level of education. After losing 20 students to follow-up, we ended up with nearly equal arms in the treatment and comparison groups by having 23 and 20 students, respectively.

Table D.2 shows the within- and between-group pre-post intervention CSE improvement

TABLE **D.2**

WITHIN- AND BETWEEN-GROUP PRE-POST INTERVENTION CSE COMPARISON IN THE TREATMENT AND CONTROL GROUPS

	0.91					
	PRE–POST TREATMENT DIFFERENCE (n = 23)		PRE–POST CONTROL DIFFERENCE (n = 20)		PRE–POST DIFFERENCE IN THE TREATMENT AND CONTROL GROUPS	
RELIABILITY OF THE CSE SCALE	MEAN (SD)	*P*-VALUE	MEAN (SD)	*P*-VALUE	MEAN (SD)	*P*-VALUE
Recognizing a Patient With No Pulse	8.04 (12.41)	.003a	2.45 (10.44)	.154	5.59 (11.54)	.060
Responding to a Patient With No Pulse	23.91 (17.38)	<.001a	−1.50 (18.57)	.639	25.41 (17.95)	<.001a
Recognizing a Patient That is Not Breathing	8.91 (16.44)	.008a	−0.50 (13.85)	.563	9.41 (15.30)	.025
Responding to a Patient That is Not Breathing	21.52 (17.28)	<.001a	−0.75 (19.62)	.567	22.27 (18.40)	<.001a
Recognizing a Patient With Dangerously Low Blood Pressure	8.48 (18.12)	.018a	−4.50 (15.12)	.900	12.98 (16.80)	.008a
Responding to a Patient with Dangerously Low Blood Pressure	18.48 (17.99)	<.001a	0.00 (17.77)	.500	18.48 (17.89)	.001a
Performing High-Quality CPR in an Adult Patient	14.78 (18.37)	.001a	−2.20 (18.96)	.695	16.98 (18.65)	.002a
Performing High-Quality CPR in a Pediatric Patient	13.91 (18.52)	.001a	2.25 (20.55)	.315	11.66 (19.49)	.029
Inserting an Oropharyngeal Airway and Using a Manual Resuscitation Bag in an Adult Patient	31.96 (24.11)	<.001a	3.00 (19.22)	.247	28.96 (21.98)	<.001a
Inserting an Oropharyngeal Airway and using a Manual Resuscitation Bag in a Pediatric Patient	31.52 (26.30)	<.001a	3.75 (21.08)	.218	27.77 (24.03)	<.001a
Responding to a Major Hemorrhage	28.26 (21.25)	<.001a	3.75 (17.46)	.175	24.51 (19.58)	<.001a

aSignificant at *p* < .05 after adjusting for multiple comparisons.

in the treatment and comparison groups. A pre-analysis of principal component analysis showed that the largest eigenvalue of the sample data set is 7.98. Therefore, we were able to calculate the Cronbach's alpha for assessing the internal reliability of the CSE items with this sample size [1]. The Cronbach's coefficient alpha was 0.91, indicating strong internal consistency among the items.

After adjusting for multiplicity, we found significant CSE improvement in all items in the treatment group after the intervention. On the contrary, there was no significant improvement in any of the items in the comparison group. When conducting between-group comparisons, we observed the treatment group has significantly higher improvements in most of the CSE items than the comparison group.

Table D.3 displays preintervention and postintervention knowledge comparison in the treatment group. From the *p*-values, we conclude that there has been a significant knowledge improvement in septic shock, myocardial infarction, and asthma after the intervention. Of note, pediatric asthma and myocardial infarction were the two virtual simulations that the treatment group completed between the high-fidelity intervention days.

Implications

The results of this study have several implications for nurse educators. First, in this population, the hybrid simulation intervention that included a total of six high-fidelity simulation cases (three pediatric and three adult) and two virtual simulation cases (pediatric asthma and adult myocardial infarction) showed statistically significant increases in clinical self-efficacy among treatment participants in all domains. Furthermore, the treatment group in comparison with the comparison group showed significant increases in knowledge on three of the six domains (myocardial infarction, pediatric asthma, and septic shock). Of interest, two of the domains, pediatric asthma and myocardial infarction were the topics of the two virtual simulations. Significant findings in this area may be important in understanding the placement of virtual simulation in scaffolding learning and may also demonstrate the cumulative effect on learning in the simulation laboratory. For instance, are virtual simulations best placed in front of high-fidelity simulation experiences or in between simulation laboratory experiences? More exploration is needed to understand the placement of virtual experiences and how they might enhance learning.

Strengths and Limitations

Limitations for this study included a small sample size due to the pilot nature of the study and that the study was conducted at a single site. A recommendation to increase the rigour of this study if repeated would be to have the performances in the simulations be observed and rated using an interrater process to see if scores increased in relation to performance as well as the students reporting increase in self-efficacy.

TABLE **D.3**

PRE–POST INTERVENTION KNOWLEDGE COMPARISON IN THE TREATMENT GROUP			
KNOWLEDGE TEST	**PREINTERVENTION**	**POSTINTERVENTION**	***P*-VALUE**
Correct Score, Median (IQR)			
Septic Shock, Out of 5	3 (1)	4 (2)	.033a
COPD, Out of 5	4 (2)	4 (1)	.500
MI, Out of 7	4 (2)	6 (2)	<.001a
Asthma, Out of 5	3 (1)	4 (1)	.029a
Seizures, Out of 5	4 (1)	4 (1)	.726

aSignificant at $p < .05$. IQR = interquartile range; MI = myocardial infarction.

Strengths of the study included the use of best practices in faculty preparation, scenario development, and debriefing practices.

DISCUSSION

This study conforms with the literature by demonstrating that simulation can enhance knowledge after simulation intervention in recognition and response to the deteriorating patient (Buckley & Gordon, 2011; Kelly et al., 2014). In addition, a new clinical self-efficacy tool was developed and demonstrated a high reliability (0.91) in this study. More studies are needed to further understand the impact of the combination of virtual simulation and high-fidelity simulation in developing competency in caring for patients who are rapidly deteriorating.

CONCLUSIONS

Simulation can be an effective strategy for teaching recognition and response to the deteriorating patient among undergraduate nursing students. The additive effect and strategic timing of virtual simulation combined with high-fidelity simulation may be an important component in acceleration of mastery of competency in responding to the deteriorating patient. Further multisite research is needed with larger sample sizes to explore the use of simulation in the recognition and response to the deteriorating patient.

ACKNOWLEDGMENT

The lead author would like to acknowledge the Faculty of Nursing, University of Calgary for the funding of this research through the Simulation Professorship (Dr. Goldsworthy).

REFERENCES

Bambini, D., Washburn, J., & Perkins, R. (2009). Outcomes of clinical simulation for novice nursing students: Communication, confidence, clinical judgment. *Nursing Education Perspectives, 30*(2), 79–82.

Bandura, A. (1986). *Social Foundations of Thought and Action: A Social-Cognitive View.* Englewood Cliffs, NJ: Prentice Hall.

Bandura, A. (2006). Guide for constructing self-efficacy scales. *Self-Efficacy Beliefs of Adolescents, 5,* 307–337.

Bogossian, F., Cooper, S., Cant, R., Beauchamp, A., Porter, J., Kain, V., & Phillips, N. M. (2014). Undergraduate nursing students' performance in recognizing and responding to sudden patient deterioration in high psychological fidelity simulated environments: An Australian multi-centre study. *Nurse Education Today, 34*(5), 691–696. https://doi.org/10.1016/j.nedt.2013.09.015.

Bogossian, F. E., Cooper, S. J., Cant, R., et al. (2015). A trial of e-simulation of sudden patient deterioration (FIRST2ACT WEB™) on student learning. *Nurse Education Today, 35*(10), e36–e42.

Buckley, T., & Gordon, C. (2011). The effectiveness of high fidelity simulation on medical–surgical registered nurses' ability to recognize and respond to clinical emergencies. *Nurse Education Today, 31*(7), 716–721.

Buykx, P., Kinsman, L., Cooper, S., McConnell-Henry, T., Cant, R., Endacott, R., & Scholes, J. (2011). Educating nurses to identify patient deterioration: A theory-based model for best practice simulation education. *Nurse Education Today, 31*(7), 687–693.

Cant, R., Young, S., Cooper, S. J., & Porter, J. (2015). E-simulation: Preregistration nursing students' evaluation of an online patient deterioration program. *Computers, Informatics, Nursing: CIN, 33*(3), 108–114.

Christian, A., & Krumwiede, N. (2013). Simulation enhances self-efficacy in the management of preeclampsia and eclampsia in obstetrical staff nurses. *Clinical Simulation in Nursing, 9*(9), e369–e377.

Cooper, S., Kinsman, L., Buykx, P., McConnell-Henry, T., Endacott, R., & Scholes, J. (2010). Managing the deteriorating patient in a simulated environment: Nursing students' knowledge, skill, and situation awareness. *Journal of Clinical Nursing, 19*(15-16), 2309–2318.

Cooper, S., Bogossian, F., Porter, J., & Cant, R. (2014). Managing patient deterioration: Enhancing nursing students' competence through web-based simulation and feedback techniques. Retrieved from https://espace.library.uq.edu.au/view/UQ:335695/UQ335695.pdf.

Cooper, S., Cant, R. P., Bogossian, F., Bucknall, T., & Hopmans, R. (2015a). Doing the right thing at the right time: Assessing responses to patient deterioration in electronic simulation scenarios using course-of-action analysis. *Computers, Informatics, Nursing: CIN, 33*(5), 199–207.

Cooper, S., Cant, R., Bogossian, F., Kinsman, L., & Bucknall, T. (2015b). Patient deterioration education: Evaluation of face-to-face simulation and e-simulation approaches. *Clinical Simulation in Nursing, 11*(2), 97–105.

Cooper, S. J., Kinsman, L., Chung, C., et al. (2016). The impact of web-based and face-to-face simulation on patient deterioration and patient safety: Protocol for a multi-site multi-method design. *BMC Health Services Research, 16*(1), 475.

Davies, J., Nathan, M., & Clarke, D. (2012). An evaluation of a complex simulated scenario with final year undergraduate children's nursing students. *Collegian, 19*(3), 131–138. https://doi.org/10.1016/j.colegn.2012.04.005.

Goldsworthy, S., & Graham, L. (2013). *Simulation Simplified: A Practical Handbook for Nurse Educators*. Philadelphia, PA: Wolters Kluwer.

Hart, P. L., Brannan, J. D., Long, J. M., Maguire, M. B. R., Brooks, B. K., & Robley, L. R. (2014a). Effectiveness of a structured curriculum focused on recognition and response to acute patient deterioration in an undergraduate BSN program. *Nurse Education in Practice, 14*(1), 30–36.

Hart, P. L., Maguire, M. B. R., Brannan, J. D., Long, J. M., Robley, L. R., & Brooks, B. K. (2014b). Improving BSN students' performance in recognizing and responding to clinical deterioration. *Clinical Simulation in Nursing, 10*(1), e25–e32.

Judge, T., Erez, A., & Bono, J. (1998). The power of being positive: The relation between positive self-concept and job performance. *Human Performance, 11*(2/3), 167–187.

Kelly, M. A., Forber, J., Conlon, L., Roche, M., & Stasa, H. (2014). Empowering the registered nurses of tomorrow: Students' perspectives of a simulation experience for recognizing and managing a deteriorating patient. *Nurse Education Today, 34*(5), 724–729. https://doi.org/10.1016/j.nedt.2013.08.014.

Liaw, S. Y., Zhou, W. T., Lau, T. C., Siau, C., & Chan, S. W. (2014). An interprofessional communication training using simulation to enhance safe care for a deteriorating patient. *Nurse Education Today, 34*(2), 259–264.

Lioce, L., Meakim, C., Fey, M., Chmil, J., Mariani, B., & Alinier, G. (2015). Standards of best practice simulation standard IX: Simulation design. *Clinical Simulation in Nursing, 11*, 300–315.

Merriman, C. D., Stayt, L. C., & Ricketts, B. (2014). Comparing the effectiveness of clinical simulation versus didactic methods to teach undergraduate adult nursing students to recognize and assess the deteriorating patient. *Clinical Simulation in Nursing, 10*(3), e119–e127.

National Institute for Health and Care Excellence. (2007). *Acutely Ill Adults in Hospital: Recognizing and Responding to Deterioration*. Retrieved from https://www.nice.org.uk/guidance/cg50/resources/acute-illness-in-adults-in-hospital-recognising-and-responding-to-deterioration-975500772037.

Prenatal Maternal Anxiety as a Risk Factor for Preterm Birth and the Effects of Heterogeneity on This Relationship: A Systematic Review and Meta-Analysis

M. Sarah Rose[1] | Gianella Pana[2] | Shahirose Premji[3]

BACKGROUND: Systematic reviews (SR) and meta-analyses (MA) that previously explored the relationship between prenatal maternal anxiety (PMA) and preterm birth (PTB) have not been comprehensive in study inclusion, failing to account for effects of heterogeneity and disagree in their conclusions.

OBJECTIVES: This SRMA provides a summary of the published evidence of the relationship between PMA and PTB while examining methodological and statistical sources of heterogeneity.

METHODS: Published studies from MEDLINE, CINAHL, PsycINFO, and EMBASE, until June 2015, were extracted and reviewed.

RESULTS: Of the 37 eligible studies, 31 were used in this MA; six more were subsequently excluded due to statistical issues, substantially reducing the heterogeneity. The odds ratio for PMA was 1.70 (95% CI 1.33, 2.18) for PTB and 1.67 (95% CI 1.35, 2.07) for spontaneous PTB comparing higher levels of anxiety to lower levels.

CONCLUSIONS: Consistent findings indicate a significant association between PMA and PTB. Due to the statistical problem of including collinear variables in a single regression model, it is hard to distinguish the effect of the various types of psychosocial distress on PTB. However, a prenatal program aimed at addressing mental health issues could be designed and evaluated using a randomized controlled trial to assess the causal nature of different aspects of mental health on PTB.

[1]Research Facilitation, Alberta Health Services, Calgary, AB, Canada, T2N 2T9
[2]Faculty of Medicine, University of Calgary, AB, Canada, T2N 1N4
[3]Faculty of Nursing and Cumming School of Medicine, Department of Community Health Sciences, University of Calgary, AB, Canada, T2N 1N4

INTRODUCTION

Preterm birth (PTB), commonly defined as delivery that occurs at a gestational age less than 37 weeks, poses a public health concern since critically underdeveloped infants are at a higher risk for neonatal mortality and survivor morbidity (Wen et al., 2004; Goldenberg et al., 2008; Dunkel-Schetter & Glynn, 2011). Preterm infants require longer hospital stays and are hospitalized more often as they are at risk for major health complications in infancy, development, and pediatric problems through childhood and chronic diseases in adulthood (Dunkel-Schetter & Glynn, 2011; Bruce et al., 2012). Substantial attention has been paid to the role of prenatal maternal mental health problems in the etiology of PTB. Theoretical models have been developed to explain the biological effect of prenatal maternal mental health problems, such as the physiological stress response of the hypothalamicpituitary axis (HPA) regulated by corticotrophin-releasing hormone (CRH) (Ruiz et al., 2003; Wadhwa et al., 2001). The pathways by which maternal mental health problems initiate a physiologic sequence of events that promote early labour, however, remain unknown (Goldenberg et al., 2008; Ruiz et al., 2003; Wadhwa et al., 2001).

Maternal mental health is a state of well-being in which a mother can cope and work productively against life stressors (Bruce et al., 2012). Maternal mental health problems include depression, anxiety, and stress. The relationship between prenatal maternal anxiety and PTB has been examined previously (SR). Two broad narrative reviews on the hypothesized and known mechanistic effects of stress on preterm labour concluded that the strongest predictor of PTB was pregnancy-specific anxiety (Dunkel-Schetter & Glynn, 2011; Shapiro et al., 2013). Although efficient and informative, such reviews are subject to selection bias (Uman, 2011). There have been two SR with meta-analysis (SRMA) (Ding et al., 2014; Littleton et al., 2007) that focused on the relationship between prenatal maternal anxiety during pregnancy and PTB with conflicting results. Ding et al. (2014) found that prenatal maternal anxiety was significantly associated with an increased risk for PTB and remained significant regardless of the timing of anxiety assessment. In contrast, Littleton et al. (2007) reported nonsignificant summary correlation coefficients between anxiety during pregnancy and gestational age at birth and between pregnancy-specific anxiety and gestational age at birth. Explicit criteria for selecting and critically appraising the primary research studies were not always evident in these reviews. Inconsistencies in the findings of the SRMA and primary studies examining the relationship between anxiety and PTB may have also arisen from potential source of heterogeneity, such as differences in the primary predictor variable measured (type of anxiety), how the predictor variable is measured, and how the outcome is determined, to name only a few. The present study was designed to be a more inclusive and comprehensive SR and MA than previous studies and the goal was to determine the effect of potential sources of heterogeneity on the relationship between PTB and anxiety, which may help to explain conflicting evidence.

The overall aim of this SR and MA is to provide a summary of the peer-reviewed published evidence regarding the relationship between maternal anxiety during pregnancy and PTB, after accounting for several potential sources of heterogeneity. The specific objectives are (1) to determine sources of heterogeneity in the methodology and analysis of the studies, (2) to assess which of the sources have an impact on the estimation of the relationship of interest, and (3) to estimate the combined effect of studies within homogenous subgroups of studies.

METHODS

Definitions

Prenatal maternal anxiety can be subdivided into three different types: trait anxiety (TA), state anxiety (SA), and pregnancy-specific anxiety (PSA). TA refers to the mother's relatively stable propensity for anxiety whereas SA refers to the temporary anxious feeling the mother develops due to a stressful event, which may or may not be related to her pregnancy (Zeidner, 2010). PSA is then considered the mental state of a pregnant woman whose concerns are specific to the pregnancy itself such as fears regarding the pregnancy, delivery, and health of the child (Blair et al., 2011).

Search Strategy

The three authors (Gianella Pana, M. Sarah Rose, and Shahirose Premji) independently searched the literature to retrieve potential studies that explored the relationship between prenatal maternal anxiety and PTB in two stages. Initially databases were searched using the exact search phrase: (prenatal OR antenatal OR pregnancy) AND (anxiety) AND (preterm OR premature OR prematurity); and the searches were limited to English, humans, and journal studies. All studies published up until June 2015 in MEDNINE (1946 to June 2015), Cumulative Index to Nursing and Allied Health Literature (1961 to June 2015), PsycINFO (1806 to June 2015), and EMBASE (1947 to June 2015) were extracted. The retrieved records were entered into Refworks and duplicates were removed. The titles of the studies were reviewed for obvious exclusion according to the study objective. Any SR or MA were separated from primary sources and screened for relevance. The abstracts of the remaining primary studies were then reviewed for relevance.

Types of Studies and Outcomes

Studies were considered relevant if they examined the relationship between any type of anxiety and PTB, measured either as a continuous (i.e., gestational age) or binary variable (PTB or spontaneous PTB).

Study Selection

Studies deemed to be appropriate were scanned in full to determine relevance. Secondly, the references lists of all relevant studies were reviewed to find additional studies that may have been difficult to detect in the database search due to nonreporting in the abstract (possibly due to nonsignificant effects). Studies published by the same team were carefully reviewed to ensure the results of a given study were not included twice in the MA.

Data Extraction

Data was extracted independently by two reviewers (Gianella Pana and M. Sarah Rose) using a standardized review form and compared for discrepancies. Any discrepancies were discussed and agreement achieved. A standardized Excel sheet was created and information from the standardized review forms was transferred in order to be readily available for the meta-analysis. The items extracted are presented in Table E.1.

Critical Appraisal

The quality and validity of each study were assessed using the critical appraisal (CASP) tool (CASP Checklist, 2014) and the included studies were summarized in tabular form. The CASP questions are also included in Table E.1.

In addition, a critical appraisal of the statistical methods used to analyze the data was done, and their relevance to the design and objectives of the study was assessed. We assessed methods used to develop multivariable models and adjusted estimates. In particular, we examined the methods used to include variables in the multivariable model (e.g., manual, forward stepwise, backward stepwise, and hierarchical). We assessed whether each included covariate was a potential confounding variable and whether it was highly correlated with the primary predictor variable. Two criteria for confounding are that the confounder must be associated with the outcome of interest and that the confounder must also be associated with the primary predictor variable. Collinearity occurs when two predictor variables in a regression model are so highly correlated that it becomes difficult or impossible to distinguish their individual effects on the outcome. Clearly a collinear variable qualifies as a confounding variable, but this is an extreme case of confounding when essentially the same variable is entered twice. Unfortunately, this may be a result of using self-report questionnaires where it may be impossible to determine participants that are depressed only, anxious only, both, or neither. Using a diagnostic tool may be

TABLE E.1

ITEMS ON THE STRUCTURED DATA EXTRACTION FORM, THE CASP TOOL FOR CRA, AND THE APPRAISAL OF THE STATISTICAL ANALYSIS

METHODS	RESULTS
First author	Age
Year of publication	Education
Other authors	SES or Poverty Index
Country	Marital status
Location	Smoking
Journal	Alcohol problem
Data collection dates	
Key words	*Primary outcome*
Type of study	Gestational age (days)
Number of and time points for observation	Preterm birth (<259 days or <37 w)
Inclusion/exclusion	
Existing study name	*Primary predictor variable*
Sample size	Descriptive analysis
Consent rate, participation rate	*Relationships*
Primary predictor variable	Unadjusted relationships
Measurement of PV	Adjusted relationships
Other predictor variables	
Outcome	Additional comments
Potential confounders	

CASP	STATISTICAL ANALYSIS
Is the clearly focused issue relevant to our study (anxiety and preterm birth)?	Unadjusted analysis:statistic and test
Was the cohort recruited in an acceptable way? That is, is the cohort representative of the population it is supposed to represent?	Appropriate?
	Numerically correct?
Was the outcome (preterm birth) accurately measured to minimize bias?	Method of adjustment; type of model Details of model development
Have the authors identified all-important confounders? (Age, marital status, ethnicity, education, income or SES, parity, previous PTB)	Appropriate confounders considered?
And have they accounted for this in the analysis?	Appropriate control of confounding? Assessment of linearity assumption
Follow-up: completeness	Methods for missing data specified
Follow-up: length (note generally not a concern in pregnancy studies)	Overall quality of adjusted analysis
Do you believe the results? (on a scientific basis and gut feeling)	Other comments

able to do this but would be much more expensive to implement. Because of the inherent difficulty of interpreting the separate effects of highly correlated variables, the adjustment was considered appropriate if the variables in the model were potential confounding variables and not highly correlated with primary predictor variable. The questions for the critical appraisal are included in Table E.1.

Potential Sources of Heterogeneity of Primary Interest

The primary sources of heterogeneity that we considered were as follows: (1) the primary predictor variable (i.e., type of anxiety, e.g., PSA, TA, SA, or anxiety disorder), (2) the primary outcome variable (gestational age, PTB, or spontaneous PTB), (3) the type of summary statistic (i.e., correlation coefficients (CC) or odds ratio (OR)), and (4) whether the estimate provided was unadjusted or adjusted and if adjusted whether this was considered an appropriate adjustment (see Section 2.6).

Statistical Methods

Data Preparation

Studies that reported the results as a relative risk (RR) were converted to OR for consistency. In order to ensure that all measures were independent when one author contributed more than one estimate due to repeated measurements of anxiety, we used a single summary estimate providing that these estimates were homogenous. When a single study reported two estimates, one for African American Women and one for White Women, these OR were combined using a Mantel-Haenszel OR.

Risk of Bias due to Confounding: Assessment and Management

Since all studies were observational in design, one of our primary concerns was the control of bias due to confounding. Some studies included only unadjusted estimates and some included only adjusted estimates. If there is substantial evidence of bias due to confounding then it would not make sense to include both unadjusted and adjusted estimates in the same meta-analysis. Consequently, we first assessed the extent of (potential) bias in the unadjusted estimates by examining the relationship between adjusted and unadjusted estimates (using a scatterplot and linear regression) including only studies that presented both estimates. We also examined the effect of inappropriate versus appropriate adjustment on the potential bias.

Meta-Analysis

The relationship between prenatal maternal anxiety and PTB was summarized using one of two statistical estimates of effect sizes: (1) the OR when the primary outcome variable was PTB or spontaneous PTB (binary variables) or (2) the CC (transformed using Fishers arc sine transformation) when the primary outcome variable was gestational age (continuous). The results are therefore reported separately for each of these two statistical estimates. Pooled estimates were based on fixed or random effects models depending on the degree of heterogeneity. Heterogeneity amongst the estimates was examined using the Q statistic (where $p < 0.05$ provides evidence against the assumption of homogeneity) and I^2 (which is the variation in the effect size due to heterogeneity). Results are illustrated using Forest Plots.

RESULTS

A total of 780 studies were identified through database searching and reviewing reference lists with 462 studies remaining after duplicates were removed (Figure E.1). After excluding by title ($N = 252$) and excluding by abstract ($N = 118$), a full-text review of 92 studies was conducted. From these 92 studies, 55 were excluded based on inclusion criteria leaving 37 studies, of which six (Roesch et al., 2004; Uguz et al., 2013; Bhagwanani et al., 1997; Bödecs et al.,

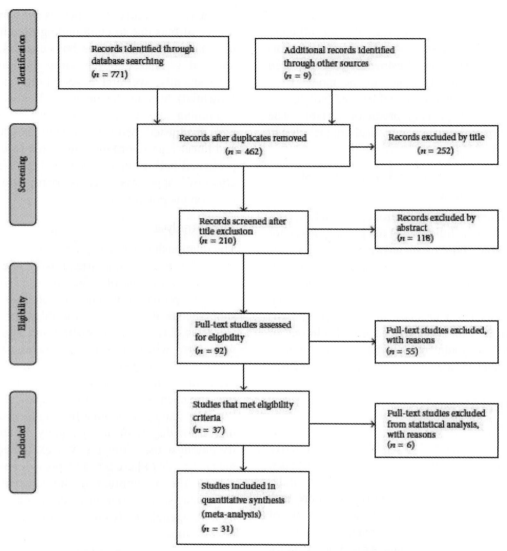

FIG. E.1   PRISMA flow diagram for inclusion of studies examining the relationship between prenatal anxiety and PTB.

2011; Levi et al., 1989; Goldenberg et al., 1996; Perkin et al., 1993; Rauchfuss & Maier, 2011; Martini et al., 2010) were excluded during data extraction since they did not provide enough information to calculate estimates, leaving 31 (Amiri et al., 2010; Andersson et al., 2004; Berle et al., 2005; Bindt et al., 2013; Catov et al., 2010, 2014; Copper et al., 1996; Dayan et al., 2006; Dole et al., 2004; Dominguez et al., 2008; Dominguez et al., 2005; Field et al., 2010; Glynn et al., 2008; Hosseini et al., 2009; Ibanez et al., 2012; Kramer et al., 2009; Latendresse & Ruiz, 2011; Lobel et al., 2008, 2000; Mancuso et al., 2004; McDonald et al., 2014; Orr et al., 2007; Pagel et al., 1990; Peacock et al., 1995; Powell et al., 2013; Rini et al., 1999; Sanchez et al., 2013; Wadhwa et al., 1993) studies eligible for the meta-analysis.

Critical Appraisal of Studies

Many of the 31 studies focused on the relationship between prenatal maternal anxiety and PTB ($N = 30$), had an unbiased measure of anxiety ($N = 25$), had an unbiased measure of gestational age and defined PTB ($N = 26$), accounted for identified confounders in their analysis ($N = 22$), and had a long enough follow-up of the subjects ($N = 34$). Many of these 31 studies, however, did not appear to have a cohort representative of the population ($N = 18$). Participants were usually recruited from hospital clinics, private practices, and walk-in clinics or were referred to the study by private practitioners. The method of sampling was not stated (e.g., sequential, systematic, random, or convenience) and participants were often selected as members of a particular subgroup (e.g., at risk of intrauterine growth restriction, low medical risk, high medical risk, low income, and availability of biomarker assays). In general, the consent rate was low, as was follow-up, so that the ratio of the size of the final sample compared to the size of the eligible sample was very low (as low as 33% in some studies). In addition, many studies did not identify all confounders ($N = 21$), and the design and methods of 18 of these studies were sufficiently flawed to make the results unreliable (Supplementary Table 1, see Supplementary Material available online at http://dx.doi.org/10.1155/2016/8312158). Overall, there were 18 studies that described the relationship between anxiety and PTB or spontaneous PTB using the OR (three studies provided two estimates) and 12 using the CC (six studies reported two estimates of the CC and five reported one only). One study provided information only in terms of the standardized mean difference and was therefore not included in the analysis. This resulted in 22 estimates of the OR and 17 estimates of the CC.

Data Management

Examination of the relationship between adjusted and unadjusted estimates of the OR in 11 estimates from eight studies indicated that there was no evidence against linearity of the relationship, deviation of the intercept from zero (estimated intercept = 0.03, 95% CI –0.06, 0.12, and $p = 0.556$ for difference from zero), or the slope from one (estimated slope = 0.93 (95% CI 0.79, 1.06), $p = 0.272$ for difference from unity). We, therefore, combined both unadjusted and adjusted estimates from the studies, and if a study provided both estimates, the adjusted estimate was used. For studies that used gestational age as the outcome variable, adjustment methods were too variable to consider combining adjusted estimates (i.e., structural equation modelling ($N = 3$), multiple linear regression ($N = 5$), and no adjusted estimate ($N = 2$)) so we focused on the CC only.

Meta-Analysis

We initially categorized the studies into five groups according to the outcome variable and the type of analysis, as illustrated in Table E.2: OR for spontaneous PTB ($N = 9$); OR for PTB ($N = 13$); correlation for PTB ($N = 3$); and correlation with gestational age ($N = 10$). These numbers do not total 31 since some studies reported more than one estimate and we had to exclude one study since we were unable to extract information (Goldenberg et al., 1996). There was substantial heterogeneity across the studies for those reporting OR for spontaneous PTB ($I^2 = 76.0\%$, $p < 0.001$) and PTB ($I^2 = 79.8\%$, $p < 0.001$). When studies that used inappropriate methods of adjustment [19–22] or reported the OR for a unit or 5-unit increase in anxiety (Copper et al., 1996; Powell et al., 2013; Dayan et al., 2002) were removed the heterogeneity was substantially reduced ($I^2 = 46.9\%$, $p = 0.094$ for spontaneous PTB and $I^2 = 0.0\%$, $p = 0.710$ for PTB). In Figure E.2 (PTB) and Figure E.3 (spontaneous PTB) we illustrate the reduction in heterogeneity in excluding these studies. There was little or no evidence of heterogeneity for the three studies reporting the CC when the outcome was PTB ($I^2 = 61.9\%$, $p = 0.073$) and for the 13 studies

TABLE E.2

(A) DETAILS OF THE STUDIES IN THE SYSTEMATIC REVIEWS INCLUSION IN THE META-ANALYSIS. THE TABLE HIGHLIGHTS THE HETEROGENEITY IN TERMS OF ETHNICITY, THE TYPE OF STATISTIC USED TO SUMMARIZE THE DATA, AND THE OUTCOME VARIABLE. (B) DETAILS OF THE PRIMARY PREDICTOR VARIABLE INCLUDED IN THE STUDIES (TYPES OF ANXIETY, MEASUREMENT TOOL, NUMBER OF ITEMS, SCORING FOR EACH ITEM, RANGE OF THE TOTAL SCALE, NUMBER OF TIMES THE PREDICTOR VARIABLE WAS MEASURED DURING PREGNANCY, THE METHOD USED BY THE AUTHORS TO DEAL WITH MULTIPLE MEASURES, AND THE TRIMESTER IN WHICH THE MEASUREMENTS WERE MOST LIKELY TO BE TAKEN). (C) THE KEY TO THE ABBREVIATIONS

(A)

AUTHOR	YEAR	INCLUSION	COUNTRY	STUDY DESIGN	ETHNICITY	W	H	B	STATISTIC	OUTCOME
Berle et al. (2005)	2005	0	Norway	CS	Norway				OR	PTB
Copper et al. (1996)	1996	2	USA	PC	B, W, H	35%	1%	63%	OR	SPTB (<35 w)
Dole et al. (2004)	2004	0	USA	PC	B, W	62%		38%	OR	PTB: SPTB
Dominguez et al. (2005)	2005	0	USA	PC	B			100%	CC	GA
Field et al. (2010)	2010	0	USA	PC	B, W, H	9%	59%	32%	OR	PTB
Glynn et al. (2008)	2008	0	USA	PC	B, W, H	48%	23%	14%	OR	PTB
Goldenberg et al. (1996)	1996	1	USA	PC	B, W	31%	69%			PTB
Hosseini et al. (2009)	2009	0	USA	PC	B, W	49%	5%	51%	CC	GA
Kramer et al. (2009)	2009	0	Canada	PC	B, W, H	80%		8%	OR	SPTB
Lobel et al. (2000)	2000	0	USA	PC	W	87%			CC	GA
Mancuso et al. (2004)	2004	0	USA	PC	B, W, H	24%	32%	43%	CC	GA
McDonald et al. (2014)	2014	0	Canada	PC	W	80%			OR	PTB
Orr et al. (2007)	2007	0	USA	PC	B, W	23%		77%	OR	SPTB
Peacock et al. (1995)	1995	0	England	PC	W	100%			OR	SPTB
Perkin et al. (1993)	1993	2	England	PC	W	100%			OR	PTB
Rini et al. (1999)	1999	0	USA	PC	W, H	48%	52%		CC	GA
Roesch et al. (2004)	2004	1	USA	PC	B, W, H	23%	35%	43%		PTB: GA
Uguz et al. (2013)	2013	1	Turkey	CS	Turkey					GA
Wadhwa et al. (1993)	1993	0	USA	PC	B, W, H	77%	13%	7%	OR, CC	PTB: GA
Bhagwanani et al. (1997)	1997	1	USA	PC	B, W, H	65%	8%	27%	OR	PTB

(A)—cont'd

AUTHOR	YEAR	INCLUSION	COUNTRY	STUDY DESIGN	ETHNICITY	ETHNICITY W	H	B	STATISTIC	OUTCOME
Andersson et al. (2004)	2004	0	Sweden	PC	Sweden				OR	PTB: SPTB
Bindt et al. (2013)	2013	0	G/C D'T*	PC	G/C D'T*				OR, CC	PTB: GA
Bödecs et al. (2011)	2011	1	Hungary	PC	Hungary					PTB
Catov et al. (2010)	2010	0	USA	PC	B, W	70%		30.0%	OR	PTB
Dayan et al. (2006)	2006	2	France	PC	W	94%			OR	PSTB
Dominguez et al. (2008)	2008	0	USA	PC	B, W	100%		100%	CC	GA
Latendresse and Ruiz (2011)	2011	0	USA	PC	B, W, H	69%	23%	4%		PTB
Lobel et al. (2008)	2008	0	USA	PC	B, W, H	65%	12%	12%	OR	SPTB: GA
Amiri et al. (2010)	2010	2	Iran	PC	Iran				OR	PTB
Rauchfuss and Maier (2011)	2011	2	Germany	PC	Germany				OR	PTB
Sanchez et al. (2013)	2013	0	Peru	CC	Peru				OR	SPTB
Martini et al. (2010)	2010	2	Germany	PC	Germany				OR	PTB
Powell et al. (2013)	2013	2	Australia	RCT	Australia				OR	PTB
Ibanez et al. (2012)	2012	0	France	PC	France				OR	PTB: SPTB
Levi et al. (1989)	1989	1	Sweden	PC	Sweden					PTB: GA
Pagel et al. (1990)	1990	0	USA	PC	B, W	78%		7%	C	GA

(B)

AUTHOR	YEAR	PPV	SCALE	# ITEMS	ITEM SCORE SCORE	RANGE	CUT-OFF	# OBS	TIMES	MMM	TRIMESTER
Berle et al. (2005)	2005	Anxiety	HADS-A*	7	1_4	0–21	≥8	1	Anytime		
Copper et al. (1996)	1996	Trait	STAI*	5	1_5	20	C	1	26 ± 0.8 w		L2/E3
Dole et al. (2004)	2004	PSA	PSIS*	6	0_3	18	ns	1	24–29 w		L2/E3
Dominguez et al. (2005)	2005	State, PSA	STAI, RD	10	1_4	10–40	ns	3	18–20 w, 24–26 w, 32–36 w	Mean	2/3

Continued

(B)—cont'd

AUTHOR	YEAR	PPV	SCALE	# ITEMS	ITEM SCORE SCORE	RANGE	CUT-OFF	# OBS	TIMES	MMM	TRIMESTER
Field et al. (2010)	2010	Anxiety	SCID	20		20–90	48	1	20 w		2
Glynn et al. (2008)	2008	PSA	Rini*	10	1_4	10–40		2	19.3 w, 31.0 w	Both	2/E3
Goldenberg et al. (1996)	1996	Trait	STAI	ns	ns	ns	ns	1	24–26 w		L2
Hosseini et al. (2009)	2009	Trait	STPI	10	1_4	10–40	NA	2	4 m, 7 m	First	2
Kramer et al. (2009)	2009	PSA	D-S*	4	1_5	16	Q	1	24–26 w		L2
Lobel et al. (2000)	2000	State	STAI	20	1_4	60		3	10–20 w, 21–30 w, >31 w	3 CC	1/E3
Mancuso et al. (2004)	2004	PSA: State	RD; STAI	4	1_5	16	NA	3	18–20 w, 28–30 w	2 CC	2/E3
McDonald et al. (2014)	2014	State	STAI	20	1_5		40	1	<25 w		L2
Orr et al. (2007)	2007	PSA	PSEI*	6	0_1	0–6	≥4	1	1st prenatal visit		1
Peacock et al. (1995)	1995	Anxiety	GHQ				Q	1	b		1
Perkin et al. (1993)	1993	Anxiety	GHQ			0–21	Q	3	b, 28 w	Max	1/E3
Rini et al. (1999)	1999	PSA	Wadhwa*	10	1_4	30		1	28–32 w		E3
Roesch et al. (2004)	2004	State	STAI	10	1_4	30		3	18 w, 28 w		L/E3
Uguz et al. (2013)	2013	PSA	PSA	4	1_5	16		1	36 w GA – 8 w PP	First	3
Wadhwa et al. (1993)	1993	PSA	PAIP*	5	0_1	0–5	C	1	28–30 w		L2/E3
Bhagwanani et al. (1997)	1997	PSA	RD	5	1_5	20		5	8–28 w, then + 6 w		1/E3
Andersson et al. (2004)	2004	AD	PRIME-MD				B	1	16–18 w		2
Bindt et al. (2013)	2013	AD	GAD-7	7	0_3	0–21	≥10	1	3 trimester		3
Bödecs et al. (2011)	2011	AD	GAD-7					1	M = 8.13		1
Catov et al. (2010)	2010	Trait	STAI-T	10	1_4	10–40	>20	1	M = 17.9		L2/E3
Dayan et al. (2006)	2006	State: Trait	STAI-Y	40	1_4	20–80	C	1	20–28 w		2
Dominguez et al. (2008)	2008	State: Trait	STAI-Y	40	1_4	60		3	18–20 w, 24–26 w, 30–32 w	Mean	2/E3

(B)—cont'd

AUTHOR	YEAR	PPV	SCALE	# ITEMS	ITEM SCORE SCORE	RANGE	CUT-OFF	# OBS	TIMES	MMM	TRIMESTER
Latendresse and Ruiz (2011)	2011	PSA	RD		1_5			1	14–20		2
Lobel et al. (2008)	2008	State	STAI					3	10–25 w, 21–30 w, >30 w	3 CC	L1/2
Amiri et al. (2010)	2010	State	STPI	10	1_4	30		1	20–28 w		L2/E3
Rauchfuss and Maier (2011)	2011	Anxiety: PSA	RD; Luke-sch*	5,3	0–5	0–6		1	13–24 w		2
Sanchez et al. (2013)	2013	Anxiety	DASS-21	4			≥10	1	PP		PP
Martini et al. (2010)	2010	AD	DSM-IV				B	1	PP		PP
Powell et al. (2013)	2013	State: Trait	STAI-6				C	1	Mean 19.7		L2/E3
Ibanez et al. (2012)	2012	State	STAI	20	1_4	20–80	≥37	1	24–28 w		L2/E3
Levi et al. (1989)	1989	S, P, C	CAI	7	?	?	?	1	36 w		3
Pagel et al. (1990)	1990	State	STAI	20	1_4	20–80	?	1	21–36 w		L2/E3

(C)

Whether the paper identified the systematic review was included in the meta-analysis

A: inclusion	0 Yes
	1 Excluded in the first stage
	2 Excluded in the second stage
A: study design	CS Cross-sectional
	PC Prospective cohort
	RCT Randomized controlled trials
	The percentages of White, Black, and Hispanic women in the sample are given where available
	B Black
A: ethnicity	W White
	H Hispanic

Continued

(C)—cont'd

Category	Description	Abbreviation	Meaning
	Where no information was given on ethnicity, the country in which the participants were recruited is given. Note that the percentages do not always add to 100%, this is due to different "other" categories		
A: statistic	Whether the data were summarized using an OR or CC or both	OR	Odds ratio
		CC	Correlation coefficient
A: outcome	Whether the outcome was measured as gestational age (GA) in weeks or as a binary PTB or SPTB	PTB	(Spontaneous) preterm birth < 37 weeks (w); GA unless otherwise stated
		SPTB	Spontaneous preterm birth < 37 weeks GA unless otherwise stated
		Anxiety	General or not otherwise specified
		Trait	Trait anxiety
B: PPV	The primary predictor variable (i.e., the type of anxiety)	State	State anxiety
		PSA	Pregnancy specific anxiety
		AD	Anxiety disorder
		HADS –A	Hospital anxiety and depression rating scale, anxiety
		STPI	State-trait personality inventory
		STAI	The Spielberger sate and trait anxiety scale and various versions of this
	The scale used to measure the type of anxiety	(-T, -Y, -6)	
	*Indicates adapted (e.g., some items were omitted such as somatic complaints)	PSIS	Prenatal social inventory scale (Orr)
B: scale	Wadhwa*, Rini*, Dunkell-Schetter*, Lukesch* all refer to PSA scales adapted from those designed by these original authors	PSEI	Prenatal social environment inventory
		GHQ	General health questionnaire
		PAIP	Psychosocial adaptation in pregnancy
		GAD-7	Generalized anxiety disorder
		DASS-21	Depression and anxiety stress scale
		CAI	Chernobyl anxiety index
		PRIME-MD	Primary care evaluation of mental disorders

(C)—cont'd		
	RD	Researcher developed
	SCID	Structured clinical interview of DSM-IV disorders
B: # items		The number of items in the scale
B: scale		The scoring for each item
	1_4	indicates 1, 2, 3, or 4
B: range		Where possible the limits of the range are given, for example, 20–80. Otherwise the width of the range is given
	N	Not clear whether the cut-point is > or ≥N
	≥N	
B: cut-off		The cut-point at which the scales was divided to indicate low compared with high anxiety
	C	The scale was used in as a continuous variable and no cut-off was used
	Q	The quartiles from the sample were used to define cut-points but were not always specified
	B	The anxiety disorder has been determined by diagnosis
B: # Obs.		Number of observations indicate the number of times that the PPV was measured during pregnancy
B: times		The times during pregnancy that the measurement was taken
		Booking (b); weeks (w)
B: MMM		The method of the author used to deal with the multiple measurements
	First	The first measurement was used
	Mean	The mean of all 3 scores was taken
	Both	Both variables were included simultaneously in the model
	Max	Maximum value at any point during a particular woman's pregnancy
	3 CC	Three correlation coefficients were calculated
B: trimester		The trimester(s) in which most of the measures in each study were probably taken
		Derived from the times
	1	First
	2	Second
	3	Third
	E	Early
	L	Late

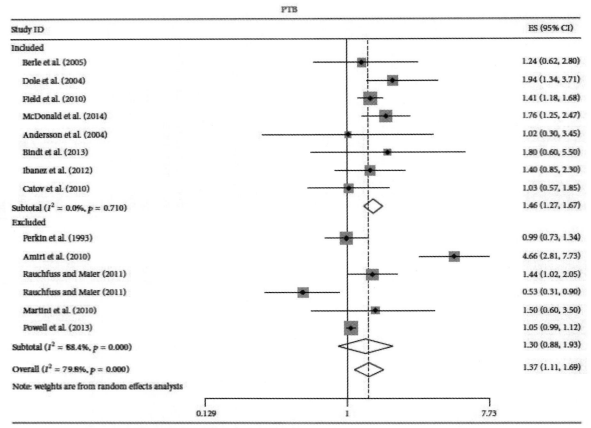

FIG. E.2   The effect of excluding estimates of dubious quality on the heterogeneity of the estimates of the OR for anxiety and PTB. There were three exclusion criteria: (1) the results of the study were numerically suspicious; (2) the authors reported the odds ratio for a continuous predictor variable; and (3) the odds ratio was inappropriately adjusted as described in Critical Appraisal.

that used gestational age as the outcome variable ($I^2 = 0.0, p = 0.570$).

For the 24 studies that remained after these exclusions, five studies used anxiety disorder for the primary predictor variable, eight used PSA, ten used SA, two used TA, and two used gestational age (note some used more than one). Since there was no evidence of heterogeneity for the OR for PTB, we combined all types of anxiety measured (anxiety disorder ($N = 4$), SA ($N = 2$) and PSA ($N = 1$)) for an overall summary OR of 1.46 (95% CI 1.27, 1.67), as illustrated in Figure E.4. When the primary predictor variable was restricted to SA and PSA the estimate was

(OR = 1.70, 95% CI 1.33, 2.18, $N = 3$) for PTB. For spontaneous PTB, the summary OR for all types of anxiety was 1.69 (95% CI 1.41, 2.02) as illustrated in Figure E.5, but when heterogeneity was reduced ($I^2 = 0.0\%, p = 0.774$) by using only estimates of SA and PSA the summary OR was almost identical 1.67 but the 95% CI was wider (95% CI 1.35, 2.07). The summary CC were almost identical −0.09 (95% CI −0.13, −0.06) for gestational age and −0.09 (95% CI −0.12, −0.06) for PTB. When restricted to SA and PSA for gestational age the CC were −0.12 (95% CI −0.17, −0.06) and −0.11 (95% CI −0.19, −0.03), respectively, as illustrated in Figure E.6. These were

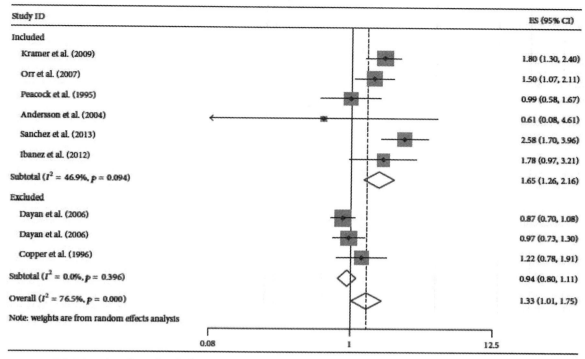

FIG. E.3 The effect of excluding estimates of dubious quality on the heterogeneity of the estimates of the OR for anxiety and spontaneous PTB. There were three exclusion criteria: (1) the results of the study were numerically suspicious; (2) the authors reported the odds ratio for a continuous predictor variable; and (3) the odds ratio was inappropriately adjusted as described in Critical Appraisal.

not combined since five of the authors contributed estimates to both.

DISCUSSION

Summary

We found the most precise estimates of the relationship between prenatal maternal anxiety and PTB when we restricted our analysis to SA (OR = 1.70 (95% CI 1.33, 2.18) for PTB, $N = 3$)) and PSA (OR = 1.67, (95% CI 1.35, 2.07) for PTB, $N = 3$)). When gestational age was the outcome variable the summary CC was −0.12 (95% CI −0.17, −0.06) for SA and −0.11 (95% CI −0.19, −0.03) for PSA. We did not combine these estimates since four of the studies included estimates for both SA and PSA. The estimates

of increased risk of PTB are almost identical for both SA and PSA. This is not surprising since these variables have been found to be very highly correlated in both validation studies (McDowell, 2006) and studies in this review (Littleton et al., 2007; Dominguez et al., 2008; Dominguez et al., 2005; Lobel et al., 2008; Lobel et al., 2000; Rini et al., 1999). There could be several reasons for this: (1) it may not be possible to separate SA and PSA using self-report questionnaires, (2) both types of anxiety have the same physiological response that may lead to PTB, and (3) SA may be a natural sequelae of PSA or vice versa. Studies suggest that PSA or fear of childbirth is more prevalent among women with high SA (Alipour et al., 2012; Arch, 2013; Hall et al., 2012). SA relates to the temporary or emotional anxiety

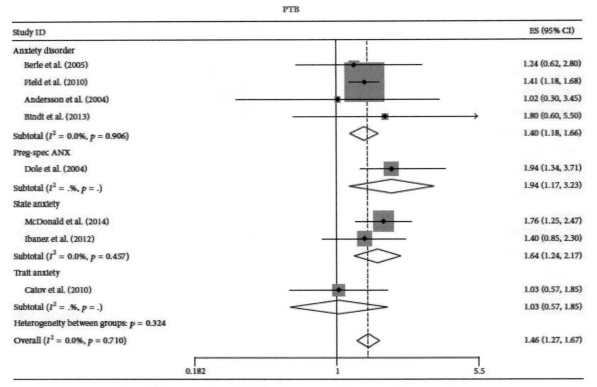

FIG. E.4   The effect of type of anxiety on the estimate of the odds ratio for the relationship between anxiety and PTB.

aroused by a situation or circumstance and is assessed using a 20-item Spielberger State and Trait Anxiety Inventory Form Y-1 (Spielberger et al., 1970; Spielberger & Vagg, 1984). PSA, on the other hand, can be assessed with a 10-item Pregnancy-Related Anxiety Scale-revised (Rini et al., 1999). and unlike the Spielberger State and Trait Anxiety Inventory Form Y-1 has no cost attached to it; thus, it is cost-effective when considering implementation of a screening program.

Comparisons with Other SRMA

There have been five reviews that have, in part, examined the relationship between prenatal maternal anxiety and PTB (Dunkel-Schetter & Glynn, 2011; Shapiro et al., 2013; Ding et al., 2014; Littleton et al., 2007; Alder et al., 2007).

Three of these have been narrative, (Dunkel-Schetter & Glynn, 2011; Shapiro et al., 2013; Alder et al., 2007) whereas two have produced summary statistics from a MA (Ding et al., 2014: Littleton et al., 2007). Dunkel-Schetter and Glynn (2011) provided a narrative review that was the most comprehensive in that her bibliography including 21/23 papers in our review published prior to 2010. They separated anxiety into anxiety (general; $N = 11$) and PSA ($N = 9$) and one situational anxiety [18]. Their conclusions were vague; "a total of 6 of the 11 studies on general or state anxiety show some impact on preterm birth or gestational age, although in all cases the effects are somehow qualified" (Dunkel-Schetter & Glynn, 2011). They also indicated that all of the eight studies, which examined PSA, showed an effect on PTB.

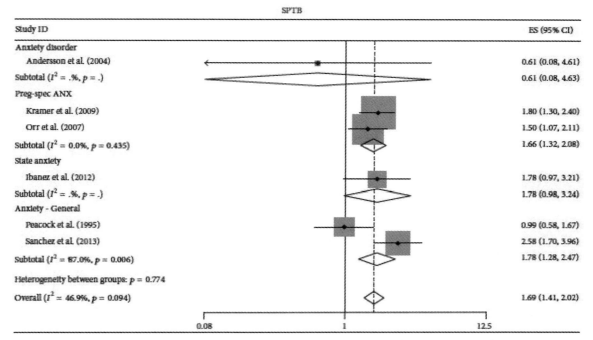

FIG. E.5 The effect of type of anxiety on the estimate of the odds ratio for the relationship between anxiety and spontaneous PTB.

Alder et al. (2007) provided a selective narrative review, in which only 5/17 studies we found prior to 2007 were included in her bibliography. Only two of these, however, were discussed in the section of the effect of maternal anxiety and depression on gestational age, from which they concluded that there was no relation to gestational age with enhanced levels of anxiety. The final narrative review (Shapiro et al., 2013). was selective with only 13/29 studies published prior to 2012 included. The authors concluded that anxiety (and general perceptions of stress) has been associated with shortened gestation in many ($N = 9/11$) studies.

Ding et al. (2014) included 12/31 studies that we found prior to 2013 in their analysis, but they purposefully omitted studies that did not include an OR; eight of these we included in the current MA, but we excluded four due to problems with the reported statistical analysis.

We also included another four studies, which were published after Ding et al.'s (2014) MA was published. Ding et al. (2014) found that prenatal maternal anxiety was significantly associated with an increased risk for PTB, but their summary relative risk (RR = 1.5 (95% CI 1.33, 1.70)) included 12 studies that had a mixture of outcome (PTB and spontaneous PTB) and types of anxiety (SA, TA, anxiety disorder, and PSA) and included both adjusted and unadjusted estimates. Surprisingly they found no evidence of heterogeneity amongst these 12 studies, whereas we found substantial evidence of heterogeneity. Littleton et al. (2007) on the other hand, provided a MA for studies that reported CC. They identified five of the studies that we found and provided a mean CC of −0.06 (95% CI −0.11 to −0.02) for 10 studies, but despite the 95% CI not including zero, they claimed that there were no associations

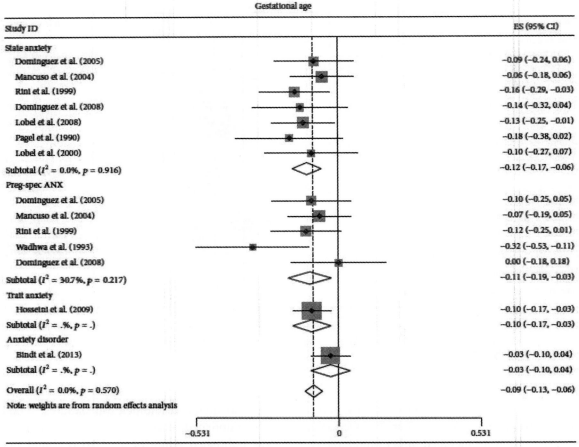

FIG. E.6 The effect of type of anxiety on the estimate of the correlation coefficient (ES) between anxiety (measured as a continuous variable) and gestational age.

between anxiety symptoms and perinatal outcomes, due to their "Fail-safe" p-values. This method has been criticized and the Cochrane handbook recommends that these methods not be used (Roesch et al., 2004). They also found a mean CC of −0.10 (95% CI −0.24, −0.06) for five studies that looked at the relationship between PSA and gestational age.

Strengths and Limitations of Our Meta-Analysis

Unlike previous narrative reviews (Dunkel-Schetter & Glynn, 2011; Shapiro et al., 2013) and meta-analysis (Ding et al., 2014), we did not find

any evidence to suggest that PSA has a greater risk than SA, although the number of studies was small but consistent. While one meta-analysis (Littleton et al., 2007) found a small relationship between PSA and PTB the estimates were below established fail state cut-off; thus, the reliability of the findings was questioned. Unlike previous meta-analysis, we separated studies that used the CC from those that used an OR, since these are inherently different statistics. We decided to investigate the summary OR and CC separately although methods exist to convert both these measures to an effect size (Borenstein et al., 2009). We did this primarily because of the potential inappropriateness of the CC, which is difficult to determine without access to the individual level data. Whether the relationship between a measure of anxiety and gestational age is linear is doubtful, which increases the difficulty of interpreting CC in this context. Another point to bear in mind is that since neither variable is known to be normally distributed the CC is in general not a good measure of the strength of the relationship. However, both the summary OR and the summary CC do have equivalent effect sizes. An OR of 1.7 with a 95% CI 1.3, 2.1 is equivalent to a CC of –0.11 with a 95% CI –0.16, –0.06. So we can conclude that our two analyses are consistent.

Heterogeneity in Meta-Analyses

Thompson makes a distinction between statistical and clinical heterogeneity (Thompson, 1994). Clinical heterogeneity arises when the included studies differ in terms of patient selection and methodological differences, such as study design and differently defined primary predictor and outcome variables. Statistical heterogeneity, as determined by a significant Q statistic or I^2, may be caused by these known clinical and methodological differences or it may be caused by unknown or unrecorded clinical and methodological differences. Thompson, among many other authors, emphasizes that sources of heterogeneity must be investigated to increase the clinical relevance of the conclusions (Thompson, 1994).

We reduced statistical heterogeneity substantially by omitting studies that were apparently numerically incorrect or had inappropriately adjusted estimates of the OR (e.g., that included another highly correlated predictor variable such as another type of anxiety or depression). In addition we did not combine estimates that did not make sense to combine, such as an OR when the predictor variable is binary with one in which the predictor variable is continuous. Although it is possible to use a random effects model to estimate the summary OR in the presence of statistical heterogeneity Thompson (1994) points out

that this is only useful if the statistical heterogeneity cannot be explained by clinical differences. In our analysis we focused on methodological differences particularly in terms of the operationalization of the primary variables and the statistical methodology.

Issues in Statistical Methodology

If we consider the situation when PTB is a dichotomous variable and anxiety as a continuous variable, it is important that the assumption of linearity between the log-odds of PTB and anxiety score is not violated. Interpretation of the OR per k-unit increase is difficult since this model assumes that the OR is the same when comparing a score of 20 with a score of 15, both of which are very low and when comparing a score of 42 with a score of 47, when both scores are around the cut-off level for high anxiety. Combining an OR expressed as a unit or 5 unit increase in the primary predictor variable with an OR when the primary predictor variable is binary is not appropriate because even within the same data these estimates will be different. Consider an example of a simulated dataset in which the CC between gestational age and anxiety is –0.2, and the variables are similarly distributed as those in the studies included in our SR and MA. The predictor variable is a measure initially on a continuous scale such as the STAI but then may be dichotomized using, for example, the 75th percentile. We could report the OR per unit or per 5-unit increase in the continuous anxiety score (e.g., in our example the coefficients would be 1.04 per unit increase or 1.25 per 5-unit increase). However, if we choose to dichotomize the predictor variable the OR will be quite different, since it is comparing one group with a range of scores to another with a different range of scores. In our example the OR for the binary predictor is 2.2.

We had to exclude four adjusted estimates from the MA (Goldenberg et al., 1996; Perkin et al., 1993; Rauchfuss & Maier, 2011; Martini et al., 2010). In these studies the authors had included anxiety as a continuous variable in the model along with a highly correlated predictor variable. Examples of highly correlated predictor variables are two measures of the same anxiety scale taken at different times during pregnancy; two different measures of anxiety (e.g., SA and PSA), and depression and anxiety. In each case the correlation between the variables is very high (in the order of 0.5 to 0.7), which will result in collinearity and difficulty in interpreting the resulting coefficients.

Limitations

Ethnicity

We would have liked to assess the effect of ethnicity on the relationship between anxiety and PTB, but it is not impossible for us to assess in the present study. In many of the North American studies the populations were a mix of Caucasian, Black, Hispanic, and Other ethnicities, some of which were not even specified. We have now included Table E.3 in the paper, which includes the percentage of White, Black, and Hispanic women in the sample for each study. Most papers did not address the issue of ethnicity and indeed would not have been powered to do so. There was only one paper in our MA that produced separate estimates of the OR for Black and White women separately. Dole et al. (2004) found an OR of 2.2 (95% CI 1.3 to 3.7) for Black women and 1.7 (95% CI 1.1, 2.5) for White; thus, there was a large overlap in the 95% CI of these estimates in spite of the large sample sizes ($N = 644$ Black women and 1098 White women). We therefore decided to combine the estimates, using the inverse variance method resulting in an estimate of 1.94 (1.34, 2.82). The estimate of I^2 was 0.0% and $p = 0.430$ for the Q statistic. We felt that it was more appropriate to combine these estimates rather than to treat them as two separate studies in the meta-analysis. Catov et al. (2014) presented estimated for Black and White women, but since this analysis was of subset of data from a previous analysis (Catov et al., 2010) we chose not to duplicate this in our MA. Interestingly in this subsequent analysis, there was no effect of anxiety

of PTB in either Black or White women and the ORs were very similar: 1.4 (95% CI 0.34, 5.0) for Black women and 1.6 (95% CI 0.6, 3.7) for White women.

Exposure

We had originally planned to examine the effect of exposure (degree of anxiety) but this became impossible to do. There were more than 13 validated scales used amongst the 37 studies, and many of these had been adapted in some form. Additionally many scales were "Researcher Developed" for the purpose of the study and others adapted from some Researcher Developed scales. Even for the validated scales, different cut-off values were used and some were intrinsically binary (such as diagnoses). We have included these in Table 3, which may help describe the sources of heterogeneity across the studies.

Other Sources of Bias

Several limitations of this MA arise from the inherent limitations of the included studies as evident in the critical appraisal conducted. Many studies did not have a cohort representative of the population, as described earlier, making it difficult to generalize the results to all pregnant women with or without anxiety. Many of the included studies did not identify and account for all confounding variables, making it difficult to determine if their results are valid, whereas other studies inappropriately adjusted their estimates with variables highly correlated with anxiety. In addition, 8 of the 35 studies that looked at the relationship between anxiety and PTB were excluded because of the limited information they provided. We did not examine publication bias using Funnel plots since it has been determined that this analysis has very little power, especially with a small number of studies (Lau et al., 2006; Tang & Liu, 2000).

Future Directions

Our investigation shows consistent findings that there is a statistically significant association

TABLE E.3

CLASSIFICATION OF STUDIES ACCORDING TO WHETHER THE PRIMARY OUTCOME VARIABLE WAS PTB, SPONTANEOUS PTB, OR GESTATIONAL AGE AND THE TYPE OF STATISTIC (ODDS RATIO OR CORRELATION COEFFICIENT) USED TO ESTIMATE THE RELATIONSHIP (TOP PANEL). THE EFFECT OF EXCLUDING ESTIMATES OF DUBIOUS QUALITY ON THE HETEROGENEITY OF THE ESTIMATES OF THE OR FOR ANXIETY AND SPONTANEOUS PTB. THERE WERE THREE EXCLUSION CRITERIA: (1) THE RESULTS OF THE STUDY WERE NUMERICALLY SUSPECT; (2) THE AUTHORS REPORTED THE ODDS RATIO FOR A CONTINUOUS PREDICTOR VARIABLE; (3) THE ODDS RATIO WAS INAPPROPRIATELY ADJUSTED AS DESCRIBED IN SECTION 2.6 (LOWER PANEL)

STATISTIC	ODDS RATIO		CORRELATION COEFFICIENT	
OUTCOME	SPTB	PTB	PTB	GA
		Berle et al. (2005)		
		Field et al. (2010)		
	Andersson et al. (2004)	Andersson et al. (2004)		Bindt et al. (2013)
	Dole et al. (2004)	Bindt et al. (2013)		Wadhwa et al. (1993)
	Kramer et al. (2009)	Dole et al. (2000)		Dominguez et al. (2005)
	Ibanez et al. (2012)	McDonald et al. (2014)	Glynn et al. (2008)	Dominguez et al. (2008)
	Peacock et al. (1995)	Ibanez et al. (2012)	Lobel et al. (2008)	Mancuso et al. (2004)
	Sanchez et al. (2013)	Amiri et al. (2010)[d]	Wadhwa et al. (1993)	Rini et al. (1999)
	Orr et al. (2007)[a]	Catov et al. (2010)		Lobel et al. (2008)
	Copper et al. (1996)[b]	Powell et al. (2013)[b]		Pagel et al. (1990)
	Dayan et al. (2006)[b]	Perkin et al. (1993)[c]		Lobel et al. (2000)
		Martini et al. (2010)[c]		Hosseini et al. (2009)
		Rauchfuss and Maier (2011)[c]		

Heterogeneity

Before exclusion	76.0%, $p < 0.001$	79.8%, $p < 0.001$	61.9%, $p = 0.073$	0.0, $p = 0.570$
After exclusion	46.9%, $p = 0.094$	0.0%, $p = 0.715$		

Goldenberg et al. (1996) was excluded since it was not possible to extract any relevant information and Latendresse and Ruiz (2011) only provided information on the mean (SD) anxiety scores in the mothers of preterm and those of term babies.

[a]Studies that provided adjusted estimates but not in the same form as the unadjusted estimate (i.e., for categorical rather than binary) so the unadjusted estimate was used.
[b]Studies that reported the OR for a continuous predictor variable (excluded).
[c]Studies that used inappropriate adjustment in the multivariable analysis and no unadjusted estimate available (excluded).
[d]Studies that were numerically suspect (excluded).

between maternal anxiety during pregnancy and PTB; the results, however, cannot assume causality. The relationship between maternal anxiety during pregnancy and PTB currently satisfies the Bradford Hill criteria (Hill, 1965) of specificity (pregnant women giving birth to preterm babies), temporality (prenatal anxiety occurs before PTB), and, with the addition of the results of this paper, consistency. In order to further satisfy the Bradford Hill criteria it would be practical to create a prenatal program designed to reduce PSA and/or SA in pregnant women. This intervention could then be utilized in a randomized-control trial (RCT) to determine if the reduction in PSA improves PTB rates. If the results of the RCT show that there is a statistically significant difference between the control group and the group with the anxiety reduction intervention, then we can begin to assume that PSA causes PTB and this would have enormous implications for health promotion in pregnant women. We identified that the OR for prenatal anxiety and PTB is of the order of 1.3 to 2.0 (considering the limits of the CI). What does this mean on a global level? We used data provided by Blencowe et al. (2013) that reports the number of births and the preterm birth rate in seven different regions of the world in 2010. If we estimate that 25% of pregnant women have some form of anxiety and take a very conservative estimate of the RR of about 1.3, then in Northern Africa and Western Asia, the number of PTB that could be prevented by treating anxiety during pregnancy (Attributable Fraction) would be very close to 44,000 and in Southern Asia would be 303,000 in one year. If we consider a less conservative RR (2.0) the number prevented in Northern Africa and Western Asia would be 150,000 and over 1,000,000 in Southern Asia.

CONCLUSIONS

There was substantial heterogeneity across the studies for those reporting OR for spontaneous PTB and PTB, but after excluding studies that used inappropriate methods of adjustment or reported the OR for a unit or 5-unit increase in anxiety, the heterogeneity was substantially reduced. Further reductions in heterogeneity were observed when the primary predictor variable was restricted to SA and PSA. Consistent findings indicate a significant association between prenatal maternal anxiety and PTB; therefore, a prenatal program designed to reduce maternal anxiety during pregnancy could decrease the burden of PTB on the healthcare system.

REFERENCES

Alder, J., Fink, N., Bitzer, J., Hösli, I., & Holzgreve, W. (2007). Depression and anxiety during pregnancy: a risk factor for obstetric, fetal and neonatal outcome? A critical review of the literature. *Journal of Maternal-Fetal and Neonatal Medicine, 20*(3), 189–209.

Alipour, Z., Lamyian, M., & Hajizadeh, E. (2012). Anxiety and fear of childbirth as predictors of post-natal depression in nulliparous women. *Women and Birth, 25*(3), e37–e43.

Amiri, F., Mohamadpour, R., Salmalian, H., & Ahmadi, A. (2010). The association between prenatal anxiety and spontaneous preterm birth and low birth weight. *Iranian Red Crescent Medical Journal, 12*(6), 650–654.

Andersson, L., Sundström-Poromaa, I., Wulff, M., Åström, M., & Bixo, M. (2004). Neonatal outcome following maternal antenatal depression and anxiety: a population-based study. *American Journal of Epidemiology, 159*(9), 872–881.

Arch, J. J. (2013). Pregnancy-specific anxiety: which women are highest and what are the alcohol-related risks? *Comprehensive Psychiatry, 54*(3), 217–228.

Berle, J.Ø., Mykletun, A., Daltveit, A. K., Rasmussen, S., Holsten, F., & Dahl, A. A. (2005). Neonatal outcomes in offspring of women with anxiety and depression during pregnancy. *Archives of Women's Mental Health, 8*(3), 181–189.

Bhagwanani, S. G., Seagraves, K., Dierker, L. J., & Lax, M. (1997). Relationship between prenatal anxiety and perinatal outcome in nulliparous women: a prospective study. *Journal of the National Medical Association, 89*(2), 93–98.

Bindt, C., Guo, N., Te Bonle, M., et al. (2013). No association between antenatal common mental disorders in low-obstetric risk women and adverse birth outcomes in their offspring: results from the CDS study in Ghana and Côte D'Ivoire. *PLoS ONE, 8*(11), e80711. Article ID.

Blair, M. M., Glynn, L. M., Sandman, C. A., & Davis, E. P. (2011). Prenatal maternal anxiety and early childhood temperament. *Stress, 14*(6), 644–651.

Blencowe, H., Cousens, S., Chou, D., et al. (2013). Born Too Soon: the global epidemiology of 15 million preterm births. *Reproductive Health, 10*, article S2.

Borenstein, M., Hedges, L. V., Higgins, J. P. T., & Rothstein, H. R. (2009). *Introduction to Meta-Analysis*. New York, NY: John Wiley & Sons.

Bruce, L., Beland, D., & Bowen, A. (2012). MotherFirst: developing a maternal mental health strategy in Saskatchewan. *Healthcare Policy, 8*(2), 46–55.

Bödecs, T., Horváth, B., Szilágyi, E., Gonda, X., Rihmer, Z., & Sándor, J. (2011). Effects of depression, anxiety, self-esteem, and health behaviour on neonatal outcomes in a population-based Hungarian sample. *European Journal of Obstetrics & Gynecology and Reproductive Biology, 154*(1), 45–50.

CASP Checklist. (2014). Critical Appraisal Skills Programme. http://www.casp-uk.net/#!checklists/cb36.

Catov, J. M., Abatemarco, D. J., Markovic, N., & Roberts, J. M. (2010). Anxiety and optimism associated with gestational age at birth and fetal growth. *Maternal and Child Health Journal, 14*(5), 758–764.

Catov, J. M., Flint, M., Lee, M., Roberts, J. M., & Abatemarco, D. J. (2014). The relationship between race, inflammation and psychosocial factors among pregnant women. *Maternal and Child Health Journal, 19*(2), 401–409.

Copper, R. L., Goldenberg, R. L., Das, A., et al. (1996). The preterm prediction study: maternal stress is associated with spontaneous preterm birth at less than thirty-five weeks' gestation. *American Journal of Obstetrics and Gynecology, 175*(5), 1286–1292.

Dayan, J., Creveuil, C., Herlicoviez, M., et al. (2002). Role of anxiety and depression in the onset of spontaneous preterm labor. *American Journal of Epidemiology, 155*(4), 293–301.

Dayan, J., Creveuil, C., Marks, M. N., et al. (2006). Prenatal depression, prenatal anxiety, and spontaneous preterm birth: a prospective cohort study among women with early and regular care. *Psychosomatic Medicine, 68*(6), 938–946.

Ding, X.-X., Wu, Y.-L., Xu, S.-J., et al. (2014). Maternal anxiety during pregnancy and adverse birth outcomes: a systematic review and meta-analysis of prospective cohort studies. *Journal of Affective Disorders, 159*, 103–110.

Dole, N., Savitz, D. A., Siega-Riz, A. M., Hertz-Picciotto, I., McMahon, M. J., & Buekens, P. (2004). Psychosocial factors and preterm birth among African American and white women in central North Carolina. *American Journal of Public Health, 94*(8), 1358–1365.

Dominguez, T. P., Dunkel-Schetter, C., Glynn, L. M., Hobel, C., & Sandman, C. A. (2008). Racial differences in birth outcomes: the role of general, pregnancy, and racism stress. *Health Psychology, 27*(2), 194–203.

Dominguez, T. P., Schetter, C. D., Mancuso, R., Rini, C. M., & Hobel, C. (2005). Stress in African American pregnancies: testing the roles of various stress concepts in prediction of birth outcomes. *Annals of Behavioral Medicine, 29*(1), 12–21.

Dunkel-Schetter, C., & Glynn, L. M. (2011). Stress in pregnancy: empirical evidence and theoretical issues to guide interdisciplinary research. In *The Handbook of Stress Science: Biology, Psychology and Health* (pp. 321–344): Springer.

Field, T., Diego, M., Hernandez-Reif, M., et al. (2010). Comorbid depression and anxiety effects on pregnancy and neonatal outcome. *Infant Behavior and Development, 33*(1), 23–29.

Glynn, L. M., Dunkel-Schetter, C., Hobel, C. J., & Sandman, C. A. (2008). Pattern of perceived stress and anxiety in pregnancy predicts preterm birth. *Health Psychology, 27*(1), 43–51.

Goldenberg, R. L., Cliver, S. P., Mulvihill, F. X., et al. (1996). Medical, psychosocial, and behavioral risk factors do not explain the increased risk for low birth weight among black women. *American Journal of Obstetrics and Gynecology, 175*(5), 1317–1324.

Goldenberg, R. L., Culhane, J. F., Iams, J. D., & Romero, R. (2008). Epidemiology and causes of preterm birth. *The Lancet, 371*(9606), 75–84.

Hall, W. A., Stoll, K., Hutton, E. K., & Brown, H. (2012). A prospective study of effects of psychological factors and sleep on obstetric interventions, mode of birth, and neonatal outcomes among low-risk British Columbian women. *BMC Pregnancy and Childbirth, 12*, article 78.

Hill, A. B. (1965). The environment and disease: association or causation? *Proceedings of the Royal Society of Medicine, 58*(5), 295–300.

Hosseini, S. M., Biglan, M. W., Larkby, C., Brooks, M. M., Gorin, M. B., & Day, N. L. (2009). Trait anxiety in pregnant women predicts offspring birth outcomes. *Paediatric and Perinatal Epidemiology, 23*(6), 557–566.

Ibanez, G., Charles, M.-A., Forhan, A., et al. (2012). Depression and anxiety in women during pregnancy and neonatal outcome: data from the EDEN mother-child cohort. *Early Human Development, 88*(8), 643–649.

Kramer, M. S., Lydon, J., Séguin, L., et al. (2009). Stress pathways to spontaneous preterm birth: the role of stressors, psychological distress, and stress hormones. *American Journal of Epidemiology, 169*(11), 1319–1326.

Latendresse, G., & Ruiz, R. J. (2011). Maternal corticotropin-releasing hormone and the use of selective serotonin reuptake inhibitors independently predict the occurrence of preterm birth. *Journal of Midwifery and Women's Health, 56*(2), 118–126.

Lau, J., Ioannidis, J. P. A., Terrin, N., Schmid, C. H., & Olkin, I. (2006). The case of the misleading funnel plot. *British Medical Journal, 333*(7568), 597–600.

Levi, R., Lundberg, U., Hanson, U., & Frankenhacuser, M. (1989). Anxiety during pregnancy after the Chernobyl accident as related to obstetric outcome. *Journal of Psychosomatic Obstetrics and Gynecology, 10*(3), 221–230.

Littleton, H. L., Breitkopf, C. R., & Berenson, A. B. (2007). Correlates of anxiety symptoms during pregnancy and association with perinatal outcomes: a meta-analysis. *American Journal of Obstetrics and Gynecology, 196*(5), 424–432.

Lobel, M., Cannella, D. L., Graham, J. E., DeVincent, C., Schneider, J., & Meyer, B. A. (2008). Pregnancy-specific stress, prenatal health behaviors, and birth outcomes. *Health Psychology, 27*(5), 604–615.

Lobel, M., DeVincent, C. J., Kaminer, A., & Meyer, B. A. (2000). The impact of prenatal maternal stress and optimistic disposition on birth outcomes in medically high-risk women. *Health Psychology, 19*(6), 544–553.

Mancuso, R. A., Schetter, C. D., Rini, C. M., Roesch, S. C., & Hobel, C. J. (2004). Maternal prenatal anxiety and corticotropin-releasing hormone associated with timing of delivery. *Psychosomatic Medicine, 66*(5), 762–769.

Martini, J., Knappe, S., Beesdo-Baum, K., Lieb, R., & Wittchen, H.-U. (2010). Anxiety disorders before birth and self-perceived distress during pregnancy: associations with maternal depression and obstetric, neonatal and early childhood outcomes. *Early Human Development, 86*(5), 305–310.

McDonald, S. W., Kingston, D., Bayrampour, H., Dolan, S. M., & Tough, S. C. (2014). Cumulative psychosocial stress, coping resources, and preterm birth. *Archives of Women's Mental Health, 17*(6), 559–568.

McDowell, I. (2006). *Measuring Health: A Guide to Rating Scales and Questionnaires* (3rd edition). Oxford, UK: Oxford University Press.

Orr, S. T, Reiter, J. P., Blazer, D. G., & James, S. A. (2007). Maternal prenatal pregnancy-related anxiety and spontaneous preterm birth in Baltimore, Maryland. *Psychosomatic Medicine, 69*(6), 566–570.

Pagel, M. D., Smilkstein, G., Regen, H., & Montano, D. (1990). Psychosocial influences on new born outcomes: a controlled prospective study. *Social Science and Medicine, 30*(5), 597–604.

Peacock, J. L., Bland, J. M., & Anderson, H. R. (1995). Preterm delivery: effects of socioeconomic factors, psychological stress, smoking, alcohol, and caffeine. *British Medical Journal, 311*(7004), 531–536. 1995.

Perkin, M. R., Bland, J. M., Peacock, J. L., & Anderson, H. R. (1993). The effect of anxiety and depression during pregnancy on obstetric complications. *British*

Journal of Obstetrics and Gynaecology, 100(7), 629–634.

Powell, H., McCaffery, K., Murphy, V. E., et al. (2013). Psychosocial variables are related to future exacerbation risk and perinatal outcomes in pregnant women with asthma. *Journal of Asthma, 50*(4), 383–389.

Rauchfuss, M., & Maier, B. (2011). Biopsychosocial predictors of preterm delivery. *Journal of Perinatal Medicine, 39*(5), 515–521.

Rini, C. K., Dunkel-Schetter, C., Wadhwa, P. D., & Sandman, C. A. (1999). Psychological adaptation and birth outcomes: the role of personal resources, stress, and sociocultural context in pregnancy. *Health Psychology, 18*(4), 333–345.

Roesch, S. C., Schetter, C. D., Woo, G., & Hobel, C. J. (2004). Modeling the types and timing of stress in pregnancy. *Anxiety, Stress and Coping, 17*(1), 87–102.

Ruiz, R. J., Fullerton, J., & Dudley, D. J. (2003). The interrelationship of maternal stress, endocrine factors and inflammation on gestational length. *Obstetrical and Gynecological Survey, 58*(6), 415–428.

Sanchez, S. E., Puente, G. C., Atencio, G., et al. (2013). Risk of spontaneous preterm birth in relation to maternal depressive, anxiety, and stress symptoms. *Journal of Reproductive Medicine, 58*(1–2), 25–33.

Shapiro, G. D., Fraser, W. D., Frasch, M. G., & Séguin, J. R. (2013). Psychosocial stress in pregnancy and preterm birth: associations and mechanisms. *Journal of Perinatal Medicine, 41*(6), 631–645.

Spielberger, C. D., & Vagg, P. R. (1984). Psychometric properties of the STAI: a reply to Ramanaiah, Franzen, and Schill. *Journal of Personality Assessment, 48*(1), 95–97.

Spielberger, C. D., Gorsuch, R. L., & Lushene, R. E. (1970). *Manual for the State-Trait Anxiety Inventory*. Palo Alto, CA: Consulting Psychologist Press.

Tang, J.-L., & Liu, J. L. (2000). Misleading funnel plot for detection of bias in meta-analysis. *Journal of Clinical Epidemiology, 53*(5), 477–484.

Thompson, S. G. (1994). Why sources of heterogeneity in meta-analysis should be investigated. *British Medical Journal, 309*(6965), 1351–1355.

Uguz, F., Sahingoz, M., Sonmez, E. O., et al. (2013). The effects of maternal major depression, generalized anxiety disorder, and panic disorder on birth weight and gestational age: a comparative study. *Journal of Psychosomatic Research, 75*(1), 87–89.

Uman, L. S. (2011). Systematic reviews and meta-analyses. *Journal of the Canadian Academy of Child and Adolescent Psychiatry, 20*(1), 57–59.

Wadhwa, P. D., Culhane, J. F., Rauh, V., & Barve, S. S. (2001). Stress and preterm birth: neuroendocrine, immune/inflammatory, and vascular mechanisms. *Maternal and Child Health Journal, 5*(2), 119–125.

Wadhwa, P. D., Sandman, C. A., Porto, M., Dunkel-Schetter, C., & Garite, T. J. (1993). The association between prenatal stress and infant birth weight and gestational age at birth: a prospective investigation. *American Journal of Obstetrics and Gynecology, 169*(4), 858–865.

Wen, S. W., Smith, G., Yang, Q., & Walker, M. (2004). Epidemiology of preterm birth and neonatal outcome. *Seminars in Fetal and Neonatal Medicine, 9*(6), 429–435.

Zeidner, M. (2010). Anxiety. *International Encyclopedia of Education*, 549–557.

Glossary

A

a priori From Latin, meaning "the former"; that is, before the study or analysis.

abstract A brief, comprehensive summary of a study at the beginning of an article.

accessible population A population that meets the population criteria and is available.

accuracy The characteristic of all aspects of a study systematically and logically following from the research problem.

after-only design An experimental design with two randomly assigned groups: a treatment group and a control group. This design differs from the true experiment in that both groups are measured only after the experimental treatment. Also known as *posttest-only control group design*.

after-only nonequivalent control group design A quasiexperimental design similar to the after-only experimental design except that participants are not randomly assigned to the treatment group or the control group.

aim of inquiry The goals or specific objectives of the research, which vary with the *paradigm*.

alpha Considered an a priori probability because it is set before the data are collected. Also considered a conditional probability because the null hypothesis is assumed to be true.

alpha coefficient See *reliability coefficient*.

alternate-form reliability A reliability measure in which two or more alternate forms of a measure are administered to the same participants at different times. The scores of the two tests determine the degree of relationship between the measures. Also called *parallel-form reliability*.

analysis of covariance (ANCOVA) A statistic that measures differences among group means and uses a statistical technique to equate the groups under study in relation to an important variable.

analysis of variance (ANOVA) A statistic that tests whether group means differ from each other; instead of testing each pair of means separately, ANOVA considers the variation among all groups.

animal rights Guidelines used to protect the rights of animals in the conduct of research.

anonymity A research participant's protection in a study so that no one, not even the researcher, can link the subject with the information given.

antecedent variable A variable that affects the dependent variable but occurs before the introduction of the independent variable.

assent An aspect of informed consent that pertains to protecting the rights of children as research participants.

assimilation The process by which a minority population is absorbed into a prevailing dominant culture.

assumptions Accepted truths, key concepts and ideas, reasons and justifications, supporting examples, parallel experiences, implications and consequences, and any other structural features of the written text used to interpret and assess it accurately and fairly.

attrition The loss of a subject from a study between time 1 data collection and time 2 data collection. Also called *mortality*.

auditability The characteristic of a qualitative study, developed by the investigator's research process, that allows another researcher or a reader to follow the thinking or conclusions of the investigator.

B

behavioural/materialist perspective In ethnographical studies, the observation of culture through a group's patterns of behaviour and customs, its way of life, and what it produces.

beneficence An obligation to do no harm and to maximize possible benefits.

benefits Potential positive outcomes of participation in a research study.

bias A distortion in the interpretation of the results of the data analysis.

biological measurement Use of specialized equipment to determine the biological status of participants in a study.

Boolean operator In a literature search, the word that defines the relationships between words or groups of words; for example, "AND," "OR," "NOT," or "NEAR."

bracketing A process by which the researcher identifies personal biases about the phenomenon of interest to clarify how personal experience and beliefs may colour what is heard and reported. The term comes from the mathematical metaphor of putting "brackets" around our beliefs so they can be put aside.

C

case study method   The study of a selected contemporary phenomenon over time to provide an in-depth description of the essential dimensions and processes of the phenomenon.

chance error   An error attributable to fluctuations in subject characteristics that occur at a specific point in time and are often beyond the awareness and control of the examiner; an error that is difficult to control, unsystematic, and unpredictable and thus cannot be corrected. Also called *random error.*

chi-square (χ^2)   A nonparametric statistic used to determine whether the frequency found in each category is different from the frequency that would be expected by chance.

citation management software   A software program that formats and stores the researcher's citations so that they are available for electronic retrieval.

clinical question   An inquiry that is the basis of evidence-informed practice. A clinical question concerns five components: population, intervention, comparison, outcome, and time (PICOT).

closed-ended item   A question that the respondent may answer with only one of a fixed number of choices.

cluster sampling   A probability sampling strategy that involves successive random sampling of units. The units sampled progress from large to small. Also known as *multi-stage sampling.*

codes   Tags or labels that are assigned to themes in a qualitative study.

coding   The progressive marking, sorting, resorting, and defining and redefining of the collected data.

cognitive perspective   In ethnographical studies, the view that culture consists of beliefs, knowledge, and ideas people use as they live.

Cohen's kappa   The level of agreement observed beyond the level that would be expected by chance alone.

cohort   The participants of a specific group that are being studied.

colonization   A state-driven process of settling an area for a variety of purposes that include labour exploitation of local inhabitants, direct resource extraction, tribute collection, and/or religious conversion. It is a form of imperialism.

community-based participatory research (CBPR)   A method by which the voice of a community is systematically accessed in order to plan context-appropriate action.

concealment   An observational method that refers to whether or not the participants know that they are being observed.

concept   An image or symbolic representation of an abstract idea.

conceptual definition   The general meaning of a concept.

conceptual framework   A structure of concepts, theories, or both that is used to construct a map for the study.

concurrent validity   The degree of correlation between two measures of the same concept that are administered at the same time.

conduct of research   The analysis of data collected from a homogeneous group of participants who meet study inclusion and exclusion criteria for the purpose of answering specific research questions or testing specified hypotheses.

confidence interval   An estimated range of values, which are likely to include an unknown population parameter calculated from a given set of sample data. Abbreviated *CI.*

confidentiality   Assurance that a research participant's identity cannot be linked to the information that was provided to the researcher.

consent   Agreement to participate in a study. See *informed consent.*

consistency   An aspect of the data-collection process that requires that data be collected from each subject in the study in exactly the same way or as close to the same way as possible.

constancy   An aspect of control in data collection that ensures that methods and procedures of data collection are the same for all participants; that is, each participant is exposed to the same environmental conditions, timing of data collection, data-collection instruments, and data-collection procedures.

constant comparative method   In the grounded theory method, a process of continuously comparing data as they are acquired during research.

constant error   See *systematic error.*

construct validity   The extent to which a test measures a theoretical construct or trait.

constructivism   The basis for *naturalistic* (qualitative) research, which developed from writers such as Immanuel Kant, who sought alternative ways of thinking about the world; a belief that reality is not fixed but rather is a construction of the people perceiving it.

constructivist paradigm   The basis of most qualitative research, which is concerned with the ways in which people construct their worlds.

consumer   A person whose activity uses and applies research.

content validity   The degree to which the content of the measure represents the universe of content or the domain of a given behaviour.

context   The personal, social, and political environment in which a phenomenon of interest (time, place, cultural beliefs, values, and practices) occurs.

context dependent   Condition in which the meaning of an observation is defined by its circumstance or the environment.

contrasted-groups approach   A method used to assess construct validity. A researcher identifies two groups of individuals who are suspected of having either an extremely high or an extremely low score on a characteristic; scores from the groups are obtained and examined for sensitivity to the differences. Also called *known-groups approach*.

control   The measures used to hold uniform or constant the conditions in a research study.

control group   The group in an experimental investigation that does not receive the experimental intervention or treatment; the comparison group.

controlled vocabulary   A selected list of words and phrases that are applied to similar pieces of information units (e.g., life skills).

convenience sampling   A nonprobability sampling strategy in which the most readily accessible persons or objects serve as participants or participants of a study.

convergent validity   A type of construct validity in which two or more tools that theoretically measure the same construct are positively correlated.

correlation   The degree of association between two variables.

correlational study   A type of nonexperimental research that examines the relationship between two or more variables.

credibility   A characteristic of qualitative research that refers to the accuracy, validity, and soundness of data.

criterion-related validity   The degree of relationship between performance on the measure and the actual behaviour, either in the present (concurrent) or in the future (predictive).

critical appraisal   A systematic process for reviewing evidence, see *critique*

critical reading   An active interpretation and objective assessment of an article, during which the reader is looking for key concepts, ideas, and justifications.

critical social theory   The use of both qualitative and quantitative research to highlight historical and current experiences of suffering, conflict, and collective struggles.

critical social thought   A philosophical orientation that suggests that reality and a person's understanding of reality are constructed by people with the most power at a particular point in history.

critical thinking   The rational examination of ideas, inferences, assumptions, principles, arguments conclusions, issues, statements, beliefs, and actions.

critique   The process of objectively and critically evaluating the content of a research report for scientific merit and application to practice, theory, or education.

critiquing criteria   The standards, appraisal guides, or questions used for objectively and critically evaluating a research article.

Cronbach's alpha   A test of internal consistency in which each item in a scale is simultaneously compared with all others.

cross-sectional study   Nonexperimental research in which data at one point in time—that is, in the immediate present—are examined.

culture   The system of knowledge and linguistic expressions used by social groups that allows the researcher to interpret or make sense of the world; the structures of meaning through which people shape experiences.

D

data   Information systematically collected in the course of a study; the plural of *datum*.

data analysis   The process of manipulating the data so that it can be used to answer the research question.

data display   Compression and organization of data that promote understanding and visualization and enable conclusions to be drawn.

data reduction   The process of selecting and transforming the data from field notes or transcriptions.

data saturation   A point when the information collected by the researcher becomes repetitive; ideas conveyed by the participant have been shared previously by other participants, and inclusion of additional participants does not result in new ideas.

debriefing   The opportunity for researchers to discuss the study with the participants and for participants to refuse to have their data included in the study.

decolonization   Undoing the effects of colonization, including many aspects, such as recovery of history, culture, language and identity; mourning continued oppression, and imagining new possibilities.

deductive   Concluded from data.

deductive reasoning   A logical thought process in which hypotheses are derived from theory; reasoning moves from the general to the particular.

degree of freedom   The number of quantities that are unknown minus the number of independent equations linking these unknowns; a function of the number in the sample. Abbreviated *df*.

delimitations   Characteristics that restrict the population to a homogeneous group of participants.

dependent variable   In experimental studies, the presumed effect of the independent or experimental variable on the outcome. Variation in the independent variable changes this effect. The dependent variable is observed but not manipulated.

descriptive/exploratory survey   A type of nonexperimental research in which descriptions of existing phenomena are collected for the purpose of using the data to justify or assess current conditions or to make plans for improvement of conditions.

descriptive statistics Statistical details used to describe and summarize sample data.

descriptive/exploratory survey Research when two methods (descriptive and exploratory) are combined in one study.

developmental study A type of nonexperimental research that is concerned not only with the existing status and interrelationships of phenomena but also with changes that occur as a function of time.

directional hypothesis A hypothesis that specifies the expected direction of the relationship between independent and dependent variables.

dissemination The communication of research findings.

divergent validity A type of construct validity in which two or more tools that theoretically measure the opposite of the construct are negatively correlated.

domains In an ethnographic study, symbolic categories that include smaller categories.

E

effect size Measurement of the magnitude of a treatment effect; how large of a difference is observed between the groups.

element The most basic unit about which information is collected.

eligibility criteria Characteristics of a population that meet requirements for inclusion in a study.

emic perspective The native's or insider's view of the world.

epidemiological study Examination of factors affecting the health and illness of populations in relation to the environment.

epistemology The theory of knowledge; the branch of philosophy concerned with how people know what they know, or what is known to be "truth."

equivalence Consistency or agreement among observers using the same measurement tool, or agreement among alternative forms of a tool.

error variance The extent to which the variance in test scores is attributable to error rather than to a true measure of behaviours.

ethics The theory or discipline dealing with principles of moral values and moral conduct.

ethnographic method A method that scientifically describes cultural groups. The goal of the ethnographer is to understand the natives' view of their world.

ethnography A qualitative research approach designed to produce cultural theory. Also called *ethnographic research*.

etic perspective An outsider's view of another's world.

evaluation The process of determining the value of data.

evaluation research The use of scientific research methods and procedures to evaluate a program, treatment, practice, or policy outcome; the analytical means used to document the worth of an activity.

evidence-based practice The conscious, explicit, and judicious use of the current best evidence in the care of patients and the delivery of health care services.

evidence-informed practice Acknowledging and considering the myriad factors beyond such evidence as local indigenous knowledge, cultural and religious norms, and clinical judgement.

evidence-informed practice guidelines Principles that help the researcher better understand the evidence base of certain practices.

exclusion criteria Criteria used to exclude individuals from participating in a study.

experiment A scientific investigation in which observations are made and data are collected by means of the characteristics of control, randomization, and manipulation.

experimental design A research design that has the following properties: randomization, control, and manipulation.

experimental group The group in an experimental investigation that receives the experimental intervention or treatment.

ex post facto study A type of nonexperimental research that examines the relationships among variables after variations have occurred. Also known as a *causal-comparative study*, a *comparative study*, and (by epidemiologists) a *retrospective study*.

external criticism A process used to judge the authenticity of historical data.

external validity The degree to which the findings of a study can be generalized to other populations or environments.

extraneous variable A variable that interferes with the operations of the phenomena being studied. Also called *mediating variable*.

F

face validity A type of content validity in which an expert's opinion is used to judge the accuracy of an instrument.

factor analysis A strategy for assessing construct validity in which a statistical procedure is used to determine the underlying dimensions or components of a variable and to assess the degree to which the individual items on a scale truly cluster around one or more dimensions.

feasibility The capability of the study to be successfully carried out.

findings The statistical results of a study and the conclusions, interpretations, recommendations, generalizations, and implications for future research and nursing practice.

Fisher's exact probability test An analysis used to compare frequencies when samples are small and expected frequencies are less than six in each cell.

fittingness The degree to which study findings are applicable outside the study situation and how meaningful the results are to individuals not involved in the research.

focus group A group of people interviewed about a phenomenon of interest in a qualitative study.

formative evaluation Assessment of a program as it is being implemented, usually focusing on evaluation of the process of a program rather than the outcomes.

frequency distribution A descriptive statistical method for summarizing the occurrences of events under study.

G

generalizability The extent to which data can be inferred to be representative of similar phenomena in a population beyond the studied sample.

"grand tour" question A question in a qualitative study that reflects a broad overview of the issue to be studied.

grounded theory method An inductive approach in which a systematic set of procedures is used to develop theory about basic social processes.

H

Hawthorne effect See *reactivity*.

hermeneutics A theoretical framework in which to understand or interpret human phenomena from the study of those phenomena.

heterogeneity Dissimilarities of a sample group, which inhibit the researchers' ability to interpret the findings meaningfully and make generalizations.

hierarchical linear modelling (HLM) A type of regression analysis that allows for analysis of hierarchically structured data simultaneously at all levels.

historical research method The systematic approach for understanding the past through collection, organization, and critical appraisal of facts.

history threat The threat to internal validity that events outside of the experimental setting may affect the dependent variable.

homogeneity A similarity of conditions. Also called *internal consistency*.

homogeneous Having limited variation in attributes or characteristics.

hypothesis A best guess or prediction about what a researcher expects to find with regard to the relationship between two or more variables.

hypothesis-testing approach A strategy for assessing construct validity in which the theory or concept underlying a measurement instrument's design is used to develop hypotheses that are tested. Inferences are made based on the findings about whether the rationale underlying the instrument's construction is adequate to explain the findings.

I

imperialism Process of territory expansion and political hegemony over another population generally through force (Beaule, 2017).

incidence The number of cases occurring in a particular period.

inclusion criteria Criteria that an individual must satisfy to participate in a study.

independent variable The antecedent or variable that has the presumed effect on the dependent variable. The independent variable is manipulated in experimental research studies.

Indigenous knowledge Ways of knowing and knowledge systems based on Indigenous peoples' communities, language, traditions, and history.

Indigenous methodologies Theory and process of conducting research that reflects Indigenous worldviews.

Indigenous peoples An umbrella term used to represent First Nations, Inuit, and Métis people.

inductive Generalizing from specific data.

inductive reasoning A logical thought process in which generalizations are developed from specific observations; reasoning moves from the particular to the general.

inferential statistics Statistical details that combine mathematical processes and logic to test hypotheses about a population with the help of sample data.

informed consent An ethical principle that requires a researcher to inform individuals about the potential benefits and risks of a study before the individuals can participate voluntarily.

instrumental case study Research undertaken to pursue insight into an issue or to challenge a generalization.

instrumentation threats Changes in the measurement of the variables that may account for changes in the obtained measurement.

internal consistency The extent to which items within a scale reflect or measure the same concept. Also called *homogeneity*.

internal criticism The process of judging the reliability or consistency of information within a historical document.

internal validity The degree to which the experimental treatment, not an uncontrolled condition, resulted in the observed effects.

interpretive description A qualitative research method that focuses on applicability in a practice setting.

interrater reliability   The consistency of observations between two or more observers; often expressed as a percentage of agreement between raters or observers or a coefficient of agreement that takes into account the element of chance; generally used with the direct observation method.

intersubjectivity   A person's belief that other people share a common world with him or her; an important tenet in phenomenology.

interval measurement   A type of measurement in which events or objects are ranked on a scale, with equal intervals between numbers but with a ranking set arbitrarily at zero (e.g., Celsius temperature).

intervening variable   A condition that occurs during an experimental or quasiexperimental study that affects the dependent variable.

intervention   An observational method that deals with whether or not the observer provokes actions from those who are being observed.

intervention fidelity   Consistency in data collection.

interview   A method of data collection in which a data collector questions a subject verbally. Such an interview may occur face to face, over the telephone, or by Skype or other electronic media, and may consist of open-ended or close-ended questions.

intrinsic case study   Research undertaken to gain a better understanding of the essential nature of the case.

item-to-total correlation   The relationship between each item on a scale and the total scale.

J

justice   The principle that human participants should be treated fairly.

K

key informants   Individuals who have special knowledge, status, or communication skills and who are willing to share their expertise with the ethnographer.

knowledge translation   A process where knowledge that has evolved from research is put into practice.

knowledge-focused triggers   Research ideas that are generated when staff read research, listen to scientific papers at research conferences, or encounter evidence-based practice guidelines published by federal agencies or specialty organizations.

known-groups approach   See *contrasted-groups approach*.

Kuder-Richardson (KR-20) coefficient   The estimate of homogeneity used for instruments in which a dichotomous response pattern is used.

kurtosis   The relative peakness or flatness of a distribution.

L

level of significance (alpha level)   The risk of making a type I error, set by the researcher before the study begins.

levels of measurement   Categorization of the precision with which an event can be measured (nominal, ordinal, interval, and ratio).

Likert-type scale   A list of statements for which responses are varying degrees of agreement or opinion; for example, "strongly agree," "agree," "no opinion," "disagree," or "strongly disagree."

limitations   The weaknesses of a study.

literature review   An extensive, systematic, and critical review of the most important published scholarly literature on a particular topic. In most cases, the literature review is not considered exhaustive.

lived experience   In phenomenological research, the focus on undergoing events and circumstances (prelingual), as opposed to thinking about these events and circumstances (conceptualized experience).

logistic regression (logit analysis)   The analysis of relationships between multiple independent variables and a dependent variable that is binary, ordinal, or polynomial.

longitudinal study   A nonexperimental research design in which a researcher collects data from the same group at different points in time. Also called *prospective study* and *repeated-measures study*.

M

manipulation   The provision of some experimental treatment, in varying degrees, to some of the participants in the study.

matching   A special sampling strategy used to construct an equivalent comparison sample group by filling it with participants who are similar to each subject in another sample group in terms of pre-established variables, such as age and gender.

maturation   Developmental, biological, or psychological processes that operate within an individual as a function of time and are external to the events of the investigation.

mean (M)   A measure of central tendency; the arithmetic average of all scores.

measurement   The assignment of numbers to objects or events according to rules.

measurement effects   Changes in the generalizability of study findings to other populations, as a result of administration of a pretest.

measures of central tendency   Descriptive statistical techniques that describe the average member of a sample (e.g., mean, median, and mode).

measures of variability   Descriptive statistical procedures that describe the level of dispersion in sample data.

median   A measure of central tendency; in a range of scores, the middle score (50% of the scores are above it and 50% of the scores are below it).

member checking   In participatory action research, sharing the findings with the participants to know whether the interpretation of their responses is accurate.

meta-analysis   A research method in which the results of multiple studies in a specific area are examined and the findings are synthesized to make conclusions regarding the area of focus.

metasynthesis   A technique for drawing inferences or synthesizing findings from similar or related studies; a type of systematic review applied to qualitative research.

methodological research   The controlled investigation and measurement of the means of gathering and analyzing data; the development and evaluation of data-collection instruments, scales, and techniques.

methodology   Discipline-specific principles, rules, and procedures that guide the process through which knowledge is acquired.

modality   The number of modes, or peaks, in a frequency distribution.

mode   A measure of central tendency; the most frequent score or result.

model   A symbolic representation of a set of concepts that is created to depict relationships.

mortality   The loss of a subject from time 1 data collection to time 2 data collection. Also called *attrition*.

multiple regression   The measure of the relationship between one interval-level dependent variable and several independent variables. Canonical correlation is used when a study has more than one dependent variable.

multistage sampling   A sampling method that involves successive random sampling of units (clusters) that progresses from large to small and meets sample eligibility criteria. Also known as *cluster sampling*.

multitrait-multimethod approach   A type of validation in which more than one method is used to assess the accuracy of an instrument (e.g., observation and interview of anxiety).

multivariate analysis of variance (MANOVA)   A test used to determine differences in group means when a study has more than one dependent variable.

N

narrative inquiry   A field of hermeneutics that focuses on the lived experience and perceptions of experience, in which materials such as in-depth interview transcripts, memoirs, stories, and creative nonfiction are used as sources of data.

naturalistic setting   The environment in which people live in every day, such as homes, schools, and communities.

network sampling   A strategy used for finding samples that are difficult to locate. It entails the use of social networks and the fact that friends tend to have characteristics in common; participants who meet the eligibility criteria are asked for assistance in getting in touch with others who meet the same criteria. Also known as *snowball effect sampling*.

nominal measurement   The level used to classify objects or events into categories without any relative ranking (e.g., gender, hair colour).

nondirectional hypothesis   A hypothesis that indicates the existence of a relationship between the variables but does not specify the anticipated direction of the relationship.

nonequivalent control group design   A quasiexperimental design that is similar to the true experiment, but participants are not randomly assigned to the treatment or the control group.

nonexperimental research design   A research design in which an investigator observes a phenomenon without manipulating the independent variable or variables.

nonparametric statistics   Statistics that are usually used when variables are measured at the nominal or ordinal level because they do not estimate population parameters and involve less restrictive assumptions about the underlying distribution. Also called *distribution-free tests*.

nonparametric tests of significance   Inferential statistics that make no assumptions about the population distribution.

nonprobability sampling   A selection technique in which elements are chosen by nonrandom methods.

normal curve   A statistical curve that is unimodal and symmetrical about the mean.

null hypothesis   A statement that no relationship exists between the variables and that any relationship observed is a result of chance or fluctuations in sampling. Also known as a *statistical hypothesis* or H_o.

O

objective   An adjective describing data that are not influenced by anyone who collects the information.

objectivity   The use of facts without distortion by personal feelings or bias.

observed test score   The actual score obtained in a measure; the true score plus error.

odds ratio   The probability of an event, which is calculated by dividing the odds in the treated or exposed group by the odds in the control group.

one-group pretest–posttest design   A study approach used by researchers when only one group is available for study; participants act as their own controls, and no randomization occurs, thus enhancing the internal validity of the study.

online database An Internet collection of journal sources (periodicals) of research and conceptual articles on a variety of topics (e.g., doctoral dissertations), as well as the publications of professional organizations and various governmental agencies.

ontology The science or study of being or existence and its relationship to nonexistence.

open-ended item A question that respondents may answer in their own words.

operational definition The description of how a concept is measured and what instruments are used to capture the essence of the variable.

operationalization The process of translating concepts into observable, measurable phenomena.

opinion leaders Individuals from the local peer group who are viewed as respected sources of influence, considered by associates to be technically competent, and trusted to judge the fit between the evidence-based practice and the local situation.

ordinal measurement A calculation to show rankings of events or objects; numbers are not equidistant, and zero is arbitrary (class ranking).

orientational qualitative inquiry A qualitative approach in which researchers begin with an ideology or orientation (e.g., feminism, Marxism, critical theory) to direct the investigation, including the research question, methodology, fieldwork, and analysis of the findings.

P

p **value** The conditional probability of obtaining, from the study data, the value of the test statistic that is at least as extreme as that calculated from the data, given that the null hypothesis is true.

paradigm From the Greek word meaning "pattern": a set of beliefs and practices, shared by communities of researchers, that guide the knowledge development process. It is a synonym of *worldview*. See also *philosophical beliefs*.

parallel-form reliability See *alternate-form reliability*.

parameter A characteristic of a population.

parametric statistics Inferential statistics that involve the estimation of at least one parameter, require measurement at the interval level or higher, and involve assumptions about the variables being studied. These assumptions usually include the fact that the variable is normally distributed.

participatory action research (PAR) A form of orientation research that seeks to change society; the researcher studies a particular setting to identify problem areas to improve practice, identify possible solutions, and take action to implement changes.

Pearson correlation coefficient (Pearson *r*) A statistic that is calculated to reflect the degree of relationship between two interval-level variables. Also called *Pearson product-moment correlation coefficient*.

percentile A measure of rank; the percentage of scores that a given score exceeds.

phenomena Occurrences, circumstances, or facts that are perceptible by the senses.

phenomenological method A process of learning and constructing the meaning of human experience through intensive dialogue with persons who are living the experience.

phenomenology A qualitative research approach with the aim of describing experience as it is lived through, before it is conceptualized.

philosophical beliefs The system of motivating values, concepts, principles, and the nature of human knowledge of an individual, group, or culture; see also *paradigm* and *worldview*.

physiological measurement The use of specialized equipment to determine the physical status of participants in a study.

pilot study A small, simple study conducted as a prelude to a larger-scale study (which is often called the "parent study").

population A well-defined set that has certain specified properties.

positivism A philosophical orientation that suggests that a material world exists; that is, things can be sensed (i.e., seen, touched, heard, tasted).

post hoc analysis Comparison of all possible pairs of means after an omnibus ANOVA to determine where the difference lies.

post-positivism The view that a "reality" exists that can be observed, measured, and understood; however, this view is tempered by the belief that science offers an imperfect understanding of the world.

posttest-only control group design See *after-only design*.

power The conditional prior probability that the researcher will make a correct decision to reject the null hypothesis when it is actually false, denoted as 1 − b.

prediction study A type of nonexperimental research design in which the investigator attempts to make a forecast or prediction on the basis of particular phenomena.

predictive validity The degree of correlation between the measure of a concept and some future measure of the same concept.

pre-experimental design The simplest form of research design where one group is studied with no control or comparison group.

prevalence The number of people affected by a disease or health problem.

primary sources Scholarly literature that is written by a person or persons who developed the theory or conducted the research; articles and books by the original author or authors. Primary sources include eyewitness accounts of historical events provided by original documents, films, letters, diaries, records, artifacts, periodicals, and tapes.

print indexes   Paper-based listings of published material, generally used to find journal sources (periodicals) of database and conceptual articles on a variety of topics, as well as publications of professional organizations and various governmental agencies. Most information is now entered into electronic (online) databases.

probability   The long-run relative frequency of an event in repeated trials under similar conditions.

probability sampling   A selection technique in which some form of random selection is used when the sample units are chosen.

problem statement   A statement in a research article in which the research question is articulated.

problem-focused triggers   Research ideas that are identified by staff through quality improvement, risk surveillance, benchmarking data, financial data, or recurrent clinical problems.

process consent   A request for the respondent's continued participation in a study.

product testing   The testing of medical devices.

proposition   A linkage of concepts that lays a foundation for the development of methods that test relationships.

prospective study   A nonexperimental study that begins with an exploration of assumed causes and then moves forward in time to the presumed effect. Also called *longitudinal study* and *repeated-measures study*.

psychometrics   The theory and development of measurement instruments.

purpose   The aims or objectives the investigator hopes to achieve with the research.

purposive sample   A group consisting of particular people who can illuminate the phenomenon they want to study.

purposive sampling   A sampling strategy in which the researcher's knowledge of the population and its elements is used to select the participants.

Q

qualitative descriptive   A method of study in which data are presented as they are and direct descriptions of phenomena are given.

qualitative research   The systematic, interactive, and subjective research method used to describe and give meaning to human experiences. Qualitative research is often conducted in natural settings and uses data that are words or text, as opposed to numerical data, to describe the experiences being studied.

quality improvement   A systematic process for improving patient care.

quantitative research   The process of testing relationships, differences, and cause-and-effect interactions among and between variables. These processes are tested with hypotheses and research questions through the use of objective, precise, and highly controlled measurement techniques to gather information that can be analyzed and summarized statistically.

quasiexperiment   Research in which the researcher initiates an experimental treatment, but some characteristic of a true experiment is lacking.

quasiexperimental design   A research approach in which random assignment is not used, but the independent variable is manipulated and certain mechanisms of control are used.

questionnaire   An instrument designed to gather data from individuals.

quota sampling   A nonprobability sampling strategy that identifies a specific strata of the population and represents the strata proportionately in the sample.

R

random error   See *chance error*.

random selection   A selection process in which each element of the population has an equal and independent chance of being included in the sample.

randomization   A sampling selection procedure in which each person or element in a population has an equal chance of being assigned to either the experimental group or the control group.

range   A measure of variability; the difference between the highest and the lowest scores in a set of sample data.

ratio measurement   The ranking of the order of events or objects that has equal intervals and an absolute zero (e.g., height, weight).

reactivity   The distortion created when those who are being observed change their behaviour because they know that they are being observed. Also known as the *Hawthorne effect*.

recommendations   An investigator's suggestions for the application of a study's results to practice, theory, and future research.

records or available data   Information that is collected from existing materials, such as hospital records, historical documents, and audio or video recordings.

refereed (peer-reviewed) journal   A scholarly journal that has a panel of external and internal reviewers or editors; the panel reviews manuscripts submitted for possible publication. The review panel uses the same set of scholarly criteria to judge whether the manuscripts are worthy of publication.

reflexivity   The situation wherein researchers must monitor whether their own perspectives are affecting their research methods, analyses, or interpretations.

relationship/difference study   A study that traces the relationships or differences between variables that can provide a deeper insight into a phenomenon.

reliability   The consistency or constancy of a measuring instrument; the extent to which the instrument yields the same results on repeated measures.

reliability coefficient   A number between 0 and 1 that expresses the relationship between the error variance, true variance, and the observed score. A correlation of 0 indicates no relationship; the closer to 1 the coefficient is, the more reliable is the tool. Also called the *alpha coefficient*.

representative sample   A sample whose key characteristics closely approximate those of the population.

research   The systematic, rigorous, logical investigation that aims to answer questions about nursing phenomena.

research ethics board (REB)   A board established in agencies to review biomedical and behavioural research involving human participants within the agency or in programs sponsored by the agency to assess whether ethical standards are met in relation to the protection of the rights of human participants.

research hypothesis   A statement about the expected relationship between variables. Also known as a *scientific hypothesis*.

research question   A presentation of an idea that forms the foundation for a study; it is developed from the research problem and results in the research hypothesis.

research utilization   A systematic method of implementing sound research-based innovations in clinical practice, evaluating the outcome, and sharing the knowledge through the process of research dissemination.

respect for persons   The idea that people have the right to self-determination and to being treated as autonomous agents; that is, they have the freedom to participate or not participate in research.

retrospective data   Data that have already been recorded, such as scores on a standard examination.

retrospective study   A nonexperimental research design that begins with the phenomenon of interest (the dependent variable) in the present and examines its relationship to another variable (the independent variable) in the past. Also known as a *causal-comparative study*, a *comparative study*, and (by social scientists) an *ex post facto study*.

rigour   The strictness with which a study is conducted to enhance the quality, believability, or trustworthiness of study findings.

risk–benefit ratio   The extent to which the benefits of the study are maximized and the risks are minimized in such a way that the participants are protected from harm during the study.

risks   The potential negative outcomes of participation in a research study.

S

sample   A subset of sampling units, or elements, from a population.

sampling   A process in which representative units of a population are selected for study in a research investigation.

sampling error   The tendency for statistics to fluctuate from one sample to another.

sampling frame   A list of all units of the population.

sampling interval   The standard distance between the elements chosen for the sample.

sampling unit   The element or set of elements used for selecting the sample.

scale   A self-report measurement tool in which items of indirect interest are combined to obtain an overall score. A set of symbols is used to respond to each item. A rating or score is assigned to each response.

scatter plots   Visual representations of the strength and magnitude of the relationship between two variables.

scientific hypothesis   The researcher's expectation about the outcome of a study. Also known as the *research hypothesis* or H_1.

scientific merit   The degree of validity of a study or group of studies.

scientific observation   The collecting of data about the environment and participants. The observations undertaken are consistent with the specific objectives of the study; the collection of data is systematically planned and recorded; all observations are checked and controlled; and the observations are related to scientific concepts and theories.

secondary analysis   A form of research in which the researcher takes previously collected and analyzed data from one study and reanalyzes the data for a secondary purpose.

secondary sources   Scholarly material written by a person or persons other than the individual who developed the theory or conducted the research. Secondary sources are usually published. Often a secondary source represents a response to or a summary and critique of a theorist's or researcher's work. Examples are documents, films, letters, diaries, records, artifacts, periodicals, and tapes that provide a view of the phenomenon from another's perspective.

selection bias   The threat to internal validity that arises when pretreatment differences exist between the experimental group and the control group.

selection effects   The threat to external validity that occurs when the ideal sample population participants are either too few or unavailable to the researcher.

semiquartile range (semi-interquartile range)   A measure of variability; the range of the middle 50% of the scores.

Sixties Scoop   The large-scale forcible removal by the Child Welfare Systems in Canada of Indigenous children from their families and placement into non-Indigenous families, homes, and institutions in the 1960s–1980s. Children were adopted into or fostered in non-Indigenous homes and suffered loss of identity, culture, and language. Abuse of the children occurred in many of the homes. Many of the adoptions did not last due to the abuse, distrust, and inability of the children to assimilate into a cultural milieu with which they were not familiar. The Sixties Scoop was devastating for Indigenous families and the children, leading to alienation, loss of culture, breakup of families, and use of unhealthy coping mechanisms.

simple random sampling   A probability sampling strategy in which the population is defined, a sampling frame is listed, and a subset from which the sample will be chosen is selected; members are randomly selected.

skew   The measure of the asymmetry of a set of scores.

snowball effect sampling   A strategy used for finding samples that are difficult to locate. This strategy entails the use of social networks and the fact that friends tend to have characteristics in common; participants who meet the eligibility criteria are asked for assistance in getting in touch with others who meet the same criteria. Also known as *snowball sampling*, *snowballing*, and *network sampling*.

snowball sampling   See *snowball effect sampling*.

social desirability   The tendency of a subject to respond in a manner that he or she believes will please the researcher rather than in an honest manner.

Solomon four-group design   An experimental design with four randomly assigned groups: the pretest-posttest intervention group, the pretest-posttest control group, a treatment or intervention group with only posttest measurement, and a control group with only posttest measurement.

split-half reliability   An index of the comparison between the scores on one-half of a test with those on the other half to determine the consistency in response to items that reflect specific content.

stability   An instrument's ability to produce the same results with repeated testing.

standard deviation   A measure of variability; measure of average deviation of scores from the mean. In equations, abbreviated SD.

standard error of the mean   The standard deviation of a theoretical distribution of sample means. It indicates the average error in the estimation of the population mean.

statistic   A characteristic of a sample, described in mathematical terms (e.g., percentage).

statistical hypothesis   A statement that no relationship exists between the independent and dependent variables. Also known as a *null hypothesis*.

stratified random sampling   A probability sampling strategy in which the population is divided into strata or subgroups; members of each strata are homogeneous with regard to certain characteristics. An appropriate number of elements from each subgroup are randomly selected on the basis of their proportion in the population.

summative evaluation   Assessment of the outcomes of a program, conducted after the program's completion.

survey study   A descriptive, exploratory, or comparative study in which researchers collect detailed descriptions of existing variables and use the data to justify and assess current conditions and practices or to make more plans for improving health care practices.

systematic   A term used when data collection is carried out in the same manner with all participants and by all persons collecting the data.

systematic error   An error attributable to the lasting characteristics of the subject that do not tend to fluctuate from one time to another. Also called *constant error*.

systematic review   A summary of research evidence from several studies.

systematic sampling   A probability sampling strategy that involves the selection of participants randomly drawn from a population list at fixed intervals.

systemic racism   When a social group has inequitable access to societal power and resources, leading to inequalities of the group in the society. This inequitable access derives from unfair policies, regulations, procedures, and rules. Social exclusion and isolation are the result, thereby further limiting political, social, and economic participation or access to social systems, programs, and activities (Indigenous Health Working Group of the College of Family Physicians of Canada, 2016).

T

t **statistic**   The test of whether two groups' means are more different than would be expected by chance. The groups may be related or independent.

target population   A population or group of individuals who meet the sampling criteria and about whom the researcher hopes to make generalizations.

testability   The ability of the variables in a proposed study to be observed, measured, and analyzed by quantitative methods.

testable   Measurable by quantitative methods.

testing effect   The effect on the scores of a posttest as the result of having taken a pretest.

test–retest reliability   The stability of the scores of an instrument when it is administered twice to the same participants under the same conditions within a prescribed time interval. The scores from the different times are paired and then compared to determine the stability of the measure.

text   Data in a contextual form; that is, narrative or words that were written from recorded interviews and then transcribed.

thematic analysis The process of recognizing and recovering the emergent themes in data.

themes Clusters of data with structured meaning that occur frequently.

theoretical framework A structure for concepts, theories, or both used to construct a map for the study based on a philosophical or theorized belief or understanding or why the phenomenon under study exists.

theoretical sampling In the grounded theory method, the sampling method used to select experiences that will help the researcher test ideas and gather complete information about developing concepts.

theory A set of interrelated concepts, definitions, and propositions that present a systematic view of phenomena for the purpose of explaining and making predictions about those phenomena.

time series design A quasiexperimental design used to determine trends before and after an experimental treatment. Measurements are taken several times before the introduction of the experimental treatment, the treatment is introduced, and measurements are taken again at specified times afterward.

transferability The extent to which findings from one qualitative research study have meaning to other studies in similar situations.

translation science The investigation of methods, interventions, and variables that influence the adoption of evidence-based practices.

triangulation The expansion of research methods in a single study or multiple studies to enhance diversity, enrich understanding, and accomplish specific goals.

true experiment A study design in which participants are randomly assigned to an experimental group or a control group, pretest measurements are performed, an intervention or treatment occurs in the experimental group, and posttest measurements are performed. Also known as the *pretest-posttest control group design* or *classic experiment*.

trustworthiness An accurate portrayal of the experience of the study's participants; a measure of rigour in qualitative research that includes the concepts of credibility, audibility, and fittingness.

type I error The researchers' incorrect decision to reject the null hypothesis.

type II error As a result of the sample data, the failure to reject the null hypothesis when it is actually false. Also known as *beta* (β).

V

validation sample The sample that provides the initial data for determining the reliability and validity of a measurement tool.

validity The determination of whether a measurement instrument actually measures what it is purported to measure.

values Personal beliefs of the researcher.

variable A defined concept; a property that takes on different values and is studied by quantitative researchers.

W

Web browser A software program used to connect to or search the World Wide Web (e.g., Internet Explorer).

worldview The way people in society think about the world; a synonym for *paradigm*. See also *philosophical beliefs*.

Z

Z score A rating used to compare measurements in standard units; an examination of the relative distance of the scores from the mean.

REFERENCE

Beaule, C. D. (2017). *Frontiers of colonialism.* Oxford: University Press Scholarship. https://www.universitypressscholarship.com/view/10.5744/florida/9780813054346.001.0001/upso-9780813054346-chapter-001.

Answers and Rationales to the Critical Judgement Questions

CHAPTER 1 THE ROLE OF RESEARCH IN NURSING

1. What is the most appropriate source of information for evidence-informed practice?
   c. Clinical practice guideline
   Rationale: These should be systematically developed and based on the most recent evidence.
2. Why are interdisciplinary networks important in research?
   a. Collaboration across disciplines improves patient outcomes
   Rationale: It is important for research to be focussed on patient outcomes, and this occurs across many disciplines.
3. What drives the priorities for healthcare research?
   c. Trends and issues in healthcare
   Rationale: Research is frequently substantiated by solving pressing problems.

CHAPTER 2 THEORETICAL FRAMEWORK

1. Nurses inform their practice through various ways of knowing. Which of the following is NOT true about how nurses use forms of knowledge in practice:
   c. Personal knowing is based on opinions rather than fact
   Rationale: Personal knowing involves an existential awareness of self and others in relationship, which goes beyond the development of opinions.

2. Which of the following statements about research methods is true?
   d. Qualitative research is more appropriate than quantitative research for questions about the meaning of an experience
   Rationale: A researcher chooses between qualitative and quantitative method, based on the question the researcher is asking. If a researcher wishes to discover and understand the meaning of an experience, a qualitative approach would be appropriate.
3. Critical social theory influences nursing because it:
   a. Shows nurses how power imbalances influence health
   Rationale: Critical social theory emphasizes that reality and our understanding of reality are constructed by people with the most power in a particular time and place.

CHAPTER 3 CRITICAL APPRAISAL STRATEGIES: READING RESEARCH

1. What level of evidence is presented in the article that appears in Appendix B?
   b. Level II
   Rationale: This was a randomized, controlled trial, but single-blinded. This means the mothers (and the nurses involved in their care) knew which mothers were in the intervention group and which were in the control group.

2. What are the key features that improve the quality of this study?

   d. Randomization and blinding

   Rationale: These reduce bias in the research.

3. Based on these findings, what would you recommend in practice?

   a. There is insufficient evidence to make recommendations for practice

   Rationale: Often more than a single study is needed to make changes in practice.

CHAPTER 4 DEVELOPING RESEARCH QUESTIONS, HYPOTHESES, AND CLINICAL QUESTIONS

1. Which of the following is the purpose of a hypothesis for any study?

   a. To provide the objective of the research by identifying the expected outcome

   Rationale: Hypothesis is a statement about the relationship between variables that suggests an answer to the research question, and hence it provides a direction to the research.

2. Which of the following identified research problems has enough significance to warrant further development?

   c. Obese males are at risk for heart attacks

   Rationale: This research problem expresses a relationship between obesity and heart attack, specifies the nature of the population to be studied, and implies a possibility of empirical testing.

3. Which part of the following research question is the dependent variable? "How does maternal employment among nurses affect infant health during the first 6 months of life?"

   a. "Infant health"

   Rationale: Infant health is affected by maternal employment of nurses.

CHAPTER 5 FINDING AND APPRAISING THE LITERATURE

1. What is an appropriate reason to use a secondary source?

b. The primary source is written in a language you do not know

Rationale: It is always best practice to go to the original source to ensure accuracy. One exception is when it is in a language you are not able to read.

2. When retrieving evidence to answer a clinical practice question, what is the most useful resource?

   d. Computerized decision support tools

   Rationale: These tools incorporate recent evidence and may also incorporate presenting conditions of the patient. They reduce human error in decision-making.

3. Which of the following sections in a research article can help you quickly decide if a research article is relevant for your purposes?

   c. The abstract and the purpose statement

   Rationale: These two pieces are the most relevant and easiest to find.

CHAPTER 6 LEGAL AND ETHICAL ISSUES

1. You are a staff nurse, and you observe a health care professional coercing a client to agree to participate in a research study. What should you do in this situation?

   a. Contact the hospital's REB

   Rationale: Principle of voluntary consent is violated. Professionals have a responsibility to conduct a study in an ethical manner without coercing the participants. Coercing clients who are under the care of healthcare professional to participate in a research study is unethical. REBs oversee the ethical conduct of a research study.

2. A woman newly diagnosed with breast cancer is asked to participate in a clinical trial for a new chemotherapy agent. Which of her human rights is protected by her freedom to choose whether or not to participate in the study?

   b. Right to self-determination

   Rationale: Autonomy or right to self-determination is an ethical principle that ensures the freedom of choice to participate or not to participate in a research study.

3. Which of the following ethical principles is violated when a potential subject refuses to participate in a clinical study and, in response, the physician takes less time to answer this patient's questions than he does with other patients?

b. Promoting Health and Well-Being

Rationale: Promoting health and well-being of the clients is a fundamental ethical duty of a physician irrespective of the behaviour of the patient. Failing to treat a patient in an unfair manner interferes with the health and well-being of the patient.

CHAPTER 7 INDIGENOUS PEOPLES: RESEARCH, KNOWLEDGES, AND WAYS OF KNOWING

1. Which of the following should be present in a research report about Indigenous peoples?

b. Evidence of established and ongoing relationships

Rationale: This is a key research principle across different Indigenous groups

2. What was one of the main effects of residential schools on Indigenous knowledge?

a. Loss of language and transmission of knowledge

Rationale: The loss of language has reduced the ability for knowledge to be shared.

3. Why is use of an Indigenous methodology important for research?

c. Many viewpoints can be represented in the methodology

Rationale: Indigenous methodology is not a prescriptive method, but represents a different worldviews.

CHAPTER 8 INTRODUCTION TO QUALITATIVE RESEARCH

1. What is a unique consideration for qualitative research?

d. There are different types of relationships developed with participants

Rationale: In quantitative research, the researcher may be blinded to the participants' identities. In qualitative research, the researcher will often speak directly to participants.

2. Why would a mixed methods approach be selected?

a. It fits the research question

Rationale: Methods are selected based on the research problem you are trying to solve.

3. Why are systematic reviews of qualitative research needed?

a. To synthesize a growing body of research

Rationale: Synthesizing qualitative research can help to develop theory and access data from different participants that would not be feasible in a single research study.

CHAPTER 9 QUALITATIVE APPROACHES TO RESEARCH

1. What needs to be considered when engaging patients in research?

a. All methods can engage patients throughout the entire research process

Rationale: Involving patients in the entire research process can improve the quality and applicability of the research.

2. Which method would be most appropriate to study processes?

b. Grounded theory

Rationale: This method is designed to examine processes.

3. What is a common critique of generic qualitative methods?

b. They can lack the rigour found in other methods

Rationale: Other methods have ties to philosophy and theory that helps to guide the analysis.

CHAPTER 10 INTRODUCTION TO QUANTITATIVE RESEARCH

1. How would an investigator ensure that the sample is homogenous?

a. Restrict eligibility criteria to limit extraneous variables relevant to the study

Rationale: Extraneous variables interfere with the operations of the phenomenon being studied. Having an eligibility criteria that limits the extraneous variables ensures homogeneity of the samples.

2. Which situation represents a threat to internal validity in an experimental study measuring the effect of an online post-op education for patients being discharged after coronary artery bypass graft surgery?

   c. Patients in the experimental group gave the link to patients in the usual care control group

   Rationale: Control is lost when the members of the control group also have the link to the intervention (manipulation) that is meant only for the experimental group. This affects the outcome of the study.

3. COVID-19 outbreak in 2020 would represent what type of threat to internal validity in a longitudinal study that started on January 1, 2018 examining mortality rates due to respiratory infection?

   d. History

   Rationale: COVID-19 outbreaks affects the dependent variable (mortality rate) in addition to the independent variable of respiratory infections.

CHAPTER 11 EXPERIMENTAL AND QUASIEXPERIMENTAL DESIGNS

1. What aspect should be the primary consideration in critiquing the research report of an experimental study and determining the validity of the conclusions presented?

   a. How well the researcher controlled for extraneous variables

   Rationale: Controlling extraneous variables ensures causality as extraneous variables affect the outcome of the phenomenon being studied.

2. In a study to help people how to avoid overdosing on opioids, one group of participants received a single supportive phone call 10 days after attending a program on harm reduction approaches. A second group received a weekly supportive phone call for 6 weeks after attending the same program, and a third group received no supportive phone calls after attending the program. What property of experimental research did the researcher employ in this study?

   c. Manipulation of the intervention

   Rationale: All three groups are receiving an intervention (manipulation) with different doses.

3. In a study to assess the effect of a videotape format teaching method on the learning of adolescent males about the warning signs of testicular cancer, why would a nurse researcher select to implement a quasiexperimental study design instead of an experimental study design?

   d. Full experimentational control is not possible

   Rationale: It will be unethical to perform experimentation.

CHAPTER 12 NONEXPERIMENTAL DESIGNS

1. Which study title suggests a cross-sectional design?

   d. Women's appraisal of the diagnosis of breast cancer within the first 48 hours after cancer diagnosis

   Rationale: In this title, the researcher is proposing to collect data only on one occasion, which is a characteristic of cross-sectional study.

2. Which title is most suggestive of a longitudinal study?

   c. Relationship between self-esteem and successful breastfeeding at 1 month, 3 months, and 6 months after birth

   Rationale: In this title, the data are collected at varying intervals, which is a feature of a longitudinal study.

3. In a study of psychosocial adjustment to breast cancer, data collection instruments were sent to the same sample of women at six different times during the first year of living with breast cancer. What type of study design does this exemplify?
   c. Longitudinal
   Rationale: In the above study, researcher is proposing to collect data at varying intervals, which is a feature of a longitudinal study.

CHAPTER 13 SAMPLING

1. Why should a researcher avoid drawing conclusions or making generalizations based on the experience of a small number of participants?
   c. Data obtained from a small number may inadequately represent the phenomenon
   Rationale: Samples have to be representative of the population.
2. What is the difference between an "accessible population" and a "target population"?
   d. The target population represents the entire set of cases the researcher wishes to study, and the accessible population represents that part of the target population that could feasibly be included in the study
   Rationale: Accessible population is drawn from the target population.
3. What is the appropriate sampling interval for drawing a systematic sample of 25 subjects who had breast enhancement surgery from 200 people who had that surgery during 1 year at a specific medical centre?
   c. Every eighth patient
   Rationale: It is through the mathematical calculation of 200/25=8. If chosen, every eighth patient would yield 25 samples from the population of 200.

CHAPTER 14 DATA-COLLECTION METHODS

1. In a study conducted at a large long-term care facility, two data collectors examined the correct use of personal protective equipment (PPE) on 100 nurses. The examinations were independently performed on the same day. A comparison of the results indicated that the data collectors scored 90 of the 100 nurses following the correct protocol for wearing and removing PPE. What can be determined from this finding?
   a. Interrater reliability between the two data collectors was high
   Rationale: High level of consistency of scores between the raters.
2. Which of the following is an example of a physiological measurement?
   c. HbA1C blood levels
   Rationale: This is a blood test and all the others are psychological tests
3. Which data-collection method is most appropriate for measuring postpartum depression?
   d. Edinburgh Postnatal Depression Scale
   Rationale: This tool is a specific and relevant tool to measure postnatal depression.

CHAPTER 15 RIGOUR IN RESEARCH

1. In testing a new scale to measure nursing students' clinical competency in simulation, the researchers administered repeatedly and obtained the same results. What is this called?
   b. Reliability
   Rationale: Reliability is the ability of an instrument to yield same results on repeated measures. It encompasses consistency, precision, and stability.
2. A newly developed instrument is found to have a Cronbach's alpha of 0.82. What is the correct interpretation of this finding?
   d. The instrument has a relatively high degree of internal consistency
   Rationale: Highest score of Cronbach's alpha is 1. The result is above 0.7, which indicates high degree of internal consistency.
3. What is the formal term for rigour in qualitative research?
   d. Trustworthiness
   Rationale: It is a combination of both repeatability and credibility of the findings.

CHAPTER 16 QUALITATIVE DATA ANALYSIS

1. Why is it important for qualitative researchers to listen to the recorded interviews?
   b. It allows for the addition of paraverbal data
   Rationale: Paraverbal data can help with the interpretation of the text.
2. Which of the following is NOT part of qualitative data analysis?
   d. Testing hypotheses
   Rationale: This is a part of quantitative research.
3. How do researchers determine that data analysis is complete?
   c. When substantial analysis has been created
   Rationale: A rigorous analysis must be completed in qualitative research and data are often collected until this is sufficient.

CHAPTER 17 QUANTITATIVE DATA ANALYSIS

1. What level of measurement would a type of nursing degree be considered?
   a. Nominal
   Rationale: Variable could be classified into categories and they are mutually exclusive and there is no ranking.
2. In a study of nurses' willingness to care for patients choosing Medical Assistance in Dying (MAID), it was found that the greater the nurses' spirituality, the lower the willingness to provide care. Which type of correlation does this finding represent?
   d. Negative correlation
   Rationale: Both variables are inversely related (spirituality and willingness to provide care to patients choosing MAID).
3. Which of the following research questions may be answered through statistical hypothesis testing?
   a. What is the relationship between perceived social support and psychological adjustment to breast cancer in unmarried women?

Rationale: This question allows the researcher to develop a null hypothesis or a statistical hypothesis and then reject or not reject the hypothesis based on the inferential statistics.

CHAPTER 18 PRESENTING THE FINDINGS

1. A researcher conducts a qualitative study that examines the lived experience of those being diagnosed with breast cancer. A reader critiquing the report would expect to find that the report:
   a. Presents the data in the form of narrative text
   Rationale: Lived experience can be better understood with the narration of that experience by the study participants.
2. Which information is appropriate to exclude from the discussion section of a research publication?
   a. Detailed data presented in tables and figures
   Rationale: This will be presented under results section.
3. Which research result is reported in an objective manner in the results section of a study?
   c. The results indicated a positive relationship between death anxiety and adherence to medication regimens in gay men with HIV/AIDS
   Rationale: This statement is very objective without any opinion/judgement by the researcher.

CHAPTER 19 CRITIQUING QUALITATIVE RESEARCH ARTICLES

1. Why is it important for researchers to publish the development of an intervention, such as Robinson et al. (2020)?
   b. Knowing the theoretical basis for an intervention improves implementation in other settings
   Rationale: This will help other researchers and healthcare leaders to better use the intervention in their own setting.
2. Why is it important to examine the authors' positions and previous work?

d. To be aware of possible motivations for presenting certain data and conclusions
Rationale: This will help you to evaluate the credibility of the research.
3. What is an appropriate application of the study by Harvey et al. (2019) in nursing practice?
a. Increased awareness of how leadership style and roles impact evidence-based practice
Rationale: Qualitative research can help in our understanding of a phenomenon.

CHAPTER 20 CRITIQUING QUANTITATIVE RESEARCH

1. The purpose of critiquing an article is to
b. Appraise the level of evidence
Rationale: Through critiquing, the nurses are able to appreciate the level of evidence produced by the study.
2. Stylistic variations of a research report might influence:
b. Ability to judge the overall quality or validity of the study
Rationale: Stylistic variations can deter from the focus of evaluating the scientific merit of a study.

3. Which of the following is the most relevant question to critique the research design of a quantitative study?
b. Does the choice of design seem logical for the proposed problem?
Rationale: This question is comprehensive, as it identifies the appropriateness of the design.

CHAPTER 21 DEVELOPING AN EVIDENCE-INFORMED PRACTICE

1. Identifying a practice issue for an evidence-informed practice project is the responsibility of:
a. All registered nurses
Rationale: This is a required competency.
2. How do you know if you should make a practice change?
c. High levels and high quality of evidence
Rationale: A substantial and compelling body of research is needed to make changes to practice.
3. What is the foundation of evidence-informed practice change?
b. Creating a spirit of inquiry
Rationale: This is important for developing a culture where questioning is supported.

Index

Page numbers followed by "*f*" indicate figures, "*t*" indicate tables, and "*b*" indicate boxes.